PRESCRIBING FOR ELDERLY PATIENTS

PRESCRIBING FOR ELDERLY PATIENTS

Edited by

Stephen Jackson
Professor of Geriatric Medicine
King's College London
London UK

Paul Jansen
Department of Geriatric Medicine
University Medical Centre Utrecht
Utrecht
The Netherlands

and

Arduino Mangoni
Department of Clinical Pharmacology
Flinders University
Adelaide
Australia

WILEY-BLACKWELL
A John Wiley & Sons, Ltd., Publication

Library of Congress Cataloging-in-Publication Data

Prescribing for elderly patients / edited by Stephen H.D. Jackson, Paul A.F. Jansen, and Arduino A. Mangoni.
    p. ; cm.
  Includes bibliographical references and index.
  ISBN 978-0-470-02428-7
  1. Geriatric pharmacology. 2. Drugs—Prescribing. I. Jackson, S. H. D. (Stephen H. D.) II. Jansen, Paul A. F. III. Mangoni, Arduino A.
  [DNLM: 1. Drug Therapy. 2. Aged. 3. Pharmaceutical Preparations—administration & dosage. 4. Pharmacokinetics. WT 166 P933 2009]
  RC953.7.P727 2009
  615′.10846—dc22
                                            2008052790

ISBN 978-0-470-02428-7

A catalogue record for this book is available from the British Library.

Set in 10/12pt Times by Laserwords Private Ltd, Chennai, India.
Printed in Singapore by Fabulous Printers Pte Ltd

First Impression   2009

We would like to dedicate this book to our parents.

Contents

List of Contributors		xix
Foreword		xxiii
Preface		xxv
Acknowledgement		xxvii

1 Clinical Pharmacology of Ageing 1
Arduino Mangoni, Paul Jansen and Stephen Jackson 1

Epidemiology	1
Age-related changes in pharmacokinetics	2
Age-related changes in pharmacodynamics	3
Adverse drug reactions and drug interactions	4
Adherence	6
Polypharmacy versus appropriate prescribing	7
Over-the-counter medicines	7
Prescribing audit	8
Medication review	9
Undertreatment	9
References	10

2 Dementia, Delirium, Agitation and Behavioural Problems 13
Catherine Bryant 13

Dementia	13
Delirium	18
Agitation and behavioural problems	22
References	25

3 Depression in Elderly Patients 27
Richard Weeks, Ross Kalucy and Jo Hill 27

Introduction	27
Aetiology	27
Signs and symptoms	28
Diagnosis	29
Therapy	30
References	33

4 Psychotic Illness in Elderly Patients 35
Ross Kalucy, Jo Hill and Richard Weeks 35

Introduction	35
Aetiology	35
Symptoms and signs	37

Diagnosis   38
Therapy   38
Key points   40
References   43

5   Sleep Disorders in the Elderly: the Pros and Cons of Prescribing   45
    R. Doug McEvoy and Karin S. Nyfort-Hansen   45

    Insomnia   45
    Restless legs syndrome and periodic limb movements of sleep   48
    Nocturnal leg cramps   50
    REM behaviour disorder   50
    References   51

6   Stroke   53
    Joseph A. Harbison and Gary A. Ford   53

    Introduction   53
    Aetiology   53
    Modifiable risk factors for stroke   53
    Therapy   54
    Key points   61
    References   61

7   Orthostatic Hypotension, Postprandial Hypotension and Syncope in Older Patients   63
    René W.M.M. Jansen   63

    Orthostatic hypotension in older patients   63
    Key points   66
    Postprandial hypotension in older patients   66
    Key points   68
    Syncope in older patients   69
    Key points   71
    Guidelines   71
    References   71

8   Parkinson's Disease   73
    Gerrit Tissingh and Erik Ch. Wolters   73

    Introduction   73
    Symptoms and signs of PD   74
    Aetiology and pathology   75
    Diagnosis   75
    Therapy   76
    Key points   81
    Links   81
    References   81

9   Epilepsy   83
    John O. Willoughby, Joseph Frasca and Emma M. Whitham   83

    Introduction   83
    Aetiology   83
    Symptoms and signs   83

Diagnosis   84
Therapy   85
Newer anti-epileptic drugs   85
Safety of anti-epileptic drugs   86
Therapy scheme of the advised drugs   87
Clinically-important drug interactions within anti-epileptic drugs   87
Clinically-important drug interactions with other drugs   87
Important adverse effects   87
Drug withdrawal   87
Key points   90
References   90

10   Hypertension   91
     Sanjeev Khindri and Stephen Jackson   91

     Introduction   91
     Aetiology   91
     Symptoms and signs   92
     Diagnosis   92
     Investigation   93
     Therapy   93
     Clinical pharmacology of antihypertensive therapy   94
     Key points   99
     Links   99
     References   99

11   Lipid-Lowering in the Elderly Patient   101
     Anthony S. Wierzbicki   101

     Introduction   101
     Aetiology   101
     Symptoms and signs   102
     Diagnosis   102
     Therapy   103
     Statins   103
     Fibrates   106
     Nicotinic acid   106
     Ezetimibe   107
     Bile acid sequestrants   108
     Omega-3 fatty acids   108
     Guidelines   108
     Key points   109
     Links   109
     References   109

12   Acute Coronary Syndrome   111
     Derek Yiu and Arduino Mangoni   111

     Introduction   111
     Aetiology   111
     Symptoms and signs   112
     Diagnosis   112

Therapy | 114
Therapy scheme of the advised drugs | 117
Key points | 117
Guidelines | 117
Acknowledgements | 117
References | 123

13 Heart Failure | 125
Arduino Mangoni | 125

Introduction | 125
Epidemiology | 125
Aetiology | 125
Clinical presentation | 127
Diagnosis | 127
Therapy | 128
Key points | 137
Guidelines | 137
Acknowledgements | 137
References | 137

14 Atrial Fibrillation and Other Rhythm Disturbances in the Elderly | 139
Abhay Bajpai, Irina Savelieva and A. John Camm | 139

Introduction | 139
Atrial arrhythmias | 139
The epidemiology and cost of AF | 139
The mechanism of atrial tachyarrhythmias | 140
Symptoms and signs | 140
Diagnosis | 140
Classification of AF | 142
Causes of AF | 142
Principles of management of AF | 142
Treatment of acute onset AF | 143
Suppression of paroxysms of AF | 143
Strategies in persistent AF—rate versus rhythm control | 145
Rate control in permanent AF | 146
Risk of stroke and antithrombotic therapy in AF | 148
Non-pharmacological techniques to prevent thrombus formation | 150
Key points | 150
References | 150

15 Valvular Heart Disease | 151
Andrew T. Elder | 151

Introduction | 151
Infective endocarditis | 151
Prevention of endocarditis | 152
Diagnosis and treatment of endocarditis | 152
Prevention of thromboembolism | 155
Prevention of progression of degenerative valvular disease | 158
References | 159

16   Anticoagulants for Thrombosis and Embolism in the Elderly   161
      Alexander Gallus and Dolly Daniel   161

      Introduction   161
      The anticoagulants   161
      Thrombosis in the elderly and indications for anticoagulants   162
      References   168

17   Haematological Disorders   171
      Bryone J. Kuss and Sabria Alhashami   171

      Introduction   171
      Anaemia   171
      Vitamin B12 and folic acid deficiencies   173
      Thrombocytopenia   173
      Myelodysplastic syndromes   175
      Acute leukaemia   176
      Lymphoproliferative conditions   177
      Multiple myeloma   180
      Key points   180
      References   180

18   COPD and Asthma in the Elderly   183
      Martin Connolly and Tina L. Davies   183

      Risk factors and triggers   183
      Presentation and diagnosis   184
      Objective tests   184
      Differential diagnoses   186
      Management of COPD and asthma   186
      Acute asthma   192
      Management of exacerbations of COPD   192
      Management of stable COPD   195
      Conclusion   195
      Key Points   196
      Learning Resources   196
      Guidelines   196
      References   197

19   Pneumonia in the Elderly   199
      Peter A. Frith and Karin S. Nyfort-Hansen   199

      Introduction   199
      Epidemiology   199
      Aetiology and pathogenesis   199
      Symptoms and signs   200
      Diagnosis   200
      Patient assessment   201
      Therapy   202
      Important considerations for drug usage   203
      Prevention   206
      References   206

20   Therapeutic Aspects of Pulmonary Tuberculosis   211
      Paul van den Brande   211

      Introduction   211
      Pathogenesis   211
      Presentation of tuberculosis in the elderly   212
      Diagnosis of tuberculosis   213
      Treatment of tuberculosis   213
      Treatment of latent tuberculosis infection   221
      Key points   222
      References   222

21   Interstitial Lung Disease in the Elderly   225
      Jeffrey Bowden   225

      Introduction   225
      Presentation of interstitial lung disease   225
      Particular problems in the elderly   227
      General comments with regard to therapy   229
      Assessing the response to therapy   229
      Drugs used in ILD   229
      Treatment for specific forms of lung disease   230
      Key points   234
      Links   234
      References   234

22   Lung Cancer in the Elderly   237
      Jeffrey Bowden   237

      Introduction   237
      Aetiology   237
      Symptoms and signs   238
      Diagnosis and staging   238
      Goals of therapy   239
      Chemotherapeutic agents   239
      Treatment protocols for NSCLC   240
      Non cytotoxic agents: EGFR Inhibitors   242
      Treatment of small cell carcinoma   244
      Treatment of mesothelioma   244
      Anti-emetic therapy   245
      Key Points   245
      Guidelines   246
      References   246

23   Nutritional Disorders and the Older Person   249
      Robert K. Penhall and Renuka Visvanathan   249

      Introduction   249
      Obesity and the older person   249
      Nutritional frailty   252
      Under-nutrition in older people   252

Screening and assessment of under-nutrition 254
The management of the under-nourished older person 257
Monitoring and change 259
Conclusion 259
References 259

24 Mouth and Dental Disorders 263
    Cees de Baat and Isaac van der Waal 263

    Introduction 263
    Periodontal disease 263
    Dental caries 264
    Odontogenic infections 265
    Alveolar osteitis 266
    Xerostomia and hyposalivation 266
    Candidiasis 267
    Angular cheilitis 268
    Denture stomatitis 268
    Burning mouth syndrome 269
    Recurrent aphthous stomatitis 270
    Recurrent herpes simplex 271
    Oral lichen planus 272

25 Swallowing Disorders and Medication in the Elderly 275
    Eddy Dejaeger 275

    Introduction 275
    Normal deglutition 275
    Changes with Age 276
    Aetiology of deglutition disorders 277
    Symptoms and signs 277
    Diagnosis 277
    Therapy 277
    Deglutition disorders and medication 278
    Key points 281
    Links 281
    References 281

26 Upper Gastrointestinal Disorders 283
    Geoffrey S. Hebbard 283

    Gastrooesophageal reflux disease 283
    Oesophageal motility disorders 286
    Non-cardiac chest pain 287
    Oesophageal infections 287
    Pill-induced oesophagitis 287
    Peptic ulcer disease 288
    Gastritis 292
    Non-ulcer dyspepsia 292
    References 293

27   Gastric Emptying in Older Patients   295
     Robert J. Fraser   295

     Introduction   295
     Aetiology of disturbed gastric motor function in ageing   296
     Symptoms and signs   296
     Diagnosis   297
     Therapy   297
     Therapy scheme of advised drugs for gastroparesis   297
     Key points   297
     Guidelines   298
     Effect of healthy ageing on appetite regulation—anorexia of ageing   298
     References   299

28   Lower Gastrointestinal Disorders   301
     Daniel L. Worthley, Graeme P. Young and Robert J. Fraser   301

     Malabsorption   301
     Inflammatory bowel disease   304
     Diverticulosis   307
     Mesenteric ischaemia   309
     Constipation   311
     Diarrhoea and faecal incontinence   313
     Haemorrhoids   317
     References   318

29   Abdominal Malignancies   321
     Sarah Zaidi and Guy Chung-Faye   321

     Introduction   321
     Epidemiology   321
     Aetiology   324
     Symptoms and signs   324
     Therapy   325
     Chemotherapy   327
     Key points   329
     Links   329
     References   329

30   Liver Diseases in the Elderly   333
     Réme Mountfield and Alan J. Wigg   333

     Introduction   333
     Physiological changes associated with ageing   333
     Drug induced liver disease   334
     Cirrhosis   335
     Alcoholic liver disease   336
     Non-alcoholic steatohepatitis (NASH)   337
     Hepatitis C   338
     Hepatitis B   340
     Liver transplantation   341
     References   341

31   Disorders of the lower urinary tract   343
     Adrian Wagg   343

     Pathophysiology   345
     Incontinence subtypes   345
     Treatment cessation   345
     Assessment with a bearing on drug addition or withdrawal   346
     Rectal examination   347
     Vaginal examination   347
     The pharmacological treatment of urinary incontinence   347
     Cognition and antimuscarincs   349
     Bladder outflow tract obstruction   349
     Other pharmacological measures   350
     Stress urinary incontinence   350
     Summary   351
     References   351

32   Management of Benign Prostatic Hyperplasia in Elderly Men   353
     Ming Liu and Gordon H. Muir   353

     Assessment   353
     Prostate specific antigen (PSA)   353
     Urinary retention   353
     Nocturnal frequency   355
     Treatment   355
     References   358

33   Management of Erectile Dysfunction in the Elderly   361
     Kevin Dennison   361

     Introduction   361
     Prevalence and aetiology of ED   361
     Physical or psychogenic?   362
     Diagnosis and assessment of ed in primary care   362
     Treatment options   363
     Key points   366
     References   366

34   Benign Gynaecological Disorders   367
     Maria Vella, James Balmforth and Linda Cardozo   367

     Urogenital atrophy   367
     Prolapse   367
     Traditional anatomical site prolapse classification   368
     Urinary incontinence   370
     Detrusor overactivity   370
     Drug therapies   373
     Lichen sclerosis   376
     Lichen planus   377
     References   377

35   Breast Cancer in Elderly Patients   381
     Bogda Koczwara   381

     Introduction   381
     Presentation and diagnosis—special considerations in elderly patients   381
     Management of breast cancer   382
     Management of early breast cancer   383
     Treatment of advanced breast cancer   383
     Supportive care during breast cancer treatment   386
     Breast cancer therapeutics in an elderly patient   386
     Conclusion   386
     Key points   386
     References   390

36   Pharmacological Management of Endocrine Conditions in the Elderly Patient   391
     Nikolai Petrovsky   391

     Introduction   391
     Diabetes aetiology   391
     Diabetes symptoms and signs   392
     Diabetes diagnosis   392
     Type 2 diabetes management   393
     Pharmacokinetic and pharmacodynamic data of diabetes medications in elderly patients   395
     Clinically important drug interactions within diabetes drugs   396
     General adverse effects of diabetes medications in elderly patients   396
     Specific adverse effects and clinically-important drug interactions of diabetes drugs   397
     Pituitary adenomas   397
     Thyroid disease   398
     Hyperparathyroidism   399
     Hormone replacement   399
     Endocrine disease in the elderly—key points   400
     Further Reading   400

37   Rheumatoid Arthritis, Osteoarthritis, Polymyalgia Rheumatica, Gout
     and Pseudogout   403
     E. Michael Shanahan and Stephen Hedger   403

     Rheumatoid arthritis   403
     Key points in rheumatoid arthritis   408
     Osteoarthritis   408
     Key points in osteoarthritis   411
     Polymyalgia rheumatica   411
     Key points in PMR   412
     Gout and calcium pyrophosphate disease (CPPD)   413
     Key points in gout and CPPD   416
     Links   416
     References   416

38 Falls, Osteoporosis, Paget's Disease and Osteomalacia   419
    Harald J.J. Verhaar and Paul Jansen   419

    Falls and osteoporosis   419
    Paget's disease   422
    Osteomalacia   425
    Key points   427
    References   427

39 Drugs and Falls   429
    Nathalie van der Velde and Tischa J.M. van der Cammen   429

    Introduction   429
    Pathophysiology   429
    Fall-risk-increasing drugs   430
    Clinical approach   432
    Treatment: drug withdrawal   432
    Key points   433
    References   433

40 Pressure Ulcers   435
    Rob J. van Marum   435

    Introduction   435
    The role of pressure in pressure ulcer development   435
    The role of nutrition in pressure ulcer development   437
    Risk assessment   437
    Prevention   438
    Local treatment   439
    Key points   439
    References   440

41 Leg Ulceration   441
    Gabrielle M. McMullin   441

    Introduction   441
    Aetiology   441
    Symptoms and signs   443
    Diagnosis   445
    Therapy   448
    Key points   452
    Guidelines   452
    References   452

42 Xerosis and Asteatotic Eczema   453
    Michael Yeung and Daniel Creamer   453

    Xerosis   453
    Actinic keratoses and Bowen's disease   453
    Bullous pemphigoid   454
    Candidiasis   455
    Erysipelas and cellulitis   456
    Contact dermatitis   457

Herpes zoster (shingles)   458
Lichen planus   459
Malignant melanoma   460
Mycosis fungoides   461
Basal cell carcinoma and squamous cell carcinoma   462
Psoriasis   463
Scabies   464
Tinea   464
Urticaria and angio-oedema   465
Venous eczema and the dependency syndrome   466

43 Age-Related Eye Diseases   469
    Genevieve Larkin   469

    Cataract   469
    Glaucoma   472
    Age related macular degeneration   476
    Diabetic retinopathy   482
    References   484

44 Ear Disorders   485
    Wynia Derks and Gerrit Hordijk   485

    Introduction   485
    Hearing loss   485
    Tinnitus   487
    External otitis   489
    Drugs causing hearing problems   490
    References   491

45 Pain   493
    Albert J.M. van Wijck   493

    Introduction   493
    Aetiology   493
    Diagnosis   494
    Therapy   494
    Key points   496
    References   498

46 Palliative Care in the Elderly   499
    Alexander de Graeff and Saskia Teunissen   499

    Introduction   499
    Symptoms   500
    Palliative care in the elderly   500
    Treatment of common symptoms in elderly patients   501
    References   503

    Index   505

List of contributors

Sabria Alhashami
Department of Haematology and Genetic Pathology
Flinders Medical Centre, Flinders University
Adelaide
Australia

Abhay Bajpai
Department of Cardiology
St George's University of London
London
UK

James Balmforth
Department of Urogynaecology
King's College Hospital
London
UK

Jeffrey Bowden
Department of Medicine
Flinders Medical Centre
Adelaide
Australia

Catherine Bryant
Department of Clinical Gerontology
King's College Hospital
London
UK

A. John Camm
Department of Clinical Cardiology
St. George's University of London
London
UK

Linda Cardozo
Department of Urogynaecology
King's College Hospital
London
UK

Guy Chung-Faye
Department of Gastroenterology
King's College Hospital
London
UK

Martin Connolly
Department of Geriatric Medicine
North Shore Hospital
Auckland
New Zealand

Daniel Creamer
Department of Dermatology
King's College Hospital
London
UK

Dolly Daniel
Department of Clinical Pathology and Blood Bank
Christian Medical College
Vellore
India

Tina L. Davies
Newcastle University
Newcastle
UK

Cees de Baat
Department of Oral Function and Prosthetic Dentistry
Radboud University Medical Centre Nijmegen
The Netherlands

Alexander de Graeff
Department of Oncology
University Medical Centre
Utrecht
The Netherlands

Eddy Dejaeger
Department of Geriatrics
University Hospital Leuven
Belgium

Kevin Dennison
King's College Hospital
London
UK

Wynia Derks
Department of Ear, Nose, Throat
Onze Lieve Vrouwe Gasthuis
Amsterdam
The Netherlands

Andrew T. Elder
Medicine of Geriatrics
Western General Hospital
Edinburgh
UK

Gary A. Ford
Institute for Ageing and Health
Newcastle University
Newcastle
UK

Robert J. Fraser
Repatriation General Hospital
Adelaide
Australia

Joseph Frasca
Department of Medicine (Neurology)
Flinders University and Medical Centre
Adelaide
Australia

Peter A. Frith
Flinders University of South Australia
Southern Adelaide Health Service
and Repatriation General Hospital
Adelaide
Australia

Alexander Gallus
Department of Haematology
Flinders Medical Centre
Adelaide
Australia

Joseph A. Harbison
Department of Medical Gerontology
University of Dublin
Dublin
Ireland

Geoffrey S. Hebbard
Department of Gastroenterology
The Royal Melbourne Hospital
Victoria
Australia

Stephen Hedger
Department of General Medicine
Flinders Medical Centre
Adelaide
Australia

Jo Hill
Department of Psychiatry
Flinders Medical Centre
Adelaide
Australia

Gerrit Hordijk
Department of Ear, Nose,Throat
University Medical Centre
Utrecht
The Netherlands

Stephen Jackson
Department of Clinical Gerontology
King's College Hospital
London
UK

Paul Jansen
Department of Geriatric Medicine
University Medical Centre
Utrecht
The Netherlands

René W.M.M. Jansen
Department of Geriatric Medicine
Meander Medical Centre
The Netherlands

Ross Kalucy
Department of Psychiatry
Flinders Medical Centre
Adelaide
Australia

Sanjeev Khindri
Department of Clinical Gerontology
King's College Hospital
London
UK

Bogda Koczwara
Department of Medical Oncology
Department of Medicine
Flinders Medical Centre
Adelaide
Australia

Bryone J. Kuss
*Department of Haematology and Genetic
Pathology
Flinders Medical Centre, Flinders University
Adelaide
Australia*

Genevieve Larkin
*Department of Ophthalmology
Kings College Hospital
London
UK*

Arduino Mangoni
*Department of Clinical Pharmacology
Flinders Medical Centre
Adelaide
Australia*

R. Doug McEvoy
*Adelaide Institute for Sleep Health
Repatriation General Hospital
Adelaide
Australia*

Gabrielle M. McMullin
*South Sydney Vascular Centre
St. George Hospital
Sydney
Australia*

Ming Liu
*Department of Urology
Beijing Hospital
Beijing
China*

Réme Mountfield
*Department of Gastroenterology
and Hepatology
Flinders Medical Centre
Adelaide
Australia*

Gordon H. Muir
*Department of Urology
King's College Hospital
London
UK*

Karin S. Nyfort-Hansen
*Pharmacy Department
Repatriation General Hospital
Adelaide
Australia*

Robert K. Penhall
*Department of Geriatric and
Rehabilitation Medicine
Adelaide
Australia*

Nikolai Petrovsky
*Department of Endocrinology
Flinders Medical Centre
Adelaide
Australia*

E. Michael Shanahan
*Department of Rheumatology
Flinders Medical Centre and Repatriation
General Hospital
Adelaide
Australia*

Irina Savelieva
*Department of Cardiology
St. George's University of London
London
UK*

Saskia Teunissen
*Department of Oncology
University Medical Centre
Utrecht
The Netherlands*

Gerrit Tissingh
*Department of Neurology
Atrium Medisch Centrum Parkstad
The Netherlands*

Paul van den Brande
*Division of Pulmonology
University Hospital Gasthuisberg
Leuven
Belgium*

Tischa J.M. van der Cammen
*Department of Internal Medicine
Erasmus University Medical Centre
Rotterdam
The Netherlands*

Nathalie van der Velde
*Department of Internal Medicine
Erasmus University Medical Centre
Rotterdam
The Netherlands*

Isaac van der Waal
Department of Oral and
Maxillofacial Surgery/Oral Pathology
Vrije Universiteit Medical Centre
Amsterdam
The Netherlands

Rob J. van Marum
Department of Geriatrics
University Medical Centre
Utrecht
The Netherlands

Albert J.M. van Wijck
University Medical Centre
Utrecht
The Netherlands

Maria Vella
Department of Urogynaecology
King's College Hospital
London
UK

Harald J.J. Verhaar
Department of Geriatric Medicine
University Medical Centre
Utrecht
The Netherlands

Renuka Visvanathan
Department of Geriatric and
Rehabilitation Medicine
Royal Adelaide Hospital
Adelaide
Australia

Adrian Wagg
University College Hospital
London
UK

Richard Weeks
Department of Psychiatry
Flinders Medical Centre
Adelaide
Australia

Emma M. Whitham
Department of Medicine (Neurology)
Flinders University and Medical Centre
Adelaide
Australia

Anthony S. Wierzbicki
Consultant Chemical Pathologist
St. Thomas' Hospital
London
UK

Alan J. Wigg
Department of Gastroenterology
and Hepatology
Flinders Medical Centre
Adelaide
Australia

John O. Willoughby
Department of Medicine (Neurology)
Flinders University and Medical Centre
Adelaide
Australia

Erik Ch. Wolters
Department of Neurology
VU Medical Centre Amsterdam
Amsterdam
The Netherlands

Daniel L. Worthley
Department of Gastroenterology
and Hepatology
Flinders Medical Centre
Adelaide
Australia

Michael Yeung
Department of Dermatology
King's College Hospital
London
UK

Derek Yiu
Department of Clinical Pharmacology, School
of Medicine, Centre for Neurosciences
Flinders University
Adelaide
Australia

Graeme P. Young
Department of Gastroenterology
and Hepatology
Flinders Medical Centre
Adelaide
Australia

Sarah Zaidi
Department of Gastroenterology
King's College Hospital
London
UK

Foreword

Across the developed and developing world, use by older people accounts for by far the largest and most rapidly growing proportion of prescribed medications.

Historically, much of the focus on this subject has been driven by the sheer scale of use and also by concerns over the propensity for older consumers to experience adverse reactions. More recently, the abandonment of inappropriate upper age limits in many major clinical trials has uncovered the failure of chronological age to diminish in any way the capacity to benefit from rational, evidence-based drug therapy. Comparable efficacy has been observed in virtually every context where this has been properly studied.

Under-prescribing, therefore, can no longer be deemed acceptable or appropriate, any more than can the excessive or inaccurate use of drugs or drug combinations (with the associated risks) where the evidence of benefit is absent or doubtful. On the contrary, the potential positive impact on the public health (and indeed the public purse!) of achieving consistent careful, informed and timely medication use across our older populations is hard to overestimate.

In spite, however, of the growth of evidence, and the recognition of safety and efficacy for older consumers as a priority within drug regulation and pharmacovigilance, the indications from audit data suggest that we, the prescribing community, still have a long way to go. This may in part reflect the sheer volume of varying information from research sources, international, national or local official guidelines and industry data that prescribers are required to digest. But it is also true that "ageing" is all too often an afterthought by comparison with the clinician's specific focus on the condition being treated. This will no longer do.

For all those concerned with prescribing for older people, therefore, this excellent and timely volume fulfills an urgent need to update and bring together an accessible and readable, but contemporary and authoritative, compilation of clear guidance from which to make sense of the therapeutic rationale and to move forward. It reflects the combined expertise of an outstanding international collaboration of contributors in the relevant specialisms, including the medicine and clinical pharmacology of ageing. The provision of a "handbook" resource for clinicians, is the clear aim. This is admirably achieved, not least for trainees (especially postgraduates) in the health care professions, as well as for those who teach them.

In an introductory chapter, the editors present relevant aspects of the effects of human ageing on drug handling and response, together with some key contemporary principles for the achievement and measurement of prescribing quality. The therapeutics of all the major disease categories and key specific disorders is thereafter covered within a clear, organ/system-based structure. The approach is didactic, but rigorously evidence based. There are many helpful flowcharts and tables, some useful bibliographies, and pointers to consensus or expert guidelines and to key websites where available.

I commend this book to all who prescribe, or who influence prescribing, for older people. A copy should be on their shelves, as well as on the shelves of all medical libraries. I hope and expect that "Jackson, Jansen & Mangoni" will make its mark in the urgent quest for optimal therapeutic medication use for this expanding age group.

Cameron G. Swift, PhD FRCP, FRCPI
Emeritus Professor of Health Care of the
Elderly, King's College School of Medicine,
London, UK
November 2008

Preface

As our population ages, clinicians are faced with an increasing number of elderly patients with multiple medical problems and prescribed medications both in the acute and in the chronic setting. The clinical presentation of common conditions often differs from other age groups and the risk of drug–drug interactions is high, leading to an increased rate of adverse drug reactions and adverse outcomes.

These difficulties prompt the need for a quick and at the same time comprehensive source of information that will assist health care professionals in diagnosing and managing common geriatric conditions effectively and safely. This handbook is designed specifically for this purpose. Unlike other products in the field, information on aetiological factors and pathophysiology is kept to a minimum whereas significant emphasis is given to diagnosis and clinical management options by experts in the field. Age-related changes in pharmacokinetics are clearly illustrated in tabular format and treatment algorithms are derived from a thorough evidence-based review of the literature and the latest guidelines. Each chapter contains key references and a list of selected websites linked to professional national and international organizations and guideline groups.

The book is primarily aimed at trainees in geriatric medicine, internal medicine, and clinical pharmacology. It also provides information useful to the busy hospital specialist and the primary care physician.

Acknowledgement

We are sincerely appreciative of the dedication, enthusiasm and cooperation of the many authors that contributed to the creation of the book.

1 Clinical pharmacology of ageing

Arduino Mangoni[1], Paul Jansen[2] and
Stephen Jackson[3]

[1]Department of Clinical Pharmacology, Flinders Medical Centre, Adelaide, Australia
[2]Department of Geriatric Medicine, University Medical Centre Utrecht,
The Netherlands
[3]Department of Clinical Gerontology, King's College Hospital, London, UK

EPIDEMIOLOGY

Trends in population ageing

In 2000, the worldwide population of those aged ≥65 years was an estimated 420 million, a 9.5 million increase from 1999. During the period 2000–2030, the worldwide population aged ≥65 years is projected to increase by approximately 550 million to 973 million, increasing from 6.9 % to 12.0 % worldwide, from 15.5 % to 24.3 % in Europe, from 12.6 % to 20.3 % in North America, and from 6.0 % to 12.0 % in Asia. The largest increases in absolute numbers of elderly people will occur in developing countries.

The ageing of the world's population is the result of two factors: declines in fertility and increases in life expectancy. Life expectancy in developed countries now ranges from 76 to 80 years and also has increased in developing countries since 1950. A higher life expectancy at birth for females compared with males is almost universal, approximately seven years in Europe and North America but less in developing countries.

The world has experienced an epidemiological transition in the leading causes of death, from infectious disease and acute illness to chronic disease and degenerative illness. Developed countries in North America, Europe, and the Western Pacific already have undergone this transition, and other countries are at different stages of progression. The epidemiological transition, combined with the increasing number of older people, represents a challenge for public health. In the United States, approximately 80 % of all people aged ≥65 years have at least one chronic condition, and 50 % have at least two.

The increased number of older people will lead to increased healthcare costs. The healthcare cost per capita for those aged ≥65 years in developed countries is three to five times greater than the cost for those aged <65 years, and the rapid growth in the number of older people, coupled with continued advances in medical technology, is expected to create increasing pressure on health and long-term care spending.

Medication use in elderly patients

Safe and effective pharmacotherapy remains one of the greatest challenges in geriatric medicine. Elderly patients often suffer from several chronic disorders and consequently use more drugs than any other age group. The diminished physiological reserve associated with ageing can be further depleted by effects of drugs and acute or chronic disease states. Ageing alters the pharmacokinetics and pharmacodynamics of many drugs. In addition, pharmacotherapy may be complicated by difficulties with obtaining drugs or complying with drug regimens.

In most developed countries, about two thirds of the population ≥ 65 years take prescription and nonprescription over the counter (OTC) drugs. At any given time, an average elderly person uses four to five prescription drugs and 2 OTC drugs and fills 12–17 prescriptions a year. The frail elderly patient uses the most drugs. Drug use is greater in hospitals and nursing homes than in the community; typically, a nursing home resident receives at least seven to eight drugs.

The type of drug used varies with the setting. Community patients use analgesics, diuretics, cardiovascular drugs, and sedatives most often; nursing home residents use antipsychotics and sedative-hypnotics most commonly, followed by diuretics, antihypertensives, analgesics, cardiac drugs, and antibiotics. Psychoactive drugs are prescribed for $\sim 65\%$ of nursing home patients and for $\sim 55\%$ of residential care patients; $\sim 7\%$ of patients in nursing homes receive $\geq$ three psychoactive drugs concurrently.

Many drugs benefit elderly patients. Some can be life-saving (i.e. antibiotics and thrombolytic therapy). Oral hypoglycemic agents can improve independence and quality of life while controlling chronic disease. Antihypertensive drugs and influenza vaccines can help prevent or decrease morbidity. Analgesics and antidepressants can control debilitating symptoms. Therefore, appropriateness, that is whether the potential benefits outweigh the potential risks, should guide therapy.

AGE-RELATED CHANGES IN PHARMACOKINETICS

Drug absorption

Pharmacokinetic studies on the effect of ageing on drug absorption have provided conflicting results. Several studies have not shown age-related differences in absorption rates for different drugs (1). However, other studies have shown a reduced absorption of vitamin B_{12}, iron and calcium and an increased absorption of the drug levodopa. For drugs absorbed by passive diffusion there is little evidence for an age related decline.

First-pass metabolism and bioavailability

There is a reduction in first-pass metabolism with advancing age. This is probably due to a reduction in liver mass and, for high clearance drugs, the consequential reduction in blood flow. The bioavailability of drugs undergoing extensive first-pass metabolism can be significantly increased. By contrast, the first-pass activation of several pro-drugs, such as the ACE inhibitors enalapril and perindopril, might be slowed or reduced (2).

Drug distribution

Significant changes in body composition occur with advancing age, such as a progressive reduction in the proportion of total body water and lean body mass (3). This results in a relative increase in body fat. Polar drugs that are mainly water-soluble tend to have smaller volumes of distribution (V) resulting in higher serum levels in older people (e.g. gentamicin, digoxin, lithium, and theophylline). By contrast, non-polar compounds (e.g. benzodiazepines, morphine and amiodarone) tend to be lipid-soluble and so their V increases with age. The main effect of the increased V is a prolongation of half-life. Increased V and elimination half life (t$^1/_2$z) have been observed for drugs such as diazepam, thiopental, lidocaine, and clomethiazole (4). The reduction in V for water-soluble drugs tends to be balanced by a larger reduction in renal clearance (CL), with a smaller effect on t$^1/_2$z, as shown in the following equation:

$$t_{1/2z} = \frac{Ln(2) \cdot V}{CL}$$

where $t_{1/2z}$ = elimination half-life, $Ln(2)$ = natural log of 2 (0.693), V = apparent volume of distribution, and CL = clearance.

Protein binding

Acidic compounds (e.g. diazepam, phenytoin, warfarin, salicylic acid) bind mainly to albumin whereas basic drugs (e.g. lidocaine, propranolol) bind to alpha-1 acid glycoprotein. Although no substantial age-related changes in the concentrations of both these proteins have been observed, albumin is commonly reduced in malnutrition or acute illness whereas alpha-1 acid glycoprotein is increased during acute illness. The main factor determining drug effect is the free concentration of the drug. Although plasma protein binding changes might theoretically contribute to drug interactions or physiological effects for drugs that are highly protein-bound, its clinical relevance is probably limited (5).

Drug clearance

Kidney

The age-related reduction in glomerular filtration rate affects the clearance of many drugs such as water-soluble antibiotics, diuretics, digoxin, water-soluble beta-blockers, lithium, and some non-steroidal anti-inflammatory drugs. The clinical importance of such reductions of renal excretion is dependent on the likely toxicity of the drug. Drugs with a narrow therapeutic index like aminoglycoside antibiotics, digoxin, and lithium are likely to have serious adverse effects if they accumulate only marginally more than intended. In elderly patients serum creatinine may be within the reference limits, while renal function is markedly diminished. The Cockcroft and Gault (6) or the Modification of Diet in Renal Disease (7) equations both use serum creatinine, age and gender and may be helpful for a better estimation of glomerular filtration rate in this situation.

Liver

Drug clearance by the liver depends on the capacity of the liver to extract the drug from the blood passing through the organ (hepatic extraction ratio) and hepatic blood flow. Drugs can be classified into three groups according to their extraction ratio (E): high (E > 0.7, such

as clomethiazole, dextropropoxyphene, glyceryl trinitrate, lidocaine, pethidine, and propranolol), intermediate (E 0.3–0.7, such as aspirin, codeine, morphine, and triazolam), and low extraction ratio (E < 0.3, such as carbamazepine, diazepam, phenytoin, theophylline, and warfarin). When E is high, the clearance is rate-limited by blood flow. When E is low, changes in blood flow produce little changes in clearance. Therefore, the reduction in liver blood flow with ageing affects mainly the clearance of drugs with a high extraction ratio. Of much greater importance is the reduction in liver volume of as much as 30% across the adult age range. This results in a reduction in clearance of a similar magnitude (8).

Several studies have shown significant age-related reductions in the clearance of many drugs metabolized by phase-1 pathways in the liver. These involve reactions such as oxidation and reduction. By contrast, phase-2 pathways (e.g. glucuronidation) do not seem to be significantly affected (8).

AGE-RELATED CHANGES IN PHARMACODYNAMICS

Studies of drug sensitivity require measurement of concentrations of drug in plasma, as well as measurement of drug effects. This is because changes in pharmacokinetics with increasing age may result in changes in response due purely to the changes in drug concentrations. Some important pharmacodynamic age-related changes are illustrated in Table 1.1.

Anticoagulants

There is evidence of a greater inhibition of synthesis of activated vitamin K-dependent clotting factors at similar plasma concentrations of warfarin in elderly compared to young patients. However, the exact mechanisms responsible for the increased sensitivity are unknown.

Cardiovascular and respiratory drugs

Although elderly subjects are less sensitive to the effects of verapamil on cardiac conduction,

Table 1.1. Selected pharmacodynamic changes with ageing

Drug	Pharmacodynamic effect	Age-related change
Adenosine	Heart-rate response	↔
Diazepam	Sedation, postural sway	↑
Diltiazem,	Acute and chronic antihypertensive effect	↑
Verapamil	Acute PR interval prolongation	↓
Diphenhydramine	Postural sway	↔
Enalapril	ACE inhibition	↔
Furosemide	Peak diuretic response	↓
Heparin	Anticoagulant effect	↔
Isoprenalin	Chronotropic effect	↓
Morphine	Analgesic effect	↑
	Respiratory depression	↔
Phenylephrine	α_1-adrenergic agonism	↔
Propranolol	Antagonism of chronotropic effects of isoprenalin	↓
Scopolamine (hyoscine)	Cognitive function	↓
Temazepam	Postural sway	↑
Warfarin	Anticoagulant effect	↑

Legend: ↑= increase; ↓= decrease; ↔= no significant change; ACE = angiotensin-converting enzyme.

the effect on blood pressure and heart rate tends to be greater in older than in younger patients. This might be explained by an increased sensitivity to the negative inotropic and vasodilator effects of verapamil as well as diminished baroreceptor sensitivity. The acute intravenous administration of diltiazem causes greater prolongation of the PR interval (dromotropic effect) in young than in elderly subjects.

Reduced β-adrenoreceptor function is observed with advancing age. Elderly patients are less sensitive to the chronotropic effect of isoprenaline. The impaired response, however, is due primarily to an age-related reduction in the influence of reflex cardiovascular effects on heart rate rather than reduced β-adrenergic sensitivity. Both salbutamol (β-agonist) and propranolol (β-antagonist) show reduced responses with age. This is secondary to impaired β-receptor function due to reduced synthesis of cyclic AMP following receptor stimulation. The total number of receptors seems to be maintained but the post-receptor events are changed because of alterations of the intracellular environment. The responsiveness of α-adrenoreceptors is preserved with advancing age.

Psychotropic drugs

Elderly patients are particularly vulnerable to adverse effects of neuroleptics, such as extrapyramidal symptoms, arrhythmias, and postural hypotension. Agents with anticholinergic effects can also impair cognition and orientation in patients with a cholinergic deficit such as those with Alzheimer's disease. Advancing age is also associated with increased sensitivity to the central nervous system effects of benzodiazepines. The exact mechanisms responsible for the increased sensitivity to these drugs with ageing are unknown, however.

ADVERSE DRUG REACTIONS AND DRUG INTERACTIONS

Adverse drug reactions (ADRs) are an important cause of morbidity and mortality in elderly patients. It is not clear however whether advancing age *per se* is a cause of increased risk of ADRs. Nursing home and frail elderly patients appear to be at high risk of ADRs (9).

Although around 10 % of the general population take more than one prescribed medicine, the incidence of combination therapy is greatest in the elderly, in females, and in those who have had a recent hospital admission. Patients aged >65 years use on average four prescribed medications. A list of common drug interactions in elderly patients is illustrated in Table 1.2.

The risk of ADRs is exponentially rather than linearly related to the number of medicines taken. More than 80 % of ADRs

Table 1.2. The most common drug interactions in elderly patients

Drug	Drug	Impact	Mechanism of interaction
Warfarin	NSAIDs	Potential for serious gastrointestinal bleeding	NSAIDs increase gastric irritation and erosion of the protective lining of the stomach and decrease platelet function during clot formation
Warfarin	Sulfa drugs	Increased effects of warfarin, with potential for bleeding	Warfarin's activity maybe prolonged due to a decreased production of vitamin K by intestinal flora during sulfa drug administration
Warfarin	Macrolides	Increased effects of warfarin, with potential for bleeding	Macrolides inhibit the metabolism of warfarin. The activity of warfarin may also be prolonged due to alterations in the intestinal flora and its production of vitamin K for clotting factor production
Warfarin	Quinolones	Increased effects of warfarin, with potential for bleeding	The exact mechanism for the warfarin-quinolone drug interaction is unknown. Reduction of intestinal flora responsible for vitamin K production by antibiotics is probable as well as decreased metabolism of Warfarin
Warfarin	Phenytoin	Increased effects of warfarin and/or phenytoin	Currently unknown, but one theory suggests a genetic basis involving liver metabolism of warfarin and phenytoin
ACE inhibitors	Potassium supplements	Elevated serum potassium	Inhibition of ACE results in decreased aldosterone production and potentially decreased potassium excretion.
ACE inhibitors	Aldosterone antagonists and potassium sparing diuretics	Elevated serum potassium	Additive effects on reduced potassium elimination
Digoxin	Amiodarone	Digoxin toxicity	Multiple theories exist, but actual mechanism is unknown. Amiodarone may decrease the clearance of digoxin, resulting in prolonged digoxin half-life. There may also be an additive effect on the sinus node activity.
Digoxin	Verapamil	Bradycardia and heart block	Synergistic effect on sinus node and atrioventricular node
Theophylline	Quinolones	Theophylline toxicity	Inhibition of hepatic metabolism of theophylline by the quinolones

causing admission or occurring in hospital are type A, i.e. they are dose related, predictable and potentially avoidable. Antibiotics, anticoagulants, digoxin, diuretics, hypoglycaemic agents, antineoplastic agents and nonsteroidal anti-inflammatory drugs are mainly responsible for type-A ADRs. Type-B ADRs (idiosyncratic reactions) are less common but can be associated with serious toxicity (e.g. hepatotoxicity with flucloxacillin and co-amoxiclav; anaphylactic shock with penicillins).

ADHERENCE

Although the term compliance has gone out of fashion, in practice the three terms compliance, concordance and adherence all refer to the extent to which patients comply with the drug regimen they agreed with the prescriber. We will use the word adherence here.

The efficacy and safety of medicines is largely determined by adherence. Adherence is defined as the extent to which a person's behaviour, taking medication, following a diet, and/or executing life-style changes, corresponds with recommendations agreed with a health-care provider (10). Poor adherence to the treatment of chronic disease is an important problem. One of the first articles pointing at the lack of adherence was published in 1957; in only 50 % of the patients who were prescribed tuberculostatics was the drug was found in urine (11). More recently a Cochrane review found 50 % non-adherence in patients using medicines for chronic diseases (12). Adherence to antihypertensives and statin therapy is often even lower. Within one year of the start of antihypertensives 50 % of the patients have stopped using these drugs (13). The adherence of elderly patients, prescribed statins, is 60 % after three months, 43 % after six months and 26 % after five years (14).

The consequences of non-adherence are considerable including hospital admissions (33–60 % of drug related hospital admissions) and higher mortality (15, 16). Even with use of placebo, high adherence had a 3.5 times greater effect on reducing mortality than the overall active treatment with candesartan in chronic heart failure (17). This finding suggests that high adherence for taking medicines, is associated with high adherence for life-style advice.

The identification of patient non-adherence is important. Factors that contribute to poor adherence are summarized in Table 1.3 (18). In general practice non-adherence is often detected by looking in the medicines cupboard at home. Another method makes use of pharmacy refill records comparing the number of dispensed doses with the number of prescribed doses. A very helpful starting point is to ask the patient and family for the problems they encountered with the drug regimen. The patient should not be blamed for poor adherence. The ability of patients to follow treatment plans is frequently compromised by several factors, including the characteristics of the disease (e.g. cognitive impairment), social system, heath care system, economic factors and patient-related factors. A tool for screening patient adherence is the Brief Medication Questionnaire (19). The Medication Event Monitoring System (MEMS) is an electronic device which records the time and date when a medication container was opened. These devices are used in controlled studies and not in daily practice, because of the expense. Other methods for detecting non-adherence are physiological markers, like low heart-rate with use of beta-blockers, or biochemical measurements in blood or urine Such as plasma angiotensin converting enzyme assays to monitor ACEI adherence.

Several methods have been shown to improve adherence. The most effective approach is multi-level targeting at several factors with several interventions. However effective interventions are often complex and not suitable for daily practice. Education in self-management of the drug regimen has limited effects. A simple and very effective method is the reduction of dose frequency. Adherence is found the highest with a dose frequency of once a day (79 %), decreasing to 69 % with b.i.d., 65 % with t.i.d and 51 % with q.i.d (20).

Integrating the patient's perspective into treatment plans is considered very important.

Table 1.3. Methods of measuring adherence (adapted from Ref (18))

Methods	Advantages	Disadvantages
Directly observed therapy	Most accurate	Patients can hide pills in mouth and then discard them; impractical for routine use
Biochemical measurement of the medicine or metabolite or measurement of a biological marker	Objective	Variations in metabolism and "white coat" adherence can give a false impression; expensive
Patient questionnaires or self-reports	Simple, inexpensive, most useful in clinical practice	Susceptible to error and distortion
Pill counts	Objective, quantifiable and easy to perform	Data easily altered by the patient (e.g. pill dumping)
Rates of prescription refills	Objective, easy to obtain data	A prescription refill is not equivalent to ingestion of medication; requires a closed pharmacy system
Assessment of the patient's clinical response	Simple; easy to perform	Factors other than medication adherence can affect clinical response
Electronic medication monitors	Precise; results are easily quantified; tracks patterns of taking medication	Expensive; requires return visits
Measurement of physiologic markers	Often easy to perform	Marker may be absent for other reasons
Patient diaries	Help to correct for poor recall	Easily altered by the patient
Questionnaire for caregiver, for patients who are cognitively impaired.	Help to correct for poor recall; simple; objective	Susceptible to error and distortion

The behaviour of prescribers is changing from a paternalistic one-way style towards concordance to improve adherence (21).

POLYPHARMACY VERSUS APPROPRIATE PRESCRIBING

Polypharmacy, often defined as the concurrent use of five or more different drugs, is common among elderly patients. Inappropriate polypharmacy contributes to unwanted and often preventable clinically relevant drug-drug and drug-disease interactions as well as adverse drug reactions (ADRs). Around 12 % of elderly patients in hospitals are admitted because of ADRs (22). It is estimated that about 47–72 % of these ADRs are avoidable (23, 25). Polypharmacy itself is not necessarily undesirable.

Polypharmacy, however, is a concept that addresses only the inappropriate use of medication. The term appropriate prescribing addresses the problems of both inappropriate use of medication as well as inappropriate non use of medication (or undertreatment).

OVER-THE-COUNTER MEDICINES

Elderly people are the largest consumers of over-the-counter (OTC) medicines. The switch of prescription drugs to OTC medicines is encouraged. Government policies make it possible to obtain increasing numbers of former prescription drugs from pharmacies, health food shops, supermarkets or by mail-order. The goal is to provide greater choice for individuals and to shift the responsibility for health care as well as the costs to individuals. The approach to OTC medicines varies between countries. In general it is considered that OTC can be used for short-term self-limiting illnesses with lower doses of commonly prescribed drugs and should have few important adverse effects.

Some consider herbal drugs, vitamins and minerals also as OTC drugs.

Older people use OTC medicines to treat minor complaints such as pain, constipation, colds and gastro-intestinal symptoms (25). The most commonly used OTCs are aspirin, paracetamol, NSAIDs, antihistamines and histamine H_2 receptor antagonists. Recently in several countries statins are also available OTC. There are concerns regarding the safety of OTC medicines, especially in elderly patients. In particular, NSAIDs may cause gastrointestinal toxicity and sedatives, increase may the risk of falls. The use of multiple medications increases the risk of drug interactions and adverse effects. Cebollero-Santamaria et al. showed that bleeding from a peptic ulcer was associated with the use of NSAIDs in 81 % of 84 patients and that 95 % had purchased their NSAIDs OTC (26). The use of recommended doses of OTC NSAIDs has a relatively good safety profile compared to presciption NSAIDs, however patients may take higher doses for a longer period with serious gastrointestinal toxicity as a result (27). Many older people use OTC drugs to improve their sleep. The risks associated with this use have not been examined (25). Also the problems in older people with OTC H_2 receptor antagonists, such as confusion, and OTC statins, such as liver and skeletal muscle toxicity, are not clearly defined.

Documentation of OTC medicines is poor. A study showed that only 5 % of OTC drugs, used by patients prior to and during hospitalization, were recorded on drug charts (28). Asking elderly patients, especially those admitted to hospitals, for their use of OTC drugs is important to prevent double-prescription and clinically relevant interactions. This applies also to herbal drugs as St. John's wort. St. John's wort is used to treat depressive symptoms. It induces the metabolism of several drugs and diminishes the absorption of digoxin (Table 1.4) (29). Other possible interactions are the diminishing effect of warfarin caused by cranberry juice and Ginseng (30, 31).

The increasing availability of OTC drugs clearly has benefits. Nevertheless, prescribers

Table 1.4. Interactions with St. John's wort (adapted from Ref (29))

amitriptyline	Steady-state concentration decreased by 22%
ciclosporine	Steady-state concentration decreased by 52%
digoxin	Steady-state concentration decreased by 25%
simvastatin	AUC decreased by 50%
tacrolimus	Steady-state concentration decreased by 80%
theophylline	Steady state concentration decreased by 50%
cumarin derivatives	INR 50% lower

AUC = Area under plasma concentration time curve

must always pay close attention to concomitant OTC medication use in order to minimize adverse drug reactions.

PRESCRIBING AUDIT

Clinical audit is fundamental to providing a high quality service. This is particularly true for prescribing. A variety of approaches have been advocated ranging from the use of purely descriptive prescribing indicators through application of consensus guidelines to strictly evidence based approaches. The use of purely descriptive approaches alone achieves little but is a useful adjunct to comparing observed prescribing to a gold standard.

Oborne et al. (1997) have described three types of prescribing indicator for use in prescribing audit (45). Purely descriptive indicators include mean numbers of drugs prescribed and numbers of drugs classified in the British National Formulary as "Black Triangle" drugs (7). These are recently introduced drugs for which all adverse events should be reported. Indicators of unnecessary or potentially harmful prescribing include duplications such as H_2 receptor blockers and proton pump inhibitors and potentially harmful drugs such as long acting hypoglycaemic agents which should no longer be used. The third category of indicator is evidence based. These indicators measure the extent to which research evidence is put into practice. Examples include the use of antithrombotic therapy in atrial fibrillation and the use of aspirin in coronory artery disease. These approaches are superceding the Beers criteria (47) which are associated with a number of problems.

MEDICATION REVIEW

Medication review is an essential process in the management of patients with chronic disease. This process should be driven by four questions and should involve the patient as much as possible:

1. Which drugs are necessary for the patient?

The first step should be to look at all the problems and diseases of the patient and to determine which drugs are indicated (32) It is important to identify indicated drugs that are missing. In making decisions, prescribers should consider the remaining life expectancy, goals of care and potential benefits of medications (33).

2. Which drugs are not necessary?

The next step is to look at the medicines the patient uses, including the OTC drugs, and to determine for which drugs there is still an indication. Unnecessary duplications with other drugs should be looked for (e.g. H_2 blockers and proton pump inhibitors), taking into account drugs that will be added to the regimen as above.

3. Are there better alternatives for the remaining drugs?

The proposed drugs should be prescribable together. It is important to look at clinically significant drug-drug and drug-disease interactions (34). It is also important to ask the patient about adverse drug reactions and, if so, to look at alternatives. Where drugs have similar efficacy/safety profiles the least expensive option should be prescribed.

4. Is the dose and the dose frequency appropriate?

Consider if the prescribed dose is still correct. Have there been any changes in the clearance of the drug, e.g. a change in renal function?

The patient should always be asked about problems with drug adherence. Adherence can be increased in several ways, but most evidence exists for reduction of the number of daily doses (20).

UNDERTREATMENT

Undertreatment is a common reason for inappropriate prescribing. It has been shown that undertreatment is frequent in elderly patients, despite the use of many medicines (35, 36). Undertreatment in elderly patients is reported in a high percentage of patients with myocardial infarction, chronic heart failure, atrial fibrillation, hyperlipidemia, osteoporosis, COPD, depression, pain and cancer (35–43). Choudhry et al. concluded that a physician's experience with bleeding events associated with warfarin in patients can cause underprescription of warfarin to other patients (39). Kuzuya et al. showed that the incidence of polypharmacy among frail community-dwelling older people is lower in the oldest members (>85 years) because of underuse of medications for chronic diseases (43). Kuipers et al. found a clear relationship between polypharmacy and underprescription (32). The probability of underprescription increased significantly with the number of medicines (Figure 1.1).

It appears that general practitioners and specialists are not willing to prescribe more drugs to frail old patients with current polypharmacy for reasons of complexity of drug regimens, fear of ADRs, interactions and poor adherence. Research has shown that for some medical problems a so-called treatment-risk paradox or risk-treatment mismatch exists meaning that patients who are at highest risk for complications have the lowest probability to receive the recommended pharmacological treatment (38, 40). The application of clinical practice guidelines

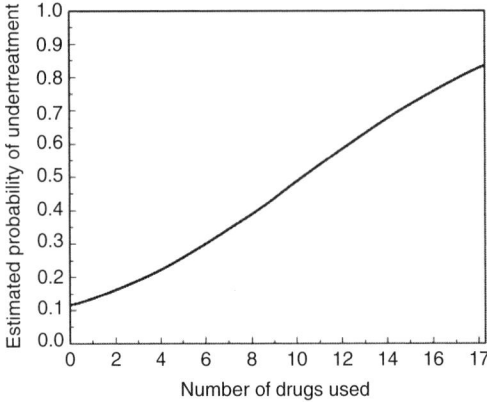

Figure 1.1. Estimated probability of underprescription related to the number of drugs (adapted from Ref (32))

(CPGs) to the care of older patients with several comorbid diseases may have undesirable effects and there could be reasons not to treat all problems. Moreover, the evidence of the benefit of CPG application in elderly patients with comorbid disease is lacking. Boyd et al. estimated that if the relevant CPGs were followed a hypothetical patient would be prescribed 12 medications (44). However, undertreatment may be harmful for the patient. In optimizing polypharmacy, attention should be directed not only to overtreatment but also to possible undertreatment. The aim is to enhance appropriate prescribing to patients with comorbid diseases. In conclusion, undertreatment is considered an important problem in elderly patients with comorbid diseases although the evidence base is lacking.

REFERENCES

1. Gainsborough N, Maskrey VL, Nelson ML, Keating J, Sherwood RA, Jackson SH et al. The association of age with gastric emptying. *Age Ageing* 1993; **22**(1): 37–40.
2. Wilkinson GR. The effects of diet, aging and disease-states on presystemic elimination and oral drug bioavailability in humans. *Adv Drug Deliv Rev* 1997; **27**(2-3): 129–59.
3. Fulop T, Jr., Worum I, Csongor J, Foris G, Leovey A. Body composition in elderly people. I. Determination of body composition by multiisotope method and the elimination kinetics of these isotopes in healthy elderly subjects. *Gerontology* 1985; **31**(1): 6–14.
4. Klotz U, Avant GR, Hoyumpa A, Schenker S, Wilkinson GR. The effects of age and liver disease on the disposition and elimination of diazepam in adult man. *J Clin Invest* 1975; **55**(2): 347–59.
5. Benet LZ, Hoener BA. Changes in plasma protein binding have little clinical relevance. *Clin Pharmacol Ther* 2002; **71**(3): 115–21.
6. Levey AS, Bosch JP, Lewis JB, Graeme T, Rogers N, Roth D. A more accurate method to estimate glomerular filtration rate from serum creatinine: a new prediction equation. Modification of Diet in Renal Disease Study Group. *Arch Intern Med* 1999; **130**: 461–70.
7. British National Formulary 54; 2007. British Medical Association and Royal Pharmaceutical Society of Great Britain.
8. Zeeh J, Platt D. The aging liver: structural and functional changes and their consequences for drug treatment in old age. *Gerontology* 2002; **48**(3): 121–7.
9. Routledge PA, O'Mahony MS, Woodhouse KW. Adverse drug reactions in elderly patients. *Br J Clin Pharmacol* 2004; **57**(2): 121–6.
10. De Geest S, Sabate E. Adherence to long-term therapies: evidence for action. *Eur J Cardiovasc Nurs* 2003; **2**(4): 323.
11. Dixon WM, Stradling P, Wootton ID. Outpatient P.A.S. therapy. *Lancet* 1957; **273**(7001): 871–2.
12. Haynes RB, Yao X, Degani A, Kripalani S, Garg A, McDonald HP. Interventions to enhance medication adherence. *Cochrane Database Syst Rev* 2005; (4):CD000011.
13. Bloom BS. Daily regimen and compliance with treatment. *BMJ* 2001; **323**(7314): 647.
14. Benner JS, Glynn RJ, Mogun H, Neumann PJ, Weinstein MC, Avorn J. Long-term persistence in use of statin therapy in elderly patients. *JAMA* 2002; **288**(4): 455–61.
15. McDonnell PJ, Jacobs MR. Hospital admissions resulting from preventable adverse drug reactions. *Ann Pharmacother* 2002; **36**(9): 1331–6.
16. Senst BL, Achusim LE, Genest RP, Cosentino LA, Ford CC, Little JA et al. Practical approach to determining costs and frequency of adverse drug events in a health care network. *Am J Health Syst Pharm* 2001; **58**(12): 1126–32.
17. Granger BB, Swedberg K, Ekman I, Granger CB, Olofsson B, McMurray JJ et al. Adherence to candesartan and placebo and outcomes in chronic heart failure in the CHARM

programme: double-blind, randomised, controlled clinical trial. *Lancet* 2005; **366**(9502): 2005–11.

18. Osterberg L, Blaschke T. Adherence to medication. *N Engl J Med* 2005; **353**(5): 487–97.

19. Svarstad BL, Chewning BA, Sleath BL, Claesson C. The Brief Medication Questionnaire: a tool for screening patient adherence and barriers to adherence. *Patient Educ Couns* 1999; **37**(2): 113–24.

20. Claxton AJ, Cramer J, Pierce C. A systematic review of the associations between dose regimens and medication compliance. *Clin Ther* 2001; **23**(8): 1296–1310.

21. Bissell P, May CR, Noyce PR. From compliance to concordance: barriers to accomplishing a re-framed model of health care interactions. *Soc Sci Med* 2004; **58**(4): 851–62.

22. Beijer HJ, de Blaey CJ. Hospitalisations caused by adverse drug reactions (ADR): a meta-analysis of observational studies. *Pharm World Sci* 2002; **24**(2): 46–54.

23. Pirmohamed M, James S, Meakin S, Green C, Scott AK, Walley TJ et al. Adverse drug reactions as cause of admission to hospital: prospective analysis of 18 820 patients. *BMJ* 2004; **329**(7456): 15–19.

24. Leendertse AJ, van den Bemt PMLA, Egberts ACG. Hospital admissions related to medication (HARM). *Arch Int Med* 2008; **168**: 1890–6.

25. Francis SA, Barnett N, Denham M. Switching of prescription drugs to over-the-counter status: is it a good thing for the elderly? *Drugs Aging* 2005; **22**(5): 361–70.

26. Cebollero-Santamaria F, Smith J, Gioe S, Van Frank T, Mc CR, Airhart J et al. Selective outpatient management of upper gastrointestinal bleeding in the elderly. *Am J Gastroenterol* 1999; **94**(5): 1242–7.

27. Lewis JD, Kimmel SE, Localio AR, Metz DC, Farrar JT, Nessel L et al. Risk of serious upper gastrointestinal toxicity with over-the-counter nonaspirin nonsteroidal anti-inflammatory drugs. *Gastroenterology* 2005; **129**(6): 1865–74.

28. Oborne CA, Luzac ML. Over-the-counter medicine use prior to and during hospitalization. *Ann Pharmacother* 2005; **39**(2): 268–73.

29. Huang SM, Hall SD, Watkins P, Love LA, Serabjit-Singh C, Betz JM et al. Drug interactions with herbal products and grapefruit juice: a conference report. *Clin Pharmacol Ther* 2004; **75**(1): 1–12.

30. Suvarna R, Pirmohamed M, Henderson L. Possible interaction between warfarin and cranberry juice. *BMJ* 2003; **327**(7429): 1454.

31. Yuan CS, Wei G, Dey L, Karrison T, Nahlik L, Maleckar S et al. Brief communication: American ginseng reduces warfarin's effect in healthy patients: a randomized, controlled Trial. *Ann Intern Med* 2004; **141**(1): 23–7.

32. Kuipers MAJ, Marum van RJ, Egberts ACG, Jansen PAF. Relationship between polypharmacy and underprescribing. *Br J Clin Pharmacol* 2008; **65**: 130–3.

33. Holmes HM, Hayley DC, Alexander GC, Sachs GA. Reconsidering medication appropriateness for patients late in life. *Arch Intern Med* 2006; **166**(6): 605–9.

34. Tamblyn RM, McLeod PJ, Abrahamowicz M, Monette J, Gayton DC, Berkson L et al. Questionable prescribing for elderly patients in Quebec. *CMAJ* 1994; **150**(11): 1801–9.

35. Sloane PD, Gruber-Baldini AL, Zimmerman S, Roth M, Watson L, Boustani M et al. Medication undertreatment in assisted living settings. *Arch Intern Med* 2004; **164**(18): 2031–7.

36. Higashi T, Shekelle PG, Solomon DH, Knight EL, Roth C, Chang JT et al. The quality of pharmacologic care for vulnerable older patients. *Ann Intern Med* 2004; **140**(9): 714–20.

37. Soumerai SB, McLaughlin TJ, Spiegelman D, Hertzmark E, Thibault G, Goldman L. Adverse outcomes of underuse of beta-blockers in elderly survivors of acute myocardial infarction. *JAMA* 1997; **277**(2): 115–21.

38. Lee DS, Tu JV, Juurlink DN, Alter DA, Ko DT, Austin PC et al. Risk-treatment mismatch in the pharmacotherapy of heart failure. *JAMA* 2005; **294**(10): 1240–7.

39. Choudhry NK, Anderson GM, Laupacis A, Ross-Degnan D, Normand SL, Soumerai SB. Impact of adverse events on prescribing warfarin in patients with atrial fibrillation: matched pair analysis. *BMJ* 2006; **332**(7534): 141–5.

40. Ko DT, Mamdani M, Alter DA. Lipid-lowering therapy with statins in high-risk elderly patients: the treatment-risk paradox. *JAMA* 2004; **291**(15): 1864–70.

41. Heston LL, Garrard J, Makris L, Kane RL, Cooper S, Dunham T et al. Inadequate treatment of depressed nursing home elderly. *J Am Geriatr Soc* 1992; **40**(11): 1117–22.

42. Turner NJ, Haward RA, Mulley GP, Selby PJ. Cancer in old age–is it inadequately investigated and treated? *BMJ* 1999; **319**(7205): 309–12.

43. Kuzuya M, Masuda Y, Hirakawa Y, Iwata M, Enoki H, Hasegawa J et al. Underuse of medications for chronic diseases in the oldest of community-dwelling older frail Japanese. *J Am Geriatr Soc* 2006; **54**(4): 598–605.

44. Boyd CM, Darer J, Boult C, Fried LP, Boult L, Wu AW. Clinical practice guidelines and quality of care for older patients with multiple comorbid diseases: implications for pay for performance. *JAMA* 2005; **294**(6): 716–24.

45. Oborne CA, Batty GM, Maskrey V, Swift CG, Jackson SHD, Development of prescribing indicators for elderly medical patients. *Br J Clin Pharmacol* 1997; **43**: 91–7.

46. Cockroft TW, Gault MW, Prediction of creatinine clearance from serum creatinine, *Nephron* 1976; **16**: 31–4.

47. Fick DM, Cooper JW, Wade WE, Waller JL, MacLean JR, Beers MH. Updating the Beers criteria for potentially inappropriate medication use in older adults: results of a US consensus panel of experts. *Arch Intern Med*. 2003; **163**: 2716–24.

2 Dementia, delirium, agitation and behavioural problems

Catherine Bryant

Department of Clinical Gerontology, King's College Hospital, London, UK

DEMENTIA

Introduction

Dementia is a syndrome due to disease of the brain, usually of a chronic or progressive nature, in which there is impairment of multiple higher cortical functions. Dementia prevalence in the United Kingdom is around 6.6 % in the population aged over 65 years and prevalence increases with age (1). The commonest form of dementia in the over 65 years is Alzheimer's disease (AD) (probably 60–70 %). Vascular dementia (VaD), either alone or co-existent with AD, (probably 15–20 %) is the second commonest with dementia with Lewy bodies (DLB) and frontotemporal dementia (FTD) also seen. Rare causes of dementia include hypothyroidism, vitamin B12 or folate deficiency, hypercalcaemia, Wernicke-Korsakoff's syndrome, progressive supranuclear palsy, neurosyphilis and Huntington's disease.

Mild cognitive impairment (MCI) is a syndrome defined as cognitive decline greater than expected for an individual's age and education level that does not interfere notably with activities of daily living (2). The prevalence is estimated to be from 3–19 % in populations aged over 65 years. Some people with MCI may remain stable or return to normal over time but more than half progress to dementia within 5 years. The commonest form of MCI is the amnestic subtype where subjects have a memory impairment but otherwise normal cognitive function and intact activities of daily living. The aetiology of this syndrome is multifactorial including genetics, vascular risk factors and use of anticholinergic drugs. The management of MCI is at present pragmatic.

Aetiology

The biggest risk factor for AD is age. Epidemiological studies have suggested associations linked to decreased capacity of the brain such as reduced brain size, low educational and occupational attainment, low mental ability in early life and reduced mental and physical activity during later life. Head injury may also be a risk factor. Vascular risk factors such as hypercholesterolaemia, hypertension, atherosclerosis, coronary heart disease, smoking and diabetes also have a role although whether they are causing silent cerebrovascular disease or are true causal factors is not known (3).

Familial AD with an onset in the under 65 years age group is an autosomal dominant disease associated with mutations in presenilin 1, presenilin 2 and amyloid precursor protein genes but is rare (less than 0.1 %). The apolipoprotein E genotype in humans has three major isoforms (apoE2, apoE3, and apoE4) which are encoded by different alleles and

Prescribing for Elderly Patients Edited by Stephen Jackson, Paul Jansen and Arduino Mangoni

regulate lipid metabolism and redistribution. The apoE ε4 allele accounts for most of the genetic risk in sporadic Alzheimer's disease in the over 65 years age group (3), increasing the risk of disease by three times in heterozygotes and 15 times in homozygotes.

The concept of VaD has historically been based on stroke and the multi-infarct model. However it now clear that vascular cognitive impairment encompasses a broader clinicopathological range of disorders including post-stroke dementia, multi-infarct dementia, subcortical ischaemic vascular dementia, strategic-infarct dementia, hypoperfusion dementia, haemorrhagic dementia and dementia caused by specific arteriopathies (4). The uniting feature is that vascular pathology causes or makes a substantial contribution to the cognitive impairment. Post-stroke dementia occurs in up to a third of patients within a year of stroke and is strongly associated with advancing age.

Symptoms and signs

Common early symptoms of AD include short-term memory impairment and disorientation in time and place. Personality changes can occur and patients have impaired judgement. In addition patients can experience aphasia (language disturbance), apraxia (inability to perform motor tasks), agnosia (failure to recognize persons or objects) and disturbance in executive function (ability to plan, organise, sequence and execute tasks). Neuropyschiatric and behavioural symptoms are common. The disease is of gradual onset and there is a progressive cognitive decline with a progressive inability to perform activities of daily living. Median life expectancy has been estimated at three to eight years after diagnosis.

The differentiation between AD and VaD can be difficult and the two may co-exist. Current diagnostic criteria for VaD focus on the presence of dementia and the presence of cerebrovascular disease (neurological signs on examination and relevant cerebrovascular disease on neuroimaging). There needs to be an association between the two (onset of dementia within three months of a recognized stroke or stepwise

progression in cognitive deficits). Gait disturbances, unsteadiness or falls, urinary symptoms and pseudobulbar palsy support a diagnosis of VaD. Neuropsychiatric symptoms can also occur. VaD probably has similar rates of decline to AD although the development of cerebrovascular disease in an AD cohort is associated with a more rapid course of illness (4).

Characteristic features of DLB are fluctuation of awareness from day-to-day and signs of parkinsonism. Visual hallucinations or delusions occur frequently and falls are common. DLB has a similar pathological basis to Parkinson's disease dementia and both are associated with progressive cognitive decline. Approximately three quarters of older people with Parkinson's disease develop dementia after 10 years.

FTD is characterized by changes in behaviour, such as disinhibition, lack of judgement, loss of social awareness and loss of insight, and these are more common than memory problems. Disturbance of mood, speech and continence are frequent. A positive family history is not uncommon.

Diagnosis

Dementia is a clinical diagnosis (Table 2.1). All patients with suspected cognitive impairment should have cognitive screening. The simplest and most widely used test is the Mini-Mental State Examination (MMSE). The Informant Questionnaire on Cognitive Decline in the Elderly (10) is a short questionnaire filled out by someone who knows the patient and provides information on pre-presentation cognitive decline. More detailed cognitive testing may be necessary if there is doubt about the diagnosis.

Therapy

Cholinergic deficiency in the brains of AD patients is well documented and linked to the cognitive deficits seen in AD. Cholinesterase inhibitors (ChEIs) are the mainstay of symptomatic treatment of cognitive symptoms. Three drugs are available donepezil, rivastigmine and galantamine (Table 2.2). The drugs inhibit acetylcholinesterase although rivastigmine and

Table 2.1. Diagnosis and assessment of dementia

Diagnosis and assessment of dementia

- Full history from patient and caregivers (onset, course, pattern of cognitive impairment and presence of non-cognitive symptoms)
- Differentiate type of dementia–diagnostic criteria may help:
  - DSM-IV (5) or NINCDS-ADRDA criteria (6) for AD
  - NINDS-AIREN criteria for VaD (7)
  - Consensus criteria for DLB (8) and FTD (9)
- Cognitive screening
- Exclude delirium and depression
- Screen for co-morbid physical disease including falls (increased in dementia) and incontinence
- Exclude B12 deficiency and hypothyroidism (neurosyphilis only if clinical suspicion)
- CT or MRI brain to look for medial temporal lobe atrophy (AD) and vascular disease

galantamine have additional pharmacological effects. The evidence of their effectiveness in treating AD is based on randomized placebo controlled trials of 6–12 months duration. Their effect has most often been measured in trials using the Alzheimer's disease assessment scale (ADAS-Cog) which assesses multiple cognitive abilities (scale of 0–70; higher scores indicating greater impairment). In the natural history of AD, patients with mild to moderate AD would be expected to deteriorate by 3–4 points and patients with moderate to severe AD by 4–6 points over a 6 month period. In clinical trials ChEIs produce improvements in cognitive function, on average of -2.7 points (95 %CI -3.0 to -2.3, $p < 0.00001$), in the midrange of the 70 point ADAS-Cog scale. Study clinicians rated global clinical state more positively in treated patients. Benefits of treatment were also seen on measures of activities of daily living and behaviour (11). However none of these treatment effects is large.

ChEIs do not work for every patient; approximately a third of patients will show improvement, a third will not deteriorate and a third will show no change. The commonest side effects of ChEIs are gastrointestinal and dose related (minimized by careful titration and taking medication with food).

Prior to starting ChEIs a baseline should be established for cognitive function, neuropsychiatric symptoms and activities of daily living. Patients should have an ECG to exclude cardiac conduction problems as ChEIs should be used with great caution in patients with conduction abnormalities due to the risk of syncope. Patients should be reassessed after they have been on a stable maintenance dose for three months and the drug should be continued if there has been a response (either improvement or no deterioration). There is some evidence that switching to another ChEI may provide benefit in about 50 % of patients who do not respond. Patients should be re-assessed at six monthly intervals to assess response to continued drug treatment.

Ultimately AD patients will continue to decline cognitively despite ChEI treatment and clinicians will be faced with a decision to stop the drugs. There is evidence from open-label extension studies that some patients continue to derive benefit from ChEIs for up to five years. In the UK the National Institute of Clinical Excellence (NICE) recommend discontinuation when the MMSE score falls below 12. However it would seem prudent that each patient is considered individually, the situation discussed with the patient and their carers and possible effects of the drugs on non-cognitive symptoms considered. If there is an unexpected deterioration on stopping the drug then it can be re-instated.

The cost effectiveness of ChEIs has been debated. The main cost of AD is the cost of institutional care and none of the randomized controlled trials addressed this. There is some open label data to suggest that ChEIs may delay institutionalisation and more robust evidence suggest that ChEIs are at least cost neutral.

Table 2.2. Drug treatment of AD

Drug	Start dose	Maintenance dose	Pharmacokinetics	Clearance	Important interactions	Important adverse effects	Other tips
Donepezil (Selective AChE inhibition)	5 mg od po (titrate up to maintenance dose after 4 weeks)	10 mg od	$Yt_{1/2}$ = 50–70 hours $Et_{1/2}$ = 100 hours	Hepatic metabolism (CYP2D6 and CYP3A4) 20% excreted unchanged in urine	Potential for increased drug levels with ketoconazole and erythromycin (inhibition of CYP3A4) and paroxetine and fluoxetine (inhibition of CYP2D6) Enzyme inducers e.g. rifampicin, phenytoin and carbamazepine may decrease levels of the drug	Nausea Vomiting Diarrhoea Anorexia Abdominal pain Headache Dizziness Tremor Weight loss Fatigue Syncope Hallucinations, agitation and aggression Urinary incontinence	Caution in hepatic impairment Caution in bradycardia or cardiac conduction disturbances Caution in asthma and COPD Caution if history of peptic ulcer disease
Rivastigmine (Slowly reversible AChE and BuChE inhibition)	1.5 mg bd po (titrate up in steps of 1.5 mg at intervals of at least 2 weeks) Available as capsules or liquid	6 mg bd	$Yt_{1/2}$ = 1–2 hours $Et_{1/2}$ = 1–2 hours (plasma levels ~ 30% higher in elderly subjects)	Hydrolysis by esterases Main metabolite has 10% activity and is renally excreted	No significant interactions known	Nausea Vomiting Diarrhoea Anorexia Abdominal pain Headache Dizziness Tremor Weight loss Fatigue Higher rate of GI side effects as BuChE found in GI tract	Give with food Avoid in hepatic impairment Caution in renal impairment Caution in bradycardia or cardiac conduction disturbances Caution in asthma and COPD Caution if history of peptic ulcer disease

Drug	Starting dose	Maintenance dose	Half-life	Metabolism	Interactions	Side effects	Cautions
Galantamine (Selective AChE inhibition and allosteric nicotine receptor modulation)	8 mg od (titrate up by 8 mg at intervals of 4 weeks-twice daily dose) Available as liquid and prolonged release capsule-once daily dose	16–24 mg daily	$Yt_{1/2}$ = 5–6 hours $Et_{1/2}$ = 8–10 hours (conventional release preparations)	Hepatic metabolism (CYP2D6 and CYP3A4) 20% excreted unchanged in the urine	Increased drug levels with ketoconazole and erythromycin (inhibition of CYP3A4) and paroxetine and fluoxetine (inhibition of CYP2D6) Enzyme inducers e.g. rifampicin, phenytoin and carbamazepine may decrease levels of the drug	Nausea Vomiting Diarrhoea Anorexia Abdominal pain Headache Dizziness Tremor Weight loss Fatigue Syncope Depression	Give with food. Avoid in moderate to severe hepatic or renal impairment Caution in bradycardia or cardiac conduction disturbances Caution in asthma and COPD Caution if history of peptic ulcer disease
Memantine (non-competitive NMDA-receptor antagonist that affects glutamate transmission)	5 mg po (titrate up by 5 mg weekly) Available as tablets or liquid	10 mg bd	$Yt_{1/2}$ = 60–80 hours $Et_{1/2}$ = 60–80 hours	80% excreted unchanged in the urine	May enhance L-dopa, dopaminergic agonists and anticholinergics. Reduced effect of neuroleptics. Do not use with amantadine or ketamine (risk of psychosis). Ranitidine, cimetidine, procainamide, quinidine, quinine and nicotine may increase plasma levels	Constipation, confusion, headache, dizziness, tiredness. Less commonly hallucinations and diarrhoea. Rarely seizures.	Avoid in renal failure Caution in patients with epilepsy

AChE = acetylcholinesterase BuChE = butyrylcholinesterase NMDA = N-methyl-D-aspartate
$Et_{1/2}$-Elderly $t_{1/2}$ (elimination half life)
$Yt_{1/2}$-Young $t_{1/2}$

Memantine is a non-competitive NMDA-Receptor antagonist that affects glutamate transmission and is licensed for the treatment of moderate to severe AD. It is predominantly used when treatment with ChEIs is no longer considered effective but could be considered in patients who cannot tolerate or have not responded to treatment with ChEIs. Memantine produces significant effects on cognition, activities of daily living, global impression of change scales and behavioural scales (12). There is also evidence that memantine added to donepezil treatment may improve activities of daily living, cognition and neuropsychiatric symptoms. It would be reasonable that memantine is prescribed within the same framework used for ChEIs (Table 2.2).

Cholinergic deficits are also found in patients with mixed AD and VaD, DLB and VaD. Although ChEIs are not yet licensed for use in these diseases they are being increasingly used on the basis of clinical research data. Donepezil and galantamine have been shown to produce significant effects on cognition and global function in VaD. Rivastigmine is now licensed for the treatment of mild to moderate dementia in Parkinson's Disease and improves global functioning and activities of daily living.

Drug therapy is only part of the overall management of patients with dementia. Patients are likely to benefit from co-ordinated management from a multidisciplinary team with experience in managing patients with dementia. Vascular risk factor control should also be part of routine clinical care.

Key Points

- Dementia is a common disease in older people for which there is as yet no cure.
- AD and mixed AD and VaD are the commonest forms in older people.
- All patients with suspected dementia need careful assessment and diagnosis.
- ChEIs and memantine provide symptomatic treatment in AD and about two-thirds of patients will have a treatment response.

Guidelines

- Scottish Intercollegiate Guidelines Network Management of patients with dementia http://www.sign.ac.uk/pdf/sign86.pdf.
- American Association for Geriatric Psychiatry Position Statement: Principles of Care for Patients With Dementia Resulting From Alzheimer Disease http://www.aagponline.org/prof/position_caredmnalz.asp.
- National Institute For Health and Clinical Excellence Dementia National Clinical Practice Guideline http://www.nice.org.uk.

DELIRIUM

Introduction

Delirium is an acute confusional state that that is common in older patients admitted to hospital. Delirium is associated with increased mortality, increased hospital stay, increased rates of institutionalization and also an increased rate of complications such as falls and pressure sores. Delirium can occur at any age but the prevalence increases with age and with the presence of dementia. It is often poorly recognized and managed. Delirium can be an unpleasant and distressing experience for patients and recall of the experience can occur with a strong relationship between distress and the presence of hallucinations and delusions (13).

Rates of delirium in older people depend on the setting of care, the characteristics of the patient population and the detection methods used. The prevalence of delirium at hospital admission ranges from 14–24 % with the incidence during hospitalisation ranging from 6–56 % among general hospital populations. Delirium occurs in 15–53 % of older patients post-operatively, 70–87 % of those in intensive care and up to 60 % of those in nursing homes. The mortality rate of hospitalized patients with delirium is 22–76 % and the one year mortality is 35–40 % (14).

As delirium may be the first presentation of an underlying dementing illness appropriate follow up of patients should be considered.

Aetiology

The cause of delirium is usually multifactorial. Predisposing and precipitating factors for delirium have been well reviewed elsewhere (15). The pathophysiology of delirium remains poorly understood, although there is widespread dysfunction of higher cortical function. There is evidence of a cholinergic deficiency in delirium (15). Drugs with anticholinergic activity can induce delirium and increased exposure to these drugs is associated with an increase in severity of the delirium (16).

Many different drugs can cause delirium in older people (Table 2.3). Drugs alone may account for 12–39 % of all cases of delirium (17).

Table 2.3. Drugs causing delirium (adapted from Alagiakrishnan and Wiens, *Postgrad Med J*. 2004; 80: 388–93)

Prescription Drugs

- Central acting agents:
  - Sedative hypnotics (for example, benzodiazepines)
  - Anticonvulsants (for example, barbiturates)
  - Antiparkinsonian agents (for example, benztropine, trihexyphenidyl)
- Analgesics:
  - Narcotics*
  - Non-steroidal anti-inflammatory drugs*
- Antihistamines (first generation – for example, hydroxyzine)
- Gastrointestinal agents:
  - Antispasmodics
  - H_2-blockers*
- Antinauseants:
  - Scopolamine (hyoscine)
  - Dimenhydrinate
- Antibiotics:
  - Fluoroquinolones*
- Psychotropic medications:
  - Tricyclic antidepressants
  - Lithium*
- Cardiac medications:
  - Antiarrhythmics
  - Digoxin*
  - Antihypertensives (ß-blockers, methyldopa)
- Miscellaneous:
  - Skeletal muscle relaxants
  - Steroids
  - Warfarin

Non prescription drugs

- Antihistamines (NB. first generation – for example, diphenhydramine, chlorpheniramine)
- Antinauseants (for example, dimenhydrinate, scopolamine)
- Liquid medications containing alcohol
- Mandrake
- Henbane
- Jimson weed
- Atropa belladonna extract

*May require dose adjustment in renal impairment

Symptoms and signs

Delirium is a syndrome of acute onset (hours and days) and has a fluctuating course. There is a change in cognition such as a memory deficit, disorientation, language disturbance or development of a perceptual disturbance. The cardinal feature is a disturbance of consciousness i.e. a reduced clarity of awareness of the environment with a reduced ability to focus, shift or sustain attention. Psychomotor disturbance occurs with hyperactive, hypoactive or mixed forms occurring. Hyperactive delirium is characterized by increased motor activity, agitation, hallucinations (often visual) and inappropriate behaviour (typical of delirium tremens). Hypoactive delirium is characterized by reduced motor activity and lethargy. Hypoactive or a mixed subtype of delirium are the commonest forms of delirium in older patients.

The main complications of delirium include falls, pressure sores, nosocomial infections, functional impairment, continence problems, over-sedation and malnutrition.

Diagnosis

The differential diagnosis of delirium includes dementia, depression, hysteria, mania, schizophrenia, dysphasia, non-convulsive epilepsy and temporal lobe epilepsy. Delirium can also arise in the presence of dementia.

Delirium should be suspected in all older patients with confusion. They require a full medical history and examination with investigations directed at identifying the underlying cause of the delirium. A corroborative history from family or carers is often needed to provide evidence of the patient's pre-admission cognitive state. Cognitive screening of patients using the MMSE can help identify confusion but not the cause. Use of the Confusion Assessment method can help differentiate delirium from dementia or detect its onset during a hospital admission (Table 2.4).

Therapy

The key therapeutic strategies in delirium are treatment of the underlying cause, management of confusion and prevention of complications. Incriminating drugs should be stopped, biochemical derangements corrected and infection treated. Thiamine should be given when alcohol abuse or under nutrition is suspected.

Patients should be nursed in a good sensory environment with a reality orientation approach and involvement of the multidisciplinary team. Non-pharmacological strategies are not only important in managing confusion but also preventing delirium in possibly up to a third of patients at high risk of the condition (19).

The use of physical restraint should be avoided. Bed rails do not prevent falls and may increase the risk of serious injury. Urinary catheters should also be avoided because of the risk of trauma and infection.

The use of sedation in delirium should be kept to a minimum and only used in patients to allow essential investigations or treatment, to prevent a patient endangering themselves or others or to relieve distress in a highly agitated patient. Drugs should be started at the lowest possible dose and titrated carefully against the patient's clinical condition. Haloperidol is the drug of choice, although benzodiazepines are the drugs of choice in patients undergoing withdrawal from drugs or alcohol (Table 2.5). Any

Table 2.4. Confusion Assessment Method (18)

Confusion Assessment Method (CAM)

To have a positive CAM result the patient must display:
Presence of acute onset and fluctuating course
and
Inattention (e.g. 20-1 test with reduced ability to shift or maintain attention)
and either
Disorganised thinking (disorganised or incoherent speech)
or
Altered level of consciousness (usually lethargic or stuperose)

Table 2.5. Drug treatment of delirium

Drug	Start dose	Maintenance dose	Pharmcokinetics	Clearance	Important interactions	Important adverse effects	Other tips
Haloperidol (Butyrophenone)	0.5–1.0 mg po with additional doses every 4 hrs 0.5–1 mg bd im	0.5–1 mg bd	$Yt_{1/2}$ = 12–38 hours $Et_{1/2}$ = 12–38 hours	Hepatic (oxidative dealkylation)	Potentiation of other psychoactive drugs Use extreme caution if patient on lithium	Extrapyramidal symptoms (dopamine D_2 blockade) especially if dose is >3 mg/day Hypotension Prolonged QT interval Anticholinergic (e.g. dry mouth, blurred vision) α_1 blockade (e.g. hypotension)	Avoid in hepatic insufficiency, neuroleptic malignant syndrome, DLB and Parkinson's disease Maximum dosage of 5 mg/24 hours Avoid intravenous use as short duration of action
Lorazepam (Benzodiazepine)	0.5–1 mg po with additional doses every 2–4 hrs 0.5–1.0 mg IV or IM	0.5–1 mg bd	$Yt_{1/2}$ = 12–15 hours $Et_{1/2}$ = 12–15 hours	Hepatic (glucuronidation)	Potentiation of other CNS depressant drugs	Sedation Respiratory depression Paradoxical excitation Postural instability	Maximum dosage of 3 mg/24 hours Caution in hepatic and renal impairment (titrate according to clinical response) Compared to younger patients there is increased sensitivity to lorazepam and hence increased risk of adverse effects

drugs used should be reviewed every 24 hours and ideally any sedation tailed off after 24–48 hours. Other drugs such as atypical antipsychotics and trazadone may have some benefit, but have only been tested in small uncontrolled studies (14).

Key Points

- Delirium is common in all hospitalized older patients and can be present on admission or develop during a hospital stay.
- Delirium is often missed by clinicians and all patients should have an assessment of cognition to help recognize confusion.
- Up to a third of delirium can be prevented by good multidisciplinary practice.
- Patients with delirium should have all incriminating drugs withdrawn and infection treated promptly.
- Use of sedatives or tranquilisers in delirium to manage confusion should be kept to a minimum and only used to treat distressing or dangerous behavioural disturbance.

Guidelines

British Geriatrics Society and Royal College of Physicians. Guidelines for the prevention, diagnosis and management of delirium in older people http://www.rcplondon.ac.uk/pubs/books/pdmd/index.asp.

AGITATION AND BEHAVIOURAL PROBLEMS

Introduction

Behavioural changes and neuropsychiatric symptoms in older patients can occur in a number of different conditions, including dementia, delirium, depression, paranoid states and drug and alcohol intoxication. More than 90 % of people with dementia develop neuropsychiatric symptoms at some stage during their illness. These symptoms can be distressing for patients and their carers and contribute to caregiver burden. They are often the precipitant for admission to institutional care.

Aetiology

Behavioural and psychological symptoms of dementia (BPSD) are common in AD and VaD, although are not required for diagnosis. In FTD and DLB they are pathognomonic and part of consensus criteria. BPSD encompass a wide range of symptoms and behaviours. In AD it is likely that they are multifactorial in aetiology and also depend on the interaction with the environment and interpersonal and familial relationships of the patient (20).

Symptoms and signs

Apathy is the most common symptom in AD and increases with disease progression (21). It is present in 50–70 % of patients with AD. Mood disorders such as anxiety and depression are also common, occurring in about 40 % of patients but may decrease with disease progression. The relationship between depression and dementia is complex as people with depression and cognitive impairment are highly likely to have dementia diagnosed during longitudinal follow up and depression is often part of a dementia prodrome.

Agitation is associated with a cluster of symptoms including irritability, motor restlessness and abnormal vocalization. These symptoms can be associated with behaviours such as pacing, wandering, aggression, shouting and nocturnal disturbance. Dementia-related causes include pain, concurrent physical illness, adverse drug effects, depression, anxiety and psychosis. Dementia-specific causes include the person's reaction to their physical and social environment arising from their cognitive deficit (22). Aggression and non-aggressive agitation probably occurs in 20 % of patients with AD who are in contact with clinical services or living in the community and up to 40–60 % of people in institutional care (23).

The most frequent psychotic symptoms in AD are hallucinations and persecutory delusions (present in about 25 % of patients). These symptoms are associated with agitation and aggression. Hallucinations usually resolve over a few months but at least 50 % patients with agitation will be experiencing these symptoms a year after onset (23). Poor visual acuity may predispose patients with dementia to visual hallucinations.

Psychiatric symptoms are as common and important in VaD as in AD. Mood symptoms such as depression, emotional lability, and apathy are particularly frequent and persistent in VaD compared with AD (4).

In DLB recurrent visual hallucinations (typically well-formed and detailed) are part of the core features in consensus criteria for the disease. Patients may also experience delusions, hallucinations in other modalities and depression (8). Neuroleptic sensitivity is a disorder characterized by the acute onset or exacerbation of parkinsonism and impaired consciousness in patients with DLB given typical neuroleptic drugs and is associated with a high mortality and morbidity (24).

The spectrum of behavioural disorders in FTD reflects frontal lobe dysfunction. They include emotional blunting and apathy, disinhibition and disruption of social conduct and lack of empathy for others. A spectrum of repetitive and compulsive behaviours can be seen including wandering, agitation and altered eating habits (9).

In dementia the sleep-wake cycle can be affected with patients becoming more agitated or active at night. "Sundowning" refers to behavioural difficulties that worsen towards the end of the day. This can be tiring and stressful for carers.

Diagnosis

A detailed assessment of the patient and a history from an informant is necessary to help identify the nature of the problem (symptoms, triggers, effects on patient and carers and time course) and to help indicate the cause. An assessment of cognition should always be done. Any concurrent physical problems (e.g. pain, constipation, fever, possible adverse drug effects) need to be considered.

The use of rating scales such as the Neuropsychiatric Inventory (NPI) may help diagnosis and management. The NPI evaluates 12 neuropsychiatric disturbances common in dementia and the amount of caregiver distress engendered

by each of the symptoms is assessed (25). The NPI is also able to show the effects of treatment.

Therapy

Management of behavioural problems in dementia is multifactorial and tailored for the individual patient. Patients should be managed by skilled multidisciplinary teams and psychiatric expertise is often needed. Delirium and depression must be treated. Physical symptoms such as pain or constipation should be treated and sensory deficits corrected. Non-pharmacological interventions should always be tried first and pharmacological interventions only considered if there is serious distress or risk to the patient.

The bulk of evidence for the use of pharmacological interventions for BPSD in dementia comes from trials of neuroleptics in AD. It should be noted that a significant placebo response is seen in trials and troublesome symptoms are likely to resolve over days or weeks. Short term use (up to 12 weeks) of atypical neuroleptics (olanzapine but particularly risperidone), are effective in the treatment of aggression in AD (Table 2.6) (23). There is also evidence that haloperidol is effective in treatment of aggression in dementia (26). However all neuroleptics are associated with adverse effects (Table 2.7) with recent data showing an increased risk of death in patients with dementia treated with atypical antipsychotics (27). An increased mortality is also seen in older patients treated with typical neuroleptics, probably related to QT prolongation. It would seem prudent that in patients with VaD or mixed disease neuroleptics are used with similar caution.

There is growing evidence that ChEIs may be helpful in treating BPSD although this has not been a primary endpoint of many of the trials of these drugs and more evidence is awaited. However rivastigmine would be the drug of choice in treatment in DLB (8) and dementia associated with Parkinson's disease.

Memantine may also be helpful for BPSD and there is evidence that it can reduce the incidence of agitation and aggression in AD (12).

Table 2.6. Drug treatment of BPSD in dementia

Drug	Start dose	Maintenance dose	Pharmcokinetics	Clearance	Important interactions	Important adverse effects	Other tips
Risperidone	0.5 mg po od Also available as liquid and oro-dispersible tablets	Up to 2 mg daily	$Yt_{1/2} = 19$ hours $Et_{1/2} = 25$ hours	Hepatic (CYP2D6)	Potentiation of other psychoactive drugs Carbamazepine may decrease plasma drug levels	Extrapyramidal symptoms Sedation Insomnia Headache Anxiety Agitation Weight gain Dizziness Orthostatic hypotension	Caution in Parkinson disease (worsening motor symptoms) Caution in renal and hepatic impairment
Olanzapine	2.5 mg po od Also available as liquid and oro-dispersible tablets	Up to 10 mg daily	$Yt_{1/2} = 33$ hours $Et_{1/2} = 52$ hours	Hepatic (CYPA12)	Carbamazepine and smoking may decrease plasma drug levels Fluvoxamine and ciprofloxacin inhibit CYPA12 and increase olanzapine levels	Weight gain Sedation Dizziness Orthoststic hypotension Anticholinergic side effects Extrapyramidal symptoms Eosinophilia Mild, usually transient, elevation of liver transaminases	Caution in Parkinson disease (worsening motor symptoms) Caution in glaucoma Caution in renal and hepatic impairment

Table 2.7. Adverse effects of neuroleptics in dementia

Adverse effects of neuroleptics in dementia
Increased mortality
Increased rate of stroke
Increased cognitive decline
Extrapyramidal symptoms
Sedation
Anticholinergic effects including delirium
ECG abnormalities potentially predisposing to arrhythmias
Risk of falls

Key Points

- Formulate a clear description of any BPSD from the patient and caregiver.
- Short term use of risperidone is indicated for aggression if there is serious distress or risk to the patient or caregiver.
- Avoid neuroleptics in DLB due to risk of neuroleptic sensitivity.

Links

The Alzheimer's Society Useful source of patient and carer information leaflets on dementias which will also be of interest to health professionals http://www.alzheimers.org.uk/.

REFERENCES

1. Medical Research Council Cognitive Function and Ageing Study. Cognitive function and dementia in six areas of England and Wales. *Psychol Med*. 1998; **28**: 319–35.
2. Gauthier S, Reisberg B, Zaudig M, Petersen RC, Ritchie K, Broich K et al. International Psychogeriatric Association Expert Conference on mild cognitive impairment. *Lancet* 2006; **367**: 1262–70.
3. Blennow K, de Leon MJ, Zetterberg H. Alzheimer's disease. *Lancet* 2006; **368**: 387–403.
4. O'Brien JT, Erkinjuntti T, Reisberg B, Roman G, Sawada T, Pantoni L et al. Vascular cognitive impairment. *Lancet Neurol*. 2003; **2**: 89–98.
5. American Psychiatric Association. *Diagnostic and Statistical Manual of Mental Disorders –*. (DSM-IV) 4th ed. Washington (DC): American Psychiatric Association; 1994.
6. McKhann G, Drachman D, Folstein M, Katzman R, Price D, Stadlan EM. Clinical diagnosis of Alzheimer's disease: report of the NINCDS-ADRDA Work Group under the auspices of Department of Health and Human Services Task Force on Alzheimer's Disease. *Neurology* 1984; **34**: 939–44.
7. Roman GC, Tatemichi TK, Erkinjuntti T, Cummings JL, Masdeu JC, Garcia JH, et al. Vascular dementia: diagnostic criteria for research studies. Report of the NINDS-AIREN International Workshop. *Neurology* 1993; **43**: 250–60.
8. McKeith IG, Dickson DW, Lowe J, Emre M, O'Brien JT, Feldman H et al. Diagnosis and management of dementia with Lewy bodies: third report of the DLB Consortium. *Neurology*. 2005; **65**: 1863–72.
9. Snowden JS, Neary D, Mann DM. Frontotemporal dementia. *Br J Psychiatry* 2002; **180**: 140–3.
10. Jorm AF. A short form of the Informant Questionnaire on Cognitve Decline in the Elderly (IQCODE): development and cross-validation. *Psychol Med*. 1994; **24**: 145–53.
11. Birks J. Cholinesterase inhibitors for Alzheimer's disease. *Cochrane Database Syst Rev*. 2006, Issue 1. Art. No.: CD005593. DOI: 10.1002/14651858.CD005593.
12. McShane R, Areosa Sastre A, Minakaran N. Memantine for dementia. *Cochrane Database Syst Rev*. 2006, Issue 2. Art. No.: CD003154. DOI: 10.1002/14651858.CD003154.pub5.
13. Breitbart W, Gibson C, Tremblay A. The delirium experience: delirium recall and delirium-related distress in hospitalized patients with cancer, their spouses/caregivers, and their nurses. *Psychosomatics* 2002; **43**: 183–94.
14. Inoye SK. Delirium in older persons. *N Engl J Med*. 2006; **354**: 1157–65.
15. Burns A, Gallagley A, Byrne J. Delirium. *J Neurol Neurosurg Psychiatry*. 2004; **75**: 362–7.
16. Han L, McCusker J, Cole M, Abrahamowicz M, Primeau F, Elie M. Use of medications with anticholinergic effect predicts clinical severity

of delirium symptoms in older medical inpatients. *Arch Intern Med*. 2001; **161**: 1099–105.

17. Alagiakrishnan K, Wiens CA. An approach to drug induced delirium in the elderly. *Postgrad Med J*. 2004; **80**: 388–93.

18. Inouye SK, van Dyck CH, Alessi CA, Balkin S, Siegal AP, Horwitz RI. Clarifying confusion: the confusion assessment method. A new method for detection of delirium. *Ann Intern Med*. 1990; **113**: 941–48.

19. Inouye SK, Bogardus ST Jr, Charpentier PA, Leo-Summers L, Acampora D, Holford TR, Cooney LM Jr. A multicomponent intervention to prevent delirium in hospitalized older patients. *N Engl J Med*. 1999; **340**: 669–76.

20. Robert PH, Verhey FR, Byrne EJ, Hurt C, De Deyn PP, Nobili F et al. Grouping for behavioral and psychological symptoms in dementia: clinical and biological aspects. Consensus paper of the European Alzheimer disease consortium. *Eur Psychiatry*. 2005; **7**: 490–6.

21. Mega MS, Cummings JL, Fiorello T, Gornbein J. The spectrum of behavioural changes in Alzheimer's disease. *Neurology*. 1996; **46**: 130–5.

22. Howard R, Ballard C, O'Brien J. Burns A. Guidelines for the management of agitation in dementia. *Int J Geriatr Psychiatry*. 2001; **16**: 714–17.

23. Ballard C, Howard R. Neuroleptic drugs in dementia: benefits and harm. *Nat Rev Neurosci*. 2006; **7**: 492–500.

24. McKeith I, Fairbairn A, Perry R, Thompson P, Perry E. Neuroleptic sensitivity in patients with senile dementia of Lewy body type. *BMJ*. 1992; **305**: 673–8.

25. Cummings JL. The Neuropsychiatric Inventory: assessing psychopathology in dementia patients. *Neurology*. 1997; **48**(Suppl 6): S10–S16.

26. Lonergan E, Luxenberg J, Colford J, Birks J. Haloperidol for agitation in dementia. *Cochrane Database Syst Rev* 2002, Issue 2. Art. No.: CD002852. DOI: 10.1002/14651858 .CD002852.

27. Schneider LS, Dagerman KS, Insel P. Risk of death with atypical antipsychotic drug treatment for dementia: meta-analysis of randomized placebo-controlled trials. *JAMA*. 2005; **294**: 1934–43.

3 Depression in elderly patients

Richard Weeks, Ross Kalucy and Jo Hill

Department of Psychiatry, Flinders Medical Centre, Adelaide, Australia

INTRODUCTION

Depressive illness is common and is associated with significant disability. According to the World Health Organisation (WHO), depression is the fourth largest contributor to the global burden of disease, and is projected to reach second position by 2020 (1). Despite a range of efficacious treatments being available, under-recognition and under-treatment of depression in elderly patients contributes to the disease burden. The lifetime prevalence of depression is in the range of 10–20 %. Over all age groups, women are roughly twice as likely as men to suffer from depressive illness.

Depression is not a normal part of the ageing process and should not be accepted as such. Anecdotal beliefs that depression is more prevalent in older persons have been challenged by the findings of some large population studies. However, it is worth noting that some of these have been challenged on methodological grounds as underestimating the extent of the problem. A large review of 34 studies of depressive illness in elderly patients reported a prevalence of all depressive syndromes of 13.5 % (2). The rate of major depression (1.8 %) was much lower than that of the general population, whilst more minor depressive syndromes (including dysthymia and "subsyndromal" depression) were more prevalent (9.8 %). Consistent with population data, elderly women were at higher risk than their male counterparts.

AETIOLOGY

The aetiology of depressive illness is usually multifactorial. A broad understanding of the biological, psychological, social and cultural factors involved in the genesis of the patient"s illness is therefore vital. Established risk factors such as a past history of depressive episodes, positive family history, female gender, stressful life events, neurotic personality traits and adverse social circumstances are equally relevant in elderly patient populations (3), although their effect size may vary. A family history of depression, for instance, is likely to be of less significance in late-onset depression than in recurrent major depression with onset at a younger age (3, 4).

Proposed biological aetiologies in depression are numerous, and have variable levels of evidence to support them. Twin, family and adoption studies have established a genetic component in the aetiology of unipolar depression, although this is much less impressive than is the case for bipolar disorder. Genetic linkage studies have further established this evidence. A theory of monoamine depletion is well accepted, although biological markers supportive of this hypothesis have remained elusive. The accumulation of small vessel ischaemic changes in key brain areas has been proposed as a vascular aetiology, and this may have particular relevance for elderly patients. Hypothalamic-pituitary-adrenal axis

Prescribing for Elderly Patients   Edited by Stephen Jackson, Paul Jansen and Arduino Mangoni
© 2009 John Wiley & Sons, Ltd

dysfunction, elevated cortisol levels and a suppressed thyroid-stimulating hormone (TSH) response to thyrotropin-releasing hormone (TRH) have, amongst many others, been proposed as having a role in depressive illness. None, however, have established clinical utility in the diagnosis or management of depressive illness.

The frequent presence of medical co-morbidities requires that organic aetiologies be considered in all cases of depression in elderly patients, particularly those with a first presentation of psychiatric symptoms at an advanced age. Neurological, endocrine and cardiac diseases may be of particular relevance. In addition, medications such as β-blockers, steroids, analgesics, digoxin, tranquilisers, and anti-parkinsonian drugs are important causes of depression in elderly patients, as is alcohol abuse.

Cognitive distortions are frequently significant. The depressed person may view themselves and their world in an unduly negative way, leading to a pattern of self-fulfilling prophecy whereby failure is expected and negative beliefs reinforced. Low self-esteem may result, predisposing to depressive illness.

Social factors are important in the aetiology of depression at any age, and may be particularly so in elderly patients. Bereavement is a frequent accompaniment to ageing, and often precipitates depressive symptoms. Normal grief is an important differential diagnosis to consider, and anniversaries of bereavements are frequently associated with a recurrence of symptoms. Stressful life events, lack of a confiding relationship and certain personality traits all predispose to depressive illness. Loss of the ability to live independently appears to have a significant impact on mood in elderly patients, with demonstrated higher levels of depression amongst those in residential care compared with those in the community. Elder abuse is an important issue to consider in certain cases.

SIGNS AND SYMPTOMS

Depressive disorders in elderly patients are under-diagnosed and under-treated in significant numbers (5), and can be clinically distinguished from normal ageing (4). Greater awareness of the problem and its various presentations is likely to result in reduced patient morbidity and mortality, in addition to reductions in carer burden and health care costs.

Depressive disorders exist on a spectrum of severity and are heterogeneous in nature. In recognition of this, classification systems include multiple diagnostic entities across the clinical spectrum. It follows, therefore, that the clinical presentation of depressive illness may vary considerably. Adding a further level of complexity to the clinical picture is the tendency of elderly patients to present with vague or atypical complaints, or symptoms overlapping with medical and psychiatric co-morbidities. These may include anxiety, somatic complaints, apathy, and memory dysfunction (6). Polypharmacy may compound the problem, and pain should never be overlooked as a potential cause of depressed mood. Premorbid personality traits may become more prominent in the setting of depressive disorders, accompanied by behaviour disorder.

Age of onset of depression has little bearing on the clinical presentation of the illness (7). Elderly females appear more susceptible to the melancholic and psychotic subtypes of depression, along with psychomotor disturbances, hypochondriasis and severe guilt (8). Subjective complaints of depressive symptoms may less severe in elderly patients, whilst observer ratings may be higher, leading to the possibility of more severe illness presenting in a group less likely to report mood disturbance.

Under-reporting of symptoms by the patient is another potential confounder in elderly patients, as is a high level of so-called "subthreshold" depressive illness, which is thought to exist in elderly patient populations. In these cases, psychological distress and some features of depression are present, but are insufficient to satisfy existing diagnostic criteria. They are clinically significant nonetheless. Despite these complexities, no specific diagnostic criteria to aid in the diagnosis of depression in elderly patients are in common use.

Depressive disorders occurring in the setting of co-morbid medical illness have the potential to add complexity to the clinical picture and may delay diagnosis. The relationship between depression and medical illness is not fully understood, but is likely to be reciprocal. Depression has been established as an independent risk factor for stroke and cardiac failure, and is a negative prognostic indicator in the recovery from a number of physical disorders including myocardial infarction (4). Conversely, many medical conditions have been shown to have causative roles in depression. Most of these are more prevalent in elderly patients, and the clinician should be aware of the possibility of a co-morbid depression developing in the setting of an established medical condition. Apathetic and hypoactive forms of delirium may mimic depression in certain circumstances, and must always be ruled out in the diagnostic work-up of elderly patients. A Cochrane meta-analysis has shown antidepressants to be effective in patients of all ages with co-morbid physical illness (9).

Depression and cognitive dysfunction

The relationship between depressive illness and cognitive dysfunction in elderly patients is particularly important in clinical practice. They are frequently present co-morbidly, and may mimic or exacerbate each other. Clarification of the underlying aetiology of the patient's presenting complaint may be difficult in some cases, but is likely to have significant implications on treatment and outcomes as depression is much more amenable to treatment than dementia.

Impaired cognitive performance in the setting of a significant depressive episode has been termed "pseudodementia" or "reversible dementia", implying that the cognitive deficits would resolve with adequate treatment of the depressive episode. However, the nature of these cognitive deficits is not fully understood, and a recent meta-analysis (10) has challenged the previously held belief that these syndromes are highly prevalent. The proposed entity of vascular depression may overlap with impaired cognitive performance in some cases, although this is not fully understood. Some authors emphasize a dysexecutive syndrome arising

from frontal-subcortical dysfunction, whilst others describe broad cognitive performance deficits attributable purely to slowed cognitive processing.

Major depression in late life may act as a risk factor for the later development of a dementia syndrome. Furthermore, major depression complicated by a reversible dementia in elderly patients may be associated with a significantly higher risk for the later development an irreversible dementia (10). It is likely that at least some of the patients in the latter group fall into the broader category of early-stage dementia. A key implication of these findings is that treatment of depressive symptoms may be beneficial to cognitive performance in the short term, but often the patient will later develop a dementia, most frequently of the Alzheimer's type.

DIAGNOSIS

The diagnostic approach to depressive illness in elderly patients should always include a thorough history, including collateral sources wherever possible. The observations of others, particularly those with a long-term relationship with the patient, may contrast significantly with the patient's own complaints.

The clinical diagnosis of depression should be made in accordance with widely accepted criteria such as ICD-10 (11) and DSM-IV (12). However, in elderly patients these criteria should not be followed slavishly, as "atypical" presentations can be the rule rather than the exception. A number of screening instruments exist which may assist in the diagnosis of depression in elderly patients. Most widely used is the Geriatric Depression Scale (13), a simple self-rating questionnaire with multiple versions of different lengths. This is probably the screening instrument of choice for depression in elderly patients. The 12-item version has been shown to maintain its validity in the setting of mild to moderate (but not severe) dementia, while the 15-item version has proven validity across cultures. A 4-item version designed for rapid screening has been shown to have almost comparable sensitivity. The Cornell Scale for

Depression in Dementia (14) may be used in cases of more advanced dementia. It has good internal validity and reliability, but its clinical utility is limited by the time needed to complete it (about 30 minutes). Despite the rigour of various instruments, they are best employed as screening tools and clinical examination should remain the gold standard in assessment. Indeed, when used alone, screening has not been shown to improve outcomes.

Cognitive screening using the Mini Mental State Examination (15) (MMSE) should be a routine part of any examination of elderly patients, and can usefully be incorporated into the cognitive domain of the mental state examination. The relative lack of sensitivity of the MMSE in detecting frontal lobe pathology can be compensated for by use of instruments targeted to the frontal lobes such as the Frontal Assessment Battery (FAB) (16). Combination of the MMSE and FAB as bedside screening tests for cognitive dysfunction in elderly patients has the potential to be particularly useful. Where indicated, neuropsychological testing can assist in further diagnostic clarification.

Vital to the diagnostic approach in elderly patients is screening for organic pathology. A thorough physical examination should be routine practice, and tailored to the individual patient. Routine blood tests should include full blood count, electrolytes, liver function, serum glucose, bone function, thyroid function, B12 and folate. Other tests, including CT head, EEG, chest x-ray and syphilis serology should be ordered if clinically indicated (3).

Exploration of suicide risk is essential in all depressed patients. Suicidal and self-harming behaviours are much more commonly genuine in their intent than similar acts in younger age groups. It is a common misconception that clinician enquiry on this subject may be counter-productive. This is not the case. Established risk factors for suicide in elderly patients include older age, isolation, male gender, previous suicide attempts, evidence of planning, recent bereavement, chronic illness or pain, alcohol and other substance abuse. Mental state findings indicative of higher risk include suicidal thoughts and plans, marked agitation, hopelessness, worthlessness, guilt, marked insomnia, marked hypochondriasis and psychosis (17). Marriage, on the other hand, is protective. Suicide risk should be assessed on an ongoing basis throughout the course of treatment, as "the risk of suicide in some patients recovering from major depressive disorder increases transiently as they develop the energy and capacity to act on self-destructive plans made earlier in the course of their illness" (18).

THERAPY

The aims of treatment are to induce remission of current symptoms, reduce the risk of suicide and self-harm, optimize function, and prevent relapse (6). A number of comprehensive, evidence-based clinical practice guidelines on the treatment of depression have been published in recent years (3, 4, 18, 19). However, most of these are not based on studies of elderly subjects.

Treatment of depression in elderly patients should be multimodal, including biological, psychological and social interventions specific to the needs of the individual patient. Psychological interventions are valuable in the treatment of depressive disorders, and may take various forms, ranging from education and supportive interventions to more structured therapies. Cognitive behaviour therapy (CBT) has a particularly strong evidence base in treating depression. A good deal of evidence supports the use of psychotherapy and antidepressants in combination, and outcomes may often be better than treatment with either alone. Factors such as hearing impairment, poor concentration, fatigue, and memory problems potentially reduce the efficacy of psychotherapeutic treatments.

Elderly patients treated with antidepressant medication have been shown to have response rates equal to those of the broader population (roughly 50–70%). Large meta-analyses (20, 21) have shown no significant difference in antidepressant effect, safety or tolerability between the major classes of antidepressants in elderly patients. Patients with co-morbid anxiety may require a longer trial of medication.

In clinical practice, issues specific to the individual patient must be considered when choosing an antidepressant. These include the nature of the current depressive illness, past treatments and their effectiveness and tolerability, medical co-morbidities, potential drug interactions, and the patient's own preferences. Given that multiple agents have demonstrated efficacy, the choice will often be made on the basis of the known side-effect profile of a medication. Depression accompanied by insomnia, agitation or anxiety may be best treated with an agent that has a mild sedating property (e.g. mirtazapine, fluvoxamine), while lethargy, apathy and amotivation may respond better to an activating agent (e.g. venlafaxine). Intolerable side-effects will invariably lead to poor compliance and failure of treatment, and in these situations an alternative agent should be employed. Some antidepressants may cause agitation and restlessness in elderly patients, and the early stages of treatment should be closely monitored for these. The very long half-life and active metabolites of fluoxetine may be clinically relevant when changing to another antidepressant as a washout period is likely to be required. The tricyclic antidepressants (TCA) may cause sedation and a range of anticholinergic side-effects including postural hypotension, which may increase the risk of falls in elderly patients.

It is useful to group the antidepressants into first line and second line agents. The first line agents are so chosen for their efficacy combined with a wide margin of safety. Each, however, has an individual profile of receptor occupancy and potential for drug interactions. Amongst the SSRIs, citalopram may be preferred for its relatively low rate of drug interactions and generally good tolerability. The second line agents are highly effective antidepressants but their clinical utility is reduced by their higher lethality in overdose, side-effect burden, and in the case of the monoamine oxidase inhibitors (MAOIs), the need for strict compliance with a tyramine-free diet to avoid a hypertensive crisis.

Recommended starting and maximum doses for most commonly used antidepressants are listed below (see Box 3.1). It should ideally be noted that a "trial" of an antidepressant requires good compliance at an effective dose for an adequate period of time. A period of 6–12 weeks is recommended initially (22). Conclusions about the efficacy or otherwise of an antidepressant should not be made until this has been achieved. Reasons for non-compliance should be explored with the patient and addressed. Clinical decision-making after the commencement of an antidepressant will be largely dependent upon the initial response to that medication. A treatment algorithm for geriatric depression which measures progress on the 24-item Hamilton Depression Rating Scale (23) (HDRS) is a useful aid to clinical decision-making (22). It may be summarized as follows:

- *Remission achieved*
  - continue medication at dose that induced remission
- *Good response (50 % improvement in HDRS or better)*
  - continue medication at current dose
- *Partial response (30–50 % improvement)*
  - increase dose of current antidepressant, or,
  - augment current antidepressant
  - trial alternative antidepressant
- *Insignificant response (<30 % improvement)*
  - discontinue current treatment
  - commence alternative antidepressant
- *Non-response*
  - discontinue current treatment
  - commence alternative antidepressant.

In the event of a good response to treatment with complete or near-complete remission of symptoms of a major depressive episode, treatment should continue for 6–12 months, with ongoing monitoring. A period of weaning off the drug under supervision could be considered at this time if indicated. Any subsequent relapse should ideally be managed with the same medication at the same dose that previously induced remission. Pharmacological management of relapsesshould ideally continue for longer (1–2 years). A second significant relapse in elderly patients may signal the need for ongoing a treatment.

Box 3.1: Antidepressant dosing guide in elderly patients

1ⁿᵈ line	Dosing Starting	Dosing Dose range	Adverse effects	CYP-450 Inhibition 1A2	CYP-450 Inhibition 2D6	CYP-450 Inhibition 3A4	Clinical tips
			(SSRI class effects)				
(Es) Citalopram	10mg	20–40mg	nausea	−	−	−	fewest drug interactions
Fluoxetine	10mg	20–40mg	diarrhoea	+ +	−	+ +	long+half-life
Fluvoxamine	50mg	100–300mg	agitation/restlessness	+ + +	+	+ +	
Paroxetine	10mg	20–40mg	insomnia	+	+ + +	+	wean slowly
Sertraline	50mg	100–200mg	sexual dysfunction	−	+ +	+ +	
Venlafaxine XR	37.5mg	150–300mg	low doses: similar to SSRI	+	+	+	often 2ⁿᵈ line agent
Duloxetine	30mg	30–60mg	high doses: similar to TCA		+		
Mirtazapine	15mg	30–60mg	sedation	+		+	may reduce insomnia / minimal data in elderly pts.
			weight gain				
Reboxetine	4mg	4–8mg	agitation/restlessness anticholinergic effects				
Moclobemide	150mg	300–450mg	headache/dizziness insomnia/agitation				minimal data in elderly patients
2ⁿᵈ line							
			(TCA class effects)				
Amitriptyline	25mg	75–100mg	sedation				all high-lethality in overdose
Clomipramine	10mg	50–150mg	postural hypotension				
Dothiepin	50mg	75–150mg	weight gain				
Doxepin	75mg	75–150mg	dizziness				
Imipramine	10mg	75–150mg	dry mouth				
Nortriptyline	20mg	20–150mg	constipation				
Trimipramine	75mg	75–150mg	blurred vision				
Phenelzine	15mg bd	30–45mg bd	postural hypotension				tyramine-free diet requires strict adherence
Tranylcypromine	5mg bd	10–15mg bd	insomnia				never combine with SSRI's
			sexual dysfunction				
Mianserin	30mg	60–120mg	similar to mirtazapine				may cause neutropenia (rare)

Treatment-resistant depression is not uncommon, and may be managed by augmenting existing antidepressants, by combining the current antidepressant with another antidepressant or formal psychotherapy, or by using electroconvulsive therapy (ECT). In the case of augmentation, the best evidence is for the use of lithium, which is effective in roughly half of cases when used in this manner. However, evidence specific to elderly patients is lacking. Some evidence also supports the use of triiodothyronine as an augmenting agent, and to a lesser extent pindolol. The atypical antipsychotics may be useful augmenting agents, particularly in psychotic depression. The use of combination antidepressants is best done under the direct supervision of a psychiatrist, and certain combinations are contraindicated. The serotonin syndrome, which can be fatal, may result from inappropriate combination therapy.

Electroconvulsive therapy (ECT) has long been employed as an effective and safe treatment for depression. It is commonly used in elderly patients, where it may be particularly effective. Absolute contraindications to its use are few, if any, and it is generally well-tolerated in elderly patients. A greater risk of post-ictal confusion is the main treatment side-effect. However, a recent Cochrane review was unable to draw any conclusions regarding the merits of ECT over antidepressants in elderly patients due to the relatively poor quality of earlier published trials (24), and further studies are needed in this area.

REFERENCES

1. Murray, C, Lopez, A. *The Global Burden of Disease: a comprehensive assessment of mortality and disability from disease, injuries and risk factors in 1990 and projected to 2020*. Harvard University Press. Boston, 1996. http://www.who.int/healthinfo/bodestimates/en/index.html.

2. Beekman, A, Copeland, J, Prince, M. Review of community prevalence of depression in later life. *British Journal of Psychiatry* 1999; **174**: 307–11.

3. World Psychiatric Association International Committee for Prevention and Treatment of Depression *Depressive Disorders in Older Persons*. NCM Publishers. New York, 1999. http://www.wpanet.org/sectorial/edu4a.html.

4. NIH Consensus Panel Diagnosis and treatment of depression in late life. *Journal of the American Medical Association* 1992; **278**: 1186–90.

5. Jeste, D, Alexopoulos, G, Bartels, S, Cummings, J, Gallo, J, Gottlieb, G, Halpain, M, Palmer, B, Patterson, T, Reynolds, C, Lebowitz, B Consensus statement on the upcoming crisis in geriatric mental health: research agenda for the next two decades. *Archives of General Psychiatry* 1999; **56**: 848–53.

6. Baldwin, R, Chiu, E, Katona, C, Graham, N *Guidelines on Depression in Older People. Practising the Evidence*. Martin Dunitz. London, 2002.

7. Brodaty, H, Luscombe, G, Parker, G, Wilhelm, K, Hickie, I, Austin, M-P, Mitchell, P. Early and late onset depression in old age: different aetiologies, same phenomenology. *Journal of Affective Disorders* 2001; **66**: 225–36.

8. Brodaty, H, Cullen, B, Thompson, C, Mitchell, P, Parker, G, Wilhelm, K, Austin, M-P Malhi, G Age and gender in the phenomenology of depression. *American Journal of Geriatric Psychiatry* 2005; **13**: 589–96.

9. Gill, D, Hatcher, S Antidepressants for depression in medical illness. *The Cochrane Database of Systematic Reviews* 2000, Issue 4. Art. No.: CD001312. DOI: 10.1002/14651858.CD001312.pub2. http://www3.interscience.wiley.com/cgi-bin/mrwhome/106568753/HOME.

10. Clarfield, A The decreasing prevalence of reversible dementias. An updated meta-analysis. *Archives of Internal Medicine* 2003; **163**: 2219–29.

11. *International statistical classification of diseases and related health problems*. World Health Organization. Geneva, 1992. www.who.int/entity/classifications/icd/en/.

12. *Diagnostic and Statistical Manual of Mental Disorders*, 4th ed. (text revision) American Psychiatric Association. Washington DC, 2000.

13. Yesavage, J, Brink, T, Rose, T, Lum, O Development and validation of a geriatric depression screening scale: a preliminary report. *Journal of Psychiatric Research* 1983; **17**: 37–9.

14. Alexopoulos, G, Abrams, R, Young, R, Shamoian, C Cornell Scale for depression in dementia. *Biological Psychiatry* 1988; **23**: 271–84.

15. Folstein, M, Folstein, S McHugh, P "Mini-Mental State": a practical method for grading the cognitive state of patients for the clinician. *Journal of Psychiatric Research* 1975; **12**: 817–98.

16. Dubois, B, Slachevsky, A, Litvan, I, Pillon, B The FAB. A frontal assessment battery at the bedside. 2000; *Neurology* **55**: 1621–6.

17. Alexopoulos, G, Katz, I, Reynolds, C, Carpenter, D, Docherty, J The expert consensus guideline series: Pharmacotherapy of Depressive Disorders in Older Patients. Postgraduate Medical Special Report (October): 1–86, Expert Knowledge Systems, LLC, McGraw-Hill Healthcare Information Programs, Minneapolis, US, 2001. http://www.psychguides.com/.

18. American Psychiatric Association: Practice Guideline for the Treatment of Patients with Major Depressive Disorder (Revision). *American Journal of Psychiatry* 2000; **157**: 1–45. http://www.psych.org/.

19. Royal Australian and New Zealand College of Psychiatrists Clinical Practice Guidelines Team for Depression Australian and New Zealand clinical practice guidelines for the treatment of depression. *Australian and New Zealand Journal of Psychiatry* 2004; **38**: 389–407. http://ranzcp.org/.

20. Mittman, N, Hermann, N, Einarson, T et al. The efficacy, safety and tolerability of antidepressants in late life depression: a meta-analysis. *Journal of Affective Disorders* 1997; 191–217.

21. Wilson, K, Mottram, P, Sivanranthan, A, Nightingale, A Antidepressants versus placebo for the depressed elderly. *The Cochrane Database of Systematic Reviews* 2001, Issue 1. Art No.: CD000561. DOI: 10.1002/14651858.CD000561 http://www3.interscience.wiley.com/cgi-bin/mrwhome/106568753/HOME.

22. Mulsant, B, Alexopoulos, G, Reynolds III, C, Katz, I, Abrams, R, Oslin, D, Schulberg, H and the PROSPECT Study Group Pharmacological treatment of depression in older primary care patients: the PROSPECT algorithm. *International Journal of Geriatric Psychiatry* 2001; **16**: 585–92.

23. Hamilton, M. A rating scale for depression. *Journal of Neurology, Neurosurgery and Psychiatry* 1960; **23**: 56–62.

24. Van der Wurff, F, Stek, M Hoogendijk, W, Beekman, A Electroconvulsive therapy for the depressed elderly. *The Cochrane Database of systematic Reviews* 2003, Issue 2. Art. No: CD003593. DOI: 1002/14651858.CD003593. http://www3.interscience.wiley.com/cgi-bin/mrwhome/106568753/HOME.

4 Psychotic illness in elderly patients

Ross Kalucy, Jo Hill and Richard Weeks

Department of Psychiatry, Flinders Medical Centre, Adelaide, Australia

INTRODUCTION

First episode psychosis in elderly patients is rarely of a non organic cause. It is most commonly sequelae to the dementias (Alzheimer's, Cerebrovascular, and Lewy Body Disease) and to delirium in this age group. An elderly patient who presents with acute, first onset psychosis, the working diagnosis of delirium until proven otherwise would prevent an important and often missed diagnosis.

Psychosis in old age is becoming a growing public health concern, as our population ages and with predicted increases in the number of patients with dementia. Psychotic symptoms cause a great deal of distress to patients, their families and their carers, interfering with their ability to look after them. Initial presentation may coincide with carers being worn out and no longer able to manage the care of the older patient with psychosis.

Psychosis is typified by the presence of delusions (irrational beliefs, such as paranoia) and/or hallucinations (visual or auditory). Persecutory beliefs of a non bizarre nature should always be investigated, given particular vulnerabilities in those patients with dementia. Patients often experience anxiety in response to their delusional beliefs and hallucinatory experiences, particularly if they are paranoid. They may even be experiencing panic symptoms, such as severe anxiety, shortness of breath, palpitations, tremor, dry mouth, gastric irritability. It is important to identify these symptoms and signs, as these are not only distressing for the patient, but may increase their likelihood of acting on their beliefs.

Deciphering the underlying cause of psychotic symptoms in elderly patients can be challenging and complex, with medical and environmental antecedents. Reversible medical causes, (such as medication side effects, urinary tract infection, occult pneumonia, transient ischaemic attacks) and physical discomfort (such as arthritic pain) should always be considered before assuming the symptoms are purely dementia related. Sensory impairment (visual and auditory) should also be taken into account prior to a diagnosis being made, as these may contribute to the patient's inability to assess their environment. Poor sleep cycles and nutrition can also adversely affect the way cognitively impaired patients can interpret the environment. Cultural factors may also play a role in the emergence of symptoms, particularly in elderly patients who have survived major wars and invasion.

AETIOLOGY

Psychosis

In order to adequately treat psychosis in elderly patients it is important to elucidate the aetiology.

Prescribing for Elderly Patients Edited by Stephen Jackson, Paul Jansen and Arduino Mangoni
© 2009 John Wiley & Sons, Ltd

It is not uncommon to find multiple aetiologies particularly in the cases of dementia with co-morbid delirium. The patients' longitudinal history (particularly of cognitive deficits or reduced function), psychiatric, medical and drug history all need to be considered, as well as thorough investigation for reversible conditions.

Delirium

Delirium is the most important diagnosis to exclude and is the most common co-morbidity in an elderly person presenting for the first time with psychosis. Advanced age is a major risk factor for delirium, with approximately 30–40 % of hospitalized patients over 65 having an episode. Around 60 % of nursing home residents over the age of 70 have repeated episodes of delirium (1). Delirium is a syndrome of many potential causes, and remains an under diagnosed and potentially life threatening disorder. Medication, particularly in elderly patients, should always be scrutinized as a potential cause of delirium. Those with underlying brain disease such as Alzheimer's Dementia, cerebrovascular disease, history of alcohol dependence are particularly vulnerable.

The Dementias

The dementias are the most common primary cause of psychosis in elderly patients. This can be explained by the ease in which older people with cognitive impairment can misinterpret their environment, particularly if there is co-morbid sensory impairment or pain. They can become more isolated and lack the ability to reality test. As well as this, they are prone to delirium, which can further impair their cognition and reasoning skills.

Parkinson's Disease

Between 20–60 % of patients with Parkinson's disease experience psychotic symptoms (2). The psychotic symptoms are most likely to be extrinsic, due to dopamine agonists (levodopa), dopamine releasers (amantadine) and monoamine oxidase inhibitors (selegiline), rather than intrinsic, due to malfunctioning dopaminergic pathways (3).

Other organic conditions

The following are less common causes that should be considered in the differential diagnosis: frontal or limbic tumours, epilepsy (particularly temporal lobe), substances (alcohol hallucinosis), Huntington's disease, B12 deficiency, Creutzfeld-Jacob disease, Herpes encephalitis, normal pressure hydrocephalus, systemic lupus erythematosus, Wernicke-Korsakoff syndrome and Wilson's disease (4).

Schizophrenia

In the over 65 year old population living in the community, less than 1 % have a diagnosis of schizophrenia. Most people with schizophrenia in old age have had their condition since early adulthood, it is much less common to present for the first time in old age.

Mood Disorders

Psychosis in old age can also present as part of a mood disorder (major depression, mania). Like schizophrenia, the causes of these syndromes are multifactorial.

Other primary psychiatric conditions

Psychosis in old age can also be due to psychiatric conditions other than mood disorders and schizophrenia. Schizoaffective disorder (which commonly has its onset in younger age groups), brief reactive psychosis and delusional disorder are less common, but should also be considered in the differential diagnosis, once organic causes are excluded.

Associated anxiety and agitation

It is important to isolate out the thought that is driving the anxiety, as it may not be psychosis related. It may be due to some medications (e.g. selective serotoninergic reuptake inhibitors, sympathomimetics), other medical conditions (eg thyrotoxicosis) or to co-morbid psychiatric disorder if there is a history. Pain can also be a major contributing factor to anxiety and agitation in elderly patients.

SYMPTOMS AND SIGNS

Due to the various underlying conditions in elderly patients that lead to psychotic symptoms, clinical presentations may vary depending on the cause.

Delirium

Patients with delirium present with disorientation, incoherence, a rapid deterioration in cognition and behaviour over hours. A diurnal fluctuation, with predominant activity in the evenings and drowsiness in the mornings and a conscious state that varies throughout the day is typical of delirium. Psychotic symptoms are usually a function of patients' inability to adequately assess their surrounds. Delusions and hallucinations are usually persecutory in nature, and not well systematised as in those patients with schizophrenia. There is usually no psychiatric history. However there may be a history of underlying cognitive disorder, use of multiple medications and co-morbid medical history. Physical signs and symptoms will be dependant on what the underlying cause is.

Dementia

In patients with dementia, the onset of psychotic symptoms appears after they have already met the criteria for dementia. Often they do not have a previous or family psychiatric history. They experience visual rather than auditory hallucinations, and their delusions are typically paranoid, simple and nonbizarre.

Frequently they describe delusions of misidentification (5). These include the belief that known others are replaced by impostors (e.g. the Gestapo disguised as nurses), that there are "phantom boarders" living in their homes, and that their reflection in the mirror represents another person with whom they can converse.

In some instances it is important to differentiate what is in fact psychotic and what can be reality based. Older people with dementia are often very vulnerable. Stories of potential emotional, physical, or financial abuse should be corroborated as thoroughly as possible, by obtaining collateral history from multiple sources.

Schizophrenia

In patients with schizophrenia of early onset, there is often a long standing history characterized by hospital admissions, use of antipsychotic medication and possible side effects such as parkinsonism and tardive dyskinesia. Schizophrenia is characterised by a history of both negative (e.g. withdrawal and apathy) and positive (e.g. hallucinations and delusions) symptoms.

Separate to the psychotic symptoms of schizophrenia, is cognitive dysfunction, and this may be difficult to differentiate from dementia later in life. As the brain ages, treatment for schizophrenia may become more challenging due to the possibility of co-morbid dementia.

In late onset schizophrenia the onset is generally more acute with fewer negative symptoms and less disorder of behaviour and speech (6). Older psychotic patients with schizophrenia are more likely to be suicidal (50 % attempting suicide, and 10 % succeeding) (7), than other elderly psychotic patients.

Mood Disorders

Patients with psychotic depression usually describe low mood often with diurnal variation, insomnia, poor appetite, anhedonia, low energy levels, and display a negative sense of self, future and world. Their delusions are usually mood congruent, in that they may focus on punishment, guilt, concerns of cancer and dying, somatization, nihilism or poverty. Auditory hallucinations may be accusative or punitive in nature. They can present with either psychomotor agitation or retardation, with flattened affect. Cognitive impairment particularly in attention and short term memory can signify the presence of depressive pseudodementia, which often resolves with antidepressant therapy. Patients with pseudodementia are more inclined to give up on memory tasks, whereas those with dementia often confabulate the answers if they are not sure. Anxiety symptoms may also be prominent.

Manic psychosis present with increased activation, decreased need for sleep, increased spending, increased risk taking behaviours due to disinhibition. Psychotic symptoms are characterized by grandiose delusions, often involving royalty or other public figure, hyper-religiosity. On mental state they exhibit pressure of speech and psychomotor agitation. There may be a personal and/or a history of recurrent depression or bipolar disorder in these patients, as well as those with psychotic depression. Like those with schizophrenia, co-morbid medical illness and evolving structural brain disease can exacerbate their condition even if it has been stable for many years. It is important to take a medication history particularly in relation to effective treatments, side effects and compliance.

DIAGNOSIS

Psychotic episodes are diagnosed purely on a clinical basis, with the presence of hallucinations and delusions that are causing considerable disruption to their functioning. The challenge here is not in the diagnosis of psychosis *per se*, but deciphering the underlying aetiologies (of which there are usually several).

Older people with first episode psychosis often present at the bequest of another, usually spouse or carer. There may be difficulties extracting a full history from the patient, due to either thought disorder, suspiciousness or memory difficulties. It is useful to initially establish rapport by asking the patient about their living circumstances, their family, what they did for a living, what they enjoy doing as hobbies, pets, for example. Once rapport is established psychotic phenomenology is more likely to be demonstrated when you ask them what is causing their distress. If information

is not so forthcoming enquiring specifically, about unusual events, things going missing, neighbours, bugging devices, home invasion, impostors and so forth might be useful. Asking about mood, sleep disturbance and appetite are also important.

A history of previous psychiatric illness, medical history (including presence of pain, and sensory deficits), medication history, substance history, family and personal history including any recent decline in function should be pursued if not from the patient, from collateral sources. A careful mental state examination paying particular attention to self care, evidence of weight loss, psychomotor agitation or retardation, coherence or pressure of speech, presence of delusions, affect, evidence of responding to auditory or visual hallucinations should be conducted. The mental state examination requires inclusion of the Folstein Mini Mental State examination looking particularly at orientation, registration and short term memory. The Frontal Assessment Battery may also be useful if frontal lobe pathology is suspected.

A full physical examination, looking for underlying causes should be carried out. Investigations should routinely include a full blood count, electrolytes, liver function tests, thyroid function tests, B12 and folate levels, urine analysis and CT head. More focused investigations (eg serology, lumbar puncture, urine drug screens, EEG, etc.) should be considered if there is clinical suspicion.

THERAPY

It may take some time between initial presentation and elucidation of underlying aetiology. In the interim patient and carer safety needs to be determined, and appropriate treatment setting needs to be established. Unless there are acute medical or safety issues, it is best to manage the patient in a familiar environment, such as in there own home with the help of a community mental health team, and close liaison with their family/carers. Safety concerns that should warrant hospitalisation include combativeness, not enabling self care, acting provocatively and homicidal/suicidal ideation and behaviours. As a last resort, use of mental health legislation may be required if the patient does not wish to be admitted to hospital. Initially psychotic patients require frequent reassurance and avoidance of confronting and overly intrusive questions and investigations. If investigations are required urgently, use of low stat dose benzodiazepines and having a familiar party available may alleviate some anxiety.

If the underlying aetiology is identified and reversible, this should be treated. Medications that are likely to worsen psychotic symptoms and confusion (e.g. anticholinergics, regular hypnotics and steroids) should be reviewed regarding their necessity and ideally weaned and/or ceased. Particular attention should be given to reducing excessive stimulation in the environment, that patients with hearing and visual impairment have access to hearing aids and glasses. Close attention should be paid to ensuring adequate night time sleep, food and fluid intake. Mobility should be assessed early by a physiotherapist due to potential falls risk, to assess the need for hip protectors, walking aids and supervision of mobility. Ideally patients should be cared for in an environment that enables mobility. Dietician involvement may be required if there has been significant weight loss due to poor self care.

Appropriate pharmacological treatment should be carefully planned in this age group. They are at increased risk of side effects, and are less inclined to report these than their younger counterparts. Lack of compliance or accidental over dosage may occur due to cognitive problems and psychotic symptoms. Age related pharmacokinetic changes such as altered oral absorption, altered volume of distribution and reduced metabolism, clearance and excretion should also be considered. Medical co-morbidity can also complicate management. Elderly patients are more likely to have cardiovascular disease and diabetes, both of which can render some antipsychotics contraindicated. Poor general health can also lead to drug toxicity in the elderly population. With co-morbid illness comes the increased likelihood of polypharmacy which

can further increase risk of adverse effects and unpredictable drug interactions.

Atypical antipsychotics such as risperidone, quetiapine and olanzapine have been increasingly used in elderly patients. They represent a safer as well as efficacious way of managing symptoms of psychosis in older people, and should always be considered as first line treatment. Short acting benzodiazepines have also shown benefit in managing anxiety and agitation in psychotic elderly patients.

The newer atypical agents have been shown to carry less risk of extra-pyramidal side effects than conventional antipsychotics, and because of their serotoninergic properties are effective against negative and positive symptoms. Patients with tardive dyskinesia who change from a conventional antipsychotic to an atypical often have resolution of their TD symptoms (8). In low doses, atypical antipsychotics are also tolerated by patients with Parkinson's disease, with minimal risk of extrapyramidal symptoms. For these reasons atypical antipsychotics should be the first line of treatment for psychosis in elderly patients (9).

For many years, psychotic symptoms in elderly patients have been treated with conventional antipsychotics, such as chlorpromazine (low potency) and haloperidol (high potency). Due to the effects on multiple receptors, low potency conventional antipsychotics carry the risk of over sedation, postural hypotension, urinary retention, constipation, visual blurring, confusion, tachycardia and mouth dryness. High potency conventional antipsychotics are more selective towards dopamine blockade and, with that, cause an increased risk in extra pyramidal symptoms (tremor, dystonia, bradykinesia). Both can lead to an increased risk in falls. Traditional antipsychotics also carry an increased risk of producing tardive dyskinesia in elderly patients, particularly with increasing cumulative dose, duration of treatment and age (10). Traditional antipsychotics are targeted specifically to positive symptoms and do not treat any of the negative symptoms of psychotic disorders.

Choice of medication and doses may also vary, for a given cause of psychosis. In psychosis secondary to Alzheimer's dementia, a limited course of low dose atypical antipsychotic, eg risperidone 1–2 mg a day, has been shown to be effective in about half nursing home patients studied by Katz and colleagues (see guidelines) (11). Care must be taken to start at a low dose of 0.5 mg and to gradually titrate upward according to tolerability. At higher doses there is an increased risk of extra pyramidal symptoms. If there are problems with hypotension or extrapyramidal symptoms, an alternative medication such as olanzapine or quetiapine may be used (see guidelines). Cholinesterase inhibitors (12), and serotoninergic antidepressants (13), have also been shown to be effective in Alzheimer's related psychosis.

In patients with Lewy Body Disease or psychotic symptoms related to Parkinson's medication, care should be taken with the use of risperidone due to its D2 antagonist properties; alternatives often chosen are olanzapine or quetiapine. Donepezil has been shown to particularly useful in treating psychotic symptoms in patients with Lewy Body Disease (14).

In either form of dementia, "as required" medication for anxiety and agitation secondary to psychotic symptoms could take the form of an intermediate acting benzodiazepine (see guidelines). Intermediate acting benzodiazepines are less likely to accumulate and increase risk of falls, than longer acting benzodiazepines such as diazepam and they are less likely to cause rebound anxiety than shorter acting benzodiazepines such as alprazolam. A regular dose of benzodiazepine in the short term may be given at times where specific intervention is required, for example with dressing and showering, if the patient is particularly resistive and agitated at these times.

Patients with schizophrenia usually require higher doses of medication, and the treatment is ongoing rather than time limited (10). Due to expected side effects, initiating an atypical antipsychotic rather than a traditional antipsychotic is important (6).

Patients with early onset schizophrenia should have their medication history reviewed, to assess previous responses, compliance and side effects. Relapse is usually due to poor physical health, the onset of dementia or cerebrovascular disease, non-compliance, concomitant substance use (e.g. alcohol) or environmental stressors (e.g. loss of parent, accommodation change). Considering a depot form of antipsychotic medication, and/or increased medication supervision in the community would be recommended for relapse due to non compliance. Risperidone now comes in depot form, and there are now current trials underway in this age group.

Reassurance, making appropriate environmental adjustments, care-giver support and multidisciplinary team approach are also important factors in managing psychosis and agitation in this age group. When treating the elderly patient with psychosis, addressing the overall care setting is very important. Often psychotic symptoms in a patient with dementia have antecedents, eg moving to a nursing home away from their spouse, discomfort in their routine, objects going missing, sensory deprivation. It is important to clarify psychotic symptoms from misinterpreted real events. As mentioned previously, this is a vulnerable group and it is important to investigate if claims are in fact reality based (e.g. stolen property). Interventions should be directed to not only the resident, but also the environment (use of familiar objects, day time activity and structure), staff members/carer (frequent introductions and orientation, friendly, positive approach), and system of care (adequate use of staff, individualize care needs to suit resident) (15).

KEY POINTS

- Delirium must always be considered as a diagnosis in psychotic elder
- Polypharmacy and medication side effects should be considered.
- Complexity in diagnosis, co-morbidity is nearly always a factor.
- Elucidation of aetiology usually made over time rather than on initial consultation.
- Treatment resistance in primary psychiatric conditions as the brain ages.

Table 4.1. First-choice medications in the treatment of psychosis in elderly subjects

Drug	Initial dose	Maintenance dose	PK in elderly subjects	Adverse drug reactions	Drug interactions	Clinical tips
Risperidone	0.5 mg/day	1–2 mg/day (dementia and delirium) 3–4 mg/day (schizophrenia)	T1/2 = 20hr	Postural hypo-tension, extra pyramidal symptoms, avoid in Parkinson disease, and Lewy Body dementia	Little clinical effect due to equal potency of parent compound and active metabolite. CYP2D6 system (SSRIs inhibit).	Dose may be increased in increments of 0.5 mg every 5–7 days, pending efficacy and tolerability. Postural blood pressure should be monitored daily after each increase.
Olanzapine	1.25–2.5 mg/nightly	5–10 mg/nightly (dementia and delirium) 10–15 mg/nightly (schizophrenia)	T1/2 = 30hr	Over sedation Tremor Raised serum glucose Weight gain	CYP2D6 and CYP1A2 inhibitors (SSRIs, grapefruit juice) can increase levels. Smoking can decrease levels due to CYP 1A2 inhibition. Little clinical effect.	Dose may be increased by increments of 2.5 mg every 5–7 days, pending efficacy and tolerability. Lower starting dose for patients with Parkinson disease or Lewy Body Dementia due to risk of extrapyramidal symptoms
Quetiapine	12.5 mg/nightly	100 mg BD for dementia and delium 500 mg BD for schizophrenia	T1/2 = 6 hr	Postural hypotension Oversedation	CYP 3A4 inhibitors (macrolide antibiotics and antifungals) may increase plasma levels and cause side effects	Dose may be increased by increments of 12.5–25 mg daily pending efficacy and tolerability. Postural blood pressure should be monitored daily after each increase.

Table 4.2. Other medications to be considered in the treatment of psychosis in elderly subjects

Drug	Indication	Dosage	PK	Adverse effects	Clinical tips
Oxazepam	Agitation and anxiety	7.5 mg–15 mg as required max 30–45 mg in 24 hours	Oral administration 30–60 min until onset of action T1/2 = 3–6 hours (no change with increased age)	Over-sedation Falls risk Hypotension	Can be given to pre-empt episodes of agitation when triggers are known. Blood pressure should be monitored when initiating, and falls risk should be established.
Midazolam	Marked agitation Refusing oral medications	1–2.5 mg as required max 5 mg in 24 hr	Intramuscular administration 30–60 seconds until onset of action. T1/2 = 1–4 hours (parent), 1–20 hours (metabolite). Hepatic clearance	Over-sedation Respiratory depression Anterograde amnesia Hypotension Falls	Liver function should be reviewed prior to use. 1/4 hourly blood pressure and respiratory rate monitoring following administration.
Haloperidol	Marked agitation, Refusing oral medications	1–2.5 mg as required Max 5 mg in 24 hours	Intramuscular administration. T1/2 = 12–36 hours	Avoid in Parkinson disease and Lewy Body Dementia. Extrapyramidal symptoms. Increased risk of Falls.	As required order of benztropine 1–2 mg should be available incase of extrapyramidal symptoms Falls risk and extrapyramidal symptoms should be assessed following use.
Mood stabilizers	Associated manic psychoses	See corresponding chapter			
Anti-cholinesterase inhibitors	Associated Dementia. Psychosis of Lewy Body Dementia particularly responsive	See corresponding chapter			
Antidepressants	Associated depressive symptoms	See corresponding chapter			

- Atypical antipsychotics are favoured over conventional antipsychotics, due to increased vulnerability to side effects in the aged population.

REFERENCES

1. Jacoby, R, Oppenheimer, C *Psychiatry in the Elderly* 2nd ed. New York,Oxford University Press, 1997.
2. Wolters, EC, Berendse, HW Management of psychosis in Parkinson's disease. *Curr Opin Neurol* 2001; **14**(4): 499–504.
3. Mintzer, J, Targum, SD Psychosis in elderly patients; classification and pharmacotherapy. *J Geriatric Psychiatry and Neurol* 2003; **16**(4): 199–206.
4. Kaplan, HI, Saddock, BJ, Sadock, VA *Kaplan and Sadock's Synopsis of Psychiatry* 8th ed. Lippincott, Williams and Wilkins, 2003.
5. Karim, S, Burns, A The biology of psychosis in older people. *J. Geriatric Psychiatry and Neurol* 2003; **16**(4): 207–12.
6. Jeste, DV, Harris, MJ, Pearlson, G., et al. Late-onset schizophrenia. Studying clinical validity. *Psychiatr Clin North Am* 1988; **11**(1): 1–13.
7. Jeste, DV, Finkel, SI Psychosis of Alzheimer's disease and related dementias. Diagnostic criteria for a distinct syndrome. *Am J Geriatr Psychiatry* 2000; **8**(1): 29–34.
8. Jeste, DV Tardive dyskinesia in older patients. *J Clin Psychiatry* 2000; **61**(suppl 4): 27–32.
9. Van De Vijver, DA, Roos, RA, Jansen, PA, et al. Use of antipsychotics in Parkinson's disease in daily practice. *Br J Clin Pharmacol* 2002; **53**(5): 551P.
10. Jeste, DV, Rockwell, E, Harris, MJ, et al. Conventional vs. newer antipsychotics in elderly patients. *Am J Geriatr Psychiatry* 1999; **7**(1): 70–6.
11. Katz, IR, Jeste, DV., Mintzer, JE, et al. Comparison of risperidone and placebo for psychosis and behavioural disturbances associated with dementia: a randomised, double-blind trial. Risperidone Study Group. *J Clin Psychiatry* 1999; **60**(2): 107–15.
12. Tariot, PN, Cummings, JL, Katz, IR, et al. A randomized, double blind, placebo—controlled study on the efficacy and safety of donepezil in patients with Alzheimer's disease in the nursing home setting. *J Am Geriatr Soc* 2001; **49**(12): 1590–9.
13. Pollock, BG, Mulsant, BH, Rosen,. et al. Comparison of citalopram, perphenazine, and placebo for the acute treatment of psychosis and behavioural disturbances in hospitalized, demented patients. *Am J Psychiatry* 2002; **159**(3): 460–465.
14. McKeith, IG Behavioural and psychological symptoms of dementia and Dementia with Lewy Bodies. *Int Psychogeriatr* 2000; **12**(suppl 1): 189–93.
15. Cohen-Mansfield, J Nonpharmacologic interventions for psychotic symptoms of dementia. *J Geriatric Psychiatry and Neurol* 2003; **16**(4): 219–24.

5 Sleep disorders in the elderly: The pros and cons of prescribing

R. Doug McEvoy[1] and Karin S. Nyfort-Hansen[2]

[1]*Adelaide Institute for Sleep Health, Repatriation General Hospital, Adelaide, Australia*
[2]*Pharmacy Department, Repatriation General Hospital, Adelaide, Australia*

INSOMNIA

Insomnia is difficulty falling asleep, staying asleep or having non-restorative sleep, resulting in distress or daytime dysfunction (1). Complaints about sleep quality are common amongst the elderly and are often incorrectly attributed to the aging process itself. Insomnia can be part of a primary sleep disorder, but in the elderly patient it is more usually a symptom associated with a co-morbid condition, or related to behavioural, environmental or pharmacological factors (2, 3). Identification of the causes of insomnia is therefore central to patient management.

Insomnia can have serious consequences in the elderly including an increased risk of falls and cognitive impairment (2, 3). Impaired attention, response times and short term memory may be mistaken for dementia and result in earlier loss of independence.

Initial assessment

A thorough sleep history should include the duration of the insomnia, usual retiring time, how long it takes to fall asleep, number of awakenings, arising time, fatigue during the day and daytime naps. The patient's beliefs about sleep and their own sleep problem and its causes may also reveal useful information.

The first step in management is to consider the potential contribution of common causes of insomnia (3–5). The patient should be questioned regarding the possible role of the following co-morbidities, medications, behavioural and environmental factors:

- Symptoms of chronic diseases and physical illnesses. This includes pain due to arthritis or leg cramps, dyspnoea due to cardiovascular or lung disease, nocturia due to BPH or reflux due to GORD.
- Psychiatric illness, such as anxiety or depression.
- Medications including sympathomimetics such as salbutamol, diuretics, SSRI antidepressants, beta blockers, corticosteroids.
- Environmental factors such as noise or intrusive light levels which may be a particular problem in institutional care.
- Behavioural factors such as caffeine or alcohol consumption in the evening or daytime naps.
- Sleep disorders such as restless legs syndrome and periodic limb movements of sleep or sleep apnoea.

Prescribing for Elderly Patients   Edited by Stephen Jackson, Paul Jansen and Arduino Mangoni
© 2009 John Wiley & Sons, Ltd

Non-drug treatment

Non-drug treatment of insomnia should always be first line (4, 5). Patients should be educated about normal sleep changes due to aging (lighter sleep with more frequent awakenings) in order to reduce anxiety about their insomnia (3).

Optimizing the symptomatic management of co-morbid conditions or physical complaints that may be contributing to insomnia should be addressed. If depression or anxiety is suspected cognitive behavioral therapy or pharmacotherapy may be considered. Suspected sleep disorders should be referred to a sleep disorders centre for further assessment.

Nocturia is a common cause of sleep disturbance in the elderly and also contributes to an increased risk of night-time falls. The possible role of BPH, diuretics, urinary tract infection, caffeine or alcohol ingestion should be considered.

If medications may be contributing to insomnia this problem can often be overcome by adjusting the dosage or the time of day when these medications are taken (Table 5.1) (2). For example most SSRIs should be taken in the morning, and if possible inhaled salbutamol should be scheduled to avoid administration at bedtime. Medications with sedating effects such as tricyclic antidepressants, mirtazapine or antihistamines should be taken in the evening to minimize daytime sleepiness. Lipid soluble beta blockers such as metoprolol and carvedilol cross the blood brain barrier and contribute to insomnia in some patients. Use of alternative agents such as bisoprolol or atenolol may improve sleep quality.

Sleep hygiene refers to daytime and night-time habits and behaviours that may affect sleep quality (3, 4). Many patients have habits which may contribute to their sleep complaints and sleep hygiene education can assist patients to change these habits. Good sleeping habits include:

Table 5.1. Commonly used drugs in the elderly which can cause CNS stimulation and insomnia (2, 5, 6)

Drug or Drug class	Possible options for minimizing sleep disruption
Adrenoreceptor agonists (e.g. salbutamol, terbutaline, salmeterol, eformoterol)	Avoid evening use via nebulizer (more systemic absorption), and within 2–4 hours of bedtime
Anticholinesterases (e.g. donepezil, galantamine, rivastigmine)	Reduce dose and/or take donepezil and controlled release formulations in the morning if patient reports insomnia/vivid dreams
Benzodiazepines	CNS stimulation and insomnia on withdrawal. Avoid chronic use, taper dose slowly if ceasing.
Beta blockers	Avoid use of lipid soluble agents (metoprolol, carvedilol, propranolol). Switch to atenolol or bisoprolol if possible.
Caffeine	Avoid caffeine-containing drinks in the evening. Check over-the-counter products for caffeine content
Glucocorticoids (e.g. prednisolone)	Taper dose if possible, take in the morning
Moclobemide	Give second dose no later than 2pm, if insomnia persists consider switch to sedating antidepressant (e.g. mirtazapine) if appropriate
Nicotine replacement therapy	Remove patch at bedtime
Selective Serotonin Receptor Inhibitors (SSRIs except fluvoxamine)	Take in the morning, reduce dose, if insomnia persists consider switch to sedating antidepressant (e.g. mirtazapine) if appropriate
Selegiline	Reduce dose, consider alternative agents for Parkinson's disease
Theophylline	Minimise dose, give last dose with evening meal
Thyroid hormones	Measure TFTs, reduce dose if indicated
Tramadol	Reduce dose, avoid evening doses, consider switch to alternative analgesic

- avoiding daytime naps;
- avoiding alcohol and caffeine consumption late in the day;
- getting up at the same time each day;
- ensuring a quiet and comfortable bedroom environment which minimizes morning sunlight and disturbances from noise or pets;
- avoiding TV programs, music and conversations in the evening which may lead to arousal, pre-occupation or anxiety.

Daytime exercise or other outdoor activities should also be encouraged where feasible.

A range of behavioural therapies such as cognitive therapy, stimulus control, sleep restriction therapy, progressive muscle relaxation and light therapy may be useful for some patients (3, 4).

In sleep restriction therapy the aim is to consolidate sleep and minimize the time spent in bed when the patient is not asleep thereby extinguishing or reducing the conditioned or anxiety component of psycho-physiological insomnia. A set retiring and arising time are adopted based on the average of total sleep time each night recorded in a two week diary. The object of this bed time restriction is to increase sleep efficiency (i.e. time asleep/time in bed × 100%) to >80%. Once this is achieved the time spent in bed is gradually increased by 20–30 minutes each week until the patient is spending about seven hours in bed. Daytime naps are not permitted. Mild sleep loss and increased fatigue are experienced in the beginning of treatment.

Drug treatment

Hypnotic agents such as benzodiazepines and related drugs should be used only when the response to non-drug treatment has been inadequate, and benefits of treatment are considered to outweigh possible risks (3–5). Therapy should be limited to the shortest possible time and a plan to discontinue the medication should be negotiated with the patient at the time of prescribing.

Benzodiazepines

Short-acting agents such as temazepam or oxazepam are preferred to avoid daytime sedation (Table 5.2). Temazepam has a faster onset of action and may be preferred if initiating sleep is a problem. Long-acting agents such as diazepam, clonazepam, nitrazepam and flunitrazepam should be avoided (3, 5).

A small dose should be used initially (e.g. temazepam 5 mg or oxazepam 7.5 mg) as the elderly are more likely to experience oversedation, memory loss, confusion, ataxia, falls, incontinence and respiratory depression (3, 5). Epidemiological evidence strongly suggests that the use of benzodiazepines in the elderly increases the risk of hip fracture by at least 50% (3, 7).

The hypnotic benefits of benzodiazepines are short-lived and more than 2–3 weeks of regular use may lead to physical and psychological dependence (5).

Benzodiazepines should be used cautiously in patients with sleep apnoea, COPD or severe hepatic impairment (3, 5).

Table 5.2. Pharmacokinetics of some commonly-used hypnotics (8, 9)

Drug	Hypnotic dose in elderly	Onset of action (mins)	Half-life* (hours)	Active metabolites
Alprazolam	Avoid	60–120	10–20	No
Clonazepam	Avoid	60–120	18–60	No
Diazepam	Avoid	60–120	>50	Yes
Flunitrazepam	Avoid	45–60	35	Yes
Nitrazepam	Avoid	30–60	15–50	No
Oxazepam	7.5–15 mg	120–180	10–15	No
Temazepam	5–10 mg	45–60	7–12	No
Zaleplon	5–10 mg	30–60	1–1.2	No
Zopiclone	3.75–7.5 mg	30–90	5–6	One with weak activity
Zolpidem	2.5–5 mg	30–90	1.5–4	No

*Marked variation between individuals

Non-benzodiazepine hypnotics

Zopiclone, zolpidem and zaleplon are nonbenzodiazepine agents which bind to the same receptors as benzodiazepines. They are short-acting hypnotics which may be associated with the same range of adverse effects and precautions as benzodiazepines (5). Zaleplon reduces sleep latency but due to its short half-life is not the agent of choice where frequent night-time awakenings are the major complaint.

Treatment should be initiated with low doses (e.g. zopiclone 3.75 mg or zolpidem 2.5 mg). Physical and psychological dependence may occur and therapy should be limited to the shortest possible duration.

Drug interactions

Additive CNS and respiratory depression with other agents such as opioid analgesics, anticonvulsants or psychotropic medication may occur. These drugs are more commonly used by the elderly and reinforce the need to use low hypnotic doses.

Both benzodiazepine and non-benzodiazepine hypnotics are hepatically metabolised and many depend on clearance via cytochrome CYP450 3A4 (9). Drugs which significantly inhibit or induce this isoenzyme may affect the clearance of these agents. For example, amiodarone, diltiazem, verapamil, azole antifungals and macrolide antibiotics may inhibit the hepatic clearance of many benzodiazepines, zopiclone, zolpidem and zaleplon and increase their sedative and adverse effects.

Other agents

A wide variety of other drugs have been used as hypnotics, including tricyclic antidepressants, antihistamines and antipsychotics. Unless these agents are being used to treat another condition, their prescribing as hypnotics should be avoided due to the risk of adverse affects.

Valerian, melatonin, German chamomile and Chinese medicines are examples of alternative medications that have been used to treat insomnia (10). Studies of melatonin in elderly patients suggest modest benefit in a limited number of patients but studies have been small and of short duration (11).

Withdrawal of hypnotics in long-term users

The benefits of benzodiazepine withdrawal include improved cognition and alertness, improved mobility, reduced risk of falls and fractures and reduced incontinence.

The major barriers to cessation of hypnotics after long-term use are physical and/or psychological dependence. The risks of continued treatment and benefits of withdrawal should be discussed with the patient or carer to secure their co-operation.

The time required to withdraw from benzodiazepines varies between individuals. In general the dose of hypnotic should be reduced gradually over six to eight weeks to minimize withdrawal effects (5). The patient should be advised that difficulty sleeping, fatigue, dizziness, anxiety and sensory or emotional disturbances may occur but are temporary effects, and do not represent a return of the original insomnia problem. Once withdrawal is completed appropriate non-drug treatment strategies should be introduced.

RESTLESS LEGS SYNDROME AND PERIODIC LIMB MOVEMENTS OF SLEEP

Restless legs syndrome (RLS), a neurological disorder first described by the Swedish neurologist Karl-Axel Eckbom in 1945 is characterized by a deep, distressing, but generally non-painful sensation in the extremities, most notably the lower legs (12, 13). In severe cases the upper limbs may also be affected. The sensation, which the subject may describe as a "crawling", "creeping" or "jittery" feeling, tends to occur at rest and follows a circadian pattern being worse in the evening. It tends to be most troublesome to sufferers when lying down to sleep or if required to remain still such as in the movie theatre, church or sitting in an aeroplane. The sufferer experiences an intense urge to move the affected limbs. However, movement such as stretching or walking brings only temporary relief. Once the movement stops the unpleasant sensation or the urge-to-move quickly returns.

The disorder, affects between 3 and 15% of the general population. It is more common amongst women and increases in prevalence and severity with age. The primary form of the disorder is by far the most common and many such patients report a positive family history. About 5% of cases are secondary and are associated with iron deficiency, pregnancy, or end-stage renal failure. The symptoms of RLS can be exacerbated by prior heavy exercise, caffeine, nicotine, alcohol and certain pharmaceuticals, e.g., antihistamines and antidepressants (both tricyclic and selective serotonin reuptake inhibitor medications).

The pathophysiology of RLS is incompletely understood but current evidence points to a disturbance of central nervous system dopamine metabolism. Most cases respond to dopaminergic medications (see below) and the association with iron deficiency may be explained by the fact that dopamine production requires ferritin as a co-factor for tyrosine hydroxylase. Idiopathic cases of RLS have been reported to have low CSF ferritin levels.

Approximately 80% of patients who experience RLS also exhibit periodic limb movements of sleep (PLMS) (12). Limb movements involving flexion at the ankle, knee and hip occur at frequent, regular intervals and are accompanied by micro arousals from sleep. The patient is usually totally unaware of sleep arousals or movements. However when severe, RLS and PLMS can lead to marked sleep disruption; both difficulty getting off to sleep and maintaining sleep. In some cases limb movements can be so severe as to prevent the patient's partner sleeping in the same bed. It is important to recognize, however, that the great majority of subjects who have symptoms of RLS are only mildly and intermittently affected.

The published literature and our own clinical experience suggests that many cases of moderate to severe RLS present late having remained undiagnosed and untreated for years. The diagnosis requires a careful history to elicit the specific features of mainly lower limb distressing sensations and urge-to-move, which are worse in the evening, exacerbated by rest and only temporarily relieved by movement. The disorder is usually easily distinguished from nocturnal cramps and pains and dysaesthesia arising from disorders such as arthritis or diabetic peripheral neuropathy.

Non-drug treatment

Careful consideration should be given to the nature and severity of the complaints before deciding on treatment. In milder cases non pharmacological therapies and advice can be beneficial. Reducing caffeine, alcohol and nicotine intake can help if these factors are temporally associated with exacerbation of symptoms. Some patients find hot baths, stretching or mild exercise prior to bed beneficial. Before embarking on drug therapy serum ferritin levels should be measured to exclude iron deficiency. Correction of iron deficiency may be curative.

Drug treatment

In more severe cases pharmaceutical treatment should be considered (13). Dopaminergic agents are first-line drug treatment for primary RLS and PLMS (13–15). Lower doses than are used for the treatment of Parkinsons disease are effective. Combination L-Dopa (100–200 mg), carbidopa (25–50 mg) taken at night is effective in suppressing restless legs sensations and periodic limb movements of sleep but tolerance (i.e. less therapeutic effect at the same dose) is common after weeks to months of therapy. Symptom augmentation and rebound are also common: intense restless legs sensations beginning earlier in the evening and recurrence of symptoms in the middle of night, respectively. The latter may be addressed by choosing a slow release formulation of levodopa: carbidopa. or levodopa:benserazide. Adverse effects of levodopa include anorexia, nausea, vomiting, postural hypotension, confusion and hallucinations.

Low-dose dopamine agonists such as pergolide, pramipexole and ropinirole (14, 15) have been shown in moderate to large scale randomized controlled trials to be superior to placebo in controlling symptoms. There is a lower risk of symptom augmentation with these agents than L-dopa:carbidopa although tolerance is still relatively common. Nausea, mental confusion/agitation, dizziness and postural hypotension are relatively common side effects, together affecting up to 40 % of patients even when using a low starting dose and slow upward titration. Confusion and hallucinations are more common than with levodopa and demented patients are most at risk. Pergolide and cabergoline, ergot derivatives, have been associated with the rare but serious side effect of valvular heart disease (16) and should therefore probably be avoided unless symptoms are debilitating and alternative medications are ineffective.

If dopamine agonists are ineffective or side effects or tolerance limit therapeutic effectiveness other medications which have been shown to have efficacy may be considered (13). These include opioids (e.g. codeine), gabapentin and clonazepam. These can be used alone, during dopamine agonist drug holidays or in combination with a dopamine agonist depending on the circumstance. To minimize over-sedation and the risk of falls treatment should be commenced with a low dose at night and titrated slowly upwards according to response.

NOCTURNAL LEG CRAMPS

The prevalence of leg cramps increases with age with about one-third of people over the age of 60 reporting at least occasional cramps (17). Cramps often occur at night and wake the subject from sleep. In most patients they occur with such a low frequency that no specific treatment is required. In some subjects they occur recurrently during sleep and are a significant cause of sleep disturbance and patient distress.

Non-drug treatment

In some instances cramps are secondary to an identified electrolyte disturbance (e.g. hyponatraemia, hypomagnesaemia) or drug therapy (e.g. salbutamol, diuretics, caffeine, nifedipine,

beta blockers) or more rarely a neurological disorder involving lower motor neurons. Most cases, however, are idiopathic.

Some patients may find benefit from exercises designed to stretch the calf muscles before bed and by adopting sleep postures that encourage foot dorsiflexion.

Drug treatment

The only treatment of proven benefit is low dose quinine sulphate (200–300 mg nocte) (17). However in some countries, including USA and Australia, leg cramps is not an approved indication for quinine due to concerns regarding the drug's toxicity. From 1969 to 2006 the United States FDA received 665 reports of serious adverse events associated with quinine use, including 93 deaths. Although serious side effects (such as thrombocytopenia, prolonged QT interval) are likely to be rare at the low doses used to treat leg cramps, the harm-benefit ratio of using medication in such a common condition which is not in itself dangerous or harmful needs careful consideration. The risk of serious drug interactions (e.g. increased serum digoxin levels, increased risk of ventricular arrythmias when taken with other drugs which prolong the QT interval such as amiodarone, some antipsychotics and quinolones) is particularly pertinent in the elderly population which is more likely to have co-morbid heart disease. Quinine should thus probably be used only in those patients experiencing distressing frequent (e.g. nightly) cramps when metabolic and electrolyte disturbances have been excluded.

REM BEHAVIOUR DISORDER

REM sleep is characterized by profound muscle hypotonia and often intense and vivid dreaming (18). The first episode typically starts 90 minutes after sleep onset, lasts 10–20 minutes and thereafter occurs repetitively at 90 minute intervals throughout the night. The sleeping subject may or may not experience dream recall the following day. Perhaps as many as one in 200 adults may lose the muscle hypotonia of REM and begin to act out their dreams by yelling out, hitting out, punching or grabbing and occasionally even leaping out of bed and participating in some violent activity which may be injurious to themselves or others in the room. This condition is termed REM Behaviour Disorder. The common form of the disorder affects older males and there is increasing recognition that it may be a harbinger of one of a group of neurodegenerative disorders known as synucleinopathies that includes Parkinson's disease, multiple system atrophy and Lewy Body dementia (19).Such disorders may develop a decade or more after the onset of REM Behaviour Disorder. REM Behaviour Disorder may also develop *after* the onset of Parkinson's Disease. Occasionally, REM Behaviour Disorder can develop as a consequence of another neurological disorder such as a brainstem astrocytoma, multiple sclerosis or cerebrovascular disease.

While uncommon, REM Behaviour Disorder is often very distressing to the patient and their bed partner. The violent behaviours are invariably quite uncharacteristic of the patient's waking behaviour which is normal, even docile and patients are often embarrassed or ashamed about their nocturnal behaviour. They may be at first reluctant to seek medical advice.

The importance of recognizing this condition is that in about 80 % of cases it resolves completely on taking a small dose of clonazepam before bed at night. A starting dose of 0.5 mg is recommended increasing up to 2 mg depending on clinical response. Another 10 % of cases will have an incomplete but nonetheless useful clinical response to this medication.

REM behaviour disorder is primarily a clinical diagnosis that is reached after taking a careful history supplemented by polysomnographic findings of increased muscle tone (tonic and/or phasic activity) in REM sleep. The acting-out behaviours occur at least 90 minutes after sleep; typically the patient can be woken readily at the time of the episode and is immediately aware of having just experienced a vivid, often frightening or violent dream. Neurological examination is usually normal unless one of the aforementioned neurodegenerative diseases has already supervened. The differential diagnosis includes non-REM sleep parasomnias such as sleep walking and talking, post traumatic stress disorder, nocturnal complex partial seizures, and unusual behaviours associated with sleep apnea. Non-REM parasomnias are usually easily distinguished from REM Behaviour Disorder because they usually occur in a younger age group and the subject is hard to awaken from the episode and has little if any dream recall. Referral to a sleep specialist for further clinical evaluation and polysomnographic assessment should be considered if REM behaviour disorder is suspected.

REFERENCES

1. *Diagnostic and Statistical Manual of Mental Disorders*, 4th ed. Washington DC, American Psychiatric Association, 2000.
2. Ancoli-Israel S, Ayalon L. Diagnosis and treatment of sleep disorders in older adults. *Am J Geriatr.Psychiatry* 2006; **14**(2): 95–103.
3. Avidan AY. Epidemiology, assessment and treatment of insomnia in the elderly patient. Medscape 2005; *Neurology and Neurosurgery* **7**(2).
4. Drug therapy is a small part of insomnia management. *Drug and Therapy Perspectives* 2000; **15**(10): 5–9.
5. Australian Medicines Handbook *Drug Choice Companion: Aged Care*. Adelaide, South Australia, Australian Medicines Handbook Pty Ltd, 2003.
6. *Meyler's Side Effects of Drugs*, 15th ed. Amsterdam, The Netherlands, Elsevier, 2006.
7. Cummin RG, Le Couteur DG. Benzodiazepines and risk of hip fractures in older people: A review of the evidence. *CNS Drugs* 2003; **17**, 825–37.
8. *Clinical Handbook of Psychotropic Drugs*. Toronto, Canada. Hogrefe & Huber Publishers, 1996.
9. *Martindale: The Complete Drug Reference*. London, United Kingdom. Pharmaceutical Press, 2005.
10. Cherniack EP. The use of alternative medicine for the treatment of insomnia in the elderly. *Psychogeriatrics* 2006; **6**, 21–30.
11. Olde Rikkert MGM and Rigaud ASP. Melatonin in elderly patients with insomnia. A

systematic review. *Z Gerontol Geriat* 2001; **34**, 491–7.

12. Montplaisir J, Allen RP, Walters AS, and Ferini-Strambi L. Restless Legs Syndrome and Periodic Limb Movements during Sleep. Meir H Kryger, Thomas Roth, and William C Dement. *Principles and Practice of Sleep Medicine*. pp. 839–52, Philadelphia, Elsevier Saunders, 2006.

13. Thorpy MJ. New paradigms in the treatment of restless legs syndrome. *Neurology* 2005; **64**(12 Suppl 3): S28–S33.

14. Bogan RK, Fry JM, Schmidt MH, Carson SW, Ritchie SY. Ropinirole in the treatment of patients with restless legs syndrome: a US-based randomized, double-blind, placebo-controlled clinical trial. *Mayo Clin Proc*. 2006; **81**(1): 17–27.

15. Walters AS, Ondo WG, Dreykluft T, Grunstein R, Lee D, Sethi K. Ropinirole is effective in the treatment of restless legs syndrome. TREAT RLS 2: a 12-week, double-blind, randomized, parallel-group, placebo-controlled study. *Mov Disord*. 2004; **19**(12): 1414–23.

16. Flowers CM, Racoosin JA, Lu SL, Beitz JG. The US Food and Drug Administration's registry of patients with pergolide-associated valvular heart disease. *Mayo Clin Proc*. 2003; **78**(6): 730–1.

17. http://www.prodigy.nhs.uk/leg_cramps/view_whole_guidance. 2006.

18. Mahowald MW and Schenck CH. REM Sleep Parasomnias. Meir H Kryger, Thomas Roth, and William C Dement. *Principles and Practice of Sleep Medicine*. pp. 897–916, Philadelphia, Elsevier Saunders, 2006.

19. Iranzo A, Molinuevo JL, Santamaria J, Serradell M, Marti MJ, Valldeoriola F et al. Rapid-eye-movement sleep behaviour disorder as an early marker for a neurodegenerative disorder: a descriptive study. *Lancet Neurol*. 2006; **5**(7): 572–7.

6 Stroke

Joseph A. Harbison[1] and Gary A. Ford[2]

[1] Department of Medical Gerontology, University of Dublin Trinity College, Dublin, Ireland
[2] Institute for Ageing and Health, Newcastle University, Newcastle, UK

INTRODUCTION

Stroke is an acute, focal neurological deficit resulting from a disruption of the blood supply to the brain. It is the third commonest cause of death in the western world and is a major cause of adult disability. Increasing age is the major risk factor for stroke. The Rotterdam Stroke study (1) demonstrated the risk of stroke comparing people in their late 50's and late 80's increased 15 fold from 1.4 to 21.7 per 1000 person years.

AETIOLOGY

Stroke is due to either cerebral infarction or intracerebral haemorrhage in a ratio of approximately 9:1. infarcts, in turn, may be divided into large vessel and small vessel strokes. Large vessel strokes occur following complete or branch occlusion of one of the arteries emergent from the Circle of Willis or occasionally the internal carotid or basilar arteries. Such occlusions may result from thrombus formation directly within the vessel or embolism from heart or the large arteries of the thorax and neck. Small vessel, or lacunar strokes result from the infarction of tissue supplied by end arteries or arterioles often secondary to hypertension but also associated with diabetes and advancing age.

Haemorrhagic stroke may be divided into primary intracerebral haemorrhage and subarachnoid haemorrhage. Haemorrhagic stroke results from rupture of a weak point in a vessel wall, most commonly in older people from hypertensive arteriopathy or amyloid angiopathy. Amyloid angiopathy is the commonest cause of intracerebral haemorrhage in non-hypertensive older subjects. It is caused by the deposition of an abnormal amyloid protein in the vessel wall resulting in a loss of structural strength. Atriovenous malformations and intracranial aneurysms also cause intracranial haemorrhage in older people although proportionately less than in young people. Occasionally cerebral infarction can undergo haemorrhagic transformation, which can be hard to distinguish from a primary intracerebral haemorrhage, particularly if scanning has not been performed early.

MODIFIABLE RISK FACTORS FOR STROKE

Hypertension

Hypertension constitutes the single biggest treatable risk factor for stroke disease, with the risk of stroke roughly doubling with every 7.5 mmHg rise in diastolic blood pressure (2). Treatment studies have shown that an average reduction in systolic blood pressure of 10 mmHg reduces stroke risk by 31 %. Isolated systolic hypertension also presents an increased risk of stroke (3).

Prescribing for Elderly Patients   Edited by Stephen Jackson, Paul Jansen and Arduino Mangoni
© 2009 John Wiley & Sons, Ltd

Anti-hypertensive therapy is discussed in detail elsewhere in this book but from the point of view of secondary prevention, the PROGRESS study (4) has demonstrated that reducing blood pressure in patients following stroke using perindopril with or without indapamide reduces stroke recurrence by 28%. Most guidelines for control of blood pressure in patients with cerebrovascular disease recommend a target of <130/80 mmHg although this is not always achievable due to tolerability problems or lack of control on maximal therapy.

Atrial Fibrillation

Atrial fibrillation affects <1% of people <65 years but over 10% of those >85 years. The risk of stroke in patients with atrial fibrillation but without rheumatic heart disease is increased five fold. About 15% of strokes are typically found associated with atrial fibrillation and there is a 35% risk of life time stroke in patients with untreated atrial fibrillation. The risk increases with age and with co-morbidities, particularly previous stroke, so that a patient over 75 years with atrial fibrillation and a history of previous strokes, diabetes and heart failure with a dilated left atrium and ventricle, may have an annual risk of stroke of 25%. In guidelines, subjects less than 65 years with uncomplicated atrial fibrillation recommend aspirin; however older patients should be anticoagulated unless contraindicated, because of an increased risk of falling or a high bleeding risk. There are a number of scoring systems such as CHADS2 (5) available to help to quantify absolute risk with more accuracy. The risk and benefits of anticoagulation in the very elderly, over 80 years, have been confirmed in the recently reported BAFTA trial (6).

Hyperlipidaemia

Lipid lowering is discussed in Chapter 44. The Stroke Prevention by Aggressive Reduction in Cholesterol Levels (SPARCL) Study (7) studied the effects of cholesterol lowering following stroke using atorvastatin 80 mg daily, with a reduced risk of recurrent cerebral infarction (Hazard ratio 0.78) but increased risk of intracerebral haemorrhage (Hazard ratio 1.66). Overall the risk of recurrent stroke was reduced (Hazard Ratio 0.84).

THERAPY

Antiplatelet Therapy

Individual antiplatelet agents reduce the risk of stroke and other cardiovascular events by about 18% amongst patients with a previous transient Ischaemic attack or stroke (8). There are three antiplatelet agents in current common use: aspirin, dipyridamole and clopidogrel.

Aspirin

Metanalysis of large trials (10) has shown that giving Aspirin 150–300 mg within 48 hours of ischaemic stroke reduces early risk of death or recurrent stroke by 9/1000 treated and later death or stroke by 13/1000. Whilst this effect is small, it is a therapy that is available and affordable to the great majority of patients with cerebral infarction. The optimal dose remains unclear. Complete platelet inhibition may take up to two weeks to occur giving aspirin at a dose of 300 mg daily but clinical trials of aspirin given for secondary prevention have shown no particular advantage of higher doses 300 mg–1.2 g daily compared to low dose 50–75 mg daily in terms of preventing recurrent stroke. Gastrointestinal side effects increase with dose and a prudent course would seem to be to give aspirin at 300 mg for a few days post event then reduce the dose to 75 mg or 150 mg daily.

Pharmacodynamics: aspirin is an inhibitor of cyclo-oxygenase (COX) enzymes, inhibiting COX 1 to a much greater extent than COX 2. The antiplatelet effect results from reduction in platelet thromboxane A2 production by COX inhibition. Thromboxane A2 causes platelet aggregation. The inhibition of COX, and thus the antiplatelet effect is irreversible until new platelets are produced by the bone marrow.

Pharmacokinetics: aspirin is absorbed rapidly from the stomach and duodenum and is both orally and parenterally active. It may also be administered rectally. Aspirin is hydrolysed in the liver to form the active salicylic acid. Following oral ingestion aspirin reaches peak serum concentrations in 15–120 minutes and the active metabolite salicylic acid has a plasma half-life of between two to three hours following administration of small doses. It is extensively bound to plasma proteins especially albumin. Salicylic acid is conjugated to either glycine or glucuronic acid and is excreted renally. This conjugation process is saturable and therefore whilst aspirin demonstrates first order pharmacokinetics at lower concentrations the kinetics become zero order with larger doses with plasma half lives of 15–30 hours (pseudo-zero order pharmacokinetics).

Drug interactions: aspirin interacts with a large number of other agents. It is associated with a higher rate of bleeding when combined with anticoagulants or clopidogrel. It also interacts with venlafaxine and selective serotonin reuptake inhibitors, which are commonly used antidepressants in older people, and both are reported as increasing the risk of gastrointestinal bleeding with aspirin use. In doses >300 mg/day aspirin increases the risk of renal impairment with ACE inhibitors and angiotensin II receptor antagonists (ARA). It enhances the effects of drugs with a high degree of protein binding such as phenytoin and valproate. Recent Studies have indicated that the antiplatelet effects of aspirin may be reduced by concomitant use of the non-steroidal anti-inflammatory ibuprofen (11).

Adverse effects: aspirin may produce bronchospasm. It is associated with a higher risk of upper gastrointestinal and other haemorrhage. At higher doses it can result in fluid retention and oedema through prostaglandin E2 and I2 mediated reduction in renal blood flow.

Using Aspirin in older patients

No clinically important differences in pharmacokinetics and pharmacodynamics have been seen in the non-frail elderly. Plasma levels of salicylic acid are more closely related to albumin levels than age and dosage is not routinely adjusted for the elderly. Older people may, however, suffer a higher rate of gastrointestinal and other NSAID related haemorrhages; through increased pharmacodynamic sensitivity. Sub-group analysis of the large International Stroke Trial (IST) and Chinese Acute Stroke Trial (CAST) has shown no significant difference in effect of aspirin as a secondary preventative measure in older people. Whilst a degree of 'aspirin resistance' has been proposed as a cause of reduced antiplatelet effect in some people this has not been found to be more common in older people although may be more frequent in subjects with type 2 diabetes.

Aspirin and dipyridamole

There is evidence that aspirin combined with modified release dipyridamole is more effective in the secondary prevention of stroke than aspirin or dipyridamole monotherapy. The addition of dipyridamole 200 mg MR BD to aspirin for all patients following cerebral infarction has been recommended in the UK by the National Institute for Clinical Excellence for two years following stroke/TIA. Until recently the evidence for the use of Dipyridamole Modified Release came primarily from the ESPS 2 study (12) which showed 12 month stroke recurrence rate of 9.5 % for a combination Aspirin 25 mg/Dipyridamole MR 200 mg BD compared to 12.5 % for aspirin 50 mg daily alone and 15.2 % for placebo. The ESPRIT study (13) (average age of subjects 63 years, 16 % 75 years and over), an open labelled trial which compared an aspirin/dipyridamole 200 mg modified release combination with aspirin monotherapy in mild strokes and TIAs showed a difference in all cause vascular mortality, non-fatal stroke or non-fatal myocardial infarction over 3.5 years of 3 %, 16 % in the monotherapy group compared to 13 % in the combination therapy. The average dose of aspirin in both groups was 75 mg. No specific mention was made of altered effect in the elderly patients.

Meta-analysis of all trials comparing aspirin and aspirin/dipyridamole combination performed as part of the ESPRIT study show a risk ratio of 0.82 for the combination therapy for combined outcome.

Dipyridamole

The mechanism of action of dipyridamole is not fully understood. It appears to act by increasing cyclic adenosine monophosphate (cAMP) by reducing red cell uptake of adenosine. Cyclic AMP inhibits thromboxane A2 formation, which in turn reduces platelet activation. Platelet inhibition by dipyridamole is not irreversible therefore compliance is important for continued effect. It may also have a mild anti-inflammatory effect.

Pharmacokinetics: following oral administration of dipyridamole peak plasma levels are reached after about 40–75 minutes. Although absorption can be variable and unpredictable in the original oral form, it appears more predictable in the newer modified release (MR) preparation. The drug is highly protein bound and is metabolised in the liver. It is conjugated to a glucuronide and excreted through the bile with negligible renal excretion. Plasma half-life is biphasic suggesting a two-compartment model. The distribution half-life is 40–60 minutes. The terminal half-life is 10–12 hours.

Important drug interactions: dipyridamole is a poorly soluble weak base and gastric absorption in the elderly has been found to be reduced in those with a high gastric pH such as those with achlorhydria or on proton pump inhibitors or antacids. There is no guidance, however, on how this should alter dosage or administration. It enhances the anticoagulant effect of warfarin, heparin and phenindione. It increases bleeding risk when combined with clopidogrel.

Adverse effects: apart from its anti-platelet effect, dipyridamole also has a vasodilator effect which gives rise to many of its side effects. The commonest side effects are gastrointestinal upset and headache. Dipyridamole may also exacerbate migraine. There is some evidence that slowly titrating the dose may reduce the incidence of side effects. Dipyridamole should be used with caution in patients with aortic stenosis, heart failure, recent myocardial infarction or unstable angina. Thrombocytopenia has been reported and hypersensitivity reactions rarely occur.

Using dipyridamole in older patients

Plasma concentrations are 30–50 % higher in patients >65 years, due probably to reduced clearance. This does not result in any recommendation to reduce dosage however.

Clopidogrel

Clopidogrel is a theinopyridine derivative. One large study the 'clopidogrel versus aspirin in patients at risk of ischaemic events' (CAPRIE) study (14), demonstrated a small benefit of the use of clopidogrel above aspirin in terms of preventing ischaemic stroke, myocardial infarction of vascular death (5.8 % vs 5.3 % over 1.9 years, relative risk reduction 8.7 %). Post hoc analysis looking at the subgroup of subjects in the CAPRIE trial with previous ischaemic stroke (15) as an entry risk factor showed a similar treatment effect (annual event rate 7.7 % vs. 7.15 %, relative risk reduction of 7.3 %). More recently the PROFESS study (16) compared clopidogrel 75 mg daily with aspirin 25 mg/dipyridamole MR 200 mg twice daily (asasantin) as a secondary prevention therapy and found an identical risk of recurrent stroke (9 % over 2.4 years) in both groups. The only difference between groups was a very small but significant increase in risk of haemorrhagic complications in the aspirin and dipyridamole group.

Large secondary prevention studies of the combination of clopidogrel and aspirin therapy in patients with high risk of stroke (MATCH (17) and CHARISMA (18) studies) have to date found no advantage in the combined therapy overall, with benefits in cardiovascular event prevention balanced by an increased hazard from haemorrhagic complications (relative Risk 7.0, compared with clopidogrel alone. Ongoing studies are examining the use of limited periods of combination treatment during high-risk periods such as the first few weeks following TIA or minor stroke.

Pharmacokinetics: clopidogrel is a prodrug with no antiplatelet activity. The antiplatelet effect resides with a minor metabolite. It appears to function by reducing adenosine diphosphate (ADP) mediated activation of the Glycoprotein IIb/IIIa complex and ADP related amplification of platelet activation induced by other agents. It does this by irreversibly modifying the platelet ADP receptor, preventing binding and activation.

Clopidogrel is absorbed rapidly following oral administration with peak plasma levels found after approximately one hour. The pharmacokinetics at therapeutic doses is linear and the drug is 98 % protein bound (94 % of the main metabolite). It is extensively metabolized in the liver. Elimination half-life of the main circulating metabolite (the carboxylic acid derivative) is eight hours, however this metabolite also has no effect on platelet aggregation. Fifty percent of the drug is excreted in the urine.

Important drug interactions: risk of bleeding is increased when clopidogrel is administered with non-steroidal anti inflammatory drugs, aspirin, dipyridamole or anticoagulants. Clopidogrel inhibits cytochrome P450 (2C0) and therefore may theoretically interfere with the metabolism of phenytoin, tamoxifen, warfarin and fluvastatin. The extent to which this happens clinically is not known.

Adverse effects: the commonest reported side effects are gastrointestinal although the risk of haemorrhage is lower than with aspirin, and a recent large surveillance study in Denmark found it to be associated with no excess of gastrointestinal bleeding when used on its own (although very substantial risk when used in combination with aspirin).

Using clopidogrel in older patients

Whilst plasma concentrations are higher in older people compared with younger, healthy controls, this does not appear to effect platelet aggregation or prolong bleeding time and dose alteration is not necessary.

Clopidogrel can cause a drop in platelet count and thrombocytopenia with thrombotic thrombocytopenic purpura reported in as many as one in 2000 patients in some studies. The population that seems to be particularly vulnerable are older people (average age 70) taking multiple drugs. There have been isolated reports of clopidogrel in older people causing ageusia (loss of taste) although this seems uncommon.

Current prescribing guidelines for antiplatelets

Current UK NICE prescribing guidelines are that patients presenting with ischaemic stroke or TIA should be commenced on aspirin 75 mg – 300 mg daily with dipyridamole MR 200 mg BD added for two years if tolerated. Where the patient is aspirin allergic or intolerant clopidogrel 75 mg daily should be given. Where the patient is both aspirin and clopidogrel sensitive, dipyridamole MR 200 mg BD should be prescribed.

Platelet glyciprotein IIb IIIa inhibitors

Platelet glycoprotein (GP) IIb/IIIa inhibitors have been shown to be effective in patients with acute coronary syndromes and those undergoing coronary stenting and a number of studies have been initiated to determine if there is a role for them in managing acute ischaemic stroke.

The majority of these studies have involved abciximab, an intravenously administered, monoclonal antibody directed at the glycoprotein (GP) IIb/IIIa receptor. The AbESTT study, a phase II safety study of Abciximab administered within six hours of cerebral infarction, showed a small, non-significant shift in favourable outcome in the intervention group. The study also showed a small increase in haemorrhagic transformation rates. However the follow up AbESTT II trial was stopped because of a high rate of intracerebral bleeding. Other studies using a combination of intravenous Abciximab and intravenous or intra arterial recombinant Tissue Plasminogen activator are underway. Currently there is no role for abciximab in acute stroke outside the context of clinical trials.

Tirofiban is a synthetic, non-peptide inhibitor of the glycoprotein IIb/IIIa receptor on the platelet. The 'Safety of Tirofiban in Acute Ischemic Stroke' (SaTIS) trial phase II examined the effect of tirofiban administered within three hours of stroke onset in patients up to 80 years of age on frequency of symptomatic intracerebral haemorrhage at 24 hours. This showed a non-significant increased risk of haemorrhagic transformation in the intervention group, however it also showed a small reduction in five to six month mortality, which was a secondary outcome measure. Phase III trials of tirofiban in stroke are awaited.

Thrombolysis

The first trials of intravenous thrombolysis for ischaemic stroke in the 1980s using streptokinase were stopped early because of increased risk of haemorrhage. In the early 1990s the National Institute of Neurological Disease and Stroke (NINDS) (20) trial established that thrombolysis using recombinant human tissue plasminogen activator (rTPA) could improve outcome of patients with ischaemic stroke although at the risk of precipitating intracerebral haemorrhage in a proportion of patients. A number of subsequent trials have confirmed this and it is now generally agreed that thrombolysis using rTPA is an effective therapy if given within three hours subject to a stringent protocol (21). Overall, the number needed to treat to prevent death or severe disability is between seven and ten. The number needed to treat to reduce disability may be as few as three. The large, observational Safe Implementation of Thrombolysis Monitoring Study (SITS-MOST) showed that the conservative risk of intracerebral haemorrhage (any bleeding with any neurological deterioration) associated with thrombolysis with rTPA is 7.2%. This compares with a risk of 1.1% found in the placebo groups of large trials of rTPA for stroke. If symptomatic haemorrhage is defined as parenchymal haemorrhage in more than one third of infarct volume with a neurobiological deterioration of four or more points on NIHSS, the rate is 1.7%.

Benefit from thrombolysis for stroke declines with time from onset. The current licence and NICE recommendation is for intravenous administration up to three hours from stroke onset. However, there is now clear evidence from the recent ECASS3 (23) study that patients may benefit from administration for up to four and a half hours and guidelines are likely to be revised accordingly. Some centres advocate thrombolysis for vertebro-baslar occlusion up to 12–24 hours post stroke onset but randomized trial evidence is lacking reflecting the rarity of this life-threatening stroke subgroup. Intra-arterial therapy using urokinase has been shown to be successful up to six hours post stroke onset in treating stroke due to MCA occlusion but the evidence base, in comparison to that for intravenous therapy, is small and only a few centres offer this as routine treatment.

Pharmacodynamics

Tissue Plasminogen activator is synthesized and released by the vascular endothelium, rTPA is structurally identical but produced by recombinant DNA technology. It is a glycoprotein, which converts plasminogen to plasmin. It is theoretically inactive in the circulation only becoming active when it binds to fibrin; however in vivo administration is associated with a more systemic lytic state and a substantial bleeding risk. RTPA produces a reduction in fibrinogen levels of about 40% and Plasminogen of about 80% over four hours. Levels increase back to near normal in 24–36 hours.

Pharmacokinetics

The drug may be administered intravenously or arterially. Standard protocol for stroke requires a dose of 0.9 mg/kg to a maximum of 100 mg. The drug is administered as a 10% bolus over two minutes followed by the remainder of the dose by infusion over one hour. There is no alteration in dose for older people. Once administered, the drug is cleared rapidly from the bloodstream by the liver, with plasma half-life of four to five minutes.

Important drug interactions: following thrombolysis for stroke antiplatelet agents or anticoagulants should not be administered for at least 24 hours. There is a higher incidence of anaphylactic reactions to rTPA reported amongst patients taking ACE inhibitors. The Canadian CASES series, but not SITS-MOST, reported oro-lingual oedema in 1.5% of treated patients.

Adverse events: the single biggest risk is of haemorrhage, either intracranially or elsewhere. Allergic or anaphylactoid reactions are uncommon but are recorded after the use of rTPA for stroke.

Thrombolysis in older patients

The outcome in older people from thrombolysis using rTPA is less good in terms of reducing mortality and significant disability in comparison to young patients. This most likely reflects that outcome from stroke in general is poorer in the elderly rather than less efficacy or more haemorrhage. Currently the licence for rTPA for stroke in the European Union extends only to subjects 80 years of age and under. However, there is increasing evidence from SITS and other trials that subjects over 80 years do not have a significantly higher rate of intracerebral haemorrhage or drug related complications than younger people, and age per-se, should not be a contraindication to therapy (22), although clearly older people are likely to have a higher incidence of other contraindications. Ongoing trials will better define risks and benefits of thrombolysis in the older stroke patient.

Anticoagulation following stroke

Anticoagulation using either heparins or other anticoagulants is not routinely indicated following acute cerebral infarction as the large International Stroke Trial found no reduction in death and disability when treatment was started within 48 hours of stroke onset (23). However, many physicians use heparin in specific circumstances where risk benefit considerations suggest anticoagulation is likely to be of benefit (vessel dissection, AF/left ventricular thrombus and associated minor stroke). As mentioned above, some patients with atrial fibrillation benefit from the use of anticoagulation in the secondary prevention of further events. The point at which anticoagulation should be commenced following acute stroke is controversial but it is common practice to commence anticoagulation seven to fourteen days post event in patients without major disability to reduce potential risk of haemorrhagic transformation of the acute infarct. Typically such patients are commenced on incremental warfarin therapy with no loading and doses slowly increased with the patient remaining on antiplatelet therapy until a satisfactory level of anticoagulation (INR 2.0–3.0)

is achieved. Immediate anticoagulation is used in other circumstances such as in the presence of carotid or vertebral artery dissection, venous stroke resulting from cerebral venous thrombosis or occasionally the presence of a large or mobile left ventricular thrombus. In these circumstances anticoagulation is commenced using heparin followed up with warfarin therapy as necessary.

Heparins

'Heparin' represents a family of molecules ranging from 5 kDa to 40 kDa in mass. They are straight chain anionic mucopolysaccharides that function by accelerating the activity of the endogenous anticoagulant antithrombin III. This antithrombin neutralizes activated coagulation factors, especially thrombin and activated Factor X. Heparin binds simultaneously to both thrombin and antithrombin III bringing them into close proximity allowing them to form a complex and also causes a conformational change in the antithrombin's structure, increasing its activity.

Pharmacokinetics

Heparin must be administered parenterally as it is not absorbed from the gastrointestinal tract. It has an almost immediate onset of action following intravenous administration. Plasma half-life is dose-dependent and variable due partly to pseudo-zero order pharmacokinetics. High molecular weight molecules are metabolised faster and the typical plasma half-life is between 30 minutes and 150 minutes. This variability necessitates regular laboratory monitoring of plasma heparin activity (Activated Partial Thromboplastin Time, APTT) throughout therapy. Sub-cutaneous administration delays onset by up to 60 minutes and peak plasma levels are achieved between two and four hours, although there is again considerable variation between individuals. Heparin is extensively bound to plasma proteins, which can limit its activity. It is metabolized predominantly by the reticuloendothelial system and to a lesser extent by the liver.

Low Molecular Weight Heparins (LMWHs) are defined as heparin salts having an average molecular weight of less than 8 kDa and for which at least 60 % of all chains have a molecular weight less than 8 kDa. They are produced by fractionating heparin or depolymerising larger heparin molecules. There are a number available including tinzaparin, dalteparin and enoxaparin that differ in their constituents, average molecular weights and relative anti-factor Xa and antithrombin activity. They have advantages over unfractionated heparin in that they have a more predictable half life and metabolism, thereby eliminating the need for regular measurement of APTT, indeed APTT ratio is generally a poor indicator of anticaogulation activity in these agents and if there is concern Factor Xa activity should be measured in preference. The TAIST study found no benefit of tinzaparin compared to aspirin in the treatment of acute ischaemic stroke when started within 24 hours. They also have a longer half-life than unfractionated heparin due to their small size permitting once daily dosing by sub-cutaneous injection. Low Molecular Weight Heparins are subject to a higher degree of renal clearance than unfractionated heparins and accordingly care needs to be taken in patients with renal dysfunction and in those with extremes of body mass.

Common adverse effects: common side effects relate to haemorrhagic complications. The anticoagulant effects of heparin can be reversed using Protamine sulphate which binds to it in vivo. Heparins may be associated with thrombocytopenia and platelet count needs to be monitored. Long term use is associated with increased bone resorption and is a risk for osteoporosis.

Heparins in older people

Whist there are no specific additional risks to the use of heparins in older people there is an increased risk of haemorrhagic complications reported in the elderly, particularly in older women. The prevalence of undiagnosed renal dysfunction in the elderly is also high and care needs to be taken to avoid over anticoagulation in older people.

Warfarin

Vitamin K is necessary for the formation of the activated forms of the clotting factors II, VII, IX and X. Warfarin is structurally similar to vitamin K and acts to inhibit the action of the enzyme vitamin K epoxide reductase in the liver, preventing formation of the active hydroquinone form of vitamin K. Accordingly, warfarin has no effect on clotting factorsbreak produced before commencement of therapy and its onset of action is dependent on the degradation of these factors which can take up to three days. It has no effect on platelet aggregation and does not cause the breakdown of pre-existing thrombus.

Pharmacokinetics

Warfarin is administered orally and is well absorbed from the gastrointestinal tract. It is extensively bound to plasma proteins and therefore shows extensive interactions with other agents. It has a plasma half-life of approximately 40 hours but the most important factor determining its duration of action is the rate of consumption and reaccumulation of reactivated clotting factors. Warfarin is metabolized in the liver and its metabolites, which are inactive and are excreted through the urine.

It has a narrow therapeutic index and activity is measured by frequent measurement of a patient's clotting time versus a normalized control sample, the International Normalised Ratio (INR). An INR in the range of 2.0–3.0 is typically recommended for patients receiving warfarin for thromboprophylaxis of atrial fibrillation. It is important to emphasize that, in people in whom anticoagulant therapy is indicated, the risk of stroke increases substantially when the INR falls below 2.0. One study (24) has demonstrated that individuals receiving warfarin for secondary prevention of stroke with an INR of 1.7 have twice the odds of stroke (95 % CI, 1.6–2.4), and those with an INR of 1.5 have 3.3 times the odds of stroke (95 % CI, 2.4–4.6) as those with an INR of 2.0. Lower levels of control may be considered, however, in patients with a higher risk of bleeding.

Adverse effects: like heparin the major adverse effects of warfarin are haemorrhagic. Activated vitamin K, in the form of phytomenadione can reverse the effects of warfarin but can take several hours or days to produce full reversal. If activated vitamin K is used in larger amounts (>5.0 mg) to reverse warfarin, it may continue to inhibit re-anticoagulation using warfarin for a number of weeks until the active vitamin depletes. In the presence of an uncontrolled INR with active bleeding, more rapid and complete reversal of warfarin induced anticoagulation can be produced with the administration of activated clotting factors in the form of fresh frozen plasma or in Pro-thrombin Complex Concentrate, e.g. Beriplex, which contains activated factors II, VII, IX and X. Warfarin may also rarely cause skin or soft tissue necrosis and can rarely cause hepatotoxicity and osteoporosis.

Warfarin in older people

There are no special precautions necessary using warfarin in the elderly, however there is probably a slightly higher incidence of haemorrhagic complications in older people. Particular care needs to be taken in assessing falls risk and in ensuring compliance and monitoring in patients with cognitive dysfunction.

Care also has to be exercised in the presence of polypharmacy, typical in older people with cardiovascular or cerebrovascular disease, in order to avoid drug interactions.

Other oral anticoagulants: In patients unable to take warfarin other vitamin K antagonists such as phenindione are occasionally used. Other alternative agents are in development. The first direct thrombin inhibitor to complete trials, ximelagatran, although effective as an anticoagulant, proved hepatotoxic and development was discontinued. Others are now under evaluation. There are also a number of oral activated factor 10 inhibitors in development as potential anticoagulants.

KEY POINTS

- Stroke is the commonest cause of disability and the third commonest cause of death in the western world.
- Eighty percent of strokes occur in people 65 years and older.
- Aspirin 150–300 mg should be administered as soon as possible after diagnosis of ischaemic stroke or TIA. Clopidogrel should be given to those who are aspirin intolerant.
- Dipyridamole 200 mg BD added to aspirin therapy probably reduces risk of future vascular events.
- Older people presenting within three hours of stroke onset should be considered for intravenous thrombolysis.

REFERENCES

1. Bots ML, Looman SJ et al. Prevalence of stroke in the general population. The Rotterdam Study. *Stroke* 1996; **27**: 1499–1501.
2. Lawes CM, Bennett DA, Feigin VL, Rodgers A. Blood pressure and stroke: an overview of published reviews. *Stroke* 2004; **35**: 776–85.
3. Rodgers A, MacMahon S, Gamble G, Slattery J, Sandercock P, Warlow C, for the United Kingdom Transient Ischaemic Attack Collaborative Group. Blood pressure and risk of stroke in patients with cerebrovascular disease. *Br Med J* 1996; **313**: 147.
4. PROGRESS Collaborative Group. Randomised trial of a perindopril-based blood-pressure-lowering regimen among 6105 individuals with previous stroke or transient ischaemic attack. *Lancet* 2001; **358**: 1033–41.
5. Gage BF, Waterman AD et al. Validation of clinical classification schemes for predicting stroke: results from the National Registry of Atrial Fibrillation. *JAMA* 2001; **285**: 2864–70.
6. Mant J, Hobbs FD et al. Warfarin versus aspirin for stroke prevention in an elderly community population with atrial fibrillation (the Birmingham Atrial Fibrillation Treatment of the Aged Study, BAFTA): a randomised controlled trial. *Lancet*. 2007; **37**: 493–503.
7. Amarenco P, Bogousslavsky J, Callahan A 3rd, Goldstein LB, Hennerici M, Rudolph AE, Sillesen H, Simunovic L, Szarek M, Welch KM,

Zivin JA; Stroke Prevention by Aggressive Reduction in Cholesterol Levels (SPARCL) Investigators. High-dose atorvastatin after stroke or transient ischemic attack. *N Engl J Med* 2006; **355**: 549–59.

8. Sandercock P, Gubitz G, Foley P, Counsell C. Antiplatelet therapy for acute ischaemic stroke. Cochrane database of systematic reviews 2006 issue 1.

9. Hankey GJ, Sudlow CL, Dunbabin DW. Thienopyridine derivatives (ticlopidine, clopidogrel) versus aspirin for preventing stroke and other serious vascular events in high risk vascular patients. The Cochrane database of systematic reviews 2006 issue 1.

10. CAST (Chinese Acute Stroke Trial) Collaborative Group. CAST: randomised placebo-controlled trial of early aspirin use in 20,000 patients with acute ischaemic stroke. *Lancet* 1997; **349**: 1641–9.

11. Catella-Lawson F, Reilly MP, Kapoor SC, Cucchiara AJ, DeMarco S, Tournier B, Vyas SN, FitzGerald GA. Cyclooxygenase inhibitors and the antiplatelet effects of aspirin. *N Engl J Med* 2001; **345**: 1809–17.

12. HC Diener, L Cunha, C Forbes, J Sivenius, P Smets and A Lowenthal, European Stroke Prevention Study 2: dipyridamole and acetylsalicylic acid in the secondary prevention of stroke, *J Neurol Sci* 1996; **143**: 1–13.

13. ESPRIT Study Group, Aspirin plus dipyridamole versus aspirin alone after cerebral ischaemia of arterial origin (ESPRIT): randomised controlled trial, *Lancet* 2006; **36**: 1665–73.

14. CAPRIE Steering Committee. A randomised, blinded, trial of clopidogrel versus aspirin in patients at risk of ischaemic events (CAPRIE). *Lancet* 1996 Nov 16; **348**: 1329–39.

15. Ringleb PA, Bhatt DL, Hirsch AT, Topol EJ, Hacke W; Clopidogrel versus aspirin in patients at risk of ischemic events investigators. Benefit of clopidogrel over aspirin is amplified in patients with a history of ischemic events. *Stroke* 2004; **35**: 528–32.

16. Sacco RL, Diener HC, Yusuf S, Cotton D, Ounpuu S, Lawton WA et al. Aspirin and extended-release dipyridamole versus clopidogrel for recurrent stroke. *N Engl J Med* 2008; **359**: 1238–51.

17. Diener HC, Bogousslavsky J, Brass LM, Cimminiello C, Csiba L, Kaste M, Leys D, Matias-Guiu J, Rupprecht HJ; MATCH investigators. Aspirin and clopidogrel compared with clopidogrel alone after recent ischaemic stroke or transient ischaemic attack in high-risk patients (MATCH): randomised, double-blind, placebo-controlled trial. *Lancet* 2004; **364**: 331–7.

18. Bhatt Dl, Fox KA, Hacke W et al. Clopidogrel and aspirin versus aspirin alone for the prevention of atherothrombotic events. *N Engl J Med* 2006; **354**: 1706–17.

19. Hallas J, Dall M, Andries A, Andersen BS, Aalykke C, Hansen JM, Andersen M, Lassen AT. Use of single and combined antithrombotic therapy and risk of serious upper gastrointestinal bleeding: population based case-control study. *BMJ* 2006; **333**: 726.

20. The National Institute of Neurological Disorders and Stroke rt-PA Stroke Study Group. Tissue Plasminogen Activator for Acute Ischemic Stroke. *N Engl J Med* 1995; **333**: 1581–8.

21. Wardlaw J, Berge E, del Zoppo G, Yamaguchi T. Thrombolysis for acute ischemic Stroke. 2004; **35**; 2914–5.

22. Wahlgren N, Ahmed N, Dávalos A, Ford GA, Grond M, Hacke W, Hennerici MG, Kaste M, Kuelkens S, Larrue V, Lees KR, Roine RO, Soinne L, Toni D, Vanhooren G; SITS-MOST investigators.Thrombolysis with alteplase for acute ischaemic stroke in the Safe Implementation of Thrombolysis in Stroke-Monitoring Study (SITS-MOST): an observational study. *Lancet* 2007; **369**: 275–82.

23. Hacke W, Kaste M, Bluhmki E, Brozman M, Dávalos A, Guidetti D, Larrue V, et al. Thrombolysis with alteplase 3 to 4.5 hours after acute ischemic stroke. *N Engl J Med* 2008; **359**: 1317–29.

24. Muir KM, Roberts M. Thrombolytic therapy for stroke: a review with particular reference to elderly patients. *Drugs Aging* 2000; **16**: 41–54.

25. International Stroke Trial Collaborative Group. The International Stroke Trial (IST): a randomised trial of aspirin, subcutaneous heparin, both, or neither among 19,435 patients with acute ischaemic stroke. *Lancet* 1997; **349**: 1569–81.

26. Hylek EM, Skates SJ, Sheehan MA, Singer DE. An analysis of the lowest effective intensity of prophylactic anticoagulation for patients with non-rheumatic atrial fibrillation. *N Engl J Med* 1996; **335**: 540–6.

7 Orthostatic hypotension, postprandial hypotension and syncope in older patients

René W.M.M. Jansen

Department of Geriatric Medicine, Meander Medical Center, The Netherlands

ORTHOSTATIC HYPOTENSION IN OLDER PATIENTS

Introduction

According to the consensus statement by the American Autonomic Society and the American Academy of Neurology orthostatic hypotension is defined as a decrease in systolic blood pressure of >20 mm Hg or a fall in diastolic blood pressure by 10 mmHg or more within 3 minutes of standing. This definition has two important clinical limitations in daily clinical practice. Following these criteria strictly may lead to missing the diagnosis of relevant orthostatic blood pressure changes. Many older patients are vulnerable to cerebral hypoperfusion at orthostatic blood pressure decreases of less than 20/10 mmHg with subsequent symptoms. Secondly, older patients may have relevant orthostatic declines in blood pressure after periods of standing longer than three minutes. There is an ongoing debate as to whether these orthostatic hypotensive periods should be included in the definition of orthostatic hypotension. However, when the history of a patient suggests orthostatic hypotension after longer periods of standing, blood pressure measurements should be performed for 10 minutes or longer.

Multiple organ systems are involved in order to maintain hemodynamic homeostasis and brain perfusion during the upright position. With age the ability to maintain homeostasis and brain perfusion during position changes becomes less effective predisposing older subjects to significant changes in blood pressure. In healthy elderly subjects a low frequency of orthostatic hypotension has been reported and most of them have no symptoms at all.

A wide range of orthostatic hypotension has been reported varying from 5 % to a prevalence rate of close to 70 % for older patients in the acute-care setting (1). The prevalence of orthostatic hypotension depends on the group of patients studied and the timing of measurements. Older people tend to be more vulnerable as a result of impaired homeostatic mechanisms.

Aetiology

A lowering of postural blood pressure is caused by the force of gravity. At standing 500 to 700 ml of blood is pooled in the lower extremities and in the gastro-intestinal and pulmonary circulation. The venous flow to the heart is decreased at standing resulting in reduction of cardiac output. The cardiopulmonary,

Prescribing for Elderly Patients Edited by Stephen Jackson, Paul Jansen and Arduino Mangoni
© 2009 John Wiley & Sons, Ltd

aortic and carotid baroreceptors are here-upon stimulated with increase of sympathetic neural outflow and sympathetically mediated increase of cardiac frequency and vasoconstriction to maintain postural blood pressure. Baroreceptor function changes with aging. The amount of beta-adrenergic receptors remains constant, however with reduced affinity at cardiac level (less increase of cardiac frequency) and at vascular level (less vasodilatation). The alpha-1-adrenergic receptors, responsible for vasoconstriction, are not influenced by the aging process. The rate of increase of cardiac frequency upon standing is diminished in the elderly and vasoconstriction becomes a more important factor in the prevention of orthostatic hypotension. Therefore blockade of the alpha-adrenergic receptors leads to significant orthostatic hypotension in the old.

The cerebral autoregulatory system limits the reduction of the cerebral perfusion pressure induced by the postural position. Age-related changes could affect the efficacy of this system and the autonomic regulation of blood pressure. The superimposition of cardiovascular diseases and the use of different medications may lead to further decrements in autonomic function with subsequent orthostatic hypotension.

Common causes of orthostatic hypotension can be divided into systemic disorders, dysfunction of the autonomic nervous system and medication-related causes. Common systemic disorders include dehydration, hypertension, diabetes mellitus, parkinsonism, deconditioning and prolonged immobility.

Symptoms and signs

All elderly patients complaining of orthostatic symptoms related to cerebral hypoperfusion should have blood pressure and heart rate measurements performed. A detailed history, including a detailed description and timing of the orthostatic symptoms and circumstances, is very important.

Elderly patients with orthostatic hypotension are often symptomatic, but the symptoms could be diverse and non-specific (1).

Dizziness, instability and a tendency to fall are the most pronounced symptoms. Older patients tolerate poorly mild brain hypoperfusion caused by orthostatic hypotension. More severe symptoms such as syncope and falls represent a clear danger for concomitant fractures and immobility.

Diagnosis

The diagnosis of orthostatic hypotension can be made simply by performing blood pressure measurements in the supine or sitting position and in the standing position. A correct diagnosis of orthostatic hypotension is dependent on an accurate technique in blood pressure measurements, however, these standardized blood pressure measurements are not followed in many clinical settings (2). Important factors affecting these blood pressure measurements are day-to-day and within-day variability, time of the blood pressure measurements and correct measurements techniques. Important deviations include arm position not at heart level during standing blood pressure measurements, wrong position of the arm cuff, and to short or to long time period following standing.

Orthostatic hypotension is highly variable during the day, but most prevalent in the morning. Because of the high variability of orthostatic hypotension, multiple blood pressure measurements should be performed, preferably in the morning, at different visits.

Therapy

Orthostatic hypotension determined by a single measurement is found frequently. When it is an asymptomatic finding it remains unknown whether this should be treated. Although orthostatic hypotension in the elderly is considered to be a risk factor for falls and syncope no clear evidence of a causal relationship is available. It should be remembered that most falls or syncope have multi-factorial causes. However, when orthostatic hypotension is confirmed on repeated examination or when it is considered to be symptomatic, orthostatic hypotension should be treated with first non-pharmacologic interventions and secondly, depending on the symptoms with pharmacologic agents (3). In many instances, orthostatic hypotension can be effectively treated by modifications of drug treatment for concomitant disorders.

The main goals of treatment are to reduce symptoms, to reduce the risk for falling, and to improve patients' functional capacity. Reducing orthostatic hypotension might fulfill these goals in daily practice and completely prevent orthostatic blood pressure reductions is normally not necessary. Even slight improvements in orthostatic hypotension can bring the arterial pressure up just enough to be within the autoregulatory zone.

Initial interventions should include the discontinuation or reduction of the dosage of any medication that could be responsible for orthostatic hypotension, such as diuretics, nitrate, antidepressants (tricyclic) (only very limited information is available about SSRI's, but orthostatic hypotension has been reported during treatment with paroxetine and fluoxetine), antipsychotics (clozapine, olanzapine), anticholinergic drugs, and selective alpha1-receptorblockers (alfuzosine, alprostadil, tamsulosin) (4, 5).

Other interventions in the elderly are chronic expansion of intravascular volume by encouraging higher fluid and salt intake, sleeping in the head-up position, and waist-high compression stockings. It should be kept in mind that these stockings should be put on before the patient leaves the bed. Often, a nurse will be required in order to perform this, thereby limiting the usefulness of these stockings. Furthermore, patients should be taught to rise slowly from beds and chairs. Patients should receive advice to avoid standing still for a prolonged period of time, straining during micturition or defaecation, hot baths or showers, and large meals. Diuretics, nitrates and drugs with vasodepressor properties should be avoided. Simply lowering the dose of a diuretic might improve orthostatic hypotension.

Orthostatic hypotension is related to baseline systolic blood pressure. Treatment of hypertension, although antihypertensive medications as a group can cause orthostatic hypotension, will reduce orthostatic hypotension. In many elderly patients, simply treating hypertension will be an effective treatment of (symptomatic) orthostatic hypotension, independent of which class of antihypertensives they were treated with (6, 7). Avoiding treating blood pressure in elderly patients with hypertension because of the fear of developing orthostatic hypotension is therefore not warranted. In patients with heart failure based on diastolic dysfunction of the left ventricle and normal ejection fraction withdrawal of diuretics and/or nitrates should be considered.

Orthostatic hypotension can develop after several days of bed rest in the elderly, as a form of deconditioning. Repeated tilt table testing might be effective in combating orthostatic hypotension induced by deconditioning.

If a patient still has symptomatic orthostatic hypotension, the use of salt retaining steroids, principally fludrocortisone, can be used (see Table 7.1). Fludrocortisone promotes reabsorption of sodium and loss of potassium from renal distal tubes. This drug expands the circulatory volume over a period of one to two weeks. This drug should be started in a low dose of 0.1 mg and slowly titrated upward in 0.1 mg increments at a two or three days intervals until mild peripheral edema develops. This drug should be used cautiously in elderly patients or patients with heart failure. Monitor orthostatic hypotension and edema. Adverse effects include supine hypertension, which is partly counter-acted by sleeping in a 30 degree upright position, hypokalemia and congestive heart failure. Contra-indications: systemic fungal infections and hypersensitivity.

Midodrine is usually most effective when used in combination with fludrocortisone. Midodrine is a prodrug and converted to desglymidodrine, a selective α_1-adrenoceptor agonist increasing blood pressure via arterial and venous vasoconstriction resulting in a rise in standing and supine blood pressure. Although midodrine is in general well tolerated, disturbing side effects have been described (8). Monitor orthostatic hypotension and renal and hepatic parameters. Contra-indications: hypersensitivity, severe

Table 7.1. Drugs used for the treatment of orthostatic hypotension

Name	Dose	Pharmacokinetics	Interactions	Precautions/adverse effects
Fludrocortisone	0.1 mg 3 times a week up to 1 mg daily	metabolism in the liver T^1/$_2$: 30–35 minutes	may antagonize effects of anticholinesterases decreases salicylate levels. Effect of fludrocortisone may be reduced by rifampicin and barbiturates.	supine hypertension, heart failure, edema, rash and bruising of the skin, muscle weakness, hypokalemia, peptic ulcer, and cataracts
midodrine	2.5 mg tid up to 10 mg tid not later than 6 pm	T^1/$_2$ is 3–4 hours of active metabolite desglymido-drine.	alpha-antagonists may antagonize effects of midrodine bradycardia may be accentuated by glycosides	supine hypertension, piloerection, pruritis, urinary urgency or retention, dysuria, paresthesis, rash, abdominal pain

heart disease, urinary retention, pheochromocytoma and thyrotoxicosis.

A variety of other drugs have been used to treat orthostatic hypotension, such as the somatostatin analog octreotide, erythropoietin, caffeine, yohimbine, clonidine, pindolol, ergot alkaloids, nonsteroidal anti-inflammatory drugs, and other agents without clear evidence of their benefits to treat orthostatic hypotension in elderly patients.

KEY POINTS

- Single measurement of asymptomatic orthostatic hypotension can frequently be found in older patients, but the clinical significance remains unknown. Repeated measurements, preferably in the morning are recommended.
- Smaller falls in standing blood pressure than the formal definition of a decrease of 20 mmHg or more may cause cerebral hypoperfusion.
- Initial treatment of orthostatic hypotension is discontinuation or reduction in dose of any medication that could be responsible for orthostatic hypotension.
- Higher salt and water intake is vital to limiting the magnitude of falls in blood pressure.

- Elastic stockings are of limited value in treating symptomatic hypotension.
- Management of orthostatic hypotension requires appropriate treatment of hypertension and limitation of the use of nitrates and diuretics.
- When non-pharmacological interventions or modifications of drug treatment is not effective, fludrocortisone and midrodine can be used.

POSTPRANDIAL HYPOTENSION IN OLDER PATIENTS

Introduction

Postprandial hypotension is defined as a decrease in systolic blood pressure of >20 mm Hg or a fall in blood pressure to less than 90 mm Hg where preprandial blood pressure is >100 mmHg within 2 hours of a meal (1, 9, 10). In healthy elderly persons, meal-induced decreases in blood pressure are common but mostly asymptomatic. Elderly persons with hypertension, heart failure, syncope, Parkinson's disease, depression, patients on dialysis or persons with autonomic dysfunction have an increased frequency of postprandial hypotension. In hospital and institutionalized populations, the prevalence of postprandial hypotension in elderly persons is higher than that in the community because of the higher frequency of co-morbid conditions and diseases and the increased number of medications, which all may have effects on blood pressure regulation. In frail elderly patients admitted to acute care hospitals, postprandial hypotension is extremely common. In a recent study, 67 % of frail geriatric patients had postprandial hypotension and 52 % were diagnosed with orthostatic hypotension (1). Eighty-one per cent of the patients had either postprandial hypotension or orthostatic hypotension. Nearly all elderly nursing home residents experience postprandial hypotension. In almost 40 % of these residents, systolic blood pressure decreases more than 20 mm Hg within 75 minutes of eating a meal.

The timing of the fall in postprandial systolic blood pressure is variable for each person (10). The time period for measuring blood pressure to detect postprandial hypotension should be at least 90 minutes. Apparent postprandial decreases in blood pressure can be found almost immediately after a meal with a nadir in blood pressure as early as 15 minutes following the meal in approximately 15 % of patients. Postprandial blood pressure usually reaches a nadir within 30–60 minutes in 70 % of patients. However, in the remaining 15 % of patients, decreases in systolic blood pressure are apparent as late as 75 minutes following the meal.

Postprandial hypotension can result in disabling symptoms such as dizziness and syncope and there is a strong association with falls (1, 10–12). The presence of symptoms depends on a reduction in the blood supply to a specific organ. In most elderly persons, falls and syncope are multi-factorial, and their resolution requires a careful evaluation. Postprandial hypotension is more common and more pronounced in elderly patients who have experienced a fall (12), and it accounts for 6 %–8 % of syncopal episodes ((1–10)). In a group of patients with unexplained syncope by conventional in-hospital evaluations, half had postprandial

hypotension (11). As a consequence, postprandial hypotension represents an important medical and economic problem.

Aetiology

The basic mechanisms by which postprandial hypotension is produced remain uncertain (10). Clearly the extent of postprandial splanchnic hyperemia is an important factor. The other major factors appear to be impairments in baroreflex function, inadequate postprandial increases in cardiac output, and inadequate sympathetic nervous system compensation.

After meal ingestion there is substantial redistribution of blood to the splanchnic circulation whose blood flow increases by up to 25 %. It is likely that this together with a reduction in autonomic (sympathetic) nerve activity and possibly changes in neurohumoral (especially serotonin and nitric oxide) mechanisms may play a role in the condition. Patients with autonomic dysfunction, either primary or secondary, are particularly at risk.

A number of factors are believed to influence the degree of hypotension. These include food related factors, such as composition, volume and timing of meals, patient co-morbidities including Parkinson's disease or diabetes mellitus and drugs especially diuretics and anti-hypertensives and selective serotonin reuptake inhibitors. The composition of the meal is of critical importance to degree of hypotension and glucose in particular is the most potent stimulator of hypotension compared to other carbohydrates, fats and proteins. The degree of gastric distension reflecting the size of the meal may also influence blood pressure (13).

Symptoms and signs

It appears that postprandial hypotension is more prevalent and more profound in the morning. Postprandial hypotension symptoms include syncope, sleepiness, nausea, headache, and chest pain (1). Remarkably, dizziness is not reported in patients with postprandial hypotension in a recent study, whereas this is the most important symptom in orthostatic hypotension (1). Patients complain frequently of feeling syncopal and needing to lie down, and if the fall in BP is sufficiently large then patients may collapse and lose consciousness. Other symptoms such as gustatory sweating may occur. The cardinal sign is a fall in serial blood pressure measurements after a meal. Although older persons may have dramatic drops in their blood pressure, the majority of them have no symptoms at all at the time of meal. Some elderly patients can tolerate extremely low levels of postprandial systolic blood pressure, especially when they are chronically exposed to low blood pressures.

Diagnosis

The condition can usually be diagnosed from history (especially of co-morbidities which are associated with autonomic nerve dysfunction) and simple blood pressure measurements following meal ingestion. Including the rest period of at least 10 minutes for preprandial blood pressure measurements, the total time of a meal test takes at least two hours, making these tests quite time-consuming. Postprandial hypotension is easily detectable by manual or automatic blood pressure measurements at intervals of 10 minutes. Ambulatory blood pressure monitoring is a valuable and useful method to investigate meal-related blood pressure changes in elderly patients.

Therapy

Although postprandial hypotension has now been recognized as a very common clinically relevant disorder in elderly persons, limited data exist about the management of this syndrome. Non-pharmacological treatments which may be of benefit include attention to fluid and electrolyte status and dietary manipulation. Reducing the glucose content of meals reduces postprandial hypotension in elderly patients with fewer and less severe symptoms compared to test meals with normal or high amounts of carbohydrates (13). Thus, reducing the size and increasing the frequency of

meals is an easy, cost-effective, and successful intervention in the management of postprandial hypotension in elderly patients.

Adequate treatment of hypertension and limitation of the use of diuretics and nitrates may improve postprandial hypotension and ameliorate symptoms (14). Appropriate fluid and salt intake are important and avoidance of dehydration due to diuretic therapy is obvious. Consumption of water (400–500 ml) as a pre-load before a meal has also been shown to attenuate the fall in blood pressure. Patients should exercise caution in standing up as orthostatic hypotension may increase the fall in blood pressure.

Although a number of drugs have been recommended as treatment for the condition, pharmacotherapy is largely unproven, associated with significant adverse effects or impractical. There is some evidence to support the use of caffeine but this is controversial. The alpha glycosidase inhibitor acarbose appears beneficial in short term use but is associated with gastrointestinal side effects, whilst use of somatostatin analogs such as octreotide are limited by cost and the need for parenteral administration (10).

KEY POINTS

- Significant hypotension after meals occurs frequently in older patients especially those with diseases associated with autonomic dysfunction.
- Postprandial hypotension can be usually diagnosed from history and serial blood pressure measurements.
- Avoidance of salt and water depletion is vital to limiting the magnitude of falls in blood pressure.
- Limitation of carbohydrate load is the major therapeutic option. Other simple measures, such water preloads, may help in management.
- Management of postprandial hypotension requires appropriate treatment of hypertension and limitation of the use of nitrates and diuretics.

- Optimal drug treatment for symptomatic postprandial hypotension requires further evaluation.

SYNCOPE IN OLDER PATIENTS

Introduction

Syncope is a common medical problem in the elderly. Distinguishing syncope from falls is often the first challenge. In the Framingham study the incidence of syncope increases sharply at the age of 70 years. In an elderly institutionalized population the incidence was 6% per year. These data are probably underestimates because of the overlap of syncopal events with episodes which present as falls. Evaluation of syncope can be difficult although recent diagnostic strategies make it possible to ascertain the contributing causes in the majority of cases (see Guidelines). Syncope is defined as a transient, self-limited loss of consciousness with a rapid onset and spontaneous recovery, usually leading to falling (15, 16). The underlying mechanism is a transient cerebral hypoperfusion. Thijs et al. presented a straightforward classification of syncope aimed at primary causes affecting the circulation and based on the ESC Task Force Guideliness on the management of syncope (15):

1. Insufficient pumping of the heart, including cardiac arrhythmia and structural heart disease.
2. Low blood pressure, including orthostatic hypotension.
3. Insufficient filling of the circulation, including dehydration and hypovolemia.
4. Inappropriate neural control over the circulation, including vasovagal syncope, carotid sinus syndrome and micturition syncope.

Syncope is an important cause of injury-related hospitalization in older persons. An important consequence of even a single syncopal event can result in restricting outdoor activities and fear of falling, reduced quality of live and independence. Even syncope that does not result in physical injuries can result in loss of confidence, loss of mobility, depression and social isolation.

Aetiology

Any factor that diminishes cerebral blood flow for a certain time may cause syncope. Cerebral perfusion is largely dependent on systemic arterial pressure. Therefore, decreases in either cardiac output or total peripheral vascular resistance reduce systemic arterial pressure and cerebral perfusion pressure.

Multiple risk factors are more common in very old subjects or frail elderly persons and the boundaries between falls and syncope are poorly delineated (17). The cause for syncope is not often obvious and over one third of older subject will have several attributable causes. Therefore, full evaluation should be performed in patients with unexplained syncope or falls, but should be modified according to the prognosis of the patient.

The commonest causes of syncope in elderly patients are cardiac arrhythmias, carotid sinus hypersensitivity, orthostatic- and post-prandial hypotension. Other causes include cardiovascular medications and vasovagal episodes. Up to 15% of syncope is vasovagal and these patients have such a history at younger ages. Micturition and defecation syncope are less common.

Symptoms and signs

A syncope without warning or with the person in the supine or sitting position is most likely to result from an arrthythmia. Syncope resulting from orthostatic hypotension is frequently associated with light headedness, dizziness, unsteadiness and occurs after standing up from bed or chair. Prolonged standing might induce syncope due to orthostatic hypotension. A syncope within 90 minutes after the start of a meal suggest postprandial syncope. A syncope during head movements or rotation suggest carotid sinus hypersensitivity (18). This might be the case for situations with pressure on the carotid sinus as in tight collars, during shaving or looking upwards. Syncope associated with exercise suggest ventricular tachycardia or aortic stenosis. Vasovagal syncope is accompanied with nausea, pallor or diaphoresis and might be related to unpleasant sight, sound, pain or smell. Venapunctures are well known events.

Diagnosis

Initial evaluation may lead to a certain diagnosis based on the history, symptoms and signs or ECG findings. The history, precipitating events and clinical features of the presentation may suggest the cause of syncope. One of the key questions is whether heart diseases is present or absent. A cardiac cause is more likely when the syncope is preceded by palpitations, occurs in the supine position or during exercise.

History taking might be complicated by cognitive impairment, which is present in at least 20 % of 80 years old. Cognitive impairment will influence the accuracy of recall for events or patients might have no recall of the syncopal event at all. Eyewitness accounts of episodes are not available in up to 40–60 % or amnesia for loss of consciousness making the diagnostic workup more complicated. Specific components in history taking are of relevance in elderly patients. The time, circumstances and what the patient was doing when events occur might be helpful for diagnosis.

In the elderly, assessments of the neurological and locomotor systems are recommended. Standing balance, gait, and cognitive examination should be performed. In each patient with syncope or unexplained falls, depending on history taking, orthostatic and postprandial blood pressure measurements and supine and upright carotid sinus massage should be performed in addition to the standard work-up as recommended by recent guidelines. Measurements of orthostatic- and postprandial measurements has been described elsewhere. Carotid sinus massage is performed in the supine position at both sides under continuous beat-to-beat blood pressure and electrocardiographic monitoring. The carotid artery is firmly massaged for

five seconds at the anterior margin of the sternocleomastoid muscle at the level of the cricoid cartilage. After two minutes the procedure is repeated at the other side of the patient. An abnormal response to carotid massage has been defined as a ventriculair pause of three seconds or more and/or a fall in systolic blood pressure of 50 mmHg or more. When carotid sinus massage shows negative results in the supine position, the same test should be repeated with the patient in the upright position.

Therapy

The need for initiating therapy depends of the likelihood that syncope will recur and the certainty that the cause of syncope is known. Therapy of syncope should address any underlying pathology if present and be directed to prevent other contributing causes. When cardiac arrhythmias or structural heart disease is considered to be the cause of syncope, the patients should be referred to a cardiologist. However, it should be kept in mind that syncope in many elderly subjects is multi-factorial.

General strategies should address avoidance of the triggering event when possible. For instance, when head rotations might trigger carotid hypersensitivity the patient can be learned not to turn their head but to rotate the whole body instead. Education and reassurance might be sufficient for many patients.

In patients with symptomatic carotid hypersensitivity based on a true cardio-inhibitory response the available studies indicate that pacing may have strong beneficial effect and prevents recurrence of syncope (16). It remains unclear as to whether pacing is also effective in patients with a mixed type of carotid hypersensitivity. There are no studies examining treatment of carotid sinus syncope in which hypotension has been involved. Medical therapy for carotid sinus syncope has largely been abandoned.

Many drugs have been investigated in the treatment of vasovagal syncope, however, the current evidence fails to show a positive effect in repeated double-blind placebo controlled trials. Recently, leg crossing has been demonstrated are able to induce significant increases of systolic blood pressure which might be applied during impending vasovagal syncope. However, the effect of this manoeuvre should be determined in older patients and frail elderly.

In postprandial syncope, small frequent meals with reduced carbohydrate content might be a very effective and an easy to use treatment (13). Syncope due to orthostatic hypotension should be treated as described elsewhere.

KEY POINTS

- Syncope should be considered in every patient with unexplained falls.
- Orthostatic and postprandial hypotension and carotid sinus hypersensitivity are common causes for syncope in elderly patients.
- Multiple factors as a cause of syncope in very old persons are more common.
- Pacing is indicated in patients with symptomatic carotid hypersensitivity based on cardio-inhibitory response. There is no medical treatment for carotid hypersensitivity based on hypotension.
- Small but frequent meals are very effective in postprandial syncope.

GUIDELINES

Task Force on Syncope, European Society of Cardiology. Guidelines on management of syncope. Update 2004. *Europace* 2004; **6**: 467–537.

REFERENCES

1. Vloet LCM, Pel-Little RE, Jansen PAF, Jansen RWMM. High prevalence of postprandial- and orthostatic hypotension among geriatric patients admitted to Dutch hospitals. *J Gerontol Med Sci* 2005; **60A**: 1271–7.

2. Vloet LCM, Smits R, Frederiks CMA, Hoefnagels WHL, Jansen RWMM. Evaluation of skills and knowledge on orthostatic blood pressure measurements in elderly patients. *Age Ageing* 2002; **31**: 211–16.

3. Ooi WL, Hossain M, Lipsitz LA. The association between Orthostatic hypotension and recurrent falls in nursing home residents. *Am J Med* 2000; **108**: 106–11.

4. Andrews C, Pinner G. Postural hypotension induced by paroxetine. *BMJ* 1998; **21**(316): 595.

5. Pacher P, Kecskemeti V. Cardiovascular side effects of new antidepressants and antipsychotics: New Drugs, old concerns? *Curr Pharm Des* 2004; **10**: 2463–2475.

6. Masuo K, Mikami H, Ogihara T, et al. Changes in frequency of orthostatic hypotension in elderly hypertensive patients under medications. *Am J Hypertens* 1996; **9**: 263–8.

7. Hajjar I. Postural blood pressure changes and Orthostatic hypotension in the elderly patient. *Drugs Aging* 2005; **22**: 55–68.

8. McClellan KJ, Wiseman LR, Wilde MI. Midodrine. A review of its therapeutic use in the management of orthostatic hypotension. *Drugs Aging* 1998; **12**: 75–86.

9. Jansen RWMM. Postprandial hypotension: Simple treatment but difficulties with the diagnosis. *J Gerontol Med Sci* 2005; **60A**: 1268–70 (editorial).

10. Jansen RW, Lipsitz LA. Postprandial hypotension: epidemiology, pathophysiology, and clinical management. *Ann Intern Med* 1995; **122**: 286–95.

11. Jansen RW, Connelly CM, Kelley Gagnon MM, Parker JA, Lipsitz LA. Postprandial hypotension in elderly patients with unexplained syncope. *Arch Intern Med* 1995; **155**: 945–52.

12. Puisieux F, Bulckaen H, Fauchais AL, Drumez S, Salomez-Granier F, Dewailly P. Ambulatory blood pressure monitoring and postprandial hypotension in elderly persons with falls or syncopes. *J Gerontol A Biol Sci Med Sci* 2000; **55**: 535–40.

13. Vloet LCM, Mehagnoul-Schipper DJ, Hoefnagels WHL, Jansen RWMM. The influence of low-, normal-, and high-carbohydrate meals on blood pressure in elderly patients with postprandial hypotension. *J Gerontol A Biol Sci Med Sci* 2001; **56**: 744–8.

14. Kraaij van DWJ, Jansen RWMM, Bouwels LHR, Hoefnagels WHL. Furosemide withdrawal improves postprandial hypotension in elderly heart failure patients with preserved left ventricular systolic function. *Arch Intern Med* 1999; **159**: 1599–1605.

15. Thijs RD, Wieling W, Kaufmann H, van Dijk JG. Defining and classifying syncope. *Clin Auton Res* 2004; **14**(suppl 1): 4–8.

16. Task Force on Syncope, European Society of Cardiology. Guidelines on management of syncope. Update 2004. *Europace* 2004; **6**: 467–537.

17. Shaw FE, Bond J, Richardson DA, et al. Multifactorial intervention after a fall in older people with cognitive impairment and dementia presenting to the accident and emergency department: randomised controlled trial. *BMJ* 2003; **326**: 73–80.

18. Claassen JA, Jansen RWMM. Carotid sinus massage and head turning in healthy aging volunteers. *J Am Geriatric Soc* 2006; **54**: 188.

8 Parkinson's disease

Gerrit Tissingh[1] and Erik Ch. Wolters[2]

[1] *Department of Neurology, Atrium Medisch Centrum Parkstad, The Netherlands*
[2] *Department of Neurology, VU Medical Center Amsterdam, Amsterdam, The Netherlands*

INTRODUCTION

James Parkinson (1755–1824) published in 1817 his celebrated *Essay on the Shaking Palsy*. He described several, typical features of what is nowadays called Parkinson's disease (PD): '*Involuntary tremulous motion, with lessened muscular power, in parts not in action and even when supported, with a propensity to bend the trunk forward, and to pass from a walking to a running pace; the senses and intellects being uninjured*'. It was Charcot who gave the disease its present name at the end of the 19th century.

PD is a progressive, neurodegenerative disease with an insidious onset. It is the most common cause of parkinsonism. Prevalence estimates vary widely and increase with age, with an overall prevalence of 10–400 per 100.000 and without a significant sex-difference. Parkinsonism is a syndrome characterized by the following cardinal features: 1) hypokinesia and bradykinesia, 2) tremor at rest, 3) rigidity and 4) postural instability. The differential diagnosis includes many other causes besides PD, such as vascular parkinsonism and multiple system atrophy (MSA) (see below).

The predominant neuropathological hallmark is a degeneration of dopaminergic neurons in the brainstem, i.e. substantia nigra and ventral tegmental area, together with the formation of Lewy bodies. This results in a marked loss of dopamine in the striatum as well as in the (pre)frontal cortex and limbic area, which receive dopamine projections from the substantia nigra respectively the ventral tegmental area. As a rule, the degeneration in the presynaptic dopaminergic system is also accompanied by a detrition of the central noradrenergic, serotonergic and cholinergic systems in the brainstem. The major motor signs will become apparent only when striatal dopamine levels are significantly reduced (about 60 %). As a consequence, the clinical course of PD can be subdivided into two different phases: the 'preclinical', or preferably 'premotor', phase and the clinical, motor phase. Extrapolating from the extent of the degeneration of the nigrostriatal dopaminergic system in PD, as visualized by functional imaging techniques, as well as post-mortem cell counts of melanoneurons in the substantia nigra, the onset of the disease process seems to antedate the clinical diagnosis of PD by about four to six years. During this premotor phase, individuals might be asymptomatic or display non-motor signs and symptoms (for example hyposmia) with, as a rule, a normal neurological examination. In this phase, though, functional imaging may already indicate a loss of the integrity of the presynaptic dopaminergic system. Better recognition of these signs as PD-related manifestations will allow earlier diagnosis and better treatment, especially when a causal/protective therapy becomes available.

Prescribing for Elderly Patients Edited by Stephen Jackson, Paul Jansen and Arduino Mangoni
© 2009 John Wiley & Sons, Ltd

SYMPTOMS AND SIGNS OF PD

Motor symptoms

PD usually presents asymmetrically. The most cardinal sign of PD is hypo- and bradykinesia (lack of spontaneous movements and slowing down of movements respectively). The poverty of blinking and the mask-like face, loss of volume of the voice, and reduction of arm movements as the patient walks are all typical manifestations.

The rest tremor is present with a frequency of 4–7 Hz, and disappears with action. It may be absent, though, both in the early and advanced stages of the disease. Rigidity, which means a resistance to passive movement of equal degree in opposing muscle groups throughout the entire range of motion ('lead-pipe rigidity'), can be detected in most patients. The well-known accompanying cogwheel phenomenon may result when the increased muscle tone is interrupted by a coexistent tremor. Pain, caused by muscle rigidity, may be the most urgent symptom which makes the patient seeks medical attention. Gait difficulties are also frequently met in this respect. Postural abnormalities and instability occur in more advanced stages of the disease. However, often a mild degree of forward flexion of the trunk is noticeable in the early phase (stooped posture).

Non-motor symptoms

Early or later in the disease, non-motor signs and symptoms, such as loss of olfaction, autonomic dysfunctions, sleep disturbances, depression, anxiety, dementia as well as psychosis, may also occur, eventually well before motor parkinsonism.

Olfactory dysfunction may be one of the earliest and most prevalent signs of PD. More than 90 % of the patients show disturbances in odor detection, discrimination and identification. Recently, it has been identified as an important risk-factor for developing PD in first degree relatives of patients. Interestingly, preserved or only mildly impaired olfactory function has been reported in patients with MPTP-induced parkinsonism and atypical parkinsonian syndromes, such as Progressive Supranuclear Palsy (PSP) and MSA.

Autonomic symptoms include orthostatic hypotension, sexual dysfunction, constipation, bladder problems, seborrhea and sweating.

Sleep disorders, such as insomnia and sleep fragmentation as well as excessive daytime sleepiness (EDS) and REM sleep behaviour disorder (RBD) have been reported in PD, even in the premotor phase. RBD is characterized by a lack of motor inhibition during REM sleep, which leads to a vigorous and potentially harmful dream-enacting behaviour. It has been shown recently that RBD patients have a profound impairment of olfactory function. Moreover, a substantial part of these hyposmic RBD patients were later found to be suffer from PD.

The relationship between depression and PD has received much attention. It may be present in as many as 40 % of the patients, with a strong variation in reported prevalence rates, depending on the sample studied and the instruments used. It reduces quality of life independently of motor symptoms and is probably underrated and undertreated.

Cognitive dysfunction in PD may be described as a progressive dysexecutive syndrome, already found at disease onset in many patients. In about 30–40 % of the patients, this syndrome may proceed to dementia with memory deficits, in the absence of aphasia, apraxia or agnosia. The main risk factor seems to be age at onset of PD. In case of dementia preceding first motor symptoms, this condition is referred to as dementia with Lewy bodies (DLB).

Psychosis can be found in up to 40 % of the patients with PD, especially in the dementing patients. Main manifestations comprise delusions (false beliefs about external reality, often paranoid in type) and hallucinations (sensory perceptions, mainly visual, in the absence of an external stimulus). Dopaminomimetic drugs seem to play an important causative role, inducing dopamine hypersensitivity in the frontal and limbic dopamine projection regions, though a cholinergic deficit may also be responsible, especially in demented patients with PD.

Pathophysiology

The pathophysiological explanation for the multilevel abnormalities in PD may be found in the fact that the basal ganglia are part of parallel neuronal cortico-subcortical circuits, connecting striatal structures (putamen, caudate, nucleus accumbens) with the prefrontal cortex and the limbic areas by way of projections through the pallidum and thalamus. Moreover, in the presence of dopamine deficiency, disturbances in central non-dopaminergic transmitter systems may contribute to the development of mental dysfunction, which varies between subjects. This diversity in cognitive disabilities, as well as the co-occurence of mood changes and psychosis in some patients, might be explained as being due to disruption of specific cortico-striatal loops in subtypes of PD, together with functional abnormalities in non-dopaminergic ascending systems.

AETIOLOGY AND PATHOLOGY

The cause of PD remains to be clarified. Both environmental and genetic factors are considered important. As a rule, main patients suffer sporadic idiopathic Parkinson's disease. Hereditary factors may play a role in, especially, young-onset PD. In recent years, several gene mutations and chromosomal loci have been identified. A great deal of current evidence suggests that oxidative mechanisms may play a key role in the processes underlying neuronal cell death.

Neuropathological examination reveals intracerebral formation of abnormal proteinaceous Lewy bodies and Lewy neurites, mainly consisting of alfa-synuclein. Recently, several stages of PD have been described by Braak et al. In (premotor) stages I and II Lewy body pathology is confined to the medulla oblongata (dorsal motor nucleus) and the olfactory bulb and anterior olfactory nucleus. Cell loss and Lewy bodies in the substantia nigra and nucleus basalis of Meynert defines the onset of stage III and IV, in which the first motor symptoms become apparent. The end-stages V and VI involve progressive involvement of the cerebral cortex.

DIAGNOSIS

Diagnostic criteria for PD have been developed (see Table 8.1). An accurate diagnosis is based on the presence of a bradykinetic syndrome with asymmetric onset, rigidity, postural instability and/or a resting tremor in the presence of a positive response to levodopa. The Unified Parkinson's Disease Rating Scale (UPDRS) can be used as a measure of the severity of symptoms and signs, both in the on and off-phase. It consists of 42 items and four sub-scores: 1) mentation, behaviour and mood, 2) activities of daily living, 3) motor examination and 4) complications of therapy. Using the UPDRS, one is able to monitor in a reliable way the clinical progress of the disease.

Other disorders that may cause primary parkinsonism are, for example, MSA, PSP and corticobasal ganglionic degeneration (CBGD). Secondary parkinsonism, due to vascular disease or drugs is also common (see Table 8.2). Discriminating the various parkinsonian disorders may be difficult, especially in the early phase. Dysautonomia (orthostatic hypotension,

Table 8.1. Diagnostic criteria for Parkinson's disease

Bradykinesia with at least one of the following signs:

Rigidity
Resting tremor
Postural instability

Supportive symptoms and signs
Asymmetric onset
Good and lasting response on levodopa
Progressive course of disease
Levodopa-induced dyskinesias

Suggestive of other parkinsonian disorder
Early postural instability and falling
(Severe) dysautonomia at onset
Supranuclear gaze palsy
Poor or not-lasting clinical efficacy of (high doses) of levodopa

Table 8.2. Main causes of parkinsonism

Primary
Idiopathic Parkinson's disease
Genetic Parkinson's Disease
Multiple system atrophy (MSA)
Progressive supranuclear palsy (PSP)
Dementia with Lewy bodies (DLB)
Corticobasal ganglionic degeneration (CBGD)
Huntington's disease

Secondary
Vascular (lower body-half) parkinsonism
Drugs (neuroleptics, anti-emetics)
Infections (postencephalitic parkinsonism)
Toxins (carbonmonoxide, MPTP)
Metabolic disorders (Wilson disease)
Other (posttraumatic, hydrocephalus)

impotence) (MSA), a supranuclear gaze palsy (PSP) or absence of any cognitive dysfunction suggest parkinsonism due to other diseases. In contrast, asymmetry of motor signs with an unilateral onset, together with an adequate response on levodopa are most typical for PD. Indeed, a good and sustained response to dopamine precursors and agonists best differentiates PD from parkinsonism due to other causes. In the end, post mortem examination remains the gold standard. Routine blood analysis or cerebrospinal fluid examination are most often not helpful. Structural neuroimaging techniques, like magnetic resonance imaging (MRI) can be used to exclude other causes of parkinsonism. Subcortical ischemic changes in the basal ganglia and the white matter are supportive for vascular parkinsonism, and in MSA, atrophy of the cerebellum and brainstem, hypointensity of the striatum or the so-called 'hot-cross bun' sign (hyperintens signal in the pons) may be seen. In PD, there are no clear structural abnormalities visible.

Functional imaging, however, with Positron Emission Tomography (PET) and Single Photon Emission Computed Tomography (SPECT) can be useful. Ligands have become available for imaging both the pre- and post-synaptic dopaminergic system. For example, [^{18}F]fluorodopa (F-dopa) PET reflects the activity of aromatic acid decarboxylase in dopaminergic neurons and is an indirect measure of nigral cell count and [^{123}I]beta-CIT (B-CIT)

SPECT is a marker for the dopamine transporter, located at the dopaminergic nerve terminal. In primary, but not in secondary parkinsonian syndromes, radioactive uptake will be decreased due to the presynaptic degeneration of the dopaminergic system. Visualization of the availability of postsynaptic dopamine receptors using IBZM-SPECT may contribute to the differential diagnosis between PD and other primary parkinsonistic syndromes as the expression of the dopaminergic receptors in these last syndromes (with both pre- and postsynaptic pathology) is decreased, which is not the case in PD, being a pure presynaptic disease. Application of these techniques may increase the accuracy of the clinical diagnosis of PD, which is estimated around 90%.

THERAPY

Non-pharmacological strategies

Initial treatment of PD should be individualized. It comprises education to patients and care-givers, physical therapy (in order to emphasize external cueing) and discussing the various pharmacological options. Sometimes, in order to obtain adequate coping with motor and non-motor symptoms of the disease, psychological help is needed. The goal is to keep the patient functioning independently as long as possible. Drug treatment can be initiated when symptoms interfere significantly with daily life. Since there are no disease modifying drugs yet, pharmacotherapy is mainly focussed on the symptomatic improvement of the motor and non-motor signs. Pharmacotherapy also reduces both morbidity and mortality of PD and has a positive effect on quality of life.

Pharmacotherapeutical strategies

Following the discovery that PD patients were suffering from a deficiency of cerebral dopamine, levodopa was successfully introduced in the late 1960s. Dopamine replacement with levodopa is still the cornerstone of symptomatic therapy in PD. It is absorbed from the duodenum and decarboxylated to dopamine and it acts on all dopamine receptors. A peripheral decarboxylase inhibitor (benserazide or carbidopa) is administered together with levodopa. The drug is very effective especially in reducing bradykinesia and rigidity and remains efficacious throughout the course of PD. Long-term use of levodopa is associated with disabling motor response complications such as wearing-off, dyskinesia (chorea and dystonia) and on-off fluctuations. Progressive loss of dopaminergic neurons required to metabolize the drug and the pulsatile stimulation of dopamine receptors (there is no convincing evidence for direct toxicity of levodopa) are most likely involved in the mechanisms causing these complications. Therefore, slow release preparations and a gel for continuous intraduodenal application have been developed. The duration of action of dopamine may also be enhanced by monoamine oxidase-B (MAO-B) inhibitors, such as selegiline and especially rasagiline (which is also claimed to have neuroprotective effects): safe, effective and well-tolerated drugs with a simple once-daily dosing scheme. The same effect on the duration of action, as well as a substantially increase of levodopa uptake in the central nervous system through the blood-brainbarrier (BBB), can be reached by the central and peripheral active catechol-O-methyltransferase (COMT) inhibitor tolcapone. The peripheral active COMT-inhibitor entacapone also promotes BBB levodopa passage.

In an attempt to overcome the adverse reactions of levodopa, dopamine agonists have been developed. They have a longer plasma half-life as compared to levodopa and interact directly with the dopamine (mostly both D_1 and D_2) receptors (see Table 8.3). As their action is independent of the presynaptic dopaminergic cells, these drugs interact in a less pulsatile way with the dopamine receptors, thus avoiding pharmacodynamic levodopa-related changes of these receptors with motor response fluctuations. The effects of dopamine agonists on the parkinsonian motor signs, however, are less dramatic than seen with levodopa. As a rule, in the long run monotherapy with agonists therefore is mostly not fully satisfying, and needs

to be combined with levodopa (after two to three years, only about 50 % of the patients is still using monotherapy). Next to oral formulations, transdermal (rotigotine patches) and subcutaneous (apomorphine) dopamine agonist are available for even better continuous receptor stimulation (Table 8.3).

Other antiparkinsonian drugs are amantadine, an antiglutamatergic and anticholinergic drug promoting the release of dopamine in the synaptic cleft, and anticholinergics, though due to potential side effects such as memory disturbances and hallucinations these last drugs should be avoided, especially in the older patient.

As mentioned earlier, levodopa is still the most effective drug in the treatment of early and advanced PD. Motor response fluctuations, especially in younger patients, however, are bothersome and limit its application. Depending on age, co-morbidity, cognitive functions and severity of disease one can decide (see Figure 8.1) to start with amantadine, followed by dopamine agonists (in the younger patients) or levodopa (in the patients >65–70 years as well as in patients with advancing cognitive deficits). Ultimately, all patients will need levodopa.

Pharmacotherapeutical complications

In the beginning, patients may complain about peripherally levodopa- and dopamine agonist-induced gastrointestinal and cardiovascular side-effects. In such situations, domperidone, a peripheral dopamine receptor antagonist, might be very useful in the treatment (and/or prevention) of the adverse events.

In the case of levodopa-induced wearing-off with predictable end-of-dose 'off' periods, exchanging levodopa standard preparations into slow release formulars, and combining levodopa with a dopamine agonist, a MAO-B or a COMT inhibitor, will reduce the duration of these off-periods. Of course, also reducing the inter-dose period and eventually add an extra dose may give the same results.

Levodopa-induced induced dyskinesias can be treated by decreasing the dose of levodopa in combination with adding (or increasing the dose of) dopamine agonists. In that case, also

Table 8.3. Drugs in Parkinson's disease

Drug	Dosing	Action	Pharmacokinetics	Metabolism	Side effects
Dopamine – precursors					
Levodopa/carbidopa (standard or sustained-release)	62.5–1250 mg/d	precursor of dopamine with decarboxylase inhibitor	T½ = 1–2 hrs	hepatic	nausea, anorexia, hypotension, psychosis, dyskinesias
Levodopa/benserazide (dispers, standard or retard)	62.5–1250 mg/d	precursor of dopamine with decarboxylase inhibitor	T½ = 1–2 hrs	hepatic	nausea, anorexia, hypotension, psychosis, dyskinesias
Levodopa/carbidopa intestinal gel	intraduodenal 500–2000 mg/d	precursor of dopamine		hepatic	nausea, anorexia, hypotension, psychosis
Dopamine - Agonists					
Apomorphine	1–5 mg s.c. up to 30–80 mg/d	dopamine D1 and D2 agonist	T½ = 15–30 min	hepatic	hypotension, nausea, psychosis, somnolence (pre-treatment with domperidone 20 mg t.i.d.)
Bromocriptine	5 mg t.i.d. up to 40 mg/d	dopamine D2 agonist (and weak D1 antagonist)	T½ = 6 hrs	hepatic	hypotension, nausea, psychosis, somnolence, ankle edema, fibrosis
Lisuride	0.2 mg q.i.d. up to 2 mg/d	dopamine D2 agonist (and weak D1 antagonist)	T½ 3–4 hrs	hepatic	hypotension, nausea, psychosis, somnolence, ankle edema, fibrosis
Pergolide	1 mg t.i.d. up to 5–6 mg/d	dopamine D1, D2 and D3 agonist	T½ 15–27 hrs	renal/hepatic	hypotension, nausea, psychosis, somnolence, ankle edema, fibrosis
Pramipexole	1 mg t.i.d. up to 5–6 mg/d	(non-ergoline) dopamine D2 and D3 agonist	T½ 7–9 hrs	renal/hepatic	hypotension, nausea, psychosis, somnolence
Ropinorole	3 mg t.i.d. up to 25 mg/d	(non-ergoline) dopamine D2 and D3 agonist	T½ = 6 hrs	renal/hepatic	hypotension, nausea, psychosis, somnolence
Rotigotine patches	transdermal 2–16 mg/d	(non-ergoline) dopamine D1, D2, D3 agonist		renal/hepatic	hypotension, nausea, psychosis, somnolence

MAO-B inhibitors					
Selegiline	5–10 mg/d	selective MAO-B inhibitor	$T\frac{1}{2}$ 35–40 hrs	hepatic/renal	insomnia, psychosis, dizziness, nausea
Rasagiline	1 mg/d	selective MAO-B inhibitor	$T\frac{1}{2}$ = 1–2 hrs	hepatic	no significant side effects compared to placebo
COMT-inhibitors					
Entacapone	200 mg t.i.d./q.i.d.	peripheral COMT inhibitor	$T\frac{1}{2}$ = $\frac{1}{2}$ hrs	hepatic	nausea, diarrhea
Tolcapone	100–200 mg t.i.d.	peripheral and central COMT inhibitor	$T\frac{1}{2}$ = 2 hrs	hepatic	nausea, diarrhea, increase of liver transaminases (monitoring of liver transaminases)
Other drugs					
Domperidone	10–20 mg t.i.d. up to 90 mg/d	peripheral dopamine receptor antagonist	$T\frac{1}{2}$ = 7–8 hrs	hepatic (renal)	increase of prolactine (rare)
Amantadine	100 mg b.i.d/t.i.d	anticholinergic antiglutamatergic dopaminergic	$T\frac{1}{2}$ = 9–37 hrs (prolonged in the elderly)	renal	nausea, confusion, memory disturbances, ankle edema, livido reticularis, urinary retention
Clozapine	6.25–50 mg/d	atypical antipsychotic	$T\frac{1}{2}$ = 6–26 hrs	hepatic/renal	somnolence, hypersalivation, agranulocytosis (rare)
Quetiapine	25–100 mg/d	atypical antipsychotic	$T\frac{1}{2}$ = 7–11 hrs	hepatic	somnolence, dizziness, dry mouth
Rivastigmine	1.5 mg b.i.d. up to 12 mg/d	central cholinesterase inhibitor	$T\frac{1}{2}$ = 6–8 hrs	hepatic/renal	nausea, vomiting, dizziness, somnolence

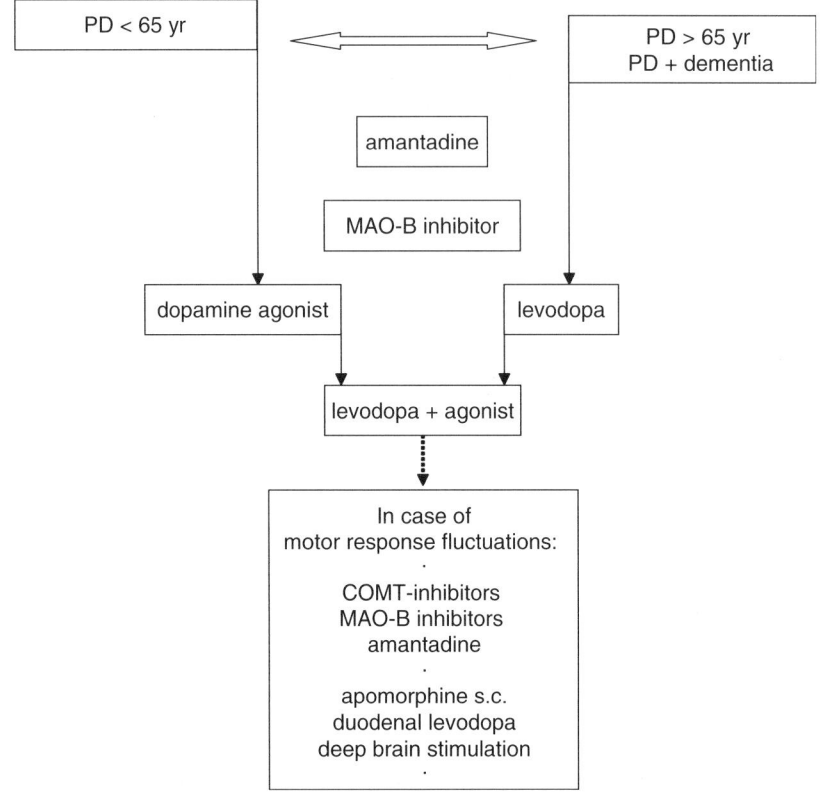

Figure 8.1. Pharmacological treatment strategy in Parkinson's disease

amantadine can be added to the medication. This drug (up to 400 mg) has a proven antidyskinetic effect. In more severe cases, continuous subcutaneous apomorfine and/or intraduodenal duodopa might be indicated as well as neurosurgical strategies (deep brain stimulation).

PD-related psychosis might be disease-related, often in combination with progressive cognitive deterioration, as well as pharmacotherapy-related. It may manifest with isolated (mainly) visual hallucinations and/or delusions with defect reality testing, often in combination with behavioural disorders and anxiety. Apart from dopaminomimetics, also anticholinergics and amantadine are significant psychotogenic factors, as well as intercurrent illnesses such as urinary infections, dehydration and social isolation or over-exposure. In these cases, amantadine and anticholinergics should always be withdrawn. The effect of tapering down the dose of dopaminomimetics is usually not very helpful: motor parkinsonism will increase and the antipsychotic effects will take considerable time to be effective. When necessary, one better treats such patients with atypical antipsychotics such as clozapine (12.5–25 mg) or quetiapine (25–50 mg). Because of a certain risk of agranulocytosis, regular monitoring of blood counts is necessary with clozapine. In demented subjects with psychosis, cholinesterase inhibitors like rivastigmine and donepezil may be also useful to treat and/or prevent psychosis.

Recently, restrictive valvular heart disease has been reported in about one third of patients treated with pergolide. This dose dependent adverse effect is also found for cabergoline and probably constitutes an adverse effect for all ergot alkoloid dopaminomimetics. To detect this adverse effect in an early stage echocardiography at regular intervals (6–12 months) is necessary.

Neurosurgical strategies

In the case of unsatisfactory treatment of levodopa-induced motor response fluctuations by continuous stimulation of the dopaminergic receptors by dopamine agonists with a long half-life and/or intraduodenal duodopa gel, one might opt for neurosurgical intervention to improve quality of life. As yet, high frequency deep brain stimulation of the subthalamic nucleus is considered the best option for these patients. This last strategy, however, may come with surgical-related (bleedings, infections) as well as stimulation-related (mood and cognition changes) complications and therefore is not suited for patients with psychiatric co-morbidity (depression, significant cognitive deficits, psychosis).

KEY POINTS

1. The differential diagnosis of parkinsonism includes many causes, PD being the most frequent.
2. A good and lasting response to dopaminergic drugs best differentiates PD from parkinsonism due to other causes.
3. The non-motor symptoms of PD have a great influence on quality of life in PD, even more than the classic motor signs.
4. Using functional imaging (PET, SPECT), one is able to increase the accuracy of the clinical diagnosis of PD.
5. Typical antipsychotics should be avoided in PD.

LINKS

http://www.ninds.nih.gov/disorders/parkinsons_disease/detail_parkinsons_disease.htm
http://www.apdaparkinson.org/user/index.asp
http://www.wpda.org/
http://pdweb.mgh.harvard.edu/

REFERENCES

1. Braak H, Del Tredici K, Rub U, et al. Staging of brain pathology related to sporadic Parkinson's disease. *Neurobiol Ageing* 2003; **24**: 197–211.
2. Charcot JM, Valpian A Revue clinique dela paralysie agitante. *Gaz Hebdomadire* 1861; **8**: 765–7.
3. Goodman RR, Kim B, McClelland S, et al. Operative techniques and morbidity with subthalamic nucleus deep brain stimulation in 100 consecutive patients with advanced Parkinson's disease. *J Neurol Neurosurg Psychiatry* 2006; **77**: 12–17.
4. Hughes AJ, Daniel SE, Ben-Shlomo Y, Lees AJ The accuracy of diagnosis of parkinsonian syndromes in a specialist movement disorder service. *Brain* 2002; **125**: 861–70.
5. Nyholm D, Nilsson Remahl AIM, Dizdar N, et al. Duodenal levodopa infusion monotherapy vs oral polypharmacy in advanced Parkinson's disease. *Neurology* 2005; **64**: 216–223.
6. Parkinson Study Group A controlled, randomized, delayed-start study of rasagiline in early Parkinson's disease. *Arch Neurol* 2004; **61**: 561–6.
7. Poewe W, Luessi F Clinical studies with transdermal rotigotine in early Parkinson's disease. *Neurology* 2005; **65**(suppl 1): S11–S14.
8. Ponsen MM, Stoffers D, Booij J, et al. Idiopathic hyposmia as a preclinical sign of Parkinson's disease. *Ann Neurol* 2004; **56**: 173–81.
9. Report of the Quality Standards Subcommittee of the American Academy of Neurology Practice Parameters for Parkinson's disease. *Neurology* 2006; **66**: 968–1002.
10. Ravina B, Eidelberg D, Ahlskog JE, et al. The role of radiotracer imaging in Parkinson disease. *Neurology* 2005; **64**: 208–15.
11. Schapira AHV Present and future drug treatment for Parkinson's disease. *J Neurol Neurosurg Psychiatry* 2005; **76**: 1472–8.
12. Schapira AHV Etiology of Parkinson's disease. *Neurology* 2006; **66**(suppl 4): S10–S23.
13. Van Camp G, Flamez A, Cosyns, B et al. Treatment of Parkinson's disease with pergolide and relation to restrictive valvular heart disease. *Lancet* 2004; **363**: 1179–83.

9 Epilepsy

John O. Willoughby, Joseph Frasca
and Emma M. Whitham

Department of Medicine (Neurology), Flinders University and Medical Centre, Adelaide, Australia

INTRODUCTION

Epilepsy is a common problem at any age and is especially so in the elderly: they are the most highly affected age group in the community, with the incidence at the age of 70 being almost double that of children (Figure 9.1). With the ageing process come several considerations making treatment and management a special challenge. The issues in the aged are coexistent disease states, concurrently administered drugs, the ageing brain and changing metabolic capacities. The concept of tailoring treatment to the individual is not foreign practice to physicians. In the elderly patient, epilepsy like many other conditions in this vulnerable population, almost always requires an individualized approach. As we discuss below, unlike childhood-onset disease in which genetic or constitutional epilepsy is frequent, epilepsy in the elderly is more likely to be symptomatic, i.e. a consequence of focal acquired lesions.

AETIOLOGY

Given the high incidence of epilepsy in the elderly, its prevalence is as high as 1–1.5%, epilepsy has become the third most common neurological condition after dementia and stroke (2). Not surprisingly, dementia and stroke both constitute independent causes of epilepsy, cerebrovascular disease leads the list.

Thus, the major causes are cerebrovascular disease, malignancy, both primary or metastatic, and trauma (Figure 9.2). Even though vascular disease (ischaemia and haemorrhage) is an important contributor to the increased incidence of epilepsy, one third have no easily defined aetiology.

In comparison to the frequent refractoriness of seizures due to structural disease in the young, it is reassuring that the prognosis for complete seizure control in the elderly is relatively favourable (4).

SYMPTOMS AND SIGNS

The key to diagnosis of epilepsy is a history of abrupt onset, brief changes in behaviour followed by prompt recovery. Features differentiating seizure from transient ischaemia, a frequent issue in the elderly, are vigorous or stereotyped motor activity of some nature rather than a deficit of function, or experiential episodes rather than deficits of experience. The presentation of epilepsy in the elderly, just as in the young, is often made difficult by the absence of reliable witnessed accounts of the episodes—in these times a more soluble problem given the ubiquity of mobile phones. All too frequently however, all the clinician has to work with is a history of collapses with impaired behaviour or consciousness—diagnosis then requires a comprehensive investigational approach.

Prescribing for Elderly Patients   Edited by Stephen Jackson, Paul Jansen and Arduino Mangoni
© 2009 John Wiley & Sons, Ltd

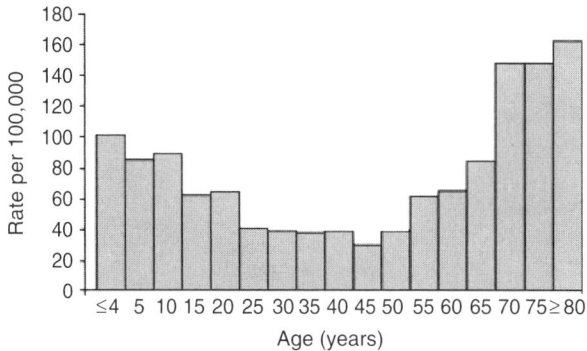

Figure 9.1. Incidence of epilepsy with age (1)

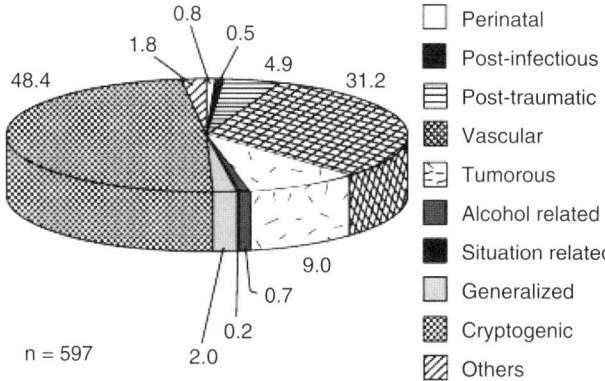

Figure 9.2. Aetiology of epilepsy (%) in elderly persons (3)

DIAGNOSIS

Numerous causes of collapses and episodes of confusion need to be considered and these commonly include transient ischaemic events, cardiac arrhythmias, syncopal disorders including impairment of vascular reflexes linked to posture, vertiginous states like benign positional vertigo, transient global amnesia, as well as hypoglycaemia. Increasingly commonly, adverse effects of therapeutic agents are being recognised as leading to episodic disturbances.

The majority of seizures are of partial onset, often complex (associated with impaired awareness and memory), which in this age group may be subtle and therefore difficult to diagnose. It is important to remember that acute confusional states or fluctuating consciousness could be due to ictal or postictal activity. In prolonged

states, non-convulsive status epilepsy should be considered routinely and an EEG in this clinical presentation is diagnostic. Non-convulsive status may occur in patients without a history of epilepsy: in a recent prospective case control study, a history of epilepsy was present in only 30% of elderly patients who developed non-convulsive status.

Some acute presentations in the elderly may be misleading, especially acute persistent neurological problems, focal or global. The states can be severe enough to mimic a flaccid hemiplegia or a very severe intellectual disorder. The commonest initial explanations are, respectively, a new stroke (ischaemic or haemorrhagic lesion) or an acute metabolic syndrome. In the absence of witnesses to the onset of such problems, it may not be clear that a seizure led to the presentation. With the passage of days, evidence of good improvement in the clinical condition makes it necessary to consider that a seizure has amplified a previously unrecognised problem, namely sub-clinical ischaemia or dementia, and both disorders may require management. The point here, is that unrecognised or clinically silent or recovered old cerebral lesions or the subtle early phase of a dementing process are all common, especially in the elderly and may cause (5, 6) or be revealed by seizures. The post-ictal metabolic consequences of seizures appear to interact with the pre-existing neural state to produce a prolonged and severe disturbance of brain function out of proportion to what would be expected.

THERAPY

Ageing is often associated with decreased clearance of many of the anti-epileptic drugs and care should be taken in slowly introducing them and aiming for lower initial maintenance doses. Given the potential for age-related variability, if drugs with a high risk of side-effects are unavoidable, blood concentrations should be assessed frequently until levels are stable.

The long established anti-epileptic drugs, especially phenobarbitone and primidone, have potentially significant effects on cognitive function and have little place in the treatment of new-onset seizures in elderly patients (7).

Benzodiazepines are rarely indicated for long term seizure control in the elderly because of their poor pharmacokinetic and pharmacodynamic profiles in this population. Clonazepam which is recommended for partial seizures has not been investigated in the older population and should be used with caution.

Carbamazepine is an enzyme-inducing drug with significant potential for drug interactions. The elderly may be more susceptible than younger patients to confusion or agitation, atrioventricular heart block, bradycardia and the syndrome of inappropriate secretion of antidiuretic hormone (SIADH). Carbamazepine clearance decreases progressively with age. It can also precipitate acute urinary retention especially in those with autonomic dysfunction, for example those with diabetes (2).

Phenytoin has zero order kinetics and age-related declines in hepatic function increase the risk of toxicity (2). Care should be taken in patients with low albumin levels and measurement of free phenytoin levels may be worthwhile.

Skeletal metabolism is affected by phenytoin, carbamazepine, phenobarbitone and primidone which cause accelerated bone loss, so that bone-density should be measured at onset of therapy. The use of these is relatively contraindicated in the elderly (8) and the use of vitamin D and calcium supplements may be required.

Increased free levels of highly bound drugs, such as phenytoin and sodium valproate can occur with hypoalbuminaemia (9) which is more common in the elderly and can lead to toxicity symptoms despite normal total serum levels.

Sodium valproate does not induce the metabolism of other drugs and this can be a relative advantage over the other older anti-epileptic drugs. The most common side effects of sodium valproate include tremor and gastro-intestinal effects.

NEWER ANTI-EPILEPTIC DRUGS

It has been observed in many studies that the elderly population are recipients of more traditional anti-epileptic drugs particularly phenytoin, despite evidence that the newer drugs are as efficacious and better tolerated in the older, as well as the general population. An ideal anti-epileptic drug has no interactions with anti-epileptic drugs or other drugs, can be introduced at therapeutic doses, absorbed orally, without hepatic metabolism or protein binding. It should lack side effects and have a good safety profile and a high therapeutic index to allow free titration of doses. In this vulnerable age group there should be minimal effects on cognition and bone mineralisation. The newer drugs are proving to match more of these requirements, with gabapentin fitting this profile

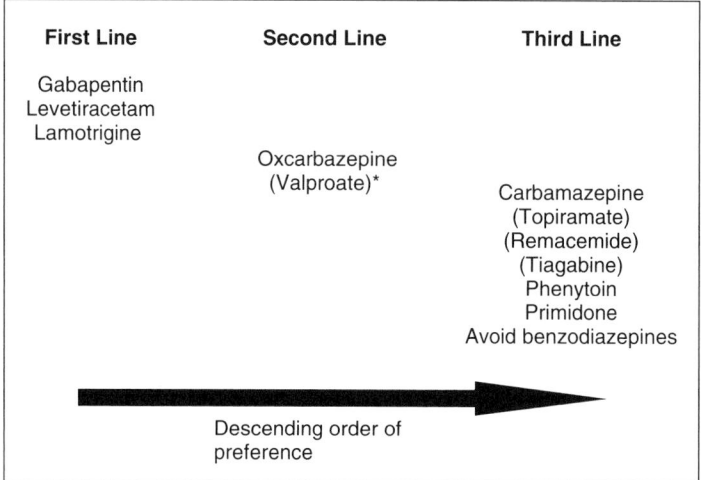

Figure 9.3. Relative preference of anti-epileptic drugs for new-onset partial seizures in the elderly.
* (brackets = untested in the elderly)

the best (although dose adjustment is needed in renal impairment), followed by levetiracetam, lamotrigine and oxcarbazepine (10). In a comparison of carbamazepine, lamotrigine and gabapentin, there were more significant side effects with carbamazepine (~30 %), than lamotrigine (~10 %) and gabapentin (~20 %) (11) and they were equally efficacious. Levetiracetam has good efficacy and tolerability with either somnolence or dizziness causing discontinuation in 20 % (12). As always when faced with using drugs with the potential for neurotoxic side effects careful titration to full dosage is recommended watching for potential adverse effects and seizure control. Often, therapeutic levels are obtained at lower dosages in the elderly, even given apparently therapeutic serum levels Again, this is not an issue with the newer agents where serum levels are unnecessary. The figure below illustrates our current recommendations for treatment of epilepsy in the elderly Figure.9.3

SAFETY OF ANTI-EPILEPTIC DRUGS

Given the relative lack of studies specifically addressing epilepsy pharmacotherapy in the elderly, we considered it helpful to examine the safety of anti-epileptic agents using evidence from studies in other age-associated disorders. There is useful information from studies in elderly subjects on the following medications:

- Levetiracetam, studied in cognitive disorder and anxiety, well tolerated in young and elderly with only slight increase in side effects of tremor and headache over young patients.
- Valproate, studied in agitation in patients with dementia, well-tolerated in 66 %. Also studied in epilepsy, no cognitive side effects, other side effects frequent and a valproate-induced parkinsonian state is now well established. No studies specific to tolerability and efficacy in the elderly.
- Topiramate, no studies of tolerability or efficacy in the elderly.
- Remacemide, trialled in Parkinson's disease: median maximum dose was low compared to younger patients, approximately one third of the maximal recommended dose: modest side effects as expected for the drug. No studies specific to efficacy in elderly.
- Tiagabine, studied in epilepsy, pharmacokinetics not age-related; in normals, promotes slow wave sleep in the elderly, no tolerability or efficacy studies in the elderly.
- Diazepam, studied in the normal population, is associated with increased heat loss besides having deleterious effects on mentation, and an increased rate of hip fracture.

THERAPY SCHEME OF THE ADVISED DRUGS

For most of the anti-epileptic drugs (AED) the pharmacokinetic properties have changed in the elderly and dose reduction is often needed. Table 9.1 shows these changes and the start and maintenance dose in the elderly.

CLINICALLY-IMPORTANT DRUG INTERACTIONS WITHIN ANTI-EPILEPTIC DRUGS

The aim of management of epilepsy is to achieve complete seizure control with the lowest possible dose, preferably of one anti-epileptic medication. This is particularly important in elderly patients likely to be taking a number of other medications. If seizure control is not achieved with the first anti-epileptic medication that is tried, then another should be introduced and the initial anti-epileptic drug should then be slowly withdrawn, keeping to the aim of monotherapy if at all possible.

Phenytoin, phenobarbitone and carbamazepine can induce the hepatic metabolism of sodium valproate, and levels can be reduced by co-medication by as much as 50 % (2). Sodium valproate is a potent inhibitor of both oxidation and glucuronidation and therefore increases the half-life and levels of lamotrigine, as well the half-life and levels of the epoxide metabolite of carbamazepine thus increasing the potential for toxicity.

CLINICALLY-IMPORTANT DRUG INTERACTIONS WITH OTHER DRUGS

Adverse drugs events are common, with many hospital admissions directly iatrogenic in nature, with incidence increasing with number of medications prescribed. Anti-epileptic drugs are commonly prescribed drugs, especially in the elderly, albeit not always specifically for epilepsy. In nursing homes as many as 56 % of adverse drug events were deemed significant with 51 % preventable (3). As with any epileptic patient the aim is for monotherapy hence reducing the risk of interactions and potential side effects. For specifics the reader is directed to the excellent and recent review in *Geriatrics* (13).

As many of the more traditional anti-epileptic drugs affect hepatic metabolism via the cytochrome P450 pathways (for example, phenytoin, phenobarbitone, carbamazepine), caution with other hepatically-cleared drugs is necessary. For example many of the cardiac antiarrhythmics, antihypertensives, antibiotics and warfarin need to be used with care. In this respect the newer anti-epileptic drugs gabapentin, lamotrigine and levetiracetam, offer advantages specifically within the elderly population.

IMPORTANT ADVERSE EFFECTS

The side effects and idiosyncratic toxic effects of anti-epileptic agents are generally well known, with sedative central nervous system effects and nausea being by far the most consistently seen with anti-epileptic drugs as well as being the most common. With the increased sensitivity of the ageing brain to medication effects, drugs with sedative effects are particularly to be avoided, and our own practice is to use the newer agents whenever possible. We are not aware of any important age-specific side effects with any anti-epileptic medication (see above). Given the diversity of medication effects on brain and body, our strategy is to introduce agents at up to half the usual rates and, in the first instance, to accept any change in health as a possible side effect of the most recently introduced agent. Routinely, an attempt would be made to change to another agent.

DRUG WITHDRAWAL

The increased incidence of epilepsy in the elderly, discussed above, is related to an increased number of structural lesions (stroke, tumours etc) and seizures due to lesions are

Table 9.1. Antiepileptic drugs (AED) in the elderly

Drug	Start dose	Maintenance dose	Pharmaco-kinetics	Metabolism	Interactions	Important adverse events	Other tips
Gabapentin	300 mg rapid titration tolerated	900–1800 mg in divided doses	young adults: t$^1/_2$ 5–7 hrs elderly: t$^1/_2$ may be prolonged	Renal Linear relation-ship with creatinine clearance	Cimetidine and antacids decrease bioavail-ability, no interactions other AED	Elderly more prone to CNS side effects	Adjustments for renal impairment
Levetiracetam	500 mg bd rapid titration possible	Max 1500 mg bd	young adults: t$^1/_2$ 6–8 hrs elderly: t$^1/_2$ 10–11 hrs	Renal	None, no interactions other AED	Somnolence possible	Adjustments for renal impairment
Lamotrigine	50 mg daily for 2 weeks increase 50 mg every 2 weeks	100–200 mg bd	young adults: t$^1/_2$ 12–50 hrs elderly: clearance decreased by 37 % and Vd by 12 %	Hepatic, no CYP450	Decreased t$^1/_2$ with hepatic enzyme inducers ie AED, rifampicin, etc.	Life threatening skin rash 1 in 500, requires cessation	Care if add on therapy with Valproate (inhibits Lamotrigine metabolism)
Oxcarbazepine	300 mg bd	Titrate to individual, 600–2400 mg/d divided doses	Active metabolite young adults: t$^1/_2$ 7–20 hrs Elderly: t$^1/_2$ 17–27 hrs	Renally cleared active metabolite Adjust-ments in renal im-pairment	Effect CYP2C19, i.e. other inducing AED, citalopram, diazepam, omeprazole, etc.	Hyponatraemia, hepatitis	Regular check LFTs, electrolytes

	Dose	Titration	Half-life	Metabolism	Interactions	Adverse effects	Monitoring
Sodium Valproate	500 mg bd	Titrate to individual	young adults: t½ 7–13 hrs elderly: t½ 15 hrs	Hepatic including CYP450	Many. Hepatic enzyme inducers and inhibitors Caution other AED, aspirin	Care with Lamotrigine may increase risk of severe skin rash. Osteoporosis, weight gain, hair loss.	Regular check electrolytes, LFTs and full blood count. Serum levels helpful for monitoring efficacy
Carbamazepine	50 mg bd and titrate very slowly	Titrate to individual, measure serum levels	Young adults: t½ 6–15 hrs elderly: not available	Hepatic	Enzyme inducer	Aplastic anaemia, hepatic toxicity, hyponatraemia, potential cardiovascular adverse effects. May worsen seizures in some epileptic syndromes	
Phenytoin	4–5 mg/kg in 2–3 divided doses	Tailor to individual based on serum levels	t½ long, but non linear kinetics therefore individualized approach required	Hepatic metabolism	Enzyme inducer CYP450 many interactions	Dose related CNS disturbances, haematological, osteoporosis	Regular check of full blood count and LFTs, serum levels helpful for monitoring efficacy.

AED = Anti-epileptic drugs
LFT = Liver function tests

less likely to remit spontaneously than seizures provoked by transient illness. Nevertheless, usual criteria (more than one unprovoked seizure) should be carefully applied in diagnosis, because for practical purposes, epilepsy will likely mean life long therapy. As for younger patients, withdrawal of medication is theoretically possible after several years of seizure freedom. This carries the usual restrictions to lifestyle such as cessation of driving during the period of transition and often in this population the choice is to continue therapy lifelong, especially if medication has been well tolerated. As a rule, any withdrawal of anti-epileptic drugs should be made slowly over months, as abrupt withdrawal has the potential to precipitate seizures.

KEY POINTS

- Epilepsy has a very high incidence in the elderly.
- The main issue is concurrent disease and concurrent medication use.
- It is best to use one agent and it should be valproate or one of three newer anti-epileptic agents gabapentin, levetiracetam and lamotrigine.
- Avoid the older anti-epileptic agents, phenobarbitone, phenytoin, carbamazepine.
- Unrecognized pre-existing brain disease is transiently amplified by seizures.

REFERENCES

1. Tallis, R, Hall, G, Craig, I, Dean, A How common are epileptic seizures in old age? *Age & Ageing* 1991; **20**: 442–8.
2. Shorvon, S *Handbook of Epilepsy Treatment*. Blackwell Science, 2000.
3. Trinka, E Epilepsy: comorbidity in the elderly. *Acta Neurologica Scandinavica Supplementum* 2003; **180**: 33–6.
4. Bergey, G.K Initial treatment of epilepsy: special issues in treating the elderly. *Neurology* 2004; **63**: S40–S48.
5. Mendez, M, Lim, G Seizures in elderly patients with dementia: epidemiology and management. *Drugs & Aging* 2003; **20**: 791–803.
6. Bogousslavsky, J, Martin, R, Regli, F, Despland, PA, Bolyn, S Persistent worsening of stroke sequelae after delayed seizures. *Archives of Neurology* 1992; **49**: 385–8.
7. Pugh, M J, Cramer, J, Knoefel, J, Charbonneau, A, Mandell, A, Kazis, L, Berlowitz, D Potentially inappropriate anti-epileptic drugs for elderly patients with epilepsy. *Journal of the American Geriatrics Society* 2004; **52**: 417–22.
8. Stephen, LJ, McLellan, AR, Harrison, J., Shapiro, D, Dominiczak, MH, Sills, G J, Brodie, MJ Bone density and anti-epileptic drugs: a case-controlled study. *Seizure* 1999; **8**, 339–42.
9. Guberman, A, Bruni, J *Essentials of Clinical Epilepsy*. Butterworth Heinemann, 1999.
10. Kutluay, E, McCague, K, D'Souza, J, Beydoun, A. Safety and tolerability of oxcarbazepine in elderly patients with epilepsy. *Epilepsy & Behavior* 2003; **4**: 175–80.
11. Rowan, AJ New onset geriatric epilepsy. A randomised study of gabapentin, lamotrigine and carbamazepine. *Neurology* 2005; **64**: 1868–73.
12. Ferrendelli, JA, French, J, Leppik, I, Morrell, MJ, Herbeuval, A, Han, J, Magnus, L Use of levetiracetam in a population of patients aged 65 years and older: a subset analysis of the KEEPER trial. *Epilepsy & Behavior* 2003; **4**: 702–9.
13. Leppik, IE, Bergey, GK, Ramsay, RE, Rowan, AJ, Gidal, BE, Birnbaum, AK, Elliott, MB Advances in anti-epileptic drug treatments. A rational basis for selecting drugs for older patients with epilepsy. *Geriatrics* 2004; **59**: 14–18.

10 Hypertension

Sanjeev Khindri and Stephen Jackson

Department of Clinical Gerontology, King's College Hospital, London, UK

INTRODUCTION

Hypertension, a sustained blood pressure above 140/90 mmHg, is a major worldwide public health burden.

Hypertension affects approximately a billion people worldwide leading to the death of 2–3 million people each year. In the United Kingdom, 32 % of men and 29 % of women over the age of 18 are hypertensive. Blood pressure (BP) rises with age, such that 50–70 % of the population over the age of 65 years are hypertensive. With the projected ageing of the population in the UK, indeed across the world, the disease burden will increase further.

Hypertension is the most modifiable risk factor for cardiovascular morbidity and mortality. Cardiovascular disease is the leading cause of death in the industrialised world. Hypertension increases the risk of cerebrovascular disease, coronary artery disease, heart failure, chronic kidney disease and occlusive peripheral vascular disease. There is an abundance of clinical trial data, in both the population as a whole and those up to the age of 80 years, clearly demonstrating a reduction in cardiovascular morbidity and mortality with blood pressure lowering. In elderly patients, these data have demonstrated a 30–40 % reduction in stroke and 16–20 % reduction in coronary heart disease. The Hypertension in the Very Elderly Trial (HYVET), an ongoing placebo-controlled, double blind, randomised trial of indapamide plus or minus perindopril to lower blood pressure to less than 150/80 mmHg in subjects over the age of 80, was published in 2008. Over two years, the mean sitting BP fell by 15/6 mmHg. This was associated with a 30% reduction in stroke, 39% reduction in rate of death from stroke, 21% reduction in rate of death from any cause, 23% reduction in rate of death from cardiovascular causes and a 64% reduction in the rate of heart failure.

Blood pressure lowering should be undertaken in the context of total cardiovascular risk and all risk factors addressed. Treatment thresholds fall for patients with higher total cardiovascular risk.

When embarking on pharmacological treatment of hypertension in elderly patients two points should be noted. First, co-morbidities, both cardiovascular and non-cardiovascular, especially those requiring drug treatment, may represent compelling indications or contraindications to particular antihypertensive agents. Second, there is greater susceptibility to postural hypotension with reduced ability to maintain an adequate BP. Postural hypotension, however, should not preclude treatment for mixed or isolated systolic hypertension.

AETIOLOGY

In over 95 % of patients, hypertension has no identifiable underlying cause. This is primary or essential hypertension. Factors that may influence the development of essential hypertension are:

- age;
- gender;

Prescribing for Elderly Patients   Edited by Stephen Jackson, Paul Jansen and Arduino Mangoni

- ethnicity;
- salt consumption;
- ethanol consumption;
- adiposity, especially central;
- insulin resistance (where hypertension is one of the defining pathophysiologies);
- family history;
- psychological factors, for example, stress.

The most important type of secondary hypertension in elderly patients is atheromatous renal artery stenosis (RAS). The role of hyperaldosteronism is controversial. Concurrent drug therapy may result in hypertension or antagonizs the effects of antihypertensives, e.g. NSAIDs, mineralocorticoids.

SYMPTOMS AND SIGNS

Hypertension is largely an asymptomatic disease. Therefore, population screening is vital in the detection and management of this silent killer.

Headache and epistaxis, and to a lesser extent nocturia and erectile dysfunction have been attributed to hypertension. Patients may present with symptoms of end-organ damage. This is seen more commonly in elderly patients. Exertional dyspnoea, orthopnoea and oedema suggest heart failure. Chest pain suggests occlusive coronary artery disease. Pain on walking suggests peripheral arterial disease. Focal weakness, speech deficits and cognitive decline signify cerebrovascular disease. Blurred vision may signify papilloedema in malignant phase hypertension. Haematuria may also be seen in the latter.

DIAGNOSIS

BP measurement in elderly patients is, in principle, no different to that of measuring BP in younger patients.

BP measurements need to be repeated over time to confirm sustained elevation of BP before diagnosing hypertension. The British Hypertension Society guidelines suggest, in the absence of end organ damage, three to four readings over three to four months.

BP should be measured using a validated, calibrated and well-maintained device. The sphygmomanometer may be mercury or aneroid and manual, semi-automated or automated. An appropriate sized cuff should be employed to avoid under (over-estimating BP) or over cuffing (under-estimating BP).

BP should be measured after a rest of least five minutes with the arm at the level of the heart. BP should be measured in both arms at the first visit, with the arm with the highest reading taken to inform treatment decisions. Older patients are more likely to have a difference in BP between the arms. Where such a difference is recorded this must be brought to the attention of the patient and others responsible for the management of the patient's BP.

BP should be measured seated and, in patients with postural symptoms, standing, immediately and at a one to three minute interval, to detect the presence of postural hypotension. A physiologically more challenging assessment is to record BP after lying for five minutes then within three minutes of standing. Older people are more prone to symptomatic postural hypotension. Only in patients with symptomatic postural hypotension should the standing BP be used to inform treatment decisions.

When measuring BP with a manual syphgmomanometer, the clinician must be aware of the auscultatory gap (between Koratkov sounds K_2 and K_3) and ensure cuff inflation to 20–30 mmHg above the systolic BP identified by palpation of the radial artery.

Pseudohypertension, a condition in which an individual's indirectly measured BP overestimates directly measured BP due to a non-compressable stiff brachio-radial artery, occurs more commonly with advancing age. Confirmation should be undertaken by comparison with beat to beat finger arterial pressure measurement. This needs to be considered and confirmed in patients with elevated clinic and ambulatory BP and no evidence of target organ damage.

"White coat hypertension" is diagnosed when BP is only elevated when attending for BP assessment. A "white coat effect" is present when BP is higher when patients attend but is persistently elevated at other times. These observations can only be made using ambulatory BP monitoring.

INVESTIGATION

All hypertensive patients should undergo evaluation to determine the existence of target-organ damage, total cardiovascular risk and potentially reversible secondary causes of hypertension.

Therefore, all patients should have determination of:

- urea, electrolytes, creatinine, liver function tests and full blood count;
- random blood glucose proceeding to a fasting sample if elevated;
- urine dipstick urinalysis;
- full lipid profile;
- 12-lead electrocardiogram.

Other investigations, particularly those aimed at identifying secondary causes, should be guided by the history, clinical examination and the results of the initial investigations.

THERAPY

All patients with hypertension should be treated to a target BP of less than 140/85 mmHg. In patients with diabetes, chronic kidney disease or stroke a lower target is appropriate. The evidence base for target BP in these situations is not strong but a target to aim for would be <135/75 if tolerated.

All patients with hypertension, whether needing pharmacological intervention or not, should be informed of the benefits of non-pharmacological approaches to blood pressure lowering. Some approaches may improve the BP-lowering effect of some drugs, for example, a low salt diet can improve the BP-lowering efficacy of angiotensin converting enzyme (ACE) inhibitors.

Non pharmacological therapy

Overweight patients should be encouraged to reduce their calorie intake. Weight reduction of 1 kilogram may sometimes result in a reduction of systolic BP (SBP) of as much as 1 mmHg.

Regular aerobic exercise, for example, a brisk 30-minute walk each day, may result in a 5–10 mmHg reduction in SBP for those that are able.

Moderation of ethanol consumption (less than 21-units per week for men and less than 14-units per week for women) can result in a modest fall in blood pressure. Binge drinking (intermittent heavy drinking) is associated with an increased risk of stroke.

Reduction in daily salt consumption to less than 6 g (100 mmol) per day can result in a 5–10 mmHg fall in SBP. This effect is at least as great in elderly patients. Clear and practical written guidelines should be given to the patient.

A diet rich in fruit, vegetables, low-fat dairy products with a reduction in total and saturated fats can reduce SBP by 8–15 mmHg. Increased consumption of oily fish is also beneficial.

Smoking is a powerful risk factor for cardiovascular risk. Therefore, smoking cessation should be a key intervention in any hypertensive patient who smokes. Pharmacological (e.g. nicotine replacement therapy) and non-pharmacological (acupuncture, hypnotherapy or cognitive behavioural therapy) strategies should be utilized, in combination as needed. First line therapy will be nicotine replacement therapy. If this fails an alternative strategy should be considered.

Pharmacological Therapy

On initiating pharmacological therapy it must be appreciated by prescribers and patients alike that more than 60 % of patients will require two or more drugs to reach blood pressure targets.

A number of different drug classes are available in the antihypertensive armamentarium. In selecting a drug, one needs to consider whether a patient has a compelling indication or contraindication for that drug or drug class (Table 10.1).

When no such compelling indication/contraindications exists, the A/CD approach should be followed as set out in the BHS/NICE collaborative guidelines of 2006 (Figure 10.1). This is based on the influence of age and ethnicity in defining two broad groups of hypertensive patients: those with high-renin and those with low-renin hypertension. The former, young patients under 55 years of age and non-black, respond better to angiotensin coverting enzyme

Table 10.1. Compelling indications and contraindications for antihypertensive drugs

Drug class	Indication		Contraindication	
	Compelling	Possible	Possible	Compelling
Alpha-blockers	BPH			Urinary incontinence Postural/postprandial Hypotension
ACE-Inhibitors	CCF, LVSD, Post-MI, Stable CAD, Type 1 DM nephropathy, 2^0 stroke prevention	Proteinuric CKD, Type 2 DM nephropathy		Bilateral RAS
ARB	ACEI intolerance, Type 2 DM nephropathy, Post-MI	CCF, CKD		Bilateral RAS
Beta-blockers	MI, CAD, CCF		PVD, COPD, Raynaud's disease	Asthma, Heart block
CCB (dihydropyridine)	ISH			
CCB (non-dihydropyridine)	CAD		Not with beta-blockers	Heart block CCF
Thiazide/Thiazide-like	CCF, 2^0 stroke prevention		Hypokalaemia, Hyponatraemia	Gout

BPH	-	Benign prostatic hypertrophy	CCF	-	Congestive cardiac failure
LVSD	-	Left ventricular systolic dysfunction	MI	-	Myocardial infarction
CAD	-	Coronary artery disease	DM	-	Diabetes mellitus
CKD	-	Chronic kidney disease	PVD	-	Peripheral vascular disease
RAS	-	Renal artery stenosis	COPD	-	Chronic obstructive pulmonary disease
ISH	-	Isolated systolic hypertension			

Adapted from the British Hypertension Society.
J Hum Hypertens 2004; **18**: 139– 85.

inhibitors (ACEIs) or angiotensin receptor blockers (ARBs) in monotherapy whereas the latter, older patients over 55 and black patients of any age, respond better to calcium channel blockers (CCBs)/diuretics. The selection of individual drugs from a given group, given equal efficacy and tolerability, should take cost into consideration.

A is ARB or ACEI; B is β blocker; C is CCB; D is diuretic.

The β-blockers, which reduce renin release from the juxta-glomerular apparatus, have been removed as first line therapy (as an alternative to the ACEI/ARB group) because of evidence showing they are less effective (compared to other groups) at reducing cardiovascular events, especially stroke and increase the risk of new-onset diabetes mellitus (especially in combination with diuretics).

In addressing global cardiovascular risk, patients with established cardiovascular disease or end-organ damage should receive lipid-lowering therapy in the form of a statin and aspirin. In patients without overt cardiovascular disease, but with a 10-year cardiovascular risk greater than or equal to 20 %, a statin and aspirin (when BP is controlled to 150/90 mmHg or less) should be considered.

CLINICAL PHARMACOLOGY OF ANTIHYPERTENSIVE THERAPY

Thiazide/Thiazide-Like Diuretics

The precise mechanism of BP-lowering is poorly understood. There is an early reduction in circulating volume and cardiac output as a

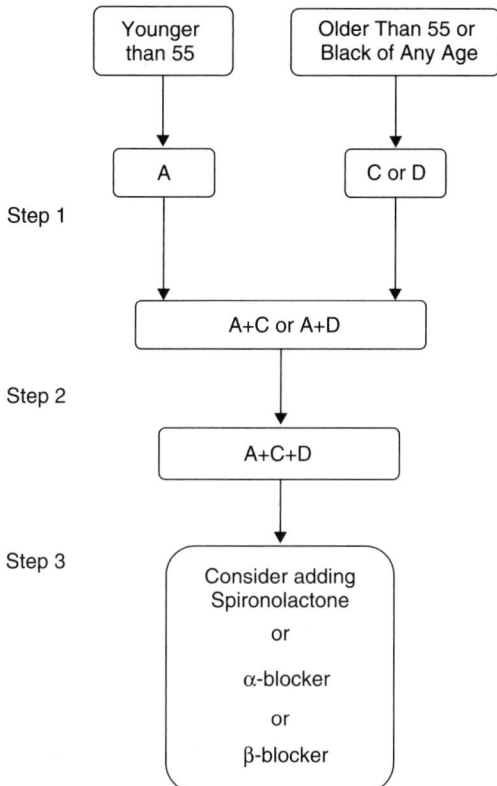

Step 1

Step 2

Step 3

Figure 10.1. Drug Treatment algorithm based on British Hypertension Society recommendations (*J Hum Hypertens* 2004; **18**: 139–85)

consequence of natriuresis. Over time there is a reduction in total peripheral vascular resistance (TPVR) because of transmembrane ion exchanges.

The thiazides are lipid soluble and well absorbed after oral administration. There is no appreciable presystemic metabolism. Elimination half-lives vary for individual drugs: bendroflumethiazide three hours, indapamide 15 to 18 hours, hydrochlorothiazide 10 to 13 hours, and chlorthalidone 90 hours. The duration of action, however, enables all to be given once daily.

The dose-response curves for BP-lowering are flat, there being little difference between that seen, for example, with 2.5 mg and 10 mg of bendroflumethiazide for most patients. However, the dose-response curves for other deleterious pharmacodynamic endpoints, for example, hyperglycaemia and dyslipidaemia

demonstrate a clear dose response relationship across this range.

There are few absolute contra-indications to thiazide diuretics. They should be avoided in patients with a history of gout and they should be used with caution in subjects with hyponatraemia or hypokalaemia. They increase the risk of insulin resistance at higher doses.

Adverse effects are: hyponatraemia, hypokalaemia, hypomagnesaemia, hypercalcaemia, hyperlipidaemia, hyperuricaemia and gout. Occasionally skin rashes and very rarely aplastic anaemia may occur.

Drug interactions: lithium salts: thiazides reduce renal excretion of lithium and therefore increase the risk of toxicity. This is a phar- macokinetic interaction and hence can be avoided using lithium therapeutic drug monitoring. Non-steroidal anti-inflammatory drugs (NSAIDs) reduce the BP-lowering effect of thiazides. Thiazides may increase the risk of NSAID-nephropathy. Usually only low doses of thiazides and thiazide like drugs are used in view of the dose response relationship (Table 10.2).

Calcium channel antagonists or blockers

The calcium channel blockers (CCBs) act on L-type calcium channels in vascular and cardiac smooth muscle to inhibit calcium entry. This results in arteriolar dilatation and hence reduction in vascular resistance. The dihydropyridines are associated with a reflex tachycardia. This occurs to a lesser degree with diltiazem. Verapamil tends to slow atrioventricular conduction. All CCBs are potentially negatively inotropic (Table 10.3).

For drugs with extensive presystemic metabolism, a careful and stepwise uptitration should occur so as to reduce the incidence

Table 10.2. Thiazide and thiazide like drugs

Drug	Dose
Bendroflumethiazide	2.5 mg/day
Chlorthalidone	12.5 mg/day
Hydrochlorothiazide	12.5 mg/day
Indapamide	1.5–2.5 mg/day

Table 10.3. Commonly used CCBs

Drug	Negative inotropism	Dose
Amlodipine	$-/+$	5–10 mg/day
Felodipine		5–10 mg/day
Nifedipine		30–60 mg/day
Diltiazem	$+ +$	120–300 mg/day
Verapamil	$+ + +$	120–480 mg/day

Note that with the exception of amlodipine, modified release preparations should be used enabling once daily dosing.

of flushing, headache and tachycardia. Slow or modified-release preparations are therefore preferred in clinical practice for agents with short elimination half lives such as nifedipine, diltiazem and verapamil.

They should be used with caution in patients with heart failure, sick sinus syndrome and second or third degree heart block. In subjects with aortic stenosis, CCBs may precipitate profound hypotension.

Adverse effects include headache, flushing, tachycardia, dependent oedema, constipation (diltiazem/verapamil), gingival hypertrophy and precipitation of heart failure.

Angiotensin converting enzyme inhibitors

The ACEIs are competitive inhibitors of the enzyme ACE. ACE catalyses the conversion of the decapeptide angiotensin-1 to the active octapeptide angiotensin-2 - a potent vasoconstrictor and stimulator of aldosterone release. Therefore, inhibition results in a reduction of peripheral vascular disease.

There is a linear relationship between plasma concentration of active drug and degree of ACE inhibition. All ACE-inhibitors, except captopril and lisinopril, are pro-drugs (Table 10.4).

The ACEIs have substantial evidence to support their use in patients with heart failure (symptomatic or not), ischaemic heart disease (post myocardial infarction and stable coronary artery disease), diabetic nephropathy and proteinuric chronic kidney disease and high vascular risk.

Adverse effects include non-productive cough (approximately 5 %), hyperkalaemia, renal dysfunction and metallic taste. The ACEIs are contraindicated in patients with hypersensitivity, angioedema and bilateral RAS. A fall in creatinine clearance is common and due to a reduction in filtration pressure. Where this fall exceeds 20 % discontinuing the drug should be considered.

Angiotensin-2 receptor antagonists or blockers

The ARBs are selective antagonists of the angiotensin-2 receptor (A2) subtype AT1. They reduce plasma aldosterone, hence, salt and water retention and result in vasodilatation by blocking A2. They do not inhibit ACE. They can be given once daily (Table 10.5).

The ARBs are effective antihypertensives and are the best tolerated of all classes of antihypertensive drugs. Of interest, most ARBs have been shown to be associated with a lower prevalence of headache than placebo. They have proven benefit in type 2 diabetic nephropathy. They also have benefit in heart failure. The contraindications are similar to those for ACE-inhibitors. Adverse effects include hyperkalaemia, renal dysfunction, fatigue and dizziness.

β-Adrenergic receptor antagonists or β-blockers

The precise mechanism of BP-lowering is incompletely understood. β_1-antagonism lowers heart rate and cardiac output therefore blood pressure. Inhibition of renin release will lower circulating levels of the potent vasoconstrictor angiotensin-2 in subjects with high-renin output hypertension.

The individual drugs vary in their solubility, beta-selectivity, intrinsic sympathometic activity and ancillary effects (Table 10.6).

The BP-lowering effects of the individual drugs are similar and therefore in this context a β_1-selective long-acting drug is preferred.

Recent evidence confirms β-blockers are the least effective agents in reducing cardiovascular mortality and increase the risk of new-onset diabetes mellitus particularly with thiazides. However, they should be used in patients with heart failure, coronary artery disease or hyperthyroidism. They also have a role in resistant hypertension.

Table 10.4. Commonly used ACEIs

Drug	Active metabolite	T1/2 (hr)	Duration of effect (hr)	Dose
Captopril	-	8	3–12	12.5–50 mg tds
Enalapril	Enalaprilat	50	24	5–40 mg/day
Lisinopril	-	30	18–30	5–40 mg/day
Perindopril	Perindoprilat	30	24	2–8 mg/day
Ramipril	Ramiprilat	17	24	5–10 mg/day
Trandolapril	Trandolaprilat	16–24	24	0.5–4 mg/day

Table 10.5. — Commonly used ARBs

Drug	Absorption (%)	$t_{1/2}$ (hr)	Dose
Candesartan	40	9	8–32 mg/day
Irbesartan	60–80	11–15	150–300 mg/day
Losartan	33	2–9	25–100 mg/day
Telmisartan	50	20	20–80 mg/day
Valsartan	23	9	80–160 mg/day

Table 10.6. Properties of commonly used β-blockers

	β_1-selectivity	Solubility	Absorption (%)	$t_{1/2}$ (hr)	Dose
Atenolol	Yes	Water	60	10	25–100 mg/day
Bisoprolol	Yes	Lipid	95	12	2.5–10 mg/day
Labetalol	No (also has $\alpha 1$ blocking properties)	Lipid	90	6	200–800 mg/day 100–400 mg/day -elderly patients
Metoprolol	Yes	Lipid	95	4	50–200 mg/day
Propranolol	No	Lipid	90	4	80–240 mg/day

They are contraindicated in asthma. They should be used with caution in subjects with chronic obstructive pulmonary disease, peripheral arterial disease, Raynaud's phenomenon and diabetes.

Common adverse effects include fatigue, cold extremities, shortness of breath on exertion, as well as depression, sleep disturbance and nightmares with lipophilic drugs.

Drug Interactions: β-blockers enhance the cardio-inhibitory response of verapamil when given intravenously but this is not a problem in hypertension management.

Centrally-Acting Vasodilating Drugs

The first used members of this group - α-methyldopa and clonidine are centrally-acting $\alpha 2$-adrenergic receptor agonists resulting in reduced efferent sympathetic tone. This results in peripheral vasodilatation and reduction in TPVR.

These drugs have been superceded by moxonidine on the basis of its better tolerability.

Moxonidine

This is a centrally-acting (venterolateral medulla) I_1-imidazoline receptor agonist resulting in reduction of efferent sympathetic tone. This results in peripheral vasodilatation and reduction in TPVR.

It has an absolute bioavailability of 90%. Peak plasma concentrations occur 3-hours post dose with an elimination half-life of 2.5 hours. Once daily dosing provides satisfactory control but at higher doses twice daily dosing minimises adverse reactions (Table 10.7). Dose reduction in renal impairment is required.

Adverse effects include dry mouth, sedation, dizziness, sleep disturbance and very rarely angioedema. The prevalence of dry mouth, the most frequent adverse effect, is sufficiently low

Table 10.7. Less commonly used vasodilators

	Drug	Dose
Centrally-Acting	**Moxonidine**	200–600 μg/day in 1 or 2 divided doses
Peripherally-Acting	**Hydralazine**	50–200 mg/day in 2 divided doses
	Minoxodil	5–50 mg/day in 2 divided doses

at low doses (200–300 μg) to make this an option for 4th line treatment.

Directly acting vasodilating drugs

These drugs are rarely used but still have a place in the management of resistant hypertension particularly when other drugs are not tolerated. They can lead to salt and water retention.

Hydralazine

Hydralazine was introduced in 1950. Whilst its vasodilator action results in reduced TPVR, it is also associated with reflex tachycardia. This can be countered, if necessary, by the concomitant use of a beta-blocker. It is rapidly and completely absorbed. Presystemic metabolism is determined by the patient's acetylator status – rapid acetylators needing higher doses. This drug is only used now in patients with multiple adverse reactions or resistant hypertension.

Adverse effects include headache, tachycardia, palpitations, oedema and a lupus-like syndrome. The latter is seen in slow acetylators at usual doses (Table 10.7).

Minoxidil

Minoxidil is a directly acting peripheral arteriolar vasodilator resulting in reduced TPVR. It is completely absorbed with a bioavailability of 90 % and an elimination half-life of 4.5-hours requiring twice daily dosing (Table 10.7). Minoxidil is only ever indicated in the treatment of resistant hypertension. As a result of its powerful salt and water retaining properties it is almost always used with a loop diuretic.

Adverse effects include oedema, tachycardia, glucose intolerance and hypertrichosis. Increased hair growth is common and precludes its use in women and some men. It is contraindicated in heart failure.

Spironolactone

Spironolactone is a competitive antagonist of aldosterone at the distal convoluted tubule. Aldosterone promotes sodium and water retention. It has a specific role in the management of hypertension in hyperaldosteronism including Conn's syndrome. Interestingly it is just as effective in patients without hyperaldosteronism.

It is highly lipid soluble. Food enhances oral absorption. Canrenone is its active metabolite with a half-life of one hour but dosing on a daily basis is effective.

There is little benefit in exceeding 100 mg/day. Usual doses are up to 50 mg daily. However, in Conn's syndrome higher doses may be required. It is also effective in resistant essential hypertension (Figure 10.1).

Spironolactone should be used with caution in patients with or prone to hyperkalaemia, for example, chronic kidney diseases and treatment with ACEIs.

Common adverse effects include hyperkalaemia, reversible gynaecomastia in men and breast tenderness in men and women, nausea and dizziness.

Alpha (α_1) adrenergic receptor antagonists or α-blockers

The α-blockers lower BP by a highly specific and competitive antagonism of peripheral post-junctional α_1-adrenoceptors resulting in a reduction in vascular resistance.

The most widely used member of this class is the modified release preparation of doxazosin. It is well absorbed with a peak plasma concentration eight to nine hours post dose. There is no significant presystemic metabolism. It is extensively metabolised with an apparent half-life of 22 hours. The dose of modified release doxazosin is 4–8 mg/day.

There is some evidence for a beneficial effect on plasma lipids and insulin resistance. This class may have a role in men with obstructive symptoms in benign prostatic hypertrophy who are not already taking a prostate selective α_1 blocker such as tamsulosin.

Although α blockers should not be considered in patients with symptomatic postural hypotension, they are useful drugs in elderly patients with resistant hypertension.

Adverse effects include weakness, ankle oedema, palpitations and urinary incontinence (mainly in women).

KEY POINTS

- Hypertension is a common, important and easily-treated modifiable risk factor for cardiovascular morbidity and mortality.
- Absolute risk reduction in cardiovascular disease with BP-lowering is seen across a wide age range including the very elderly.
- BP-lowering should be undertaken within the context of an individual's total cardiovascular risk.
- Non-pharmacological methods for BP-lowering should be explored in all patients.
- Selection of drugs for BP-lowering should take into consideration an individual's co-morbidity, concomitant drug-therapy and age.
- Most patients will require two or more drugs to achieve their blood pressure targets.

LINKS

http://www.bhsoc.org British Hypertension Society Guidelines

http://www.nice.org.uk National Institute for Health and Clinical Excellence

http://www.heartstats.org/homepage.asp British Heart Foundation. 2005 Coronary Heart Statistics

http://www.eshonline.org European Society of Hypertension

http://www.ish-world.com International Society of Hypertension

http://www.hbprca.com.au High Blood Pressure Research Council of Australia

Patient Information

http://www.heartfoundation.org.au Heart Foundation, Australia

http://www.bpassoc.org.uk Blood Pressure Association, UK

REFERENCES

1. British Hypertension Society guidelines for hypertension management 2004 (BHS-IV): Summary. *Brit Med J* 2004; **328**: 634–40.
2. Brown MJ. Matching the right drug to the right patient in essential hypertension. *Heart* 2001; **86**: 113–20.
3. Chobanian AV, Bakris GL, Black HR. Seventh report of the Joint National Committee on prevention, detection, evaluation and treatment of high blood pressure (JNC-7). *Hypertension* 2003; **42**: 1206–52.
4. Dahlöf B, Sever PS, Poulter NR, Wedel H, Beevers DG, Caulfield MJ, Collins R, Kjeldsen SE, Kristinsson A, McInnes GT, Mehlsen J, Nieminen M, O'Brien E, Östergren J and for the ASCOT investigators. Prevention of cardiovascular events with an antihypertensive regimen of amlodipine adding perindopril as required versus atenolol adding bendroflumethiazide as required, in the Anglo-Scandinavian Cardiac Outcomes Trial-Blood Pressure Lowering Arm (ASCOT-BPLA): a multicentre randomised controlled trial. *Lancet* 2005; **366**: 895–906.
5. Gueyffier F, Bulpitt C. Boisell J-P, Schron E, Ekbom T, Fagard R, Casiglia E, Kerlikowske K, Coope J, INDANA Group. Antihypertensive drugs in very old people: a subgroup meta-analysis of randomised controlled drugs *Lancet* 1999. **353**: 793–6.
6. Kearney PM, Whelton M, Reynolds K et al. Global burden of hypertension:analysis of worldwide data. *Lancet* 2005; **365**: 217–23.
7. Primatesta P, Brookes M, Poulter NR. Improved hypertension management and control: results from the health survey of England 1998. *Hypertension* 2001; **38**: 827–32.
8. Staessen JA, Gasowski J, G Wang G, Thijs L, Den Hond E, Boisesel J-P, Coope J, Ekbom T, Gueyffier F, Liu L, Kerlikowske K, Pocock S, Fagard RH. Risks of untreated and treated

isolated systolic hypertension in the elderly: meta-analysis of outcome trials. *Lancet* 2000; **355**: 865–72.

9. Wing LMH, CM, Ryan P, Beilin LJ, Brown MA, Jennings GLR, Johnston CI, McNeil JJ, Macdonald GJ, Marley JE, Morgan TF, West MJ, for the Second Australian National Blood Pressure Study Group A Comparison of Outcomes with Angiotensin-Converting-Enzyme Inhibitors and Diuretics for Hypertension in the Elderly Volume. *New Eng J Med* 2003; **348**: 583–92.

10. Beckett NS, Peters R, Fletcher AE, Staessen JA, Lia L, Damitrasen D, Stoyanousky V, Antikainen RL, Nikitin Y, Andersan C, Belhani A, Forette F, Rajkumar C, Thijs L, Banya W, Bulpitt CJ. Treatment of Hypertension in Patients 80 years of age or older. *New Eng J Med* 2008; **358**: 1887–1898.

11 Lipid-lowering in the elderly patient

Anthony S. Wierzbicki

Consultant Chemical Pathologist, St. Thomas' Hospital, London, UK

INTRODUCTION

Atherosclerosis is a disease of aging. Numerous epidemiological studies have shown that age is the principal unmodifiable risk factor for events (1–3). The modifiable risk factors include ratio of total cholesterol: HDL-cholesterol (which can be expressed in terms of particle protein composition as apolipoprotein B : A-I), diabetes and blood pressure (4). Both diabetes and hypertension are strongly age-related risk factors. In parallel with these risk factors levels of total cholesterol rise with age especially after middle age or the menopause. The increasing incidence of metabolic syndrome and obesity with age means that HDL-C levels tend to fall and triglyceride levels rise. Thus hyperlipidaemia is an increasing risk factor for coronary events, aortic valve disease, stroke, peripheral vascular disease including abdominal aortic aneurysm and possibly dementia (multi-infarct type). As many elderly patients have suffered one cardiovascular event they are at high risks of another often in a different vascular bed. Thus patients with strokes more often have coronary events than second strokes.

AETIOLOGY

Most hyperlipidaemia in the elderly is caused by dietary and lifestyle choices. The slowly declining metabolic rate of the elderly patient, associated with reduced levels of activity due to concurrent aging or osteological problems, means that many show feature of the metabolic syndrome. Dietary conservatism also tends to mean that currently elderly subjects are less likely to consume a diet rich and fruit and vegetables ands more likely to eat a diet rich in saturated fat.

Secondary causes of hyperlipidaemia are commoner in the elderly. The commonest cause of mixed hyperlipidaemia is insulin resistance and/or type 2 diabetes. Other causes that tend to be associated with aging include alcohol-induced hyperlipidaemia, which is commoner due to a reduction in liver-related detoxification in the elderly and its frequent association with depression, especially in single males. Alcohol-induced hyperlipidaemia may show a profile varying between mixed hyperlipidaemia to pure hypercholesterolaemia depending on the frequency of alcohol intake. Non-alcoholic steatitic hepatitis, often associated with a mixed hyperlipidaemia, is commoner in the centrally obese elderly.

The commonest cause of pure secondary hypercholesterolaemia is hypothyroidism. The significance of this is that prescription of a lipid lowering drug (statin > fibrate > nicotinic acid > ezetimibe) to a grossly hypothyroid patient massively increases their risk of drug-associated rhabdomyolysis.

Prescribing for Elderly Patients   Edited by Stephen Jackson, Paul Jansen and Arduino Mangoni
© 2009 John Wiley & Sons, Ltd

SYMPTOMS AND SIGNS

Hyperlipidaemia is an asymptomatic condition picked up on general screening. Specific screening for lipids in the elderly is recommended as part of general cardiovascular health assessment in the National Service Frameworks for Coronary Heart Disease and the Elderly. Some lipid-related signs associated with hyperlipidameia in the young are potentially misleading in the elderly. Arcus is associated with familial hypercholeserolaemia in the young but not in the elderly. In some patients tendon xanthomata may be confused with gout tophi and or Heberden's nodes. Unlike these, xanthomata move with the underlying tendons. Xanthelasma are commoner with age and retain their association with mixed hyperlipidaemia but also mark autoimmune disease especially primary biliary cirrhosis.

DIAGNOSIS

Lipid screening in the elderly should comprise a full profile of total cholesterol, triglycerides and HDL-cholesterol. LDL-Cholesterol can usually be calculated by the Friedwald formula. Levels of total cholesterol > 7.5 mmol/L justify automatic treatment. At lower levels of total cholesterol, current recommendations from the Joint British Societies guidelines recommend risk assessment using the Framingham (1991) equation assuming the elderly are aged 60 years (1). The purpose of this adjustment is to reduce prescribing in the otherwise fit elderly given the strong association of risk with age. Treatment is recommended for any cardiovascular risk factor at 15 %/future decade risk of cardiovascular disease (20 %/future decade risk of coronary heart disease). This approach differs from European (2) and US guidelines (3) where risk is assessed at the chronological age and treatment instituted at 20 % coronary heart disease risk. It should be noted that risk assessment is an imprecise art and that the results of the algorithm, even before modifications for obesity, ethnicity or family history, show considerable variation with a risk estimate of 30 % subject

to a 95 % confidence interval of 6 % on single point estimates.

The risk assessment biochemical profile should include measurement of transaminases (AST/ALT), thyroid function tests and a baseline creatine kinase. Lipid-lowering therapy with a statin or fibrate is contra-indicated if AST/ALT exceeds 3 × upper reference limit of normal (ULN) (usually > 150 iu/L). The actual contra-indication is to persistent elevations in transaminases as many elevations turn out to be transient and caused by either infections or to be secondary to other drug therapies (e.g opiate-containing analgesics). If gamma-glutamyl transferase is measured it level is irrelevant to starting or continuing lipid-lowering therapies.

The thyroid function test should be measured. Gross hypothyroidism (TSH > 20 mU/L) is associated with a hypercholesterolaemia and this should be treated prior to re-measurement of the lipid profile due to the risk of lipid-lowering therapy associated rhabdomyolysis. The risk factors for rhabdomyolysis are age, creatinine, muscle mass, female sex and hypothyroidism. Mild hypothyroidism is common and not a contra-indication to lipid-lowering therapies though some reports suggest that reports of myalgia may be commoner in patients with borderline hypothyroidism.

The significance of creatine kinase (CK) measurement in the elderly is debated. Lipid-lowering therapies are contra-indicated in patients with CK > 10 × ULN though most clinicians are reluctant to prescribe if 5 × ULN. Recent data from the SEARCH trial has suggested that myopathy with simvastatin can be predicted by prior elevations in response to statin therapy in alanine aminotransaminase (ALT) (× 1.7) and creatine kinase (× 5) over baseline values and/or 3 × upper reference limit of normal (5) (1). Some elevated CK measurements, e.g in Africans or Afro-Caribbeans represent normal variants. In other patients a mildly elevated CK allied with a mild adverse reaction to lipid-lowering therapies should prompt investigation for rheumatological causes of disease as the lipid-lowering therapy may have uncovered either fibromyalgia or polymyalgia rheumatica.

THERAPY

Most lipid-lowering trials are conducted in middle-aged patients though some studies include a significant proportion of the elderly, e.g. Heart Protection Study though one trial did specifically recruit an elderly population aged > 70 years: PROSPER. The results of the statin studies are consistent in all age groups, both genders and for all atherosclerotic disease. Treatment with a statin delivering a 1 mmol/L reduction in LDL-cholesterol will result in a 20–25 % reduction in cardiovascular events depending the exact endpoint counted (6). Statins are accepted first-line therapy for all patients with cardiovascular disease or at risk of developing cardiovascular disease. Other drug classes are used second-line or for specific indications.

STATINS

General overview

Statins are used to lower LDL-cholesterol (7). Statins reduce LDL-C by 20–55 % depending on the drug and dose. All statins reduce triglycerides in proportion to their efficacy in lowering LDL-C and to baseline triglyceride levels. They have variable and modest effects on levels of HDL-cholesterol. Six drugs are available (Table 11.1). All agents, except rosuvastatin which has only shown benefits to date on surrogate endpoints, have shown benefits in hard endpoint trials if used at sufficient dose- sufficient to lower LDL-C by 1 mmol/L.

Dose adjustment

No specific dose reduction is advised or necessary for the elderly with statins though many general practitioners worldwide initiate therapy at low doses but unfortunately do not titrate the dose to efficacious levels resulting in a persistent under-treatment of lipids in the elderly.

Drug interactions

Drug interactions vary between compound in the class. The most significant interaction is of cytochrome P450 CYP 3A4 metabolized statins (lovastatin, simvastatin, atorvastatin) with other dugs metabolized by this pathway-conazole anti-fungals, erythromycin, and in specialist practice ciclosporin and HIV protease inhibitors. Simvastatin interacts with amiodarone at doses > 20 mg and other statins should be used if amiodarone therapy is necessary (e.g. for atrial fibrillation). A weaker interaction CYP 3A4 can occur with diltiazem through this pathway but is not usually clinically significant. Drug interactions of this type are less significant for the other statins. Recently one of the pathways involved in this interaction has been described as 40–60 % of the variance in statin myopathy in the SEARCH trial was caused by a single nucleotide poymorphism rs4149056 in SLC 01B1 gene encoding the Organic Acid Transporter Protein 1b1 (OATP1B1) that transports statin acids and other drug acids (e.g. fibric or nicotinic acid) (5) (1).

Adverse events

All statins frequently cause gastrointestinal disturbance by a transient dysregulation of bile acid metabolism through the farnesoid-X receptor pathway. This maybe accompanied by a transient increase in bilirubin and transaminases. This problem is usually self-limiting within two to three weeks and on repeat measurement liver profiles have usually normalized.

Similarly, myalgia occurs in 5 % of patients and is not associated with any change in CK. Again often it is self limiting but if symptoms persist than the statin therapy should be changed to the weaker agents that show predictably better side-effect profiles (pravastatin, fluvastatin).

Myositis (raised CK, muscle pain) and rhabdomyolysis (CK > × 20 ULN; muscle pain; myoglobinuria) are rare side effects of statin therapy. The risk factors for rhabdomyolysis are age, creatinine, muscle mass, female sex, hypothyroidism and concomitant therapy with drugs interacting through the relevant cytochrome pathway (usually CYP 3A4); likely to displace statins from plasma proteins; or sharing a

Table 11.1. Pharmacokinetics and pharmacodynamics of lipid-lowering drugs

Drug	Start dose	Usual dose	Pharmaco-kinetics	Metabolism	Important interactions	Important adverse events	Other tips
Atorvastatin	10 mg	20 mg (10–80)	Y $t_{1/2}$ = 14 hrs E $t_{1/2}$ > 16 hrs AUC +30%	CYP3A4	Conazoles Erythromycin Ciclosporin	GI disturbance Myalgia-myositis-rhabdomyolysis	
Fluvastatin	80 mg	80 mg (20–80)	Y $t_{1/2}$ = 0.6 hrs E $t_{1/2}$ = 0.6 hrs AUC–nil	CYP2C9	Nil	GI disturbance Myalgia-myositis-rhabdomyolysis	
Lovastatin	40 mg	80 mg (20–80)	Y $t_{1/2}$ = 3 hrs E $t_{1/2}$ >3 hrs AUC +45%	CYP3A4	Conazoles Erythromycin Ciclosporin	GI disturbance Myalgia-myositis-rhabdomyolysis	
Pravastatin	40 mg	40 mg (10–40)	Y $t_{1/2}$ = 2 hrs E $t_{1/2}$ >2 hrs AUC– +19–27%	3 − α-isomer	Nil	GI disturbance Myalgia-myositis-rhabdomyolysis	
Rosuvastatin	10 mg	10 mg (10–20; [40])	Y $t_{1/2}$ = 19 hrs E $t_{1/2}$ = 19 hrs AUC–nil	CYP2C19 (10%)	Nil	GI disturbance Myalgia-myositis-rhabdomyolysis	
Simvastatin	40 mg	40 mg (10–80 mg)	Y $t_{1/2}$ 1.9 hours E $t_{1/2}$ –3 hours AUC +45%	CYP3A4	Conazoles Erythromycin Amiodarone Ciclosporin	GI disturbance Myalgia-myositis-rhabdomyolysis	
Bezafibrate	400 mg	400 mg	Y $t_{1/2}$ = 4 hrs E $t_{1/2}$ = 8 hrs AUC +160%	Glucuronide	Warfarin Statins	GI disturbance, rash Myalgia-myositis-rhabdomyolysis	
Ciprofibrate	100 mg	100 mg	Y $t_{1/2}$ = 81 hrs E $t_{1/2}$ = NA AUC = NA	Glucuronide	Warfarin Statins	GI disturbance, rash Myalgia-myositis-rhabdomyolysis	

Fenofibrate	Various 122/160/200 mg	Various 122/145/160/200 mg (122–267)	Y $t_{1/2}$ = 20 hrs E $t_{1/2}$ > 20 hrs AUC +10%	Glucuronide UGT A2	Warfarin Statins	GI disturbance, rash Myalgia-myositis-rhabdomyolysis	Avoid with statin combination therapy
Gemfibrozil	300 mg bd	600 mg bd	Y $t_{1/2}$ = 3.0 hrs E $t_{1/2}$ = 3.0 hrs AUC = +10%	Glucuronide UGT A1 & UGT A3 **NB CYP 2C8 inhibitor**	Warfarin Statins	GI disturbance, rash Myalgia-myositis-rhabdomyolysis	
Nicotinic acid (Niacin)	375–500 mg	1000–2000 mg (500–2000)	Y $t_{1/2}$ = 0.5 hrs E $t_{1/2}$ = NA AUC = NA	10% nicotinuric acid	-	Flush, rash, hyperglycaemia Hypophosphataemia Gout	Reduce flush with aspirin/indomethacin
Ezetimibe	10 mg	10 mg	Y $t_{1/2}$ = 22 hrs E $t_{1/2}$ > 22 hrs AUC +200%	Glucuronide	Ciclosporin	GI disturbance, rash	Add to low dose statin in myalgia
MaxEPA	1 g	10 g	Y $t_{1/2}$ = NA E $t_{1/2}$ = NA	Beta-oxidation	-	Bloating, weight gain	-
Omacor	1 g	1–2 g	Y $t_{1/2}$ = N/A E $t_{1/2}$ = N/A	Beta-oxidation	-	Bloating	-

Y = Young E = Elderly

myopathic tendency (e.g. other lipid-lowering drugs).

FIBRATES

General overview

Fibrates are used to lower triglycerides and raise HDL-C though their principal action is to increase lipoprotein particle sizes (which is well marked by triglycerides). They reduce triglycerides by 30–50 %, raise HDL-C by 2–15 % and reduce LDL-C by 0–10 % depending on the drug and dose. Four drugs are available (Table 11.2). The evidence base for fibrates is contradictory (8). Initial studies showed benefits with clofibrate but the later World Health Organisation trial showed decreased cardiovascular events but an increase in total mortality due mostly to an excess of pancreatits/cholecystitis. Clofibrate is not used any more. Later fibrate trials with gemfibrozil in primary prevention (Helsinki Heart Study) and in secondary prevention patients with low HDL-C (< 0.95 mmol/L) (VA-HIT) showed reductions in cardiovascular events. Data with bezafibrate in the BIP study showed a non-significant slight reduction in events concentrated in a high triglyceride group (> 2.3 mmol/L) though this was not reproduced in the patients with peripheral vascular disease in the Northwick Park Study. Fenofibrate reduced coronary events non-significantly in patients with type 2 diabetes in the FIELD study but did reduce overall cardiovascular events. The benefits of fenofibrate in FIELD were attenuated by concomitant asymmetric statin therapy. There are no outcome studies with ciprofibrate.

Dose adjustment

No specific dose reduction is advised or necessary for the elderly with fibrates. Fibrate therapy needs to be used with caution in patients with creatinine > 150 μmol/L (eGFR < 30 mls/min) as these drugs are renally cleared.

Drug interactions

Fibrates show a significant interaction with warfarin such that warfarin dose needs to decreased by 33 %. Fibrates can interact with other lipid-lowering therapies to increase the risk of rhabdomyolysis. This is a particular problem with gemfibrozil, which has a unique mechanism of glucuronidation and this causes increases in free statin acid concentrations (lovastatin, simvastatin) as well as causing problems with other drugs (e.g. pioglitazone). Gemfibrozil is not recommended to be used in combination therapy (especially statins) for any lipid disorder (9).

Adverse events

All fibrates frequently cause gastrointestinal disturbance by a transient dysregulation of bile acid metabolism through the farnesoid-X receptor pathway. This maybe accompanied by a transient increase in bilirubin and transaminases. This problem is usually self-limiting within two to three weeks and on repeat measurement liver profiles have usually normalised. In general fibrates reduce transaminases and are used to treat NASH. Though fibrates are used as first-line therapy to treat hypertriglyceridaemia-induced pancreatitis their lithogenic actions in patients with typical lipid profiles lead to an increase in gallstones and all are associated with a slight increase in pancreatitis. Fibrates can be associated with skin rashes. Myalgia occurs in 0.5 % of patients on fibrates and is not associated with any change in CK. Again often it is self-limiting but if symptoms persist than the therapy should be changed to another drug class. Myositis (raised CK, muscle pain) and rhabdomyolysis (CK > × 20 ULN; muscle pain; myoglobinuria) are very rare side effects of fibrate therapy. The risk factors for rhabdomyolysis are similar to those described for statins.

NICOTINIC ACID

General overview

Nicotinic acid is used to raise HDL-C and reduce triglycerides. It raises HDL-C by 10–25 %, reduces triglycerides by 20–40 %, and reduces LDL-C by 10–20 % depending on the dose. It can also reduce lipoprotein (a) levels by 10–25 % (10). There is endpoint evidence with the immediate release formulation used a 3 g/day in the Coronary Drug Project where is reduced cardiovascular evens by 22 %. Given the problems with flushing and hyperglycaemia with the immediate release form a modified release formulation (up to 2 g/day) is commonly used these days. This has similar lipid-lowering efficacy but lesser rates of flushing, no transaminase effect and causes less hyperglycaemia. A novel form of niacin co-formulated with a flush suppressant—laropiprant—a prostaglandin D2 DP1 receptor antagonist is in development.

Dose adjustment

No specific dose reduction is advised or necessary for the elderly with nicotinic acid. Nicotinic acid therapy needs to be used with caution in patients with creatinine > 150 μmol/L (eGFR < 30 mls/min) as this drug is renally cleared.

Drug interactions

Nicotinic acid shows a significant interaction with warfarin such that warfarin doses need to decreased by 20 %. Nicotinic acid can interact with other lipid-lowering therapies to increase the risk of rhabdomyolysis but the effect is less than with statin or fibrate monotherapy.

Adverse events

The principal side effect of nicotinic acid is facial flushing. This can extend beyond erythema to a burning sensation. Though spectacular this is not a serious side effect. It occurs in 80 % of patients commencing nicotinic acid therapy and the frequency and intensity of flushes habituates with time. Flushing can be decreased by slow dose titration, concurrent aspirin therapy (150 mg) or by indomethacin (200 mg) and by slowing absorption using a snack. Occasionally a photosensitive rash may be seen with nicotinic acid.

Nicotinic acid has variable effects on glycaemic control in diabetes (11). In most patients it has no or a transient effect though in some patients increases of up to 1 mmol/L in glucose (0.5 % in HbA_{1c}) are seen.

Transient increases in bilirubin and transaminases are rare with nicotinic acid than other lipid-lowering agents.

Myalgia occurs in 0.1 % of patients on nicotinic acid and is not associated with any change in CK. Again often it is self-limiting but if symptoms persist than the therapy should be changed to another drug class. Myositis (raised CK, muscle pain) and rhabdomyolysis (CK > × 20 ULN; muscle pain; myoglobinuria) are very rare side effects of nicotinic acid therapy. The risk factors for rhabdomyolysis are similar to those described for statins.

EZETIMIBE

General overview

Ezetimibe is a specific cholesterol absorption inhibitor reducing LDL-C by 15–20 % (12). It can be used in monotherapy or combination therapy with any lipid-lowering drug. It reduces triglycerides in proportion to their efficacy in lowering LDL-C and to baseline triglyceride levels. It has modest effects on levels of HDL-cholesterol. A combination of ezetimibe and low dose stain is often used to treat patients that have developed side effects on moderate dose statin therapy. There is no endpoint evidence with ezetimibe as yet.

Dose adjustment

No specific dose reduction is advised or necessary for the elderly with ezetimibe.

Drug interactions

Ezetimibe has few drug interactions. The only significant interaction is with ciclosporin, which raises ezetimibe levels eight to16 fold.

Adverse events

Ezetimibe causes gastrointestinal disturbance by a transient dysregulation of bile acid metabolism through the farnesoid-X receptor pathway. This maybe accompanied by a transient increase in bilirubin and transaminases. This problem is usually self-limiting within two to three weeks and on repeat measurement liver profiles have usually normalised. Ezetimibe can be associated with skin rashes. Myalgia, myositis (raised CK, muscle pain) and rhabdomyolysis (CK > × 20 ULN; muscle pain; myoglobinuria) are rare side effects of ezetimibe therapy and usually occur when it is prescribed with a concomitant statin.

BILE ACID SEQUESTRANTS

General overview

Bile acid sequestrants reduce cholesterol absorption and reduce LDL-C by 15–20 %. They can be used in monotherapy or combination therapy with any lipid-lowering drug except ezetimibe. They may raise triglycerides levels and have modest positive effects on levels of HDL-cholesterol. They are not often used in the elderly as gastrointestinal side effects are common and interact with irritable bowel syndrome and diverticulitis to cause bloating, diarrhea and constipation. Endpoint evidence exists for bile acid sequestrants from the Lipid Research Clinics trial where they reduced coronary events by 15 %.

Dose adjustment

No specific dose reduction is advised or necessary for the elderly with bile acid sequestrants.

Drug interactions

Bile acid sequestrants have multiple drug interactions as they interfere with the absorption of all lipid-soluble drugs. A four-hour clear interval is recommended between taking these drugs and taking any other medication.

Adverse events

Bile acid sequestrants cause gastrointestinal disturbance in 20–40 % of patients. This may be accompanied by a liver-X-receptor (LXR) induced hypertriglyceridaemia.

Myalgia, myositis (raised CK, muscle pain) and rhabdomyolysis (CK > × 20 ULN; muscle pain; myoglobinuria) are rare side effects of

bile acid sequestrant therapy and usually occur when it is prescribed with a concomitant statin.

OMEGA-3 FATTY ACIDS

General overview

Omega-3 fatty acids reduce triglycerides by 20–25 % at high doses. At moderate doses they have proportionally lesser effects but seem to reduce cardiovascular events especially sudden cardiac death. They can be used in monotherapy or combination therapy with any lipid-lowering drug. The endpoint evidence with omega-3 fatty caids is controversial. In the GISSI-P (secondary prevention), JELIS (primary and secondary prevention) GISSI-HF (heart failure) and DART-1 one studies they reduced coronary events and sudden death but in the DART-2 study an increase in cardiovascular events was seen (13) (2).

Dose adjustment

No specific dose reduction is advised or necessary for the elderly with omega-3 fatty acids.

Drug interactions

Omega-3 fatty acids have few significant drug interactions.

Adverse events

Omega-3 fatty acids can cause gastrointestinal disturbance and bloating. They may be associated with weight gain if given in preparations that require taking multiple capsules as they contain relatively low levels of docosahexaenoic acid and eicosapentanenoic acid.

GUIDELINES

Treatment of lipid-associated atherosclerosis risk forms a key part of the National Service Frameworks for Coronary Heart Disease, Diabetes, Renal Disease and the Elderly in the UK. Lipid screening in the elderly should comprise part of cardiovascular risk assessment in all elderly patients. Levels of total cholesterol

> 7.5 mmol/L justify automatic treatment. At lower levels of total cholesterol, current recommendations from the Joint British Societies guidelines recommend risk assessment using the Framingham (1991) equation assuming the elderly are aged 60 years (1). The purpose of this adjustment is to reduce prescribing in the otherwise fit elderly given the strong association of risk with age. Treatment is recommended for any cardiovascular risk factor at 15 %/future decade risk of cardiovascular disease (20 %/future decade risk of coronary heart disease). This approach differs from European (2) and US guidelines (3) where risk is assessed at the chronological age and treatment instituted at 20 % coronary heart disease risk. It should be noted that risk assessment is an imprecise art and that the results of the algorithm, even before modifications for obesity, ethnicity or family history, show considerable variation with a risk estimate of 30 % subject to a 95 % confidence interval of 6 % on single point estimates.

KEY POINTS

- Hyperlipidaemia is a common risk factor for atherosclerosis in the elderly.
- Cardiovascular risk assessment should be performed in all elderly patients with risk factors.
- Statin therapy is recommended for all patients at significant risk (> 20 % cardiovascular disease risk/future decade) with the aim of reducing LDL-C by 1 mmol/L or more.
- Fibrates or nicotinic acid are used second line after statins with the primary aims of reducing triglycerides or raising HDL-C respectively.
- Ezetimibe can be added to lipid lowering therapies to increase LDL-C reduction by 15–20 %.

LINKS

American Heart Association http://www.americanheart.org

European Society of Cardiology http://www.escardio.org

Hyperlipidaemia Education and Atherosclerosis Research Trust- UK http://www.heartuk.org.uk

Department of Health (UK) http://www.doh.gov.uk

National Institute for Clinical Excellence http://www.nice.org

REFERENCES

1. British Cardiac Society, British Hypertension Society, Diabetes UK, HEART UK, Primary Care Cardiovascular Society, The Stroke Association. JBS2: Joint British Societies' guidelines on prevention of cardiovascular disease in clinical practice. *Heart* 2005; **91**(Suppl V): V1–V52.
2. De Backer G, Ambrosioni E, Borch-Johnsen K, Brotons C, Cifkova R, Dallongeville J, et al. European guidelines on cardiovascular disease prevention in clinical practice. Third Joint Task Force of European and Other Societies on Cardiovascular Disease Prevention in Clinical Practice. *Eur Heart J* 2003; **24**(17): 1601–10.
3. Executive Summary of The Third Report of The National Cholesterol Education Program (NCEP) Expert Panel on Detection, Evaluation, And Treatment of High Blood Cholesterol In Adults (Adult Treatment Panel III). *JAMA* 2001; **285**(19): 2486–97.
4. Yusuf S, Hawken S, Ounpuu S, Dans T, Avezum A, Lanas F, et al. Effect of potentially modifiable risk factors associated with myocardial infarction in 52 countries (the INTERHEART study): case-control study. *Lancet* 2004; **364**(9438): 937–52.
5. Link E, Parish S, Armitage J, Bowman L, Heath S, Matsuda F, et al. SLCO1B1 variants and statin-induced myopathy–a genomewide study. *N Engl J Med* 2008 Aug 21; **359**(8): 789–99.
6. Baigent C, Keech A, Kearney PM, Blackwell L, Buck G, Pollicino C, et al. Efficacy and safety of cholesterol-lowering treatment: prospective meta-analysis of data from 90,056 participants in 14 randomised trials of statins. *Lancet* 2005; **366**(9493): 1267–78.
7. Wierzbicki AS, Poston R, Ferro A. The lipid and non-lipid effects of statins. *Pharmacol Ther* 2003; **99**(1): 95–112.

8. Wierzbicki AS. FIELDS of dreams, fields of tears: a perspective on fibrate trials. *Int J Clin Pract* 2006; **60**(4): 442–9.

9. Wierzbicki AS, Mikhailidis DP, Wray R, Schacter M, Cramb R, Simpson WG, et al. Statin-fibrate combination: therapy for hyperlipidemia: a review. *Curr Med Res Opin* 2003; **19**(3): 155–68.

10. Chapman MJ, Assmann G, Fruchart JC, Shepherd J, Sirtori C. Raising high-density lipoprotein cholesterol with reduction of cardiovascular risk: the role of nicotinic acid–a position paper developed by the European Consensus Panel on HDL-C. *Curr Med Res Opin* 2004; **20**(8): 1253–68.

11. Vogt A, Kassner U, Hostalek U, Steinhagen-Thiessen E. Evaluation of the safety and tolerability of prolonged-release nicotinic acid in a usual care setting: the NAUTILUS study. *Curr Med Res Opin* 2006; **22**(2): 417–25.

12. Mikhailidis DP, Wierzbicki AS, Daskalopoulou SS, Al-Saady N, Griffiths H, Hamilton G, et al. The use of ezetimibe in achieving low density lipoprotein lowering goals in clinical practice: position statement of a United Kingdom consensus panel. *Curr Med Res Opin* 2005; **21**(6): 959–69.

13. Wierzbicki AS. A fishy business: omega-3 fatty acids and cardiovascular disease. *Int J Clin Pract* 2008; **62**(8): 1142–6.

12 Acute coronary syndrome

Derek Yiu and Arduino Mangoni

Department of Clinical Pharmacology, Flinders Medical Centre, Adelaide, Australia

INTRODUCTION

Acute Coronary Syndrome (ACS) encompasses three separate clinical entities:

1. ST segment elevation myocardial infarction (STEMI).
2. Non-ST segment elevation myocardial infarction (NSTEMI).
3. Unstable angina (UA).

Elderly patients constitute about 60 % of emergency presentations with ACS. Despite this, as a group, they have often been excluded from the major trials in this field (1). Even when trials are conducted in elderly patients, there tends to be a bias towards carefully selected "healthy" elderly subjects, or those with fewer comorbidities. As a result, the volume of evidence that is applicable to the elderly population in general is minuscule in comparison to that which can be applied to younger patients. In addition, there are numerous known and suspected differences in the way elderly patients present and respond to therapy, that make generalization of trial evidence questionable.

Foremost amongst the concerns regarding this generalization, is the increased prevalence of co-morbid conditions. Some prevalent conditions (e.g. renal dysfunction, diabetes mellitus) have a direct or indirect effect upon coronary risk, and peri- and post-procedural complications, whereas others may limit the choice or effectiveness of therapy (e.g. peptic ulcer disease, cardiac conduction defects).

Cadaveric studies have shown that the prevalence of anatomic coronary artery disease is about 50 % at age >50, rising to 70 % during the eighth decade. The severity and number of stenoses also increases. Despite this, reported prevalence of symptomatic coronary disease is 20–30 %. This is probably because the condition is under-recognised, due to atypical presentation, physician apathy, or being masked by activity levels which are insufficient to produce ischaemia-related symptoms.

AETIOLOGY

Coronary artery disease tends to be more severe and diffuse with advancing age. The magnitude of risk attributable to a family history of coronary artery disease is relatively less than in younger presenters. However, there is a tendency for a larger number of atherogenic risk factors (e.g. diabetes mellitus, hypercholesterolaemia, hypertension, cigarette smoking) to be present.

Hypertension is the most important of these, due to a prevalence of almost 60 %. Of elderly subjects with hypertension, about 65 % have isolated systolic hypertension. Observational data suggest that isolated systolic hypertension is more likely to be poorly controlled than other types of hypertension.

Prescribing for Elderly Patients   Edited by Stephen Jackson, Paul Jansen and Arduino Mangoni
© 2009 John Wiley & Sons, Ltd

Fortunately, in the majority of cases, these modifiable atherogenic risk factors may be addressed far more effectively than previously has been the case. For example, in terms of absolute benefit, treated elderly patients have a 3–4 % reduction in cardiovascular mortality, a 1–2 % reduction in coronary events, a 1–2 % reduction in stroke, and a 1–4 % reduction in all cardiovascular events.

SYMPTOMS AND SIGNS

In young to middle-aged males with ACS, clinical presentations are often dramatic. By far the most common presentation is of central crushing chest pain, accompanied by profuse sweating and perhaps pain radiating down the arm(s) or to the back, neck or jaw. Accordingly, this syndrome has been labelled "typical". Many variants on this presentation are still considered to fall within the spectrum of "typical", but usually only if there is frank crushing chest pain.

If the character of the pain justifies different qualitative description, such as "sharp", "stabbing", or "burning", or if indeed, there is no pain at all, then often the syndrome is labelled "atypical".

Traditionally, it has been taught that "atypical" presentations are much more common in the elderly population than the young. However, given that elderly patients essentially represent the majority of those who present with ACS, it may be more practical to consider that the spectrum of "typical" presentations in the elderly should include painless presentations and "ischaemic equivalents", rather than just the "typical" syndrome. Dyspnoea may be the most common "ischaemic equivalent", followed by shoulder or back pain, weakness, fatigue, or acute confusion.

Presentations are often further clouded by the presence of other co-morbid conditions (eg. dyspnoea or fatigue may be due to anaemia or pulmonary disease). In addition ACS may be precipitated by concurrent illness, especially pneumonia or a systemic infection. The risk is highest in the first three days of an acute illness, and may be three to four times higher than the patients risk factor profile may otherwise suggest.

The incidence of cognitive impairment increases with age, which may limit the utility of the history for recognising ACS. This may only be countered by maintaining an increased level of suspicion for the presence of cardiac ischaemia.

Finally, it is thought that up to 40 % of myocardial infarctions in this age group may be silent, i.e. there is no indication whatsoever, but unequivocal evidence of localised myocardial damage is subsequently discovered.

DIAGNOSIS

The electrocardiogram (ECG) is considered to be the critical diagnostic test in the patient presenting with chest pain–in fact, we define the condition and its treatments based upon the ECG changes or lack thereof (i.e. STEMI vs. non-STEMI) (Figure 12.1). However, the sensitivity of the ECG in detecting ischaemia has been reported to be as low as 50 % (2), and interpretation is made more difficult by the increasing likelihood that the baseline ECG will be abnormal in elderly patients.

The presence of persistent ST-elevation in the presence of symptoms indicates the need for immediate thrombolysis or percutaneous coronary intervention (PCI) to open the affected artery (Figure 12.1).

However, less definitive ECG changes have much less bearing on prognosis (and therefore management)–in fact amongst those with no ECG changes, there is still about 4 % mortality within 42 days (3).

The next phase of assessment, ie the use of biochemical markers for diagnosis and risk stratification in elderly patients, is similar to younger patients (Figure 12.1).

Cardiac-specific troponins are now used to stratify the risk of all patients with non-ST elevation ACS (NSTE-ACS). In patients who present with rest angina in the last 48 hours, a raised cardiac troponin indicates a 30-day risk of MI or death of 15–20 %, compared with <2 % for a negative test. "False positive"

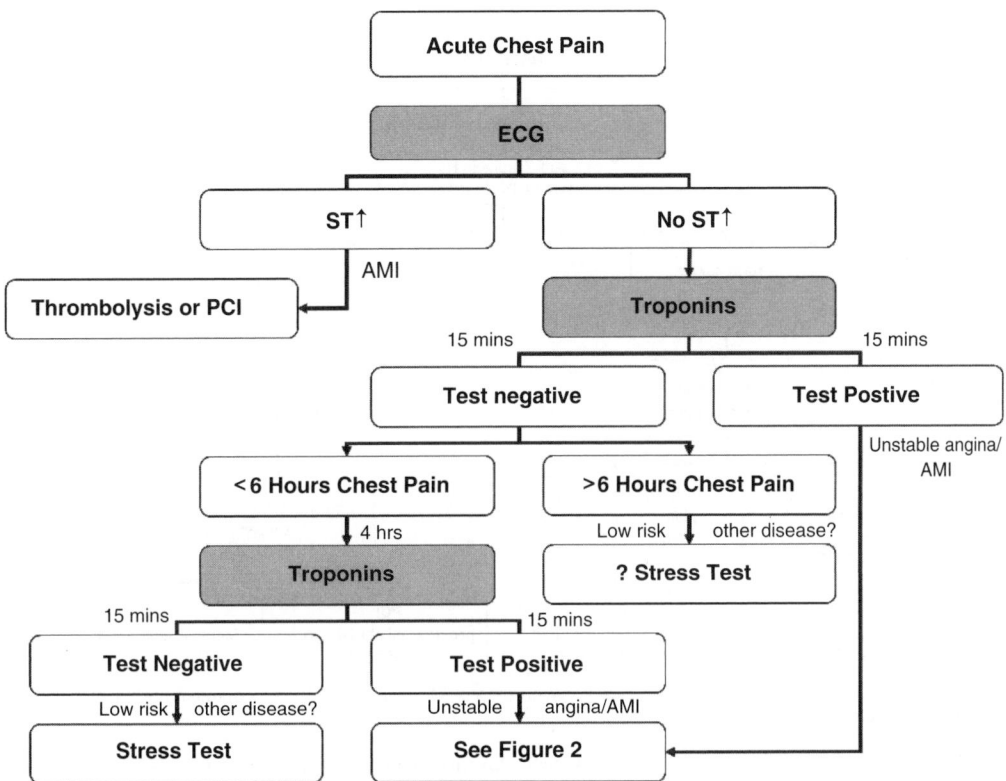

ECG = Electrocardiogram; PCI = percutaneous coronary intervention; AMI = acute myocardial infarction

Figure 12.1. Diagnostic algorithm for acute chest pain.
Adapted from Hamm C.W., Braunwald E. *Circulation* 2000; **102**:118–122. A classification of unstable angina revisited. Figure 12.2, p 120

elevations in troponins (particularly troponin T) can occur more frequently in patients with reduced glomerular filtration. Whilst this may limit their utility in this setting, some studies have demonstrated that even asymptomatically elevated troponins in patients with reduced GFR predict for poor prognosis.

Non-ACS causes for cardiac troponin elevation are listed in Table 12.1.

The final step in risk stratification is the use of PCI. Patients with NSTE-ACS at high risk should have an angiogram within 48 hours (Figure 12.2). These criteria are listed in Table 12.2.

There has been debate about delaying intervention to allow the thrombotic milieu to "cool" but this is no longer recommended. The use of glycoprotein IIb/IIIa inhibitors is recommended in these cases, and they are discussed in the next section.

Although they have been evaluated, and may have some role to play, resting myocardial perfusion imaging and echocardiography are not

Table 12.1. Non-ACS causes of cardiac troponin elevation

Critical illness	Trauma
Tachycardia	Heart failure
Coronary vasospasm	Myocardial strain
Acute stroke	Myocyte death (eg, myocarditis)
Direct myocardial damage (eg cardiac surgery)	Pulmonary embolism
Chronic kidney disease	Pulmonary hypertension

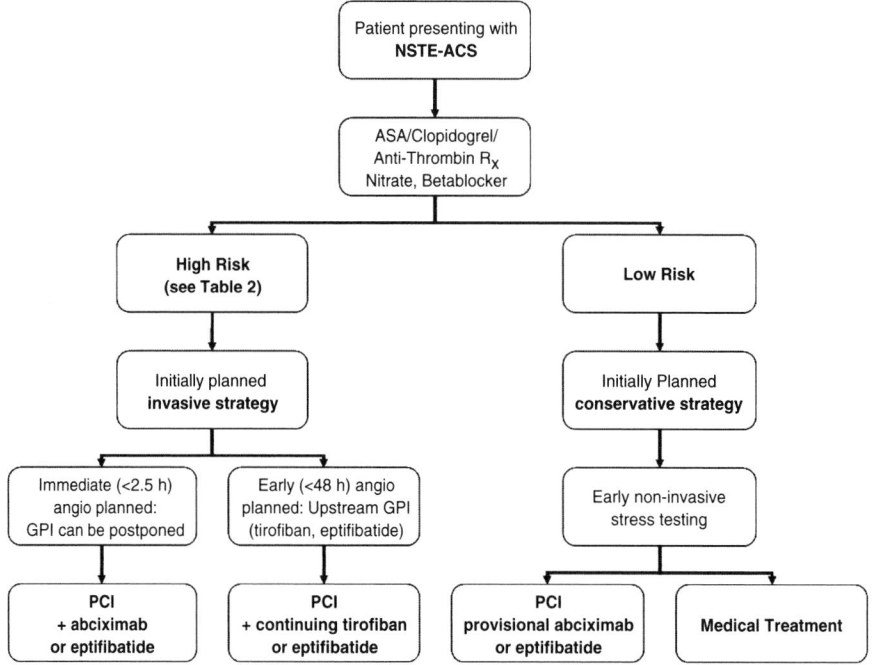

NSTE-ACS = non-ST elevation acute coronary syndrome: ASA = aspirin; GPI = glycoprotein IIb/IIIa inhibitor; PCI = percutaneous coronary intervention

Figure 12.2. Management of non-ST segment elevation acute coronary syndrome.
Adapted from the ESC Guidelines for Percutaneous Coronary Interventions, *European Heart Journal* (2005) **26**: 804–847, Figure 12.1, p 811

currently included in European and American guidelines for the acute assessment of ACS.

THERAPY

Antiplatelet agents

Aspirin

Aspirin is indicated in all patients – unfortunately, the most common contraindication to aspirin use (peptic ulcer) has a much higher prevalence in elderly patients. The recommended initial dose varies from 300–325 mg. In order to facilitate rapid absorption, this first dose should be administered in soluble form. If this is not available, standard aspirin may be chewed. The maintenance dose is 75–150 mg daily.

Clopidogrel

Clopidogrel has been shown to be beneficial in combination with aspirin in ACS, but has not been trialled as acute monotherapy. As an adjunct to aspirin, it should be continued for 9–12 months. The CURE trial showed

Table 12.2. Criteria for high risk in ACS

Recurrent ischaemia despite intensive anti-ischaemic therapy
Elevated troponin level
New ST-segment depression
Symptoms of cardiac failure or new or worsening mitral regurgitation
Depressed left ventricular systolic function
Haemodynamic instability
Sustained ventricular tachycardia
PCI within 6 months
Prior coronary artery bypass grafting

benefit in NSTE-ACS, immediately and up to 12 months later (and included patients with a mean age of 64.2 ± 11.3 years) (4). The COMMIT trial demonstrated the benefit of the addition of clopidogrel to the usual management of STEMI. It had no upper age limit—in fact, 26.0 % of the trial population was aged ≥ 70 years (5). Whilst this did demonstrate that the effects were concordant in elderly subjects, caution must still be exercised in generalizing this conclusion to non-Chinese populations, as the trial was undertaken only in China.

Pre-treatment with clopidogrel >6 hours prior to PCI is also beneficial, unless cardiac surgery is expected within five days. When stents are implanted, it is recommended that clopidogrel be continued for at least one month for bare metal stents, and three to six months for drug-eluting stents (because of delayed endothelial coverage). There is however evidence that supports the use of clopidogrel for at least 1 year following stenting (PCI-CURE, CREDO). The studies in this area included subjects >65 years of age, but had population means of ~ 61 years.

Clopidogrel can be used as an alternative for any patients intolerant of aspirin.

Intravenous GPIIb/IIIa inhibitors

Agents such as abciximab, tirofiban, eptifibatide, and lamifiban have reduced death, MI and target vessel re-intervention when given during and after PCI. A GPIIb/IIIa inhibitor is therefore recommended in all patients with troponin-positive ACS who are to undergo PCI, and should continue for 12–24 hours post procedure. However, there has been a documented increase in bleeding events with these agents in elderly patients, with a substudy of GUSTO-IV ACS showing an almost threefold increase in both minor and major bleeding events in subject aged >65 years (6).

Anti-thrombin therapy

Unfractionated and low molecular weight heparin

Until recently there has been much debate about the use of unfractionated (UFH) vs. low

molecular weight heparins (LMWH) in ACS. The weight of evidence and the ACC/AHA (American College of Cardiology, American Heart Association) guidelines now support the use of LMWH in all patients with ACS, except where there is significant renal impairment (calculated creatinine clearance <30 ml/min). Once again, because of the prevalence of renal impairment rises with age, care needs to be taken in the elderly population.

Factor Xa inhibitors

Fondaparinux was evaluated in NSTE-ACS in the OASIS-5 trial, a large (>20, 000 subjects) multicentre/multinational head-to-head comparison with enoxaparin. The number of patients with primary outcome events (death, myocardial infarction, or refractory ischaemia at nine days) was similar in the two groups (5.8 % fondaparinux vs. 5.7 % enoxaparin). However, the rate of major bleeding at nine days was significantly reduced with fondaparinux (absolute risk reduction 1.9 %, P < 0.001). OASIS-6, the parallel arm in STEMI, showed that fondaparinux significantly reduced the primary endpoint (composite of death or reinfarction at 30 days) compared to placebo or unfractionated heparin (absolute risk reduction 1.5 %, P = 0.008). No significant differences were detected in terms of major bleeding rates.

Beta blockers

Despite, or more likely because of their ubiquity, there is limited RCT data on the use of beta blockers in unstable angina. Recommendations for their use have been extrapolated from data gathered in MI. Their efficacy in NSTEMI has been shown in multiple trials, and in large meta-analyses. However, the majority of the data in STEMI were gathered prior to the advent of thrombolytic therapy. Since then, only one (very) large randomized controlled trial has been published, demonstrating that there was no mortality benefit. Twenty six per cent of the study population was aged ≥ 70 years. There were significant reductions in re-infarction and ventricular fibrillation, but these were offset by an increase in cardiogenic shock (7).

Intravenous administration has not been demonstrated to be more beneficial than oral administration.

Thrombolytics and Primary PCI

Patients who present within 12 hours of symptoms onset, and ST elevation or new bundle branch block on ECG should be considered for reperfusion therapy. There has been a demonstrated benefit of timely primary PCI over thrombolysis in all age groups, but this is most marked over the age of 75 years. Whilst the single trial to demonstrate this was small (87 patients), numerous subgroup analyses of much larger trials support this finding. In this small trial, primary PCI was compared to streptokinase. At 30 days it reduced the composite endpoint of death, reinfarction, or stroke to 9 % (vs. 29 %). At one year the benefit was magnified (13 vs. 44 %) and mainly due to reduced mortality (11 vs. 29 %).(8) There is insufficient evidence to support an upper age limit for primary PCI.

Primary PCI should therefore be the preferred treatment of STEMI, in all cases where:

1. primary PCI is appropriately available (see ACC guidelines);
2. the door-to-balloon time is expected to be <90 min;
3. there is a contraindication to thrombolysis; or
4. the patient is in shock.

Age should not preclude PCI – on the contrary, according to the available evidence, the benefit over thrombolysis is more marked in elderly patients.

Nitrates

As with beta blockers, the evidence for the use of nitrates in ACS is limited. There is no evidence that outcome is altered. They are therefore used for symptom relief. They should be avoided in right ventricular MI, and when the patient is hypotensive.

Calcium channel blockers

There is no trial evidence to support the use of calcium channel blockers in ACS. There is a consensus opinion that diltiazem may offer some protection in NSTEMI. There may also be a role in symptom control, or in those with a contraindication to beta blockers. Short acting nifedipine should not be used, as pooled observational data suggests an increase in mortality.

Additional Post-ACS Management

Angiotensin Converting Enzyme Inhibitors (ACEI) and Angiotensin Receptor Antagonists (ARA)

Inhibitors of the renin-angiotensin system have a beneficial effect in post-infarct remodelling and in reduction of subsequent ischaemic events. The evidence for this is stronger in STEMI than NSTEMI, but the use of ACEI is still recommended by the ACC/AHA guidelines. There is no evidence for their use following unstable angina per se.

Statins

There is unequivocal evidence that statin therapy is beneficial following ACS, via multiple large secondary prevention trials (4S, CARE, LIPID, HPS, PROSPER). Many statins have been proven in this setting. In elderly patients, the benefits are similar in magnitude to those seen in younger patients. The reduction in cardiovascular endpoints has been 20–50 %, with onset of benefit in 6–24 months.

There is also emerging evidence that greater benefit can be obtained from early initiation of high dose therapy following ACS. Currently, only atorvastatin has been proven to be effective in this context.

It is now believed that the benefit from early statin therapy results from plaque stabilization, reversal of endothelial dysfunction, decreased thrombogenicity, and reduced inflammation. These benefits can be seen as early as three days after initiation of therapy. Therapy should continue indefinitely, even in the setting of "normal" cholesterol. There is debate about the use of inflammatory and other markers to guide therapy, but at this stage the recommendation is that therapy should be sufficient to lower LDL-C to less than 80 mg/dL (2.1 mmol/L).

THERAPY SCHEME OF THE ADVISED DRUGS

See Table 12.3.

KEY POINTS

- Patients aged >65 with Acute Coronary Syndrome often present with "ischaemic equivalents" rather than typical angina.
- Risks, dose modifications and contraindications should, in general, take into account co-morbidities rather than age per se. However, "normal" creatinine levels can mask an age-related decline in glomerular filtration rate, which may require dose modification or selection of an alternate agent. This is particularly relevant in the use of antithrombotics and angiotensin active agents.
- Percutaneous coronary interventions should not be withheld because of age – elderly patients have the greatest marginal benefit from primary angioplasty compared with thrombolysis or conservative management in ST elevation myocardial infarction.

GUIDELINES

European Society of Cardiology

- The Task Force on the management of ST-segment elevation acute myocardial infarction of the European Society of Cardiology. Management of acute myocardial infarction in patients presenting with persistent ST-segment elevation. Eur Heart J 2008; 29: 2909-45.
- The Task Force for the diagnosis and treatment of non-ST-segment elevation acute coronary syndromes of the European Society of Cardiology. Guidelines for the diagnosis and treatment of non-ST-segment elevation acute coronary syndromes. Eur Heart J 2007; 28: 1598-660.

American College of Cardiology/American Heart Association

- ACC/AHA 2007 Guidelines of the Management of Patients with Unstable Angina/Non-ST-Elevation Myocardial Infarction. J Am Coll Cardiol 2007; 50: e1-e157.
- Antman EM, Anbe DT, Armstrong PW, Bates ER, Green LA, Hand M, Hochman JS, Krumholz HM, Kushner FG, Lamas GA, Mullany CJ, Ornato JP, Pearle DL, Sloan MA, Smith SC Jr. ACC/AHA guidelines for the management ©2004 by the American College of Cardiology Foundation and the American Heart Association, Inc. of patients with ST-elevation myocardial infarction: a report of the American College of Cardiology/American Heart Association Task Force on Practice Guidelines (Committee to Revise the 1999 Guidelines for the Management of Patients With Acute Myocardial Infarction). 2004. Available at http://www.acc.org/clinical/guidelines/stemi/index.pdf.
- 2007 Focused Update of the ACC/AHA 2004 Guidelines of the Management of Patients With ST-Elevation Myocardial Infarction. J Am Coll Cardiol 2008; 51: 210-47.

ACKNOWLEDGEMENTS

We wish to thank Karli Goodwin for her excellent technical support.

Table 12.3. Selected drugs for acute coronary syndrome

Drug	Start dose	Maintenance dose	Pharmacokinetics (and PK in elderly)	Metabolism	Interactions/ ADRs	Practice tips	Dose adjustment?
Aspirin	300 mg	75–150 mg daily	$T_{1/2}$ 30 min, salicylate 2–3 hrs Saturable at very high doses Aspirin is an irreversible inhibitor of thromboxane A_2, and therefore has a duration of action dependent upon platelet turnover	ASA – Hepatic Salicylate – Renal	Increased bleeding risk with anti-coagulants	Elderly more prone to bleeding side effects Can exacerbate gout	None
Clopidogrel	300 mg	75 mg daily	$T_{1/2}$ 8 hrs Clopidogrel is an irreversible inhibitor of ADP binding, and therefore has a duration of action dependent upon platelet turnover	**Renal**/hepatic	Increased bleeding risk with anti-coagulants	Cease at least 5 days prior to cardiac surgery	None
Tirofiban (for ACS)	0.4 mcg/kg/ min for 30 min	0.1 mcg/kg/ min	$T_{1/2}$ 1.4–2.2 hrs	Renal	Major risk of bleeding Thrombocy-topaenia	Check Hb, plts at baseline, 6 hrs, and daily thereafter	Halve dose for CrCL <30 ml/min Current guidelines do not recommend dose reduction in the elderly, although CL is known to be reduced by 19-26%
Eptifibatide (for ACS)	180 mcg/kg bolus	2 mcg/kg/ min	$T_{1/2}$ 2.5 hrs	**Hepatic**/Renal	Major risk of bleeding	Check Hb, plts at baseline, 6 hrs, and daily thereafter	Contraindicated if CrCL<30 ml/min

	Bolus/initial dose	Maintenance	Pharmacokinetics	Metabolism/ elimination	Major risks	Cautions	Elderly
Abciximab (for ACS)	0.25 mg/kg	10 mcg/min	$T_{1/2}$ 30 min $T_{1/2}$ is shorter in subjects with an active thrombotic episode than in healthy volunteers	Platelet binding	Major risk of bleeding Thrombocytopaenia	Complex heparin protocol Check plts at baseline, 2–4 hrs, and 24 hrs	None
Heparin (unfractionated)	Bolus: 60–70 units/kg (max 5000u) Initial: 12–15 units/kg/hr (max 1000 units/hr)	Maintenance: adjust according to aPTT	$T_{1/2}$ 1–5 hrs saturable	**Reticulo-endothelial** and renal	Increased bleeding risk Can cause thrombocytopaenia +/− prothrombotic state		Dose reduction for elderly is recommended
Enoxaparin	1 mg/kg BD (max 100 mg BD)	1 mg/kg BD (max 100 mg BD)	$T_{1/2}$ 4 hrs, elderly 6–7 hrs saturable	Renal	Increased bleeding risk Lesser risk of thrombocytopaenia cf UFH	Can accumulate with prolonged use	Once daily dosing if CrCL<30 ml.min No reduction in elderly per se
Streptokinase	1.5×10^6 IU over 30–60 min	none	$T_{1/2}$ 23 min	Unknown	Major risk of bleeding	Do not use if >5 days and <12 months since previous streptokinase therapy, or after serious streptococcal infections	None
Tenecteplase	6000–10000 IU over 10 sec (weight based)	none	$T_{1/2}$ 24 min	Hepatic	Major risk of bleeding	Must have heparin concomitantly and for 24 hours following	None

(continued overleaf)

Table 12.3. (*Continued*)

Drug	Start dose	Maintenance dose	Pharmacokinetics (and PK in elderly)	Metabolism	Interactions/ADRs	Practice tips	Dose adjustment?
Alteplase (accelerated)	10–15 mg bolus (weight-based)	0.75 mg/kg (max 50 mg) over 30 min 0.5 mg/kg (max 35 mg) over 60 min	$T_{1/2}$ 5 min	Hepatic	Major risk of bleeding	Must have heparin concomitantly and for 24 hours following	None
Reteplase	10 U bolus over 2 min	10 U bolus over 2 min at 30 min	$T_{1/2}$ 18 min	Unknown	Major risk of bleeding	Must have heparin concomitantly and for 24 hours following	None
Glyceryl trinitrate	5 mcg/min	titrate	$T_{1/2}$ 1–4 min	Hydrolysis in plasma	Elderly more prone to dose-related side effects, eg headache, hypotension, bradycardia	Use non-PVC tubing Alcohol intoxication has been seen at very high doses	None
Metoprolol (oral)	25–50 mg BD	12.5–100 mg BD	$T_{1/2}$ 3–5 hrs	Hepatic	Bradycardia Impotence Nightmares Elderly more prone to postural symptoms, lethargy		None
Atenolol (oral)	12.5–25 mg daily	25–50 mg daily	$T_{1/2}$ 7–9 hrs	Renal	Bradycardia Impotence Elderly more prone to postural symptoms, lethargy	Accumulation may occur in severe renal impairment	None

Drug	Starting dose	Dose range	T½	Elimination	Side effects	Monitoring	Notes
Perindopril	1–2 mg daily	2–4 mg daily	T$_{1/2}$ 25–30 hrs	Renal	Cough, Hyperkalaemia, Renal Failure, Postural hypotension, Angioedema	Electrolytes should be checked within 1 week	Lower starting dose in the elderly and in renal impairment
Ramipril	1.25–2.5 mg daily	1.25–10 mg daily	T$_{1/2}$ 9–18 hrs	Renal	Cough, Hyperkalaemia, Renal Failure, Postural hypotension, Angioedema	Electrolytes should be checked within 1 week	Lower starting dose in the elderly and in renal impairment
Enalapril	2.5–5.0 mg daily If possible discontinue diuretics prior	10–40 mg daily (divided doses required in some)	T$_{1/2}$ 35–38 hrs	Renal	Cough, Hyperkalaemia, Renal Failure, Postural hypotension, Angioedema	Electrolytes should be checked within 1 week	Lower starting dose in the elderly and in renal impairment
Captopril	6.25 mg daily	25–50 mg TDS	T$_{1/2}$ 1–2 hrs	Renal	Cough, Hyperkalaemia, Renal Failure, Postural hypotension, Angioedema	Electrolytes should be checked within 1 week	Lower starting dose in the elderly and in renal impairment
Fosinopril	10 mg daily	10–40 mg daily	T$_{1/2}$ 11.5–14 hrs	**Renal/Hepatic** (minor)	Cough, Hyperkalaemia, Renal Failure, Postural hypotension, Angioedema	Electrolytes should be checked within 1 week	Lower starting dose in the elderly and in renal impairment

(continued overleaf)

Table 12.3. (*Continued*)

Drug	Start dose	Maintenance dose	Pharmacokinetics (and PK in elderly)	Metabolism	Interactions/ ADRs	Practice tips	Dose adjustment?
Trandolapril	0.5–1 mg daily	1–4 mg daily	$T_{1/2}$ 22 hrs	Renal	Cough Hyperkalaemia Renal Failure Postural hypotension Angioedema	Electrolytes should be checked within 1 week	Lower starting dose in the elderly and in renal impairment
Lisinopril	2.5–5 mg daily	5–10 mg daily	$T_{1/2}$ 11–12 hrs	Renal	Cough Hyperkalaemia Renal Failure Postural hypotension Angioedema	Electrolytes should be checked within 1 week	Lower starting dose in the elderly and in renal impairment
Quinapril	2.5–5 mg daily	10–20 mg daily	$T_{1/2}$ 25 hrs	Renal	Cough Hyperkalaemia Renal Failure Postural hypotension Angioedema	Electrolytes should be checked within 1 week	Lower starting dose in the elderly and in renal impairment
Atorvastatin	80 mg daily	10–80 mg daily	$T_{1/2}$ 14 hrs	Hepatic CYP 3A4	Hepatitis Myopathy	Baseline LFTs and periodically thereafter	None

REFERENCES

1. Lee PY, Alexander KP, Hammill BG, Pasquali SK, Peterson ED. Representation of elderly persons and women in published randomized trials of acute coronary syndromes. *JAMA* 2001; **286**: 708–13.
2. Erhardt L, Herlitz J, Bossaert L et al. Task force on the management of chest pain. *Eur.Heart J*. 2002; **23**: 1153–76.
3. Hamm CW, Braunwald E. A classification of unstable angina revisited. *Circulation* 2000; **102**: 118–22.
4. Yusuf S, Zhao F, Mehta SR, Chrolavicius S, Tognoni G, Fox KK. Effects of clopidogrel in addition to aspirin in patients with acute coronary syndromes without ST-segment elevation. *N.Engl.J Med* 2001; **345**: 494–502.
5. Chen ZM, Jiang LX, Chen YP et al. Addition of clopidogrel to aspirin in 45,852 patients with acute myocardial infarction: randomised placebo-controlled trial. *Lancet* 2005; **366**: 1607–21.
6. James S, Armstrong P, Califf R et al. Safety and efficacy of abciximab combined with dalteparin in treatment of acute coronary syndromes. *Eur.Heart J* 2002; **23**: 1538–45.
7. Chen ZM, Pan HC, Chen YP et al. Early intravenous then oral metoprolol in 45,852 patients with acute myocardial infarction: randomised placebo-controlled trial. *Lancet* 2005; **366**: 1622–32.
8. de Boer MJ, Ottervanger JP, van't Hof AW, Hoorntje JC, Suryapranata H, Zijlstra F. Reperfusion therapy in elderly patients with acute myocardial infarction: a randomized comparison of primary angioplasty and thrombolytic therapy. *J.Am.Coll.Cardiol*. 2002; **39**: 1723–8.

13 Heart failure

Arduino Mangoni

Department of Clinical Pharmacology, Flinders Medical Centre, Adelaide, Australia

INTRODUCTION

Heart failure (HF) is defined traditionally as an inability of the heart to deliver blood and oxygen at a rate commensurate with the requirements of the peripheral tissues despite normal or increased cardiac filling pressures. This abnormality may be acute or chronic and usually arises as a consequence of a myocardial, valvular, pericardial, endocardial or electrical problem (or some combination of these) (1).

EPIDEMIOLOGY

HF affects mainly the elderly population. The prevalence of symptomatic HF ranges from 0.4 to 2.0 % but it increases from < 1 % in adults < 50 years to > 10 % in persons over > 80 years (2). In Europe, the mean age of the HF population is 74 years. As the proportion of the elderly population is increasing, this partly accounts for the rising prevalence of HF. Unlike other common cardiovascular disorders, the age-adjusted mortality attributed to HF is also increasing. In USA, HF is currently the leading indication for hospitalization among elderly subjects, as well as the most costly cardiovascular disorder in the Medicare population. Over the next 30 years, the number of persons > 65 years is expected to double, with the largest relative growth occurring in the population over age 85. As a result, it may be anticipated that the social burden of HF in the elderly population will increase

dramatically, especially among the subjects > 85 years (Figure 13.1).

The prognosis of HF is poor. Once symptomatic, the two-year mortality is about 35 %. Over the next six years, it increases to 80 % for men and 65 % for women. The presence and severity of symptoms predict outcome. The yearly risk of death with mild to moderate symptoms is 5–10 %, vs. 30–40 % with severe symptoms. After an episode of pulmonary oedema, only 50 % survive one year or longer. Following cardiogenic shock, 50–85 % of patients die within one week. The New York Heart Association (NYHA) HF class is the most widely used prognostic scale. Despite poor sensitivity and high inter-observer variability, the scale is useful for predicting mortality (Table 13.1). Elderly patients, once rated as NYHA class IV, have a one-year mortality > 50 %.

AETIOLOGY

The age-related increase in HF is attributable to 1) the effects of ageing on the cardiovascular system and other organ systems; and 2) the high prevalence of hypertension, ischaemic heart disease, and valvular heart disease in elderly subjects. Increasing age is associated with significant changes in cardiovascular structure and function, such as arterial stiffening and an increase in ventricular wall thickness and myocardial interstitial collagen content. These abnormalities significantly impact on diastolic

Prescribing for Elderly Patients   Edited by Stephen Jackson, Paul Jansen and Arduino Mangoni

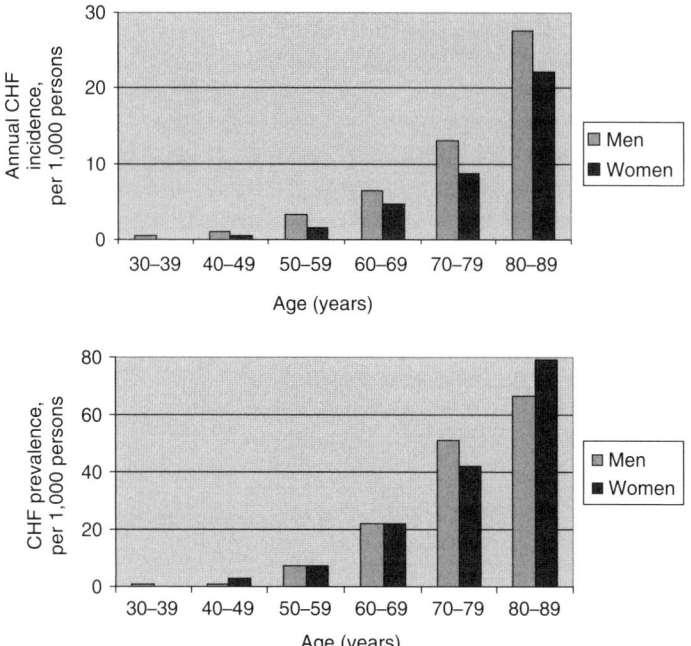

Figure 13.1. Incidence (upper panel) and prevalence (lower panel) rates of congestive heart failure (CHF) among Framingham Heart Study subjects, by gender and age

function, resulting in impaired ventricular relaxation and increased left ventricular wall stiffness. Resting systolic function is well preserved and measures of cardiac function are unaffected by age in healthy patients. However, there is a significant reduction in cardiovascular reserve, such that the ageing heart is less able to compensate in response to stressful stimuli (i.e. ischaemia, hypoxia, infection, vigorous exercise), thus predisposing to the onset and progression of HF. In addition, there is an increasing prevalence of systolic hypertension and ischaemic heart disease with advancing age. Systolic hypertension is the most important risk factor for

HF in elderly women, accounting for up to 60 % of cases. In elderly men, hypertension and ischaemic heart disease, singly or in combination, account for over 70 % of HF cases. Aortic stenosis, mitral regurgitation, and cardiac amyloidosis are also important causes of HF in elderly subjects.

Traditionally, abnormal systolic function with impaired contractility and left ventricular ejection fraction (LVEF) < 40 % have been regarded as the hallmark of HF. However, an important feature which often differentiates HF in elderly subjects from HF in young and middle-aged adults is the increasing proportion

Table 13.1. The New York Heart Association classification of heart failure symptoms

Class I	No limitations. Ordinary physical activity does not cause fatigue, breathlessness or palpitation. (Asymptomatic left ventricular dysfunction is included in this category).
Class II	Slight limitation of physical activity. Such patients are comfortable at rest. Ordinary physical activity results in fatigue, palpitation, breathlessness or angina pectoris (symptomatically 'mild' heart failure).
Class III	Marked limitation of physical activity. Although patients are comfortable at rest, less than ordinary physical activity will lead to symptoms (symptomatically 'moderate' heart failure).
Class IV	Inability to carry on any physical activity without discomfort. Symptoms of heart failure are present even at rest. With any physical activity increased discomfort is experienced (symptomatically 'severe' heart failure).

of cases that occur in the setting of normal left ventricular systolic function. This syndrome, often referred to as 'diastolic HF', accounts for about 30–50 % of all HF cases. Diastolic HF is relatively rare in persons under age 65 (< 10 % of HF cases), whereas more than 50 % of HF patients ≥ 70 years have preserved left ventricular systolic function (Table 13.2). Diastolic HF exhibits a particular predilection for older women, among whom it accounts for about two thirds of prevalent HF cases. This reflects in part the dominant role of hypertension as the causative factor of HF in this group. Although diastolic HF is somewhat less common in older men, it still accounts for about 40 % of cases. The high prevalence of diastolic HF in the elderly population has important implications for HF management as only a minority of the HF trials reported to date have specifically focused on this syndrome (3).

CLINICAL PRESENTATION

Exercise-induced dyspnoea, orthopnoea, and fatigue are the typical symptoms of HF. However, they may be difficult to interpret in elderly patients because of the frequent coexistence of co-morbidities that render the 'typical' symptoms of HF relatively nonspecific.

In addition, atypical symptoms such as cognitive impairment, confusion, irritability, nausea, and anorexia become increasingly common presentation of HF in elderly subjects. In some cases, they may be the sole manifestation of HF. Inter-observer agreement on the presence or absence of symptoms of HF is often low. Moreover, there is no standard questionnaire available for the diagnosis of HF. The available scoring systems have not yet been validated and cannot be recommended for clinical practice.

The presence of S_3 gallop rhythm, respiratory crepitations, elevated jugular venous pressure, and leg oedema are the most common physical findings in patients with HF. However, as with symptoms, the sensitivity and specificity decreases with advancing age. For example, respiratory crepitations may be secondary to chronic obstructive pulmonary disease or bronchiectasis, and leg oedema may be caused by venous insufficiency or posture.

DIAGNOSIS

The clinical suspicion of HF must be confirmed by objective tests assessing cardiac structure and function.

Electrocardiogram (ECG)

Electrocardiographic abnormalities are common in patients with HF. The negative predictive value of a normal ECG to rule out left ventricular systolic dysfunction is > 90 %. At the same time, the presence of anterior Q-waves and left bundle branch block in patients with ischaemic heart disease are good predictors of reduced LVEF. ECG signs of left atrial overload and/or left ventricular hypertrophy may be associated with systolic as well as isolated diastolic dysfunction but they have a low predictive value.

The ECG is a crucial tool for the detection of atrial fibrillation or flutter, and sometimes ventricular arrhythmia, all of which are considered causative or contributive factors for HF.

Chest X-ray (CXR)

CXR is useful to detect the presence of pulmonary venous congestion as well as other respiratory conditions causing dyspnoea. A cardiothoracic ratio > 0.50, in addition to pulmonary venous congestion, is a useful indicator

Table 13.2. Prevalence of systolic and diastolic dysfunction according to age

Variable	45–64	55–64	65–74	≥ 75
Mild diastolic dysfunction	4.8	13.2	34.2	52.8
Moderate diastolic dysfunction	1.4	6.0	9.9	14.6
Severe diastolic dysfunction	0	0.4	0.7	3.4
Systolic dysfunction, ejection fraction ≤ 50 %	3.0	4.8	7.1	12.9
Systolic dysfunction, ejection fraction ≤ 40 %	0.8	1.3	2.7	4.4

of abnormal cardiac function with decreased ejection fraction and/or elevated left ventricular filling pressure. Unilateral or bilateral pleural effusions are also common. Interstitial/alveolar pulmonary oedema is a reliable sign of severe left ventricular dysfunction. However, it must be stressed that the CXR findings must be interpreted in the context of the clinical and ECG findings.

Natriuretic peptides

An important advance in the diagnostic evaluation of patients with suspected HF is the measurement of the blood concentration of B-type natriuretic peptide (BNP) (4). BNP is a neurohormone released from the cardiac ventricles in response to increased wall tension. BNP measurement has been shown to be useful in ruling out HF in patients with dyspnoea in primary care and emergency departments. Although the diagnostic potential of BNP is less clear-cut when systolic function is normal, there is increasing evidence that elevated levels occur in the presence of diastolic dysfunction. Importantly, female gender and advancing age are also associated with elevated BNP levels. Nonetheless, a BNP level < 100 pg/mL makes the presence of HF unlikely. A BNP level ≥ 400 pg/mL strongly suggests the presence of HF whereas levels in the range of 100–400 pg/mL are non-diagnostic. Elevated BNP levels are also observed in subjects with left ventricular hypertrophy, valvular heart disease, acute or chronic ischaemic heart disease, hypertension, pulmonary embolism, and renal failure (4).

Elevated BNP levels are associated with an increased risk of morbidity and mortality in HF. However, the role of serial BNP measurements to monitor the response to treatment has not yet been established, but is presently being investigated.

Echocardiography

Transthoracic Doppler Echocardiography is the preferred method to document the presence of cardiac dysfunction. The most important measurement of cardiac function is represented by the LVEF, which allows distinguishing between patients with systolic dysfunction (LVEF ≤ 40 %) from patients with preserved systolic function. The diagnosis of 'diastolic' HF is generally based on the presence of symptoms and signs of HF in a patient who is shown to have normal LVEF and no valvular abnormalities on echocardiography. Further research in this area is required though (5).

Exercise or pharmacologic stress testing with echocardiographic imaging should be considered in ambulant patients with moderate or high likelihood for having concomitant ischaemic heart disease, especially those who are suitable candidates for revascularization procedures.

THERAPY

The optimal management of HF in elderly patients involves control of risk factors, patient education and self-management, and the judicious use of medications. The goals of therapy are to relieve symptoms, improve quality of life, reduce the need for hospitalization, and prolong survival (1).

General measures

Hypertension, diabetes, and dyslipidaemia must be treated aggressively in accordance with established guidelines. Use of tobacco products must be discontinued and alcohol should be used in moderation (no more of one to two standard drinks daily) or not at all. Elderly patients with severe ischaemic heart disease confirmed by noninvasive testing should undergo coronary angiography and, if needed, percutaneous or surgical revascularization. Patients with other treatable conditions that may exacerbate HF (i.e. anaemia, thyroid disease, arrhythmias) should be managed appropriately (Table 13.3). Several classes of drugs can exacerbate HF and should be avoided whenever possible (Table 13.4).

Serum potassium should be monitored carefully as both hypo- and hyperkalaemia adversely affect cardiac excitability and conduction and increase the risk of malignant arrhythmias and sudden death. Correction of hypokalaemia may require supplementation of magnesium and potassium. However, this strategy may be

Table 13.3. Factors potentially contributing to worsening heart failure

Cardiovascular factors
  Superimposed ischaemia or infarction
  Uncontrolled hypertension
  Unrecognized primary valve disease
  Worsening secondary mitral regurgitation
  New onset or uncontrolled atrial fibrillation
  Arrhythmias
  Pulmonary embolism

Systemic factors
  Inappropriate medications
  Superimposed infection
  Anaemia
  Uncontrolled diabetes
  Thyroid dysfunction
  Electrolyte disorders

Patient-related factors
  Medication non-compliance
  Diet
  Alcohol consumption

potentially risky in patients treated with angiotensin converting enzyme (ACE) inhibitors, angiotensin receptor blockers (ARBs) and/or aldosterone antagonists (6).

Non-adherence with diet and medications can significantly affect the clinical status of HF patients. Increases in body weight and minor changes in symptoms commonly precede by several days the occurrence of major clinical episodes requiring hospitalization. Patient education and close supervision, which includes surveillance by the patient and his or her family, can reduce the likelihood of non-adherence and lead to the detection of changes in body weight or clinical status early enough to allow the initiation of treatments that can prevent clinical deterioration. Supervision need not be performed by a physician and may ideally be accomplished by a nurse with special training in the care of patients with HF.

Pharmacological treatment of systolic HF

Symptomatic improvement has been demonstrated with digoxin, diuretics, beta blockers, ACE inhibitors, and ARBs. Prolongation of patient survival has been documented with ACE inhibitors, beta blockers, ARBs, and, in selected patients, aldosterone antagonists (i.e. spironolactone and eplerenone).

Order of therapy

The introduction of drugs for the treatment of overt HF requires a specific approach that includes both the order of therapy and attention to the clinical response as therapy is titrated. Current guidelines recommend the following sequence, with allowance for variations depending upon clinical response (Figure 13.2 and Table 13.5):

1. ACE are usually started at low doses and then titrated to goals based upon trial data as described below.
2. Beta blockers are initiated after the patient is stable on ACE inhibitors, again beginning at low doses with titration to trial goals as tolerated.
3. Diuretics can be introduced to control symptoms of fluid overload.
4. ARBs can be added to the above regimen in patients with NYHA class II-III. ARBs are also recommended in patients intolerant to ACE inhibitors.
5. Spironolactone or eplerenone should be added to the above regimen in HF patients with NYHA class IV.
6. Digoxin may be considered in: 1) patients who continue to have symptoms of HF despite the above regimen; and 2) patients with atrial fibrillation (rate control).
7. The combination of hydralazine and nitrates may be an alternative to ARBs in black patients.

ACE inhibitors

ACE inhibitors improve survival in patients with different severities of HF, ranging from asymptomatic left ventricular dysfunction to moderate or severe HF, with or without ischaemic heart disease. These drugs should be prescribed to all patients with HF unless they have a contraindication to their use or have been shown to be unable to tolerate the treatment (7).

Beginning therapy with low doses reduces the risk of hypotension and pre-renal failure, particularly if the concomitant diuretic therapy

Table 13.4. Drugs that should be avoided in patients with HF

- Anti-arrhythmic agents
  - Cardiodepressant and pro-arrhythmic effects (only amiodarone and dofetilide have been shown not to affect survival).
- Calcium channel blockers
  - Worsening HF and increased risk of cardiovascular events
- Nonsteroidal anti-inflammatory drugs
  - Sodium retention and peripheral vasoconstriction
  - Attenuate the efficacy of diuretics and ACE-inhibitors
- Thiazolidinediones
  - Fluid retention
- Metformin
  - Increased risk of lactic acidosis, especially in the presence of haemodynamic instability, renal and/or liver failure, or severe infection with decreased tissue perfusion
- Sildenafil
  - Potentially hazardous in HF patients with low blood pressure and/or volume depletion

is stopped 24–48 hours before the first dose of ACE inhibitor and re-instated thereafter. If the initial therapy is tolerated, the dose is then gradually increased to a maintenance dose unless side effects occur.

Maintenance doses are recommended because they have been used in clinical trials, although there is some uncertainty if these doses are more beneficial than lower doses. Renal function should be assessed within one to two weeks of initiation of therapy and periodically thereafter, especially in patients with pre-existing hypotension, hyponatraemia, diabetes, or in those taking potassium supplements.

Although most large-scale randomized trials with ACE inhibitors have included highly selected elderly patients without significant co-morbidities, community-based observational studies support a benefit from ACE inhibitors in elderly patients with HF that is similar in magnitude to that seen in younger patients. The benefit is significant even in those who have a perceived contraindication to ACE inhibitors (i.e. systolic blood pressure ≤ 90 mmHg, serum creatinine ≥ 220 μmol/L, *serum potassium* ≥ 5.5 mmol/L, and severe aortic stenosis). Treatment with ACE inhibitors induces a significant increase in serum creatinine (e.g. > 0.03 mmol/L) in 15–30 % of patients with severe HF, but only in 5–15 % of patients with mild-to-moderate symptoms. Renal function usually improves after a reduction in the dose of concomitantly administered diuretics. Therefore, these patients can generally be managed

without the need to withdraw treatment with ACE inhibitors. However, if the dose of diuretic cannot be reduced because of fluid retention, a mild-moderate degree of azotemia can be tolerated in order to maintain therapy with ACE inhibitors.

Although it is generally recommended that therapy with an ACE inhibitor should be instituted before beta blockade is implemented, the results of a recent trial in patients ≥ 65 years (CIBIS-III) show that treatment with the beta-blocker bisoprolol before commencing ACE inhibitor therapy provides similar benefits (8).

Beta blockers

The beta blockers carvedilol, metoprolol, bisoprolol, and nebivolol improve overall and event-free survival in HF patients with NYHA class II–III and, probably, class IV. The benefits of nebivolol in elderly patients have been recently demonstrated (9). The different beta blockers have distinct pharmacologic properties; metoprolol has a high degree of specificity for the β_1 adrenergic receptor, while carvedilol blocks β_1, β_2, and α_1 adrenergic receptors, and nevibolol selectively blocks the β_1 adrenergic receptor and exerts vasodilator effects (10).

The controlled trials on beta-blockers in HF, however, excluded patients with the following relative contraindications to beta blocker therapy.

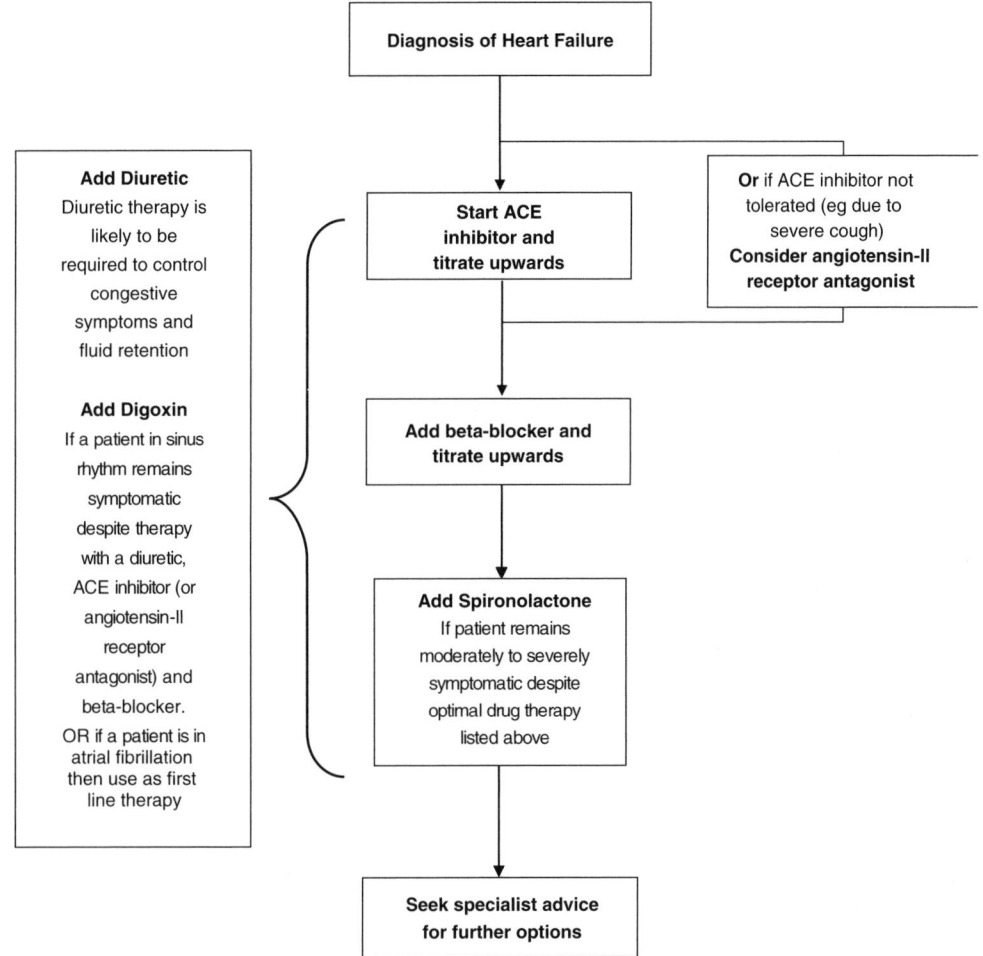

Figure 13.2. Pharmacological treatment of systolic HF

- Heart rate < 60 b/min.
- Systolic blood pressure < 100 mmHg.
- Severe peripheral vascular disease.
- PR interval > 0.24 sec on ECG.
- Second- or third-degree atrioventricular block.
- Severe chronic obstructive pulmonary disease.
- History of asthma.

Because of these issues and the risk of transient worsening of symptoms, it is recommended that beta blocker therapy be initiated under strict clinical guidance. Among inpatients, initiation of therapy prior to hospital discharge improves beta blocker use without an increase in side effects or drug discontinuation. Prior to initiation of therapy, the patient should have no or minimal evidence of fluid retention and should not have required recent intravenous inotropic therapy. The patient should be informed that beta blockers may lead to worsening of symptoms for four to 10 weeks before any improvement is noted. Therapy should start at very low doses and the dose doubled every two to three weeks, until the target dose is reached or symptoms become limiting.

Every effort should be made to achieve the target dose since the improvement appears to be dose-dependent. The proportion of patients who reach the target dose is higher in clinical trials than in the general population. However,

Table 13.5. Pharmacological treatment of HF

Drug	Start dose	Maximal dose	Pharmacokinetics t1/2	Metabolism	Interactions	Important adverse events	Other tips
Chlorthalidone	12.5–25 mg od	50 mg od	Y: ~50 hrs E: ~110 hrs	Renal	↑lithium levels	Gout[a]	Avoid if creatinine clearance <30 ml/min
Hydrochlorothiazide	12.5–25 mg od	100 mg od	Y: 6–15 hrs E: 10–11 hrs	Renal	↑lithium levels	Postural hypotension[a]	Avoid if creatinine clearance <30 ml/min
Metolazone	5–10 mg od	80 mg od	Y: 8–14 hrs E: NA	Renal	↑lithium levels	Urinary urgency[a]	May produce diuresis even if clearance <20 ml/min
Bumetanide	0.5–1 mg od or bd	10 mg od	Y: ~1.5 hrs E: ~1.7 hrs	Renal	↑lithium levels	Hypokalaemia[a]	Beware of renal impairment if ACE inhibitor is coadministered
Frusemide	20–40 mg od or bd	1000 mg od	Y: ~1.5 hrs E: ~1.7 hrs	Renal	↑lithium levels	Hyponatraemia[a]	Beware of renal impairment if ACE inhibitor is coadministered
Torasemide	5 mg od	40 mg od	Y: 3.5 hrs E: NA	Hepatic CYP2C9	↑lithium levels	Hyperuricaemia[a]	Beware of renal impairment if ACE inhibitor is coadministered
Eplerenone	25 mg od	50 mg od	Y: 3.2–6.8 hrs E: NA	Hepatic CYP3A4	↑levels with CYP3A4 inhibitors ↓levels with CYP3A4 activators	Hyperkalaemia[b] Diarrhoea[b] Hypotension Nausea[b]	Check blood chemistry at 1, 4, 8, and 12 weeks; 6, 9, and 12 months, 6 monthly thereafter If K^+ rises between 5.5 and 5.9 mmol/L or creatinine rises to 200 μmol/L reduce dose to 25 mg on alternate days and monitor blood chemistry closely[b]
Spironolactone	25 mg od	50 mg od	Y: 13–24 hrs (canrenone) E: NA	Hepatic	↑digoxin levels	Gynaecomastia[b]	

Drug	Starting dose	Target dose	Half-life	Metabolism	Interactions	Side effects	Comments
Captopril	6.25 mg tds	25–75 mg bd	Y: 1–2 hrs E: 1.4 hrs	Renal	↑lithium levels	Hypotension Cough Hyperkalaemia Nausea[c]	An increase in creatinine of up to 50% above baseline, or to 200 μmol/L, whichever is the smaller, is acceptable[d]
Enalapril	2.5 mg od	10–20 mg od	Y: 11 hrs E: ~19 hrs		↑lithium levels		An increase in K^+ <5.9 mmol/L is acceptable[d]
Lisinopril	2.5 mg od	20 mg od	Y: 12.6 hrs E: NA		↑lithium levels	Renal impairment[c]	Advise patients that the treatment is likely to improve symptoms within a few weeks to a few months[d]
Ramipril	1.25 mg od	10 mg od	Y: 13–17 hrs E: NA		↑lithium levels		Assess for hyperkalaemia during treatment Onset of ACE inhibitor associated angioedema may not occur for several years[d]
Bisoprolol	1.25 mg od	10 mg od	Y: 10–12 hrs E: NA	Renal and hepatic	-	Bronchospasm, Dyspnoea[e]	Advise patients that symptomatic improvement may develop slowly (over 3–6 month or longer)[f]
Carvedilol	3.125 mg bd	25–50 mg bd	Y: 6–10 hrs E: 5–14	Hepatic	-	Cold extremities[e] Bradycardia Heart block Hypotension[e]	Before starting beta-blocker therapy, optimise conventional treatments[f]
Metoprolol XL	23.75 mg od	190 mg od	Y: 4 hrs E: 8 hrs	Hepatic CYP2D6	↓lercanidipine concentrations ↓levels with phenobarbitone	Fatigue[e]	Reduce dose if heart rate is <55 beats/minute Treat transient worsening of HF with increased doses of diuretics Do not stop beta-blockers abruptly; halve dose each week[f]
Candesartan	4–8 mg od	32 mg od	Y: 9 hrs E: 9–12 hrs	Renal	-	Hypotension and hyperkalaemia	-

(continued overleaf)

Table 13.5. (*Continued*)

Drug	Start dose	Maximal dose	Pharmacokinetics t1/2	Metabolism	Interactions	Important adverse events	Other tips
Valsartan	40 mg bd	160 mg bd	Y: 9 hrs E: 7–9 hrs	Hepatic		Hypotension and hyperkalaemia	Consider lower dose in mild to moderate hepatic impairment
Digoxin	62.5–125 μg od	125–250 μg od	Y: 34–44 hrs E: 55–85 hrs	Renal	↑levels with amiodarone, diltiazem, verapamil, and spironolactone ↓levels with St John's Wort	Anorexia, nausea, vomiting, diarrhoea, visual disturbances, cognitive impairment, drowsiness, dizziness, nightmares, agitation, depression, arrhythmias	Assess renal function before and during treatment
Hydralazine	25 mg tds or qds	50–75 mg qds	Y: 2–3 hrs E: NA	Liver	–	Flushing, headache, dizziness, tachycardia, palpitations, oedema	Prolonged treatment may induce a lupus-like syndrome; check antinuclear factor before and during treatment
Isosorbide dinitrate	20–40 mg tds or qds	20–40 mg tds or qds	Y: 1.1–7.7 hrs E: NA	Liver	–	Headache, flushing, palpitations, orthostatic hypotension, syncope, peripheral oedema	Tolerance to nitrates occurs with frequent or continuous exposure; avoid by ensuring a nitrate-free interval of 10–12 hours each day

[a]These adverse events are common with Chlorthalidone, Hydrochlorothiazide, Metolazone, Bumetanide, Frusemide, Torasemide.
[b]These are common with both eplerenone and spironolactone.
[c]These are common to captopril, enalapril, lisinopril, ramipril.
[d]These are common to captopril, enalapril, lisinopril, ramipril.
[e]These are common to bisoprolol, carvedilol, metoprolol XL.
[f]These are common to bisoprolol, carvedilol, metoprolol XL.

although not optimal, even low doses appear to be of benefit and should be used when higher doses are not tolerated.

The patient should monitor his/her body weight daily and contact the physician if there has been a 1–1.5 kg weight gain. Weight gain alone may be treated with diuretics, but resistant oedema or more severe decompensation may require dose reduction or cessation, possibly transient, of the beta blocker.

The beta blocker trials in HF were carried out in patients receiving therapy with an ACE inhibitor; thus, the improvement in survival is additive to that induced by ACE inhibitors.

Although data about the duration of beta blocker therapy in HF are lacking, it has been suggested that patients who are doing well should not have the beta blocker withdrawn, since clinical deterioration and sudden death or death from progressive HF has been observed in these circumstances.

Diuretics

Diuretic therapy can typically control fluid overload and improve symptoms at any stage during the treatment of elderly patients with HF. These effects occur within hours to days. In comparison, the clinical effects of ACE inhibitors and beta blockers may require weeks or months to become fully apparent. There have been no long-term studies of diuretic therapy in HF and their effects on morbidity and mortality are not known.

Diuretic usage may affect the efficacy of other drugs given for the treatment of HF. Inappropriately low doses will result in fluid retention, which can diminish the response to ACE inhibitors and ARBs and increase the risk of decompensation with the use of beta blockers. Conversely, excessive diuresis will lead to volume contraction with 1) increased risk of hypotension and renal insufficiency with ACE inhibitors, ARBs, and beta blockers; and 2) reflex activation of the sympathetic nervous system and the renin-angiotensin system with an increased risk of arrhythmias and ischaemia.

Loop diuretics have significant advantages over thiazide diuretics in the treatment of HF

because they increase sodium excretion up to 20–25 % of the filtered load (compared with the 5–10 % increase observed with thiazides), enhance free water clearance, and maintain their efficacy unless renal function is severely impaired. However, thiazide diuretics may be the preferred option in hypertensive HF patients because of their longer half-life, provided that the creatinine clearance is ≥ 40 ml/min.

Frusemide is the most commonly used loop diuretic for the treatment of HF. However, some patients respond better to bumetanide or torasemide because of superior bioavailability and longer duration of action. A reasonable goal is weight reduction of 0.5–1.0 kg/day. If a patient does not respond, the diuretic dose should initially be increased to find the single effective dose, rather than giving the same dose twice a day. Diuretics are usually combined with moderate dietary sodium restriction (3–4 g daily).

Intravenous loop diuretics, both as a bolus or a continuous infusion, are effective in the presence of significant interstitial oedema of the gastrointestinal tract and may be required for severe HF. In this context, thiazide diuretics can be added for a synergistic effect.

An excessive reduction in intra-cardiac filling pressure during diuretic therapy may lower the cardiac output via the Frank-Starling relationship. This effect is usually minor and does not interfere with therapy. However, an otherwise unexplained rise in serum urea and creatinine should be viewed as a sign of a potentially important reduction in tissue perfusion. Further diuresis should be performed only with careful monitoring for signs and symptoms attributable to hypoperfusion.

Over the long term, diuretic therapy should be maintained to prevent recurrent oedema. In many cases, this adjustment can be facilitated by having the patient record his or her weight each day and allowing him or her to make changes in dose if the weight increases or decreases beyond a specified range.

Angiotensin receptor blockers (ARBs)

The experience with ARBs in controlled clinical trials of patients with HF is considerably less than that with ACE inhibitors (11). Current guidelines state that ARBs should not be used in preference to an ACE inhibitor for the treatment of HF in patients who have no prior use of an ACE inhibitor and should not be substituted for ACE inhibitors in patients who are tolerating ACE inhibitors without difficulty. ARBs should be used in patients with NYHA class II–III who cannot tolerate ACE inhibitors. Data from large-scale randomized clinical trials have demonstrated that both valsartan and candesartan are effective in this setting.

Combined therapy with candesartan and an ACE inhibitor has been shown to reduce mortality and hospitalization rates in patients with NYHA class II–III. Therefore, if tolerated, ARBs should be added to a regimen including ACE inhibitors and beta blockers in patients with NYHA class II–III.

Digoxin

The use of digoxin is recommended 1) in patients with left ventricular systolic dysfunction who continue to have NYHA functional class II-IV symptoms despite therapy with ACE inhibitors, beta blockers, and, if necessary for fluid control, diuretics; and 2) in the presence of co-existing atrial fibrillation, to control the ventricular rate. Digoxin therapy reduces hospitalization for HF but does not provide significant survival benefits. Recent evidence suggests that the effects on survival depend on serum digoxin concentrations (i.e. improved survival for concentrations between 0.5 and 0.8 ng/mL). However, these data have been obtained retrospectively from a male population and need confirmation (12).

Aldosterone antagonists

Spironolactone and eplerenone prolong survival in selected patients with HF (13). Current guidelines recommend the use of spironolactone in patients with either current class IV HF or class III HF with a history of class IV HF within the previous six months treated with an ACE inhibitor and a loop diuretic. Eplerenone is indicated in patients with LVEF $\leq 40\%$ post-myocardial infarction. The endocrine side effects of spironolactone result from nonselective binding to androgen and progesterone receptors; eplerenone has greater specificity for the mineralocorticoid receptor and therefore has a lower incidence of endocrine side effects (1 versus 10 %). Hyperkalaemia is a common complication during treatment with aldosterone antagonists.

Hydralazine and isosorbide dinitrate

The combination of the arterial vasodilator hydralazine and the venodilator isosorbide dinitrate has been shown to reduce all-cause mortality and first HF-related hospitalization and improve quality of life in black patients with NYHA class III-IV receiving standard therapy including ACE inhibitors, beta blockers, and aldosterone antagonists. Clinical trials, however, included only a small percentage of people > 65 years (mean age 58 years). It is not clear whether the addition of hydralazine plus isosorbide dinitrate is preferable to an ARB in this setting or whether hydralazine plus isosorbide dinitrate would be beneficial in patients treated with ACE inhibitors and ARBs.

There is at present no evidence that hydralazine plus isosorbide dinitrate should be added to ACE inhibitors and beta blockers in white patients or members of other ethnic populations, although it may be reasonable to use such therapy in patients who have received the standard HF regimen and are still hypertensive.

Additional measures

Cardiac resynchronization therapy (CRT)

The current evidence supports the use of CRT in HF patients who are in sinus rhythm, have an LVEF $\leq 35\%$, a prolonged QRS duration (> 120 msec), and NYHA class III-IV despite optimal medical therapy (14). Mean patients' age in the clinical trials assessing the efficacy and safety of CRT was 64 years.

Anticoagulation

The incidence of thrombosis and embolization from the left ventricle increases as left ventricular function deteriorates. Although there are no controlled trials of warfarin or other antithrombotic agents in HF, risk models derived from large clinical trials of anticoagulation in patients with atrial fibrillation have identified HF as an important risk factor for embolization and an indication for warfarin therapy. Current guidelines recommend warfarin therapy in patients with HF who have experienced a previous embolic event or who have paroxysmal or chronic atrial fibrillation or atrial flutter. Warfarin therapy may be of benefit in selected stable patients in sinus rhythm with LVEF < 30 percent and in those with evidence of a left ventricular thrombus.

Exercise training

Cardiac rehabilitation should be offered to patients with stable NYHA class II-III HF who do not have advanced arrhythmias and who do not have other limitations to exercise. Exercise training should be used in conjunction with drug therapy. The beneficial effects of exercise are seen with high or low levels of training, and are apparent as early as three weeks after training. There are not enough data at present to recommend cardiac rehabilitation for patients with NYHA class IV HF.

Pharmacological treatment of diastolic HF

At present, the treatment of HF due to diastolic dysfunction remains empiric, since trial data do not support a specific drug or class of drugs (3). Some small short-term studies indicate that calcium channel blockers, ACE inhibitors, and ARBs might be useful in improving exercise capacity and quality of life (3). However, two large studies using the ARBs candesartan and irbesartan have failed to demonstrate any significant benefit in this population in terms of survival (15, 16). The available evidence supports the following strategies:

- Control of systolic and diastolic hypertension.
- Control of ventricular rate in patients with atrial fibrillation.
- Control of pulmonary congestion and peripheral oedema with diuretics.

- Coronary revascularization in patients with ischaemic heart disease in whom ischaemia is judged to have an adverse effect on diastolic function.

KEY POINTS

- The burden of heart failure in the elderly population will increase dramatically in the next few years, especially among subjects > 85 years.
- More than 50 % of elderly patients with heart failure have preserved left ventricular function (i.e. 'diastolic' heart failure).
- Diuretics, ACE inhibitors, and beta-blockers, if tolerated, represent the mainstay of treatment in 'systolic' heart failure.
- At present, the treatment of 'diastolic' heart failure remains largely empiric.

GUIDELINES

The Task Force for the Diagnosis and Treatment of Acute and Chronic Heart Failure 2008 of the European Society of Cardiology. ESC Guidelines for the diagnosis and treatment of acute and chronic heart failure 2008. Eur Heart J 2008; 29: 2388–442.

American College of Cardiology/American Heart Association Guidelines for the Diagnosis and Treatment of Chronic Heart Failure in the Adult (2005). http://content.onlinejacc.org/cgi/reprint/46/6/e1

ACKNOWLEDGEMENTS

I wish to thank Karli Goodwin for her excellent technical support.

REFERENCES

1. McMurray JJ, Pfeffer MA. Heart failure. *Lancet* 2005; **365**: 1877–89.
2. Ho KK, Pinsky JL, Kannel WB, Levy D. The epidemiology of heart failure: the Framingham Study. *J Am Coll Cardiol* 1993; **22**: 6A–13A.

3. Aurigemma GP, Gaasch WH. Clinical practice. Diastolic heart failure. *N Engl J Med* 2004; **351**: 1097–1105.

4. Costello-Boerrigter LC, Burnett JC, Jr. The prognostic value of N-terminal proB-type natriuretic peptide. *Nat Clin Pract Cardiovasc Med* 2005; **2**: 194–201.

5. Mottram PM, Short L, Baglin T, Marwick TH. Is 'diastolic heart failure' a diagnosis of exclusion? Echocardiographic parameters of diastolic dysfunction in patients with heart failure and normal systolic function. *Heart Lung Circ* 2003; **12**: 127–34.

6. Macdonald JE, Struthers AD. What is the optimal serum potassium level in cardiovascular patients? *J Am Coll Cardiol* 2004; **43**: 155–61.

7. McMurray JJ, Pfeffer MA, Swedberg K, Dzau VJ. Which inhibitor of the renin-angiotensin system should be used in chronic heart failure and acute myocardial infarction? *Circulation* 2004; **110**: 3281–8.

8. Willenheimer R, van Veldhuisen DJ, Silke B et al. Effect on survival and hospitalization of initiating treatment for chronic heart failure with bisoprolol followed by enalapril, as compared with the opposite sequence: results of the randomized Cardiac Insufficiency Bisoprolol Study (CIBIS) III. *Circulation* 2005; **112**: 2426–35.

9. Flather MD, Shibata MC, Coats AJ et al. Randomized trial to determine the effect of nebivolol on mortality and cardiovascular hospital admission in elderly patients with heart failure (SENIORS). *Eur Heart J* 2005; **26**: 215–25.

10. Satwani S, Dec GW, Narula J. Beta-adrenergic blockers in heart failure: review of mechanisms of action and clinical outcomes. *J Cardiovasc Pharmacol Ther* 2004; **9**: 243–55.

11. Erhardt LR. A review of the current evidence for the use of angiotensin-receptor blockers in chronic heart failure. *Int J Clin Pract* 2005; **59**: 571–8.

12. Rathore SS, Curtis JP, Wang Y, Bristow MR, Krumholz HM. Association of serum digoxin concentration and outcomes in patients with heart failure. *JAMA* 2003; **289**: 871–8.

13. Tang WH, Parameswaran AC, Maroo AP, Francis GS. Aldosterone receptor antagonists in the medical management of chronic heart failure. *Mayo Clin Proc* 2005; **80**: 1623–30.

14. Kass DA. Cardiac resynchronization therapy. *J Cardiovasc Electrophysiol* 2005; **16** Suppl 1: S35–S41.

15. Yusuf S, Pfeffer MA, Swedberg K, Granger CB, Held P, McMurray JJ, Michelson EL, Olofsson B, Ostergren J. CHARM Investigators and Committees. *Effects of candesartan in patients with chronic heart failure and preserved left-ventricular ejection fraction: the CHARM-Preserved Trial*. Lancet 2003; **362**: 777–81.

16. Massie BM, Carson PE, McMurray JJ, Komajda M, McKelvie R, Zile MR, Anderson S, Donovan M, Iverson E, Staiger C, Ptaszynska A. I-PRESERVE Investigators. Irbesartan in patients with heart failure and preserved ejection fraction. *N Engl J Med* 2008; **359**: 2456–67.

14 Atrial fibrillation and other rhythm disturbances in the elderly

Abhay Bajpai[1], Irina Savelieva[1] and A. John Camm[2]

[1] *Department of Cardiology, St George's University of London, London, UK*
[2] *Department of Clinical Cardiology, St George's University of London, London, UK*

INTRODUCTION

The population is aging and the elderly heart is vulnerable to the development of a wide range of arrhythmias which result not only from age-related physiological changes, but also from prolonged exposure to conditions such as hypertension, coronary atherosclerosis and left ventricular dysfunction. With age, there is deposition of amyloid, collagen and fibrous tissue amongst the atrial myocardium and the ventricular conduction tissue which leads to the development of both slow and fast arrhythmias such as, sick sinus syndrome, conduction blocks, atrial tachyarrhythmias and ventricular tachycardia. The following chapter focuses on the issues arising when pharmacological management of atrial fibrillation and other atrial tachyarrhythmias is undertaken.

ATRIAL ARRHYTHMIAS

Atrial fibrillation (AF) is the most commonly encountered arrhythmia in clinical practice. Atrial ectopics and short bursts of atrial tachycardia (AT) are also common findings in the elderly. Atrial flutter (AFl) occurs infrequently and is generally managed similarly to AF except that cardiac ablation strategies

are very easily used to cure this arrhythmia permanently.

THE EPIDEMIOLOGY AND COST OF AF

The Framingham Heart Study revealed a high lifetime risk for development of AF (one in four) for men and women aged 40 years or older which increased rapidly with advancing age despite the absence of antecedent structural heart disease (1). Men are 1.5 times more likely to develop AF. The number of patients with AF is likely to increase 2.5-fold during the next 50 years, reflecting the growing proportion of elderly individuals many of whom have survived cardiovascular diseases that have proved fatal in previous times. Much AF is relatively asymptomatic until complications arise. The increased use of routine electrocardiograms for the diagnosis of an irregular pulse or for pre-operative or general health checks has revealed that almost as many elderly patients have the silent form of AF as are symptomatic with this arrhythmia.

The presence of AF increases morbidity and mortality approximately two-fold, the most serious complications being stroke and heart failure.

Prescribing for Elderly Patients Edited by Stephen Jackson, Paul Jansen and Arduino Mangoni
© 2009 John Wiley & Sons, Ltd

AF and its associated morbidity represent a significant socio-economic burden on the health-care system. Presence of heart failure, concomitant coronary disease, hypertension, metabolic disease, use of class III antiarrhythmic drugs and hospitalizations are the major determinants of cost in the treatment of AF. Both AF and heart failure are recognised as modern epidemics predominantly afflicting the elderly population in western societies.

THE MECHANISM OF ATRIAL TACHYARRHYTHMIAS

The exact electrophysiological mechanisms of initiation and maintenance of AF remain controversial. AF appears to be a micro re-entry arrhythmia with multiple wavelets and daughter wavelets that randomly collide with each other. Progressive structural changes in the atria with aging are the most common cause of AF. These include atrial dilatation, atrophy or hypertrophy of atrial myocardial fibres, degenerative changes with increase in fibrous tissue and senile amyloidosis. These are associated with the genesis of atrial ectopics, paroxysmal AF or AT, which eventually results in chronic AF or AFl. The majority of AF originates from the left atrium. Recent evidence shows that "sleeves" of atrial tissue extend into the pulmonary veins and are frequently involved in the initiation of atrial arrhythmias (the basis of pulmonary vein isolation procedure for termination of AF). With advancing age, these remnants of atrial tissue may become active and trigger AT or AF. AFl, on the other hand, mostly conducts over a single anatomically distinct and therefore more organised form of re-entrant circuit and unlike AF, arises predominantly from the right atrium.

SYMPTOMS AND SIGNS

The clinical presentation of a patient varies from a chance finding of asymptomatic AF to incapacitating hemiplegia or sudden death due to thromboembolism or ventricular arrhythmia. In most instances patients notice nothing more than a general fatigue or malaise coupled with increased breathlessness and a reduction of exercise tolerance. Palpitations and chest pain are relatively infrequent symptoms in the elderly. Patients may not notice symptoms and their degraded quality of life may only be recognised after effective treatment of the condition has been instituted. Examination reveals a completely irregular pulse without any repetitive pattern (unlike that seen when frequent atrial or ventricular extrasystoles are present). Physical examination may also reveal underlying causes of AF (valvular heart disease, hypertension, hyperthyroidism, pulmonary disease, etc.). Similarly one of the potential consequences of this arrhythmia such as heart failure or stroke may also be detected.

AF is associated with a seemingly completely irregular ventricular response and when untreated the heart rate is often rapid. In the elderly, disease or damage to the atrioventricular node often causes AF to present with a normal or possibly slow heart rate even in the absence of treatment with AV nodal blocking drugs.

AFl can be triggered by AF or can arise during treatment of AF with antiarrhythmic drugs, especially class I agents such as flecainide or propafenone and sometimes with class III compounds such as amiodarone. AFl is usually stable but can degenerate into AF. It is not uncommon for the pattern to change back and forth between AF and AFl.

DIAGNOSIS

AF is easily recognized from the electrocardiogram. It is usually a narrow QRS complex arrhythmia characterized by the absence of organised P waves on the ECG which are replaced by fibrillatory (f) waves. These waves may be coarse (large amplitude) or fine (seen especially in association with longstanding AF and an enlarged heavily fibrosed left atrium). When the fibrillation is intermittent ambulatory ECG monitoring or event monitoring may be needed. Regular R-R intervals are possible when an accelerated ventricular or junctional rhythm dominates, during periods of atrioventricular

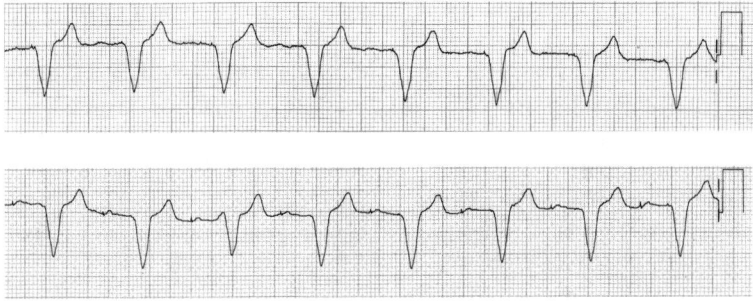

Figure 14.1. Atrial fibrillation in a patient with a permanent pacemaker (no P waves visible on the surface ECG or on the device atrial electrode). In the lower strip, note the re-appearance of atrially paced P waves following cardioversion

block or when the ventricles are permanently paced (Figure 14.1). In these situations the underlying atrial fibrillatory waves may not be noticed and AF may not be recognized. Appropriate assessment and treatment may then be overlooked. A wide QRS complex occurs when bundle branch block is present or when the ventricular rhythm arises in the ventricles (idioventricular rhythm, ventricular tachycardia or paced ventricular rhythm).

In contrast to AF, *atrial flutter* is a more organized and regular form of atrial activation due to re-entry or circular movement around the tricuspid valve ring. On the electrocardiogram this typically results in a saw-tooth pattern of flutter (F) waves at a rate of around 300 beats/minute, particularly apparent as negative waves in leads II, III and aVF, and positive deflections in lead V1. The ventricular response to atrial flutter is usually regular since every two or four flutter waves conduct to the ventricles. Occasionally a rapid rhythm (2:1 or even 1:1 AV conduction ration) may be encountered and sometimes the rhythm is "irregular" because the AV conduction ratio varies for moment to moment.

In *atrial tachycardia* the P wave rate usually ranges from 130 to 240 bpm, but unlike AFl, the P waves are separated by an isoelectric segment due to their slower rate and faster atrial depolarization (Figure 14.2). Short asymptomatic episodes of AT are common in the elderly and do not require treatment unless they begin to trigger AF. In multifocal atrial tachycardia (MAT), the P waves have varying morphology as the complexes originate from different foci. This can result in an irregularly irregular pulse mimicking AF. MAT is also associated with chronic obstructive airway disease and toxicity

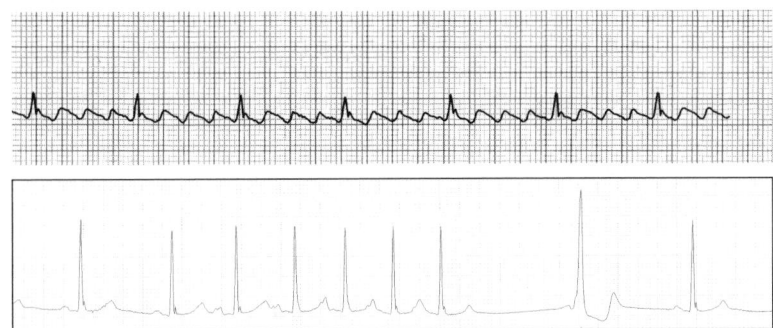

Figure 14.2. Atrial flutter and atrial tachycardia. In the top panel, flutter waves are clearly seen (saw-tooth appearence) with a consistent 4:1 conduction into the ventricles giving rise to a regular pulse. The lower panel shows a short burst of atrial tachycardia-the morphology of the P waves is different from those during sins rhythm and as the rate of tachycardia increases, P waves become superimposed over the preceding T waves

from certain drugs (digoxin, tricyclic antide-pressants and theophyllines).

In most cases an echocardiogram is advised in order to search for any underlying cause of AF, to complete the risk stratification for potential thrombo-embolic consequences and to provide a baseline estimate of left atrial size and left ventricular function. However, in the very old or incapacitated this investigation may not be essential, especially since it is usually obvious on age grounds alone that prophylactic therapy against thrombo-embolism is needed. Thyroid function tests are necessary especially in the elderly since underlying, otherwise clinically silent (apathetic) hyperthyroidism is not infrequently present.

CLASSIFICATION OF AF

The most widely accepted classification of AF is based on its temporal pattern of occurrence (2). *First detected* AF is the first clinical presentation, the onset of which may be unknown. *Paroxysmal* AF is a recurrent form that typically last minutes to hours, occasionally days (not more than seven), but eventually self-terminates. *Persistent* AF is present when arrhythmia has lasted for more than seven days, is not self-terminating and pharmacological or electrical cardioversion is required to restore sinus rhythm. AF is regarded as *permanent* when all attempts to restore sinus rhythm have been abandoned due to physician or patient decision, frequent recurrence, or inability to cardiovert the patient.

The longer AF persists, the more difficult it becomes to achieve and maintain sinus rhythm. This is due to time-dependent remodelling of the electrical and structural properties of the atrium, making the atria more susceptible to initiation and maintenance of arrhythmia. AF tends to recur after the first detected episode unless a transient or reversible cause is identified and corrected. Initially the episodes are brief, rare and self terminating (paroxysmal) but then become longer lasting more frequent and require active intervention (persistent). Finally the arrhythmia may be accepted as permanent if the patient cannot tolerate interventions to restore sinus rhythm or the physician cannot offer any more successful therapy. This classical natural history may be abbreviated or unnoticed in the elderly and often the patient is discovered to be in asymptomatic AF. In such cases the physician may choose not to intercede except to safeguard the patient against inappropriate ventricular rates and thromboembolic complications.

CAUSES OF AF

Most patients in the western world develop AF against a background of coronary artery disease and/or systemic hypertension, whilst in developing countries rheumatic valvular disease remains the most common heart disease underlying AF. Other clinically important causes include heart failure, chest infection, pulmonary neoplasm, chronic obstructive airways disease, pulmonary embolism, obesity, sleep apnoea syndrome and hyperthyroidism. Cardiac or thoracic surgery may provoke AF but this is readily reversed if diagnosed and treated promptly.

AF may occur in patients with structurally normal hearts and no signs of any demonstrable cardiovascular or other underlying disease. This is described as "*idiopathic*" or "*lone*" atrial fibrillation implying that there is no known cause but the arrhythmia may be due to an imbalance of cardiac autonomic innervation or sub-clinical hyperthyroidism or alcohol toxicity. In the elderly it is difficult to make a diagnosis of lone AF since other co-morbidities such as hypertension or coronary artery disease are either evident or suspected. Although these conditions may encourage the development of AF it may still be an "unknown" factor, such as disturbed autonomic innervation, that first or repetitively initiates the arrhythmia.

PRINCIPLES OF MANAGEMENT OF AF

The main aspects of managing AF are:

1. Urgent control of the ventricular rate during paroxysmal or persistent AF.

2. Restoration of sinus rhythm by pharmacologic or electrical means.
3. Prevention of recurrence of AF following successful restoration of sinus rhythm.
4. Long term rate control in those with permanent AF.
5. Prevention of thromboembolic complications.

TREATMENT OF ACUTE ONSET AF

In an emergency setting the priority is to maintain haemodynamic stability which can be achieved either by urgently restoring sinus rhythm or by controlling the ventricular rate in a patient presenting with AF and a rapid ventricular response. Immediate direct-current cardioversion (DCC), irrespective of the duration of AF, is indicated in patients who are haemodynamically unstable or have evidence of life-threatening acute myocardial ischaemia or heart failure. If DCC is not urgently available, amiodarone or digoxin can be given parenterally. In unstable patients, amiodarone is more effective than digoxin by initially providing rapid rate control because of its action on the AV node, followed by cardioversion to sinus rhythm. If the arrhythmia is of recent onset (<48 hours) and the patient is haemodynamically stable, pharmacological cardioversion can be effective. Class IC agents, such as intravenous or oral flecainide or oral propafenone, are commonly used for terminating acute-onset AF in stable patients. These agents act within minutes when given intravenously or several hours if given orally. Amiodarone, by contrast, achieves cardioversion much more slowly by oral or intravenous routes. Usually, but without any compelling evidence, class IC agents are avoided in the elderly in favour of amiodarone due to the possibility of co-morbidities such as coronary artery disease and left ventricular dysfunction. Class III agents such as dofetilide and ibutilide (not available for use in the UK) have high success rates in cardioverting atrial flutter (AFl) but are less useful for cardioversion of AF. For example, intravenous ibutilide has shown higher success in cardioverting AFl

(65–80%) than AF (35–50%). However, all class III agents may be more effective than IC drugs when the arrhythmia has persisted more than a few days. Most agents which are useful for acute pharmacological cardioversion of AF can also be used orally for longterm maintenance of sinus rhythm. AF associated with chest infections and electrolyte disorders usually settles with adequate treatment of the primary disorder, but may require elective cardioversion if it persists. In less acute situations, rate-control using intravenous or oral digoxin, beta-blockers or rate-limiting calcium channel antagonists (diltiazem and verapamil) is indicated as most patients with paroxysmal episodes will spontaneously revert to sinus rhythm within 24 hours and the control of ventricular rate may be all that is necessary. Patients should be anticoagulated using heparin and subsequently with warfarin if AF has persisted for >48 hours, if cardioversion is anticipated or if the patient is at risk for thromboembolism. However, it is often difficult to ascertain the exact duration of AF even when presenting acutely. Long-term continuation of oral anticoagulation (discussed below) is guided by the presence of risk factors for thrombo-embolism and does not depend on the frequency or duration of paroxysms.

SUPPRESSION OF PAROXYSMS OF AF

Antiarrhythmic agents are frequently required for effective maintenance of sinus rhythm following successful cardioversion (CV) (Table 14.1). These drugs may improve the success rates of elective CV but may need to be prescribed for several weeks prior to the procedure to provide optimal effect. Drugs commonly used in the UK to prevent future paroxysms are conventional beta-blockers, class IC agents (flecainide and propafenone) and class III agents (sotalol and amiodarone). Class IC and class III agents are given only if standard beta-blocker therapy has failed to prevent paroxysms or is contraindicated.

Amiodarone is highly effective in achieving long-term maintenance of sinus rhythm, but is

Table 14.1. Drugs used for acute pharmacological cardioversion of AF or for longterm maintenance of sinus rhythm

Name	Dose	Pharmacokinetics	Action	Precautions/adverse effects
Amiodarone (class III)	1200–1800 mg i.v or oral loading until total of 10 g; Oral maintenance–200–400 mg daily	Elimination half-life 30–60 days. Metabolised largely via liver	Prolongs atrial and ventricular APD; Reduces heart rate; Prolongs ventricular repolarisation **Uses:** Cardioversion and prophylaxis of AF, PAF, AFL; PSVT: ventricular arrhythmias (VT or VF)	Hypotension, liver and hyper/hypothyroidism, skin discolouration, corneal deposits, pulmonary fibrosis, phlebitis; propensity to QT prolongation (though lower than class I); avoid combining with agents affecting cardiac repolarisation
Flecainide (class Ic)	1.5–3.0 mg/kg i.v over 10–15 min. Oral loading–200-300 mg single dose Oral maintenance– 100–300 mg daily.	Elimination half-life 13–19 hours; 75 % metabolised by liver, 25 % renal	Powerful blocker of sodium channels; prolongs atrial repolarisation and ERP; significant negative inotropy at high doses. **Uses:** Cardioversion and prophylaxis of AF, PAF, AFL; PSVT; idiopathic (primary) ventricular arrhythmias	Prolongation of QRS duration and polymorphic ventricular tachycardia, TdP; contraindicated in patients with structural heart disease or coronary ischaemia; can also allow rapid conduction of atrial flutter (combine with AV nodal blocking agents during chronic use)
Propafenone (class Ic)	1.5–2.0 mg/kg i.v loading; Oral loading- 450–600 mg single dose; Oral maintenance- 150–300 mg thrice daily	Elimination half-life 2–10 hours (12–32 hours in poor metabolisers)	Actions as for flecainide. **Uses:** Cardioversion and prophylaxis of AF, PAF, AFL; idiopathic ventricular arrhythmias	As above
Sotalol (class III)	Orally 80 mg initially; 160–320 mg in divided doses thereafter (usually given to prevent recurrences)	Plasma half-life in the young 7 hours, in the elderly 10–15 hours; mainly eliminated by kidneys	Prolongs atrial and ventricular APD; slows sinus node activity **Uses:** Prophylaxis AF, PAF; PSVT; sometimes used for ventricular arrhythmias	QT prolongation; TdP; symptomatic bradycardia; avoid with other QT prolonging drugs; avoid if ventricular hypertrophy
Procainamide (class Ia)	100–1000 mg over 30 min i.v (33 mg/min followed by 2– 6 mg/min infusion); Oral loading- 1000 mg; Oral maintenance- 500 mg every 3–6 hours	Elimination half-life 4–6 hours; 40 % liver metabolism and 60 % renal excretion	Prolongs APD and ERP in atrial and ventricular tissue; no effect on nodal tissues **Uses:** Conversion or prophylaxis of AF; WPW; ventricular arrhythmias	QRS widening; TdP; rapid AFL; hypotension, agranulocytosis and features of systemic lupus
Disopyramide (class Ia)	100–200 mg 6 hourly orally (usually given to prevent recurrences)	Elimination half-life 7–8 hours; renal excretion	As for procainamide; also has strong anticholinergic action (useful for vagally mediated AF); negative inotropic action (useful for patients with hypertrophic cardiomyopathy developing AF) **Uses:** Prophylaxis of AF, PAF; WPW; PSVT; VT	QRS prolongation; TdP; aggravates heart failure

[a]AF-atrial fibrillation; AFL-atrial flutter; PAF-paroxysmal atrial fibrillation; PSVT-paroxysmal supraventricular tachycardia; VT-ventricular tachycardia; VF- ventricular fibrillation; WPW-Wolf-Parkinson-White syndrome; TdP-torsades de pointes; APD-action potential duration; ERP-effective refractory period

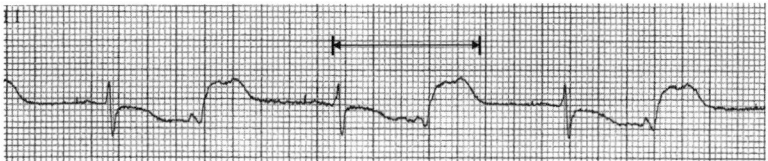

Figure 14.3. Abnormal repolarisation and severe prolongation of QT interval in a 75 year old female patient receiving oral sotalol therapy

limited by side effects from chronic use and should therefore be less frequently prescribed in those with structurally normal hearts (3). Class IC agents are contraindicated in the presence of ischaemic heart disease and/or ventricular dysfunction because of their proarrhythmic and negative inotropic effects. Sotalol is best avoided in those with heart failure or ventricular hypertrophy (or depressed renal function) due to increased risk of QT prolongation and proarrhythmia. (Figure 14.3). Since ischaemic heart disease and myocardial dysfunction are common in the elderly, amiodarone generally becomes the drug of preference in such situations. Amiodarone is also associated with potentially dangerous prolongation of the QT interval, although less commonly than with sotalol, regular monitoring of the QT interval (and QRS duration with class IC agents) on the 12-lead ECG is important during outpatient review.

Patients with infrequent and brief paroxysms of AF need not require regular therapy or may be controlled on low doses of antiarrhythmic agents. Such patients may be best suited for the strategy of suppressing the arrhythmia by taking a single dose or an extra dose of the antiarrhythmic medication (sotalol or class I agents) at the time of experiencing a paroxysm (the 'pill-in-the-pocket' approach). This approach however, is less preferred in the elderly unless they have a structurally normal heart, normal resting heart rate and blood pressure and an understanding of how and when to take the extra medication.

STRATEGIES IN PERSISTENT AF—RATE VERSUS RHYTHM CONTROL

The most appropriate initial treatment strategy depends on individual patient circumstances and comorbid conditions. Recent data suggests, contrary to expectations raised in previous trials (4), that patients with heart failure can be equally well treated using rate or rhythm control. (4a)

Factors favouring rhythm or rate-control are based on evidence from recent trials (4–7).

Rhythm control	Rate control
• Symptomatic patients • Younger age group • Presence of lone AF • AF secondary to known precipitant cause (e.g. thyrotoxicosis, chest infection, alcohol, excessive caffeine intake)	• Asymptomatic patients • Age > 65 years • Contraindication or side effects from antiarrhythmic therapy Unsuitable for cardioversion (e.g. AF > 1 year, large left atrium >5.5cms, relapses or failed multiple attempts at cardioversion despite use of antiarrhythmic agents)

Patients considered suitable for rhythm-control require electrical or pharmacological cardioversion to achieve sinus rhythm. Pharmacological cardioversion (PCV) as discussed above, commonly involves the same agents that are to be used for long-term maintenance of sinus rhythm. The decision to adopt either strategy usually depends on symptoms, age, the risk-benefit ratio of chronic therapy (efficacy versus proarrhythmia, negative inotropism and non-cardiac side effects) and on factors that predict future recurrences of AF:

• Failed attempts at cardioversion.
• AF duration > 1 year.
• Enlarged left atrium.
• Ventricular dysfunction.
• Valvular dysfunction (especially mitral).

There is increasing evidence that inflammation and fibrosis is in large part responsible for the maintenance of AF. Post hoc, retrospective analyses of several recent clinical trials suggest that statins, angiotensin converting enzyme inhibitors (ACE-I) and angiotensin receptor blockers (ARB) are effective in preventing episodes of AF. Several small prospective controlled randomized trials of statins, ACE-I and ARBs also support their value specifically for the treatment of AF (i.e., independent of their effect on lipids, blood pressure, heart failure, etc.). Statins may achieve some efficacy through an anti-inflammatory mechanism or antioxidant effect, while ACE-I and ARB reduce apoptosis and fibrosis. In a recent sub-analysis of the LIFE trial, ARB and beta blockade appeared to be equally effective at reducing blood pressure whilst ARBs were superior to beta-blockers in preventing episodes of new-onset AF in hypertensive patients with left ventricular hypertrophy (8).

RATE CONTROL IN PERMANENT AF

Once the decision has been made to leave AF permanent, optimal control of the ventricular rate is necessary to reduce rate-related symptoms as well as to prevent the development of tachycardia associated cardiomyopathy. What should be the optimal heart rate in AF remains controversial. Heart rate should neither be too high (leading to reduction of exercise tolerance and development of tachycardia induced cardiomyopathy) nor too slow (reduced exercise tolerance, dizziness, pre-syncope, etc). AF is generally considered to be well controlled when the ventricular rate at rest is 60–80 bpm and 90–115 bpm during exercise although less strict criteria (<100 beats/minute at rest and <115 beat/minute during exercise) are also used.

Rate control is achieved by drugs which predominantly affect conduction through the AV node. Commonly used agents are digoxin, beta-blockers and non-dihydropyridine calcium channel blockers such as verapamil and diltiazem (Table 14.2). In permanent AF digoxin usually provides adequate rate control at rest, but does not prevent excessive heart rates during exercise or other high adrenergic states such as fever, thyrotoxicosis, volume loss and following surgery. Digoxin should thus be reserved for sedentary patients. Beta-blockers or calcium antagonists may be given as monotherapy as first line agents for rate control. Combination therapy using digoxin with a beta-blocker or calcium antagonist is often necessary for adequate rate control (Figure 14.4). If such combinations are ineffective, an oral beta-blocker may be used together with diltiazem (less negatively inotropic than verapamil) or amiodarone may be used for its powerful AV nodal blocking properties.

However, in the elderly AF frequently co-exists with periods of bradycardia (sick sinus disease or AV block) and caution must be exhibited when combining AV nodal blocking agents that may also suppress sinus node activity. Such patients usually require support from a permanent pacemaker when therapy involves combinations or higher doses of these drugs. Permanent pacing also becomes necessary when it is difficult to control the ventricular rate and symptoms in certain patients despite drug therapy. The option then is to completely block the AV conduction by radiofrequency or cryo-ablation of the AV node followed by implantation of a permanent ventricular pacemaker.

Table 14.2. Drugs commonly used for acute or chronic rate-control in the elderly

Name	Dose	Pharmacokinetics	Action	Precautions/adverse effects
Digoxin	1–1.5 mg iv or po over 24 hrs; maintenance 62.5ug–500ug po od	Elimination half-life in the young 1.5 days in the elderly 3 days; renal excretion	Central and peripheral actions to increase vagal activity; prolongs AV nodal refractory period; may at times induce AF by shortening atrial refractory period; positive inotropic effect on the myocardium	Gastrointestinal upset, bradycardia and conduction blocks, paroxysmal atrial tachycardia at times, interaction with amiodarone, propafenone, verapamil, quinidine; adjust dose if renal impairment.
Metoprolol	5 mg iv over 5 min; maintenance- 25–100 mg po bd	Elimination half-life in the young 3–4 hours in the elderly 8 hours. Liver metabolism. 40 % bioavailability from hepatic first pass effect	Prolongs refractory period within AV and SA nodes	
Esmolol	0.5 mg/kg i.v over 1 min	Elimination half-life 8 min. rapid attenuation of effects after stopping infusion	Prolongs refractory period within AV and SA nodes	Additive effects with digoxin and calcium channel blockers
Verapamil	5-20 mg i.v over 20 min; Oral dose- 80–120 mg 3–4 times daily; long-acting preparations- 240–480 mg od	Elimination half-life 3–4 hours in the young, 4–10 hours in the elderly (longer for slow-release preparations); renal excretion	Prolongs refractory period within AV and SA nodes. Peak effect at 10–15 min after iv and at 3 hrs after oral administration	Hypotension with i.v route; bradycardia, conduction blocks, constipation, drug-drug interaction with amiodarone and digoxin
Diltiazem	20 mg i.v bolus over 2 mins followed by 5–15 mg/hour infusion; oral dose- long acting preparations 60, 90, 120, 180, 240, 300 mg once or twice daily)	Elimination half-life 4–7 hours; renal excretion	Prolongs refractory period within AV and SA nodes. Peak effect in 1–2 hours	As for verapamil

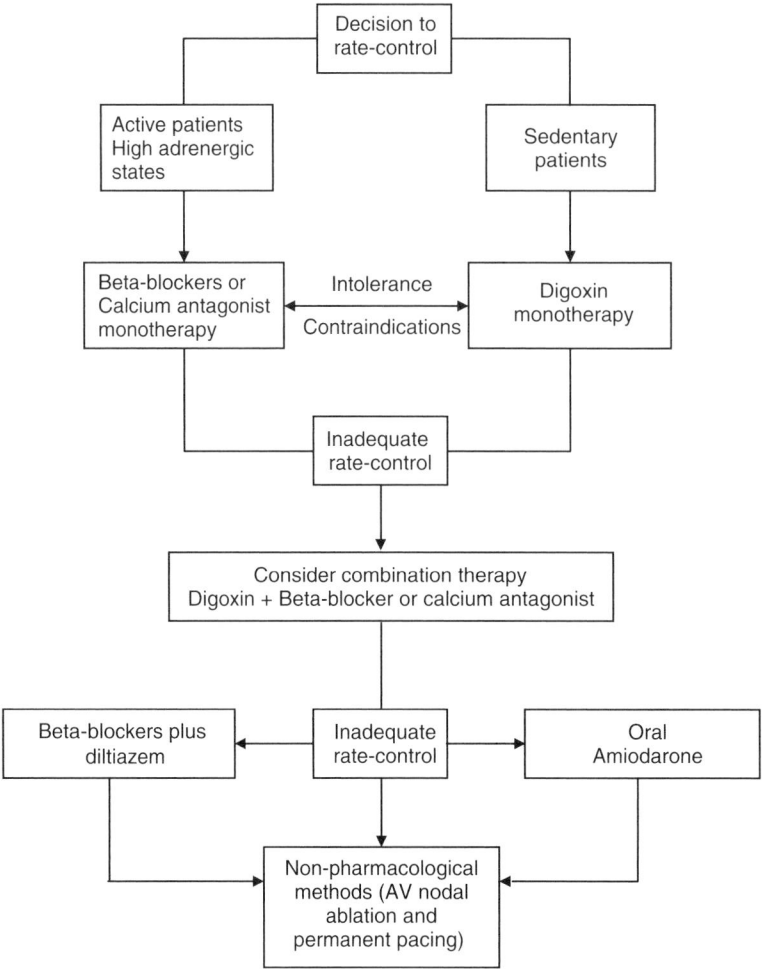

Figure 14.4. Algorithm for rate-control in permanent AF

RISK OF STROKE AND ANTITHROMBOTIC THERAPY IN AF

Atrial fibrillation once controlled causes little direct damage, but the risk of peripheral thromboembolism remains significant and increases with age from 1.5 % in patients less than 60 years to 24 % in those over 80 years of age (1). The rate of ischaemic stroke in AF is related to coexistent cardiovascular disease and is similar in those with recurrent (including paroxysmal) and permanent AF.

Warfarin remains underprescribed in clinical practice. More than 40 % of those at high risk of thromboembolism may not be receiving adequate

anticoagulation. This is particularly true for the most vulnerable group, the elderly and institutionalized patients, who are denied anticoagulation on the basis of an assumed increased risk of haemorrhagic complications (9), (9a).

All patients with AF lasting >48 hours who are selected for elective cardioversion require at least 3 weeks of adequate anticoagulation (INR of 2.5; range 2.0–3.0) regardless of what method of cardioversion is employed. In practice this usually involves anticoagulating patients for six to eight weeks until sufficiently well controlled INR values have been achieved. In selected patients, pre-cardioversion transoesophageal echocardiography (TOE) can be used to exclude the presence of intra-atrial thrombi. TOE guided elective cardioversion is of comparable efficacy and is probably cost-effective when compared to the conventional anticoagulation strategy. Patients with confirmed AF of <48 hours duration have the least risk of thromboembolism during cardioversion and can be safely cardioverted with heparin cover. The atria remain 'stunned' and may not achieve full mechanical function for several days following electrical cardioversion, despite the presence of P waves on the surface ECG. Unless contraindicated, all patients subjected to DCC and those with AF >48 hrs duration require at least four weeks of full anticoagulation (INR2.0–3.0) in the post-cardioversion period.

Long term continuation of antithrombotic therapy with anticoagulant or antiplatelet agents is guided by the patient's risk of thrombo-embolism (10). Risk stratification guidelines differ between various expert groups particularly for those falling in the 65–75 year age group. The box provides a simplified and practical approach to guide prophylactic antithrombotic drug usage by combining views from three major groups-the ACCP, the ACC/AHA/ESC consensus and the CHADS$_2$ risk stratification scheme (11). CHADS$_2$ is an acronym which describes the major risk factors: Congestive heart failure, Hypertension, Age equal to or above 75 years, Diabetes, and previous stroke or transient ischemic attack. At any age a previous stroke or transient ischemic attack will warrant anticoagulation. Above 65 years stroke or any two other risk factors indicate the need for warfarin. At 75 years or above one additional risk factor mandates formal anticoagulation.

Stratification of thromboembolic risk in AF

Clinical features	Antithrombotic treatment
Age < 65, structurally normal heart, no other risk factors	Aspirin 300 mg/day (low risk)
Age 65– 75 years, structurally normal heart, no other risk factors	Aspirin 300 mg/day or oral anticoagulation[†] (intermediate risk)
Age > 75 years	Oral anticoagulation[†] (high risk)
Any age < 75 years with structurally abnormal heart,* presence of stroke/TIA or more than one other risk factor**	Oral anticoagulation[†] (high risk)

* = Moderate to severe left ventricular impairment; mitral valve disease; prosthetic heart valves; left atrial dilatation
** = Previous stroke or TIA; hypertension (controlled or uncontrolled); coronary arterial disease; diabetes; clinical heart failure; thyroid dysfunction; atherothrombotic vascular disease.
† = unless contra-indicated

Antithrombotic therapy should be prescribed on an individual basis after assessing the risks and benefits of warfarin or aspirin (12). On the risk-benefit ratio, adjusted-dose warfarin is given to AF patients at moderate to high risk of thromboembolism with an aim to maintain a target INR of 2.5 (range 2.0–3.0). When the INR is >3.0, the risk of intracranial haemorrhage increases significantly. Patients at low risk, or those with contraindications or intolerance to warfarin, can be treated with 300 mg of aspirin. Decision to initiate antithrombotic therapy depends on the presence or absence of risk factors for stroke and not on the frequency or severity of paroxysms. Antiplatelet combinations such as aspirin plus clopidogrel or aspirin plus dipyridamole are only acceptable in situations where warfarin cannot be given. Since thrombin plays a key role in propagation of thrombus formation, the safety of orally administered direct and indirect thrombin inhibitors is also currently under investigation.

NON-PHARMACOLOGICAL TECHNIQUES TO PREVENT THROMBUS FORMATION

In patients with AF, more than 90 % of thrombi form in the left atrial appendage. Surgical closure or removal of the left atrial appendage has previously been tried, mainly in patients undergoing valve surgery. Newer techniques allow the percutaneous deployment of left atrial appendage transcatheter occlusion devices.

KEY POINTS

- Morbidity and mortality from atrial fibrillation predominantly results from the increased risk of stroke and aggravation of heart failure.
- Both rate control and rhythm control are important strategies for the management of atrial fibrillation, but each approach should be chosen according to individual patient circumstances.
- Most elderly patients will benefit from ventricular rate control.
- Rhythm control can be achieved with class Ic and class III antiarrhythmic drugs.
- Anticoagulation with warfarin remains underprescribed, especially in elderly people.

REFERENCES

1. Lloyd-Jones DM, Wang TJ, Leip EP, et al. Lifetime risk for development of atrial fibrillation. The Framingham Heart Study. *Circulation* 2004; **110**: 1042–46.
2. Levy S, Camm AJ, Saksena S, Aliot E, Breithardt G, Crijns H et al. International consensus on nomenclature and classification of atrial fibrillation. *Europace* 2003; **5**: 119–22.
3. Kochiadakis GE, Marketou ME, Igomenidis NE et al. Amiodarone, sotalol or propafenone in atrial fibrillation: which is preferred to maintain normal sinus rhythm? *PACE* 2000; **23**: 1883–7.
4. Wyse DG, Waldo AL, DiMarco JP, et al. Atrial fibrillation follow-up investigation of rhythm management (AFFIRM) investigators. A comparison of rate control and rhythm control in patients with atrial fibrillation. *New Eng J Med* 2002; **347**: 1825–33.
4a. Roy D, Talajic M, Nattel S et al. Rhythm control versus rate control for atrial fibrillation and heart failure. *New Engl J Med* 2008 Jun 19; **358**(25: 2667–77.
5. Hagens VE et al. RACE study group. Effect of rate or rhythm control on quality of life in persistent atrial fibrillation. Results from the Rate Control Versus Electrical Cardioversion (RACE) Study. *J Am Coll Cardiol* 2004 Jan 21; **43**(2): 241–7.
6. Carlsson J, Miketic S, Windeler J, et al. STAF Investigators. Randomized trial of rate-control versus rhythm-control in persistent atrial fibrillation: the Strategies of Treatment of Atrial Fibrillation (STAF) study *J Am Coll Cardiol.* 2003; **41**(10): 1690–6.
7. Gronefeld GC, Lilienthal J, Kuck et al. Pharmacological – Intervention-in-Atrial-Fibrillation- Impact of rate versus rhythm control on quality of lifein patients with persistent atrial fibrillation. Results from a prospective randomised study (PIAF) *Eur Heart J* 2003; **24**: 1430–6.
8. Watchtell K, Lehto M, Gerdts E, et al. Angiotensin II receptor blockade reduces new-onset atrial fibrillation and subsequent stroke compared to atenolol: the Losartan Intervention For End Point Reduction in Hypertension (LIFE) study. *J Am Coll Cardiol* 2005 Mar 1; **45**(5): 712–9.
9. Brophy MT, Snyder KE, Gaehde S, et al. Anticoagulant use for atrial fibrillation in the elderly. *J Am Geriatr Soc* 2004; **52**: 1151–56.
9a. Savelieva I, Bajpai A, Camm AJ. Stroke in atrial fibrillation: update on pathophysiology, new antithrombotic therapies, and evolution of procedures and devices. *Ann Med* 2007; **39**(5): 371–91.
10. ACC/AHA/ESC 2006 Guidelines for the management of patients with atrial fibrillation: Executive summary. *Circulation* 2006; **114**: 700–52.
11. Rockson SG, Albers GW. Comparing guidelines: Anticoagulation therapy to optimize stroke prevention in patients with atrial fibrillation. *J Am Coll Cardiol* 2004; **43**: 929–35.
12. Fang MC, Chang Y, Hylek EM, et al. Advanced age, anticoagulation intensity, and risk for intracranial hemorrhage among patients taking warfarin for atrial fibrillation. *Ann Intern Med.* 2004 Nov 16; **141**(10): 745–52.

15   Valvular Heart Disease

Andrew T. Elder

Medicine of Geriatrics, Western General Hospital, Edinburgh, UK

INTRODUCTION

Although the incidence of rheumatic fever has declined in Western populations, valvular heart disease predominantly caused by degenerative changes and/or calcification, remains a significant clinical problem. Such degenerative valvular disease is particularly prevalent amongst ageing populations, and can occur in congenitally abnormal or previously normal cardiac valves, or in those damaged by previous rheumatic fever or infective endocarditis. A smaller proportion of valvular disease relates to rupture or dysfunction of the mitral papillary muscle apparatus due to coronary artery disease, or to dilation of the right or left ventricle as a consequence of cardiac failure.

Valvular disease resulting in significant haemodynamic compromise or lifestyle limiting symptoms is best managed surgically. Recent improvements in surgical and anaesthetic techniques have produced dramatic improvements in surgical mortality and longer-term outcomes. Accurate prediction of the optimal timing of valve repair or replacement is vital if deterioration in myocardial function is to be avoided. Currently, advanced age in itself should not be regarded as a contraindication to assessment for surgical treatment.

The precise indications for, and timing of, surgery in valvular heart disease in older patients are not considered in detail in this chapter.

Medical management is appropriate for patients with lesser degrees of haemodynamic compromise, milder symptoms, or for those in whom surgery is not an option, either because of personal preference, or the presence of co-morbidity that increases surgical risk to an unacceptable level.

Six major issues in the medical care of elderly patients with native valvular disease or prosthetic cardiac valves following surgery can be identified. Two of these, the management of heart failure, and arrhythmias, are covered elsewhere.

This chapter will therefore focus on four major issues:

(a) Prevention of infective endocarditis.
(b) Treatment of infective endocarditis.
(c) Prevention of thromboembolism.
(d) Prevention of the progression of native degenerative valvular disease.

INFECTIVE ENDOCARDITIS

Infective Endocarditis may affect previously normal or abnormal native or prosthetic valves and continues to carry a significant mortality in older patients partly due to the difficulty that may surround diagnosis. In native valvular disease, the mitral valve is most commonly affected, but infection of both mitral and aortic valves can occur in up to a quarter of all cases. A wide range of organisms may be implicated. *Streptococcus* sp and Enterococci account for up to 70 % and 25 % of cases in elderly patients, respectively. This is probably due to the higher prevalence of urinary infection and urethral instrumentation in this group. *S. bovis*, is

Prescribing for Elderly Patients   Edited by Stephen Jackson, Paul Jansen and Arduino Mangoni

isolated in up to 25 % of older patients, and an association with underlying colonic disease, especially cancer, has been demonstrated. Staphylococci, particularly *Staphylococcus aureus*, are found in up to 30 % of older patients. *S. epidermidis* is relatively uncommon in native valve endocarditis, but is the commonest cause of early prosthetic valve endocarditis. Late prosthetic endocarditis is most commonly due to streptococci, with entry sites similar to that found in native valve endocarditis. Other organisms are rarely encountered and up to 20 % of cases prove to be culture negative, in part due to prior antibiotic administration in older patients.

PREVENTION OF ENDOCARDITIS

Although no data from prospective randomised controlled trials exist to conclusively demonstrate the value of antibiotic prophylaxis of endocarditis in any specific clinical situation, it remains standard clinical practice in at risk patients (1).

The need for prophylaxis and choice of specific regime should be guided by assessment of the risk of the specific procedure to be undertaken, the nature of the underlying cardiac disease, the patient's comorbidites and the presence of drug allergies.

The risk of bacteraemia and subsequent endocarditis is greatest following some dental procedures. Invasive genitourinary procedures and gastrointestinal procedures are associated with lower risk.

The risk of endocarditis is greatest in patients with prosthetic valves and/or a past history of endocarditis. Patients with a history of prior rheumatic heart disease, congenital valvular heart disease, native valve repair surgery, and mitral valve prolapse with regurgitation or other acquired valvular dysfunction should also be considered for antibiotic prophylaxis.

Risk is generally regarded as low in patients with "physiologic", "functional", or "innocent" heart murmurs; mitral valve prolapse without associated regurgitation; valvular leaflet thickening; mild or haemodynamically insignificant tricuspid regurgitation; and previous rheumatic fever without valvular dysfunction. In the absence of a past history of endocarditis such patients would not normally be considered for antibiotic prophylaxis.

Table 15.1 summarizes recommended prophylaxis for patients judged to be at risk of endocarditis.

DIAGNOSIS AND TREATMENT OF ENDOCARDITIS

The modified Duke criteria remain the standard criteria for diagnosis. Presentation may however be cryptic and a high level of diagnostic suspicion is necessary in older patients, particularly given the high prevalence of cardiac murmurs in this age group.

In patients with prosthetic valves the development of systemic embolisation or perivalvular leaks should prompt intensive investigation for endocarditis preferably including transoesophageal echocardiography. Transoesophageal echocardiography is a more sensitive method of detecting vegetations than transthoracic echocardiography particularly in patients with prosthetic valves. Echocardiography by either route cannot exclude the diagnosis of infective endocarditis.

In all patients with suspected endocarditis, blood cultures should be taken before commencement of treatment, with three pairs taken over two hours in the acutely unwell patient who needs early treatment and three pairs taken over 24 hours in stable patients. Blood cultures should be incubated for seven days, and will be positive in 75–95 % of infective endocarditis patients. If blood cultures are negative and a diagnosis of infective endocarditis is still felt possible, infection with the HACEK group, *Bartonella* spp., *Brucella* spp., *Chlamydia* spp., *Coxiella burnetii* (Q-fever), *Legionella* spp., mycobacteria and fungi, should be considered.

The timing of commencement of antibiotic treatment is determined by the clinical situation. Patients without heart failure, sepsis, evidence of progressive valvular damage or haemodynamic compromise should preferably have treatment delayed until the diagnosis can be confirmed bacteriologically.

Table 15.1. Summary of recommended antimicrobial prophylaxis for patients at risk of infective endocarditis

	Recommended regime	Alternative if penicillin allergic	Timing of administration	Comment
Dental extractions, scaling, periodontal surgery	Amoxicillin 2–3 g oral	Clindamycin 600 mg oral Or Erythromycin 1.5 g oral	1 hour before procedure	If under general anaesthesia, amoxicillin 3 g oral 4 hours before, repeated immediately post procedure
Invasive genitourinary or gastrointestinal procedures	Amoxicillin 1 g IV And Gentamicin 1.5 mg/kg IM	Vancomycin 1 g IV And Gentamicin 1.5 mg/kg	30 minutes before the procedure	If genitourinary tract actively infected extend cover appropriately This regime may also be preferred in patients with a past history of endocarditis or prosthetic valves.
	Followed by Amoxicillin 500 mg oral	No post procedure dose	6 hours after the procedure	

Antibiotic choice

The choice and duration of antimicrobial treatment depend upon the type of microorganism, its susceptibility profile, patient allergy to antimicrobials and whether infection involves a native or prosthetic valve (2).

A bactericidal antimicrobial, or combination of antimicrobials, is required to eradicate infection. The minimum inhibitory concentration (MIC) of the chosen antimicrobial should be established by a standardized laboratory method to ensure susceptibility. Routine measurement of MBC (minimum bactericidal concentration) is not recommended in current guidelines.

Table 15.2 shows the recommended antimicrobial treatment in the event of a specific organism being isolated. In situations where empirical therapy is necessary, either before culture results are fully available, or when cultures are negative, current consensus guidelines recommendations are as follows.

For patients presenting with an acute illness, flucloxacillin (8–12 g iv daily in four to six divided doses) plus gentamicin (1 mg/kg body weight iv 8 hourly, modified according to renal function). If the patient has a more indolent presentation, penicillin (7.2 g iv daily in 6 divided doses) or ampicillin/amoxicillin (2 g iv 6 hourly) plus gentamicin (1 mg/kg body weight 8 hourly iv, modified according to renal function).

In patients with prosthetic valves or suspected MRSA infection who require "blind" treatment, vancomycin (1 g 12 hourly iv, modified according to renal function *plus* rifampicin (300–600 mg 12 hourly by mouth) *plus* gentamicin (1 mg/kg body weight 8 hourly iv, modified according to renal function).

Duration of treatment

The table indicates broad guidelines for duration of treatment in different situations. Although some evidence exists to support the use of brief two week regimes for some penicillin sensitive streptococcal infections, in most situations a minimum of four weeks treatment is necessary, extended to six weeks in patients with prosthetic valves or resistant organisms or when symptoms have been prolonged before diagnosis had been made. Treatment should be intravenous throughout.

Monitoring of treatment

In addition to monitoring of drug trough levels as appropriate and MIC at outset of treatment,

Table 15.2. Recommended antimicrobial regimes in infective endocarditis

Organism	Antibiotic	Dosing	Comment
Staphylococci			***Treat for at least 4 weeks, or 6 weeks in the presence of prosthetic valve***
Methicillin sensitive	Flucloxacillin	2 g iv 4–6 hourly	
Methicillin resistance or Penicillin Allergy	Vancomycin	1 g iv 12 hourly	Dosage modified according to renal function Target trough 10–15 mg/L
	plus		*Two antibiotic combination recommended*
	Rifampicin *Or*	300–600 mg oral 12 hourly	
	Gentamicin		Dosage modified according to renal function.
	Or Sodium Fusidate	1 mg/kg IV 8 hourly 500 mg IV 8 hourly	Ideally use 8 hourly dose regime. Target trough < 1 mg/L
Prosthetic Valve (methicillin sensitive or resistant)	Flucloxacillin **or** Vancomycin	2 g IV 4–6 hrly 1 g IV 12 hrly	Dosage modified according to renal function
	plus Rifampicin	300–600 mg oral 12 hrly	For the first 2 weeks of therapy at least
	And gentamicin **or** Sodium fusidate	1 mg/kg IV 8 hourly 500 mg Oral 8hrly	*Three agents may be beneficial if organism sensitive*
Streptococci Native valve	Penicillin alone	1.2—2.4 g 4hrly	Modify dosage according to renal function. 4 weeks for *Viridans*, *Bovis*, or Group A streptococci with MIC < 0.5 mg/L and Pneumoniae spp with MIC < 0.1 mg/L.
	Or Penicillin and Gentamicin		
	Or Ceftriaxone		2 weeks Viridans or bovis spp with MIC < 0.1 mg/l
	Or Vancomycin		4 weeks Viridans, bovis, Group A and pnuemoniae spp
	Or Vancomycin and Gentamicin		4 weeks Viridans, bovis, Group A and pnuemoniae spp 4–6 weeks Organisms with high MIC > 0.5 mg/l
Prosthetic valve	Vancomycin **Or** Penicillin		6 weeks
	And Gentamicin		For first 2 weeks at least an up to 6 weeks if MIC > 0.1 mg/l

Table 15.2. (Continued)

Organism	Antibiotic	Dosing	Comment
Penicillin allergic patients	Vancomycin		If MIC > 0.1 < 0.5 mg/L for 4 weeks
	Vancomycin plus Gentamicin		If resistant organism. Two drugs for two weeks, Gentamicin alone for further two weeks.
Enterococci	Ampicillin plus Gentamicin	2 g 4hrly IV 1 mg/kg 12 hourly IV	4 weeks treatment at least. Substitute teicoplanin or vancomycin if penicillin allergic or ampicillin resistant organism. Substitute streptomycin if gentamicin resistant organism.

Notes:
These are guidelines only.
Expert microbiological advice should always be sought to select optimal treatment for individual patients.
Adapted from (2).

clinical monitoring in the form of assessment for signs of clinical heart failure, embolism, or worsening systemic infection should be undertaken. ECG monitoring is appropriate in cases where development of septal abscess is possible, with PR interval lengthening the cardinal manifestation.

Embolic complications in endocarditis

There is no evidence that oral anticoagulation reduces the incidence of embolisation in patients with native valve endocarditis. Prompt establishment of appropriate antibiotic therapy does however do so.

The situation is more complex in patients with prosthetic valve endocarditis when many patients will already be on anticoagulants. Limited evidence suggests that continuation of anticoagulation in the setting of prosthetic valve endocarditis increases the incidence of haemorrhagic transformation of embolic cerebral infarction. Expert consensus is divergent. Some authorities recommend discontinuation of oral anticoagulants in patients with prosthetic valve endocarditis as soon as the diagnosis is made, and until evidence of infection resolves. Others recommend discontinuation only if the patient develops a stroke.

In general, introduction of oral anticoagulants in anticoagulant-naïve patients with native or prosthetic valve endocarditis is not recommended unless a concurrent indication develops (e.g. deep venous thrombosis). In such situations some authorities recommend the use of heparin rather than warfarin in the hope that tighter control of anticoagulation can be achieved.

Potential interactions with antimicrobial drugs should always be considered in any patient receiving oral anticoagulants.

There is no evidence that aspirin therapy reduces the incidence of embolic stroke in patients with native or prosthetic valve endocarditis.

PREVENTION OF THROMBOEMBOLISM

Patients with diseased, congenitally abnormal or prosthetic valves are at enhanced risk of developing valvular and intracardiac thrombus and subsequent peripheral or cerebral embolism.

The risk of thromboembolic complications is enhanced by the presence of several commonly associated cardiac abnormalities, particularly atrial fibrillation, left atrial enlargement and left ventricular systolic dysfunction.

The relative risk of morbidity and mortality associated with oral anticoagulant therapy or oral antiplatelet treatment increases with age, particularly in association with the occurrence of haemorrhage. Decisions regarding appropriate use of such treatment in patients with native valvular disease and prosthetic valves should include an individualised assessment of thrombotic risk and haemorrhagic risk and include consideration of likely drug adherence, anticipated life expectancy, severity of comorbidites and extent of coexisting polypharmacy.

A fuller discussion of the relative risks of anticoagulation in patients with atrial fibrillation is included in Chapter 14.

Mitral valve disease

Patients with rheumatic mitral valve disease have been recognized to have an enhanced risk of embolism for many years, with lifetime risk estimated at one in five.

The risk is greater in dominant mitral stenosis compared to mitral regurgitation; in the presence of atrial fibrillation or left ventricular dysfunction; and in older age. Importantly, embolism may be the presenting feature of what is subsequently found to be relatively mild valvular disease.

Current guidelines suggest, despite the lack of evidence from randomised trials, which have focussed predominantly on *non-valvular* atrial fibrillation, that patients with rheumatic mitral valve disease and atrial fibrillation or a history of previous embolism are treated with oral anticoagulant therapy. If the risk of bleeding is judged to be too great with anticoagulant therapy, some benefit will be gained from the use of aspirin. The benefit of alternative antiplatelet agents in aspirin intolerant patients in this setting is unclear but is generally recommended.

Those patients with rheumatic mitral valve disease who remain in sinus rhythm should be treated with oral anticoagulants if there is a history of previous embolism. In addition, some authorities recommend anticoagulation in those patients with dilated left atria (> 5.5 cm) on echocardiography. In the absence of atrial fibrillation, a history of embolism or atrial dilatation there is no evidence to support oral anticoagulation in other patients with rheumatic mitral valve disease causing either mitral regurgitation or stenosis.

The risk of embolism in other forms of mitral valve disease, specifically mitral valve prolapse and mitral annular calcification syndrome are lower than in rheumatic valvular disease. In the absence of atrial fibrillation or prior embolism, oral anticoagulation is not recommended and antiplatelet treatment is of unknown value. Patients with mitral valve prolapse and otherwise unexplained transient ischaemic attacks may benefit from aspirin treatment.

Aortic valve disease

Patients with pure aortic valvular disease due to congenital, rheumatic or degenerative heart disease are at low risk of systemic embolism. Calcific microemboli from severely calcified aortic valves are however well described but rarely clinically significant. There is no evidence that oral anticoagulant or antiplatelet therapy is of benefit in such patients in the absence of any other indication and such treatment is not therefore generally recommended.

Antithrombotic treatment is summarized in Table 15.3.

Prosthetic valves

The need for oral anticoagulants or antiplatelet therapy must be considered in all elderly patients with prosthetic cardiac valves, taking into consideration an overall assessment of hemorrhagic risk, and embolic risk relating to factors such as the presence of atrial fibrillation, prior history of embolisation, left atrial size, and left ventricular function (3).

The overall risk of embolisation for all prosthetic valves *without* anticoagulants is around 4 % per annum, with antiplatelet agents 2.2 % per annum and with anticoagulants 0/7−1.0 % per annum. In general, the risk of embolisation is higher with prosthetic valves in the mitral position than in the aortic position, and with mechanical rather than bioprosthetic valves. Of the three types of prosthetic valve, risk is highest with ball cage, intermediate with tilting disk, and lowest with bileaflet valves.

The risk of bleeding in association with both anticoagulant and antiplatelet agents increases with age and estimation of bleeding risk should

Table 15.3. Summary of embolic prophylaxis in native valvular heart disease

Valve lesion	Recommendation
Rheumatic Mitral stenosis (MS) or regurgitation (MR)	If history of systemic embolism, unexplained TIA; paroxysmal or persistent atrial fibrillation; dilated left atrium (5.5 cm) then warfarin to INR 2.5 (2, 3). If thromboembolism occurs with therapeutic INR **either** increase target INR to 3.0 (2.5–3.5) **or** add aspirin 75–100 mg/day **or** dipyridamole 400 mg/day **or** clopidogrel 75 mg/day.
Mitral valve prolapse with MR	If history of systemic embolism, unexplained TIA; paroxysmal or persistent atrial fibrillation; then warfarin to INR 2.5 (2, 3).
Mitral annular calcification	If history of systemic embolism, unexplained TIA; paroxysmal or persistent atrial fibrillation; then warfarin to INR 2.5 (2, 3).
Aortic stenosis (rheumatic or degenerative)	No anticoagulation recommended unless a comorbid indication exists.
Aortic regurgitation (rheumatic or degenerative)	No anticoagulation recommended unless a comorbid condition exists.

be individualized in the light of previous known tolerance to warfarin or antiplatelets, comorbidity, coprescription, mobility, risk of falling and likely drug compliance.

In the first three months following valve replacement all patients, irrespective of the position of the valve, or whether it is mechanical or bioprosthetic, should be anticoagulated to a target INR of 3 (range 2.5–3.5). In the immediate post operative period low molecular weight or unfractionated heparin should be used until the INR is in required therapeutic range for two days. Elderly post-operative patients are particularly sensitive to warfarin and require careful monitoring.

Thereafter it is generally recommended that all patients with mechanical prostheses are anticoagulated long term unless absolute contraindications exist. In that instance antiplatelet therapy should be used. Patients with bioprosthetic valves should be anticoagulated in the immediate postoperative period and for three months thereafter. They do not however necessarily require long-term anticoagulation but this should be considered in patients with additional risk factors for thromboembolism, such as atrial fibrillation, left ventricular systolic dysfunction or left atrial dilatation.

When oral anticoagulants are used the general target INR is 2.5–3.0 although the intensity of anticoagulation should be balanced according to the risk of valve related embolic events and individual risk of haemorrhage (see Table 15.4).

The addition of antiplatelet treatment in the form of aspirin 75–100 mg daily to oral anticoagulants further reduces the risk of embolism, but at the expense of an increase in the risk of hemorrhagic complications. Such treatment should be based on careful assessment of individual patient risk.

Management of anticoagulation in patients undergoing non-cardiac surgery

Many patients with prosthetic valves are required to undergo further non-cardiac procedures. In minor surgery, withdrawal of anticoagulation is often not necessary. In major surgery, patients at relatively low risk of embolization (for example sinus rhythm with tilting disk or bileaflet mechanical prostheses) can have anticoagulation withdrawn 72 hours before the procedure. In high-risk patients (for example those with older generation mechanical valves or atrial fibrillation), most authorities recommend withdrawal of oral anticoagulation 72 hours before surgery to lower the INR to < 1.5 and substitute intravenous or low molecular weight heparin. Heparin should be started when the INR is < 2.5 in high-risk patients and < 2.0 in

Table 15.4. Antithrombotic Treatment for patients with prosthetic valves

Position	Type of prosthesis	Target INR	Comment
Mitral	Tilting disc	3.0 (2.5–3.5)	Add aspirin 75-100 mg in presence of additional risk factors such as AF, LV dysfunction, previous thromboembolism, enlarged left atrium (> 5 cm)
	Bileaflet	3.0 (2.5–3.5)	As above
	Caged ball.	3.0 (2.5–3.5)	As above
	Bioprosthetic	2.5 for first three months	Continue long term with target INR 3 (2.5–3.5) in presence of AF, LV dysfunction, previous thromboembolism, enlarged left atrium (> 5 cm). If no additional risk factor present aspirin 75-100 mg per day is recommended. Aspirin intolerant patients may benefit from dipyridamole.
Aortic	Tilting disc (Medtronic)	2.5 (2, 3)	Increase target INR to 3.0 (2.5–3.5) if additional risk factors such as AF, LV dysfunction, previous thromboembolism, enlarged left atrium (> 5 cm). Some authorities recommend increasing INR to 3.0 **and** adding aspirin 75–100 mg in presence of risk factors.
	Bileaflet	2.5 (2, 3)	As above
	Other tilting disc, or caged ball.	3.0 (2.5–3.5)	Add aspirin 75–100 mg in presence of additional risk factors such as AF, LV dysfunction, previous thromboembolism, enlarged left atrium (> 5 cm) **or** if systemic embolism occurs in presence of a therapeutic INR
	Bioprosthetic	2.5 for first three months	Continue long term with target INR 2.5 (2.0–3.0) in presence of AF, LV dysfunction, previous thromboembolism, enlarged left atrium (> 5 cm). If no additional risk factor present aspirin 75–100 mg per day is recommended. Aspirin intolerant patients may benefit from dipyridamole.

Notes:

1. If thromboembolism occurs when a patient has INR within target range for their prosthesis then either increase target INR by 0.5–1.0 **or** add aspirin **or** both **or** increase aspirin dose.
2. If additional risk factors but patient intolerant of aspirin consider either increasing target INR by 0.5, or adding dipyridamole.

those at lower risk, with a target activated partial thromboplastin time of twice the control value. Heparin should be discontinued four to six hours before surgery and resumed as soon as possible thereafter, and continued until the INR is > 2.5 in high risk patients and > 2.0 in those at lower risk, for 48 hours. Oral anticoagulation should ideally be resumed on the day of the procedure although this may be delayed in exceptional circumstances, e.g. following neurosurgery.

A similar strategy, with withdrawal of oral anticoagulation, and substitution with intravenous or low molecular weight heparin, may be adopted during times of severe intercurrent illness.

PREVENTION OF PROGRESSION OF DEGENERATIVE VALVULAR DISEASE

A significant proportion of older adults develop calcific change in cardiac valvular and perivalvular structures in association with advancing age. This occurs most frequently in the aortic valve leaflets and the mitral annulus.

In recent years it has been recognized that although a frequent accompaniment of ageing, this change is not ubiquitous, and as such is likely to represent a disease process rather than an inevitable accompaniment of "normal" ageing. An association between atherosclerosis and its risk factors, including hypercholes-terolaemia, and calcific aortic valve disease has been demonstrated. The renin-angiotensin system is also known to influence the progression of atherosclerosis. In addition, histologic studies demonstrate similarities between the changes seen in atherosclerosis and degenerative valvular disease. This has raised the question of whether drugs that influence the progression of *vascular* atherosclerotic change (particularly statins) may also modify the progression of valvular disease (4, 5).

Large randomized controlled trials are underway but smaller studies to date have produced negative or inconclusive results. At present therefore no specific treatment to retard disease progression can be recommended.

REFERENCES

1. Dajani AS; Taubert KA; Wilson W; Bolger AF; Bayer A; Ferrieri P; Gewitz MH; Shulman ST; Nouri S; Newburger JW; Hutto C; Pallasch TJ; Gage TW; Levison ME; Peter G; Zuccaro G JrSO Prevention of bacterial endocarditis. Recommendations by the American Heart Association. *JAMA* 1997 Jun 11; **277**(22): 1794–801.

2. Elliott TSJ, Foweraker J, Gould FK, Perry JD, Sandoe JAT. Guidelines for the antibiotic treatment of endocarditis in adults: report of the Working Party of the British Society for Antimicrobial Chemotherapy. *J Antimicrob Chemother* **54**: 971–81.

3. ACC/AHA guidelines for the management of patients with valvular heart disease. A report of the American College of Cardiology/American Heart Association. Task Force on Practice Guidelines (Committee on Management of Patients with Valvular Heart Disease). *J Am Coll Cardiol* 1998; **32**: 1486.

4. Baumgartner H, Aortic Stenosis: Medical and Surgical Management. *Heart* 2005; **91**: 1483–8.

5. Bellamy, MF, Pelikka, PA, Klarich, KW, et al. Association of cholesterol levels, hydroxymethylglutaryl coenzyme-a reductase inhibitor treatment, and progression of aortic stenosis in the community. *J Am Coll Cardiol* 2002; **40**: 1723.

16 Anticoagulants for thrombosis and embolism in the elderly

Alexander Gallus[1] and Dolly Daniel[2]

[1]Department of Haematology, Flinders University, SA Pathology at Flinders Medical Centre, Adelaide, Australia
[2]Department of Clinical Pathology and Blood Bank, Christian Medical College, Vellore, India

INTRODUCTION

The annual incidence of thromboembolic disorders increases with age. So do the benefits and the bleeding risks of anticoagulant therapy; the balance is age-dependent and differs greatly between individuals. A common reason for under-use of anticoagulants in the elderly is a reflex and often excessive fear of bleeding (1).

THE ANTICOAGULANTS

There are now two classes of widely used anticoagulants: injectable heparins and orally active vitamin K antagonists like warfarin (Table 16.1).

Unfractionated heparin is composed of sulphated glycosaminoglycan chains. Only the heparin chains that contain a specific pentasaccharide sequence can bind plasma antithrombin to greatly accelerate antithrombin dependent inactivation of several activated clotting factors, especially factor IIa (thrombin) and factor Xa. Anticoagulant activity also depends on chain length; below 18 saccharide units the effect is limited to factor Xa alone. Unfractionated heparin is given by intravenous (iv) injection or infusion and by subcutaneous (sc) injection. Absorption after sc injection is dose-dependent. Elimination half-life increases with dose, but

not with age or diminishing renal function. Anticoagulant effect is measured using the activated partial thromboplastin time (aPTT), although the test response to heparin is blunted by illness, surgery, pregnancy and insensitive laboratory reagents (2)

Low molecular weight heparins (LMWH; enoxaparin, dalteparin and others) are derived by degrading and/or fractionating heparin chains until factor Xa inhibition predominates. Their predictable pharmacodynamics permits fixed but weight-adjusted dosing without measuring anticoagulant effect except in kidney failure (since excretion is largely renal) and perhaps in pregnancy or extreme obesity. Anticoagulant effect is measured using a factor Xa inhibition assay (not the aPTT). LMWHs differs in their factor Xa:IIa inhibition ratio (about 6–10:1) and elimination half-life (about two to four hours), are given by daily or twice-daily sc injection, but have mostly similar clinical effects (2).

Vitamin K antagonists (warfarin and other coumarins) are rapidly and well absorbed after oral administration. In the liver, they block interconversion between vitamin K1 and its 2, 3 epoxide and so prevent the vitamin K dependent γ-carboxylation of glutamate residues found at the N-terminal ends of clotting factors II, VII, IX and X (and also the natural anticoagulant proteins C and S). Without γ-carboxyl groups, these

Prescribing for Elderly Patients   Edited by Stephen Jackson, Paul Jansen and Arduino Mangoni
© 2009 John Wiley & Sons, Ltd

Table 16.1. Mode of action and anticoagulant effects of anticoagulants now in wide clinical use

Anticoagulant	Action	Route	Pharmacodynamics and kinetics
Unfractionated heparin	Factor IIa and Xa inhibition, mediated through plasma antithrombin	sc or iv	Complex
			Variably prolonged aPTT and TCT (rising bioavailability with increasing sc dose); equal inhibition of factor Xa and IIa
			$t^1/_2$ rises from 30 to 150 mins with increasing iv bolus dose
			Cmax about 3 hours after sc injection
Low molecular weight heparins (LMWH)	Mainly factor Xa (some factor IIa) inhibition, mediated through plasma antithrombin	sc	Predictable absorption and reproducible time-course of factor Xa inhibition
			$t^1/_2$ 3–6 hrs independent of dose
			Clearance mainly by kidney (prolonged $t^1/_2$ in renal failure)
Vitamin K antagonists	Prevent conversion of vitamin K to its 2, 3 epoxide; reduce the activity of factors II, VII, IX and X	oral	Good and rapid oral absorption (Cmax about 90 mins).
			Warfarin: $t^1/_2$ 40–70 hrs
			Phenprocoumon: $t^1/_2$ 90–140 hrs
			Acenocoumarol: $t^1/_2$ 3–10 hrs

clotting proteins cannot bind to phospholipid surfaces through calcium bridges and remain inactive. The anticoagulant effect is reversed by vitamin K1 (3).

Warfarin and other coumarins have different half-lives (Table 16.1) and dose regimens but share a narrow therapeutic window, variable dose response, multiple interactions with other drugs and concurrent illness, and a critical need for excellent communications between doctor and patient (3). Their anticoagulant effect is measured using a standardised prothrombin time ratio (the INR or International Normalised Ratio) and dosing is generally adjusted to maintain a target INR of 2.5 (range 2.0–3.0). Warfarin, like other coumarins, contains R- and S- isomers metabolized by the hepatic CYP enzyme complex, with CYP2CP most relevant to the more potent S-form (4). Dose requirement varies greatly between individuals. Genetic polymorphisms of CYP2CP and of the gene encoding the warfarin target enzyme (vitamin K epoxide reductase complex 1; VKORC1) explain more than half the variability in warfarin dose (5).

Newer and New Anticoagulants: Fondaparinux is a synthetic pentasaccharide that replicates the antithrombin binding site of heparins, has a much longer elimination half-life of about 18 hours (further prolonged in renal failure) and is given by daily sc injection. Fondaparinux inactivates only factor Xa. A number of newly developed orally active anticoagulants specifically inhibit thrombin or factor Xa without needing a plasma cofactor. The first was ximelagatran, a direct antithrombin which was clinically effective but had unacceptable liver toxicity. It is hoped that others still under clinical development will be effective, safe and have no need for dose-adjustment using laboratory tests.

THROMBOSIS IN THE ELDERLY AND INDICATIONS FOR ANTICOAGULANTS

Reasons for long-term anticoagulant therapy include atrial fibrillation (AF), other heart diseases, venous thromboembolism (VTE), and artery surgery. Short-term indications include preventing VTE during times of high risk. Two very high priorities for clinical practice improvement are better oral anticoagulant management and improved prevention of venous thromboembolism.

Atrial Fibrillation reduces cardiac output, predisposes to thrombus formation in the dysfunctional left atrium, and is a major cause of systemic embolism in the elderly. AF affects roughly 5 % of people aged over 65 with prevalence rising from < 0.1 % at 55 years to 10 % above age 80, and accounts for about 15 % of all ischaemic strokes (7 % at age 50–59, but one third in octogenarians). Risk of stroke is similar in paroxysmal and persistent AF. Stroke in AF tends to be severe, leaving 15–30 % of victims permanently disabled (6).

The $CHADS_2$ score is widely used to estimate the likelihood of systemic embolism and allots two points for a previous stroke or TIA, and one point each for age $\geq$ 75 years, previous hypertension, diabetes or heart failure. The annual stroke rate rises from 2 % to 18 % as the score increases from 0 to 6 (6, 7). Nearly 85 % of people with AF present with a high risk of a future stroke and are candidates for antithrombotic therapy (1).

Vitamin K antagonists reduce stroke rates in AF by almost 70 %. Reduction by aspirin is only 20 % but serious bleeding is much less likely. Warfarin is greatly superior to aspirin when AF has already led to a previous transient cerebral ischaemic attack or minor stroke.

Meta-analysis suggests that one year of warfarin would prevent 23 more ischaemic strokes per 1000 patients than one year of aspirin but cause 9 extra bleeding events (8). Treatment must balance these opposing outcomes. Based on the likelihood of future embolism, warfarin is preferred if the risk is high (e.g. age $\geq$75, other risk factors). If risk is moderate (age 65–75 without risk factors) then warfarin or aspirin is appropriate, depending on bleeding risk. Aspirin is preferred if risk is low (age $\leq$65 without risk factors) (6). Treatment continues for life, unless stopped for bleeding or bleeding risk.

It was hoped that adding a second antiplatelet drug to aspirin in AF would improve efficacy and retain safety, but adding clopidogrel has proved disappointing. In a recent comparison, the annual stroke rate was 5.6 % with combined antiplatelet therapy and 3.9 % with warfarin;

the corresponding rates of major bleeding were 9.4 % and 2.2 % (9).

Prosthetic heart valves: The life-long risks from valve thrombosis and systemic embolism are much reduced by vitamin K inhibitors. Adding aspirin to warfarin increases efficacy but adds to gastrointestinal bleeding. Aspirin is ineffective when given alone.

Deep vein thrombosis (DVT) and pulmonary embolism (PE): Annual risk of developing VTE increases exponentially with age to 50 per 1000 above 80 years. Common predispositions include major surgery, trauma, severe immobility and medical illness but about two thirds of cases develop in the community and 25–50 % have no apparent cause. A low threshold for diagnostic suspicion must be combined with reliable confirmatory testing, since the typical signs and symptoms are notoriously misleading. An underlying cancer is usually obvious at presentation and is more likely with increasing age. There is, however, need for simple cancer screening in people aged over 60 years with apparently unprovoked VTE, since 5–10 % subsequently present with a malignancy. A careful clinical examination, chest X-ray, blood tests, stool haemoglobin, urinalysis and perhaps pelvic ultrasound examination or CT scanning are enough, since a more intensive search has not improved outcomes. Inherited or acquired thrombophilias contribute little to VTE in the elderly, where screening for these disorders has negligible benefit.

Anticoagulants reduce the chances of extension or recurrence by at least 90 %. Untreated pulmonary embolism recurs in 50 % of people, causing death in 25 %. This compares with recurrence rates of about 3 % during three to six months of standard anticoagulant therapy (fatal in < 1 %) and major bleeding in 2–4 %. The usual treatment is at least 4 days of a heparin coupled with ongoing warfarin, but continued treatment with a LMWH is more effective if thrombosis complicates an active cancer (10, 11). The planned treatment duration should balance the relative risks of a recurrence without continued therapy and of bleeding during warfarin. Recurrence rates are high during the first two to four weeks after presentation and then diminish during three to six months of treatment.

Unprovoked late recurrence is unlikely when the predisposition was transient (surgery, injury or acute medical illness) but reaches 25–30 % during three to five years after idiopathic (unprovoked) venous thromboembolism. Risk persists indefinitely when there is active cancer or the phospholipid antibody syndrome, or after repeated recurrences, and in rare cases of familial thrombosis. Bleeding risk permitting, treatment should continue for three to six months after VTE with a transient cause, and at least six to 12 months after idiopathic thrombosis (10). It remains uncertain if thrombus resolution and/or a normal D-Dimer level after three to six months of therapy can predict low recurrence rates in people with idiopathic thrombosis.

Preventing Venous Thromboembolism: Systematic VTE prophylaxis during and soon after a major surgical or medical illness is highly effective. The choice between unfractionated or low molecular weight heparin, graded compression stockings and warfarin depends on predisposition and clinical profile (decreased renal function requires LMWH dose reduction). Aspirin has limited benefit. Prophylaxis is underused especially during medical admissions, which are no less prone to cause VTE than surgery or trauma.

Artery thrombosis: Anticoagulants have little value in thrombotic artery occlusion. Any benefit from warfarin after surgery for peripheral vascular disease is limited to patients at high risk of postoperative occlusion and limb loss.

Warfarin and bleeding risk

The reported annual incidence of major bleeding during treatment with coumarins in atrial fibrillation is about 1.3 % compared with 1 % in untreated controls (intracranial bleeding rates were 0.3 % and 0.1 %). Reported bleeding rates soon after VTE are a little higher (12).

The most important predictor of bleeding is INR. Other determinants are age over 65 or 70 years, female gender, comorbidities like cancer, renal failure, diabetes and severe anaemia, previous bleeding or stroke, and concomitant treatment with antiplatelet drugs like aspirin and clopidogrel, stomach irritants like nonsteroidal anti-inflammatory drugs, or drugs that prolong the INR. A simple risk assessment counts two points for previous bleeding and one point each for hepatic or renal disease, ethanol abuse, malignancy, age over 75 years, reduced platelet count or function, uncontrolled hypertension, anaemia, and a high risk of falling or of stroke. Each point raises the annual bleeding risk: from 1.9 % when the score is zero to > 12 % with five or more points (13). Warfarin-induced bleeding may unmask urogenital or gastrointestinal pathology. The chances of intracranial bleeding are raised by pre-existing cerebrovascular disease or uncontrolled hypertension, by increasing INR > 3.0, and probably by concomitant antiplatelet therapy.

Likely benefit and probable hazard

Choices between warfarin or aspirin in AF and of treatment duration after VTE are coloured by the perceptions about efficacy, risks and inconvenience. *Clinicians* increasingly accept the need for evidence-based decisions but add subjective assessments (cognitive status and predicted treatment compliance). Their prescribing may also be distorted by recent treatment complications (clinicians are 20–40 % less likely to recommend warfarin for AF during the three to six months after a patient has suffered major anticoagulant-related bleeding, but tend to take less notice of patients who suffer a stroke while not taking warfarin) (14). *Patients* often have higher thresholds for accepting warfarin in AF than the expert guidelines suggest, and tend to reject warfarin unless the annual risk of stroke with aspirin exceeds 2–6 % (15). Treatment preferences of patients with VTE are often unrelated to the likelihood of a recurrence: regardless of the predicted long-term recurrence rate, 23 % would continue warfarin while 25 % would stop. They also differ greatly when valuing treatments and outcomes like 'no anticoagulant therapy' or 'non-fatal haemorrhagic stroke' (16).

Special concerns in the elderly: In AF, old age raises the risks of both stroke and the chances of major bleeding with warfarin. Net benefit of warfarin extends into extreme old age if the likelihood of an embolic stroke is high, since this often causes long-term disability while non-fatal bleeding usually resolves (17). Net benefit persists despite moderate alcohol intake, previous stroke or gastro-intestinal bleeding, a tendency to fall, or treatment with non-steroidal anti-inflammatory drugs if combined with a proton-pump inhibitor (18). Nevertheless, the safe use of warfarin in the very old is often limited by significant contra-indications.

How to treat

Unfractionated heparin: Usually, iv injection of 5000 units (U) is followed by iv infusion of 1250 U/hour (30,000 U/24 hours), adjusted to prolong the aPTT to 1.5–2.5 times normal (or more correctly, a range that correspond to 0.3–0.7 IU/mL of factor Xa inhibition) (2). At first, the aPTT is measured at least twice-daily because many patients need higher than average doses, circulating half-life is short and anticoagulant response varies. An early target effect is important, since delay is associated with recurrence after VTE and poor outcomes in coronary artery disease. In DVT, heparin is effective by sc injection (5000 U iv, then 17 500 U 12 hourly sc, adjusted to achieve a mid-interval APTT of 1.5 to 2.5 times normal, or 333 U/kg iv, followed by 250 U/kg 12 hourly sc without adjusting for aPTT)(10;19). Much smaller doses of 5000 U given sc 12 or 8 hourly are effective for preventing VTE in elderly medical inpatients and after general surgery but are suboptimal after major joint surgery (hip or knee replacement and hip fracture) where LMWH are preferred. Preventive therapy should continue until the acute predisposition has passed. No laboratory monitoring is needed.

Antidote: protamine sulphate (1 mg neutralizes 100 IU of unfractionated heparin).

Low molecular weight heparins (LMWHs) after DVT or submassive PE are equally or more effective and safe than unfractionated heparin and seem to be superior after ACS without ST-elevation (20). Their predictable anticoagulant effect allows home therapy. LMWHs are more effective than unfractionated heparin in preventing VTE after hip replacement and hip fracture, where prophylaxis should usually continue for four to five weeks, and after knee replacement where 10 days of prophylaxis are usually enough (21). The LMWHs differ in dosage (mg or units of factor Xa inhibiting

activity) and approved treatment regimen, and are not all available in all countries. Readers should consult relevant product guidelines. Table 16.2 summarizes dosing for two widely approved LMWH (enoxaparin and dalteparin). Clinical trials find few if any differences in efficacy or safety.

LMWHs are cleared mainly by the kidney, and renal failure in the elderly seems to increase the bleeding risk. Enoxaparin dose-reduction is recommended if derived creatinine clearance is < 30 mL/min, but unfractionated heparin is often preferred in renal failure. LMWHs are less likely than standard heparin to cause heparin-induced thrombocytopenia (HIT), an infrequent but potentially devastating immune-mediated thrombotic syndrome, but cross-react with the causal antibody and should not be given to people with this condition.

Antidote: Protamine sulphate reverses about 50 % of the factor Xa inhibition by LMWHs. Its clinical utility for arresting bleeding remains untested.

The vitamin K antagonists: warfarin, phenprocoumon and acenocoumarol

The target INR for most clinical indications is 2.5 (range 2.0–3.0). In AF, the stroke rate is increased when INR falls below 2.0 (Odds Ratio 5.07 for all ischaemic events) or when INR ≤ 1.6 is compared with INR of 2–3 (relative risk 2.0 for any thrombosis, and 2.2 for ischaemic stroke) (22). After VTE, about 30 % of effectiveness is lost if target range is reduced to 1.5–2.0 after six to 12 months of standard therapy (10). Raising the range to 3.0–4.5 does not add efficacy even in the phospholipid antibody syndrome, although some mechanical prosthetic heart valves may benefit. The likelihood of major bleeding increases progressively above an INR of 3.0. Typically, the times spent within, above or below the recommended INR during long-term therapy are about 60 %, 15 %, and 25 %, although these results are suboptimal and can be improved.

Dose regimens are quoted for warfarin, the most widely used vitamin K antagonist.

Starting warfarin. The rate and extent of rise in INR vary greatly when starting warfarin.

Table 16.2. Dosing with the LMWHs enoxaparin and dalteparin

	Indication	Usual dosing regimen	Comments
Enoxaparin	Treatment	1 mg/kg bid sc or 1.5 mg/kg od sc	1 mg/kg od if derived creatinine clearance < 30 ml/min.
	VTE Prevention	20 mg sc od, or 40 mg sc od	Low to medium risk surgery. High risk surgery (major joint replacement) and medical VTE prevention; 20 mg sc od if creatinine clearance < 30 ml/min. Consider post-discharge prophylaxis if continued risk (recommended after hip replacement and in many patients after cancer surgery).
Dalteparin	Treatment	200 IU/kg od sc	6 months of sc dalteparin (dose reduced to 150 IU od after 4 weeks) more effective than warfarin for VTE with active cancer
	VTE prevention	2500 IU sc od, or 5000 IU sc od	Low to medium risk surgery. High risk (eg cancer) surgery and high risk medical inpatients. Consider post-discharge prophylaxis if continued risk (recommended after hip replacement and in many patients after cancer surgery).

Warfarin has a delayed effect because it takes time for circulating vitamin K dependent clotting factors to clear. Factor VII is lost first (t^1/$_2$ six hours), followed by factors IX (t^1/$_2$ 24 hours), X (t^1/$_2$ 36 hours) and II (t^1/$_2$ 72 hours) (23), and it takes some days after dose alteration to reach a new steady state. Warfarin also reduces protein C and S levels. The eight hour half-life of protein C means it can be depleted before the effects on factors II, X and IX are fully expressed. Rarely, this may cause a prothrombotic state which is countered by four to five days of initial overlap with a heparin. The slower onset of warfarin effect with starting doses of 5 mg/day or less (as in atrial fibrillation) avoids the need for initial heparin.

A popular regimen for hospital inpatients begins with 10 mg/day and aims for a rapid INR effect (larger doses are often excessive). It is more usual to begin with 5 mg/day or less if the expected dose requirement is low or when there is no urgency (as in community patients with AF). At first, INR is measured every one to two days, although starting doses of 3–4 mg/day need less frequent testing. A randomised comparison of starting with 10 mg or 5 mg daily found that 10 mg/day achieved its target INR 1.4 days sooner, with similar chances of an INR > 5.0 and of adverse events during the first four weeks

(24). Once INR has reached 2.0–3.0 for several days, the frequency of testing can be reduced; to once weekly and then to once in—three to six or even eight to 12 weeks depending on clinical need. The clinical value of identifying fast or slow warfarin metabolisers by testing for genetic polymorphisms remains under investigation.

Computer based dosing algorithms or simple nomograms are widely used when starting warfarin. These derive the evening's warfarin dose from that morning's INR and tend to perform as well or better than experienced clinicians. There is a rough correlation between dose-response when starting warfarin and subsequent maintenance dose, but the need to frequently monitor the INR during the first weeks of therapy remains.

Adjusting warfarin dose for age: median daily dose-requirement decreases from 5–5.5 mg at age 50–59 to 3–3.5 mg above 90 years; women need about 0.5 mg/day less than men and are more prone to overanticoagulation. Starting doses of 5 mg/day are too high in about 65 % of men and over 80 % of women aged > 75 years(25). Reasons include an age-related decrease in warfarin clearance, comorbidities (heart failure and liver dysfunction) and nutritional status. Elderly patients may bleed at lower INR levels than younger people, suggesting the need for an earlier response to excessive INR.

Table 16.3. Examples of important drug interactions with warfarin (adapted from (3))

Mechanism	Drug or Comorbidity	Effect on INR
Reduced warfarin absorption	cholestyramine	decrease
Inhibition of S-warfarin metabolism	metronidazole, trimethoprim-sulphamethoxazole, amiodarone	increase
Inhibition of R-warfarin metabolism	cimetidine, omeprazole	Modest increase
Increased hepatic metabolism of warfarin	Barbiturates (CYP3A), rifampicin and carbamazepine (CYP3A4)	decrease
Effect on vitamin K—vitamin K epoxide	Some cephalosporins	increase
Metabolism of factors II, VII, IX, X	Hyperthyroidism	Increase
Unknown	clofibrate	Increase
Known to have no interaction	Alcohol, antacids, atenolol, diltiazem, famotidine, ibuprofen, ketoconazole, metoprolol, naproxen, paracetamol (probably), ranitidine, vancomycin	

Drug Interactions: Many drugs can change warfarin absorption or metabolism, although relatively few cause a predictable and important increase or decrease in INR (Table 16.3). In case of doubt, it is important to check a current database for known interactions and also to check INR weekly for several weeks when starting or stopping other medications. For instance, it can take six weeks for the inhibitory effects of barbiturates or carbamazepine to resolve (3). It seems likely that an association of excessive INR during warfarin therapy with large daily doses of paracetamol (acetaminophen, > 6 gm/d) was due to the comorbidities requiring analgesia rather than a major drug interaction (12).

Intake of dietary vitamin K or alcohol: A small effect on INR can follow very large serves of vegetables (400 gm with 700–1500 microgram of Vitamin K1) but is unlikely with more typical helpings of < 100 gm (26). Small daily doses of vitamin K1 can help to stabilize INR in people with an otherwise erratic anticoagulant effect. Moderate alcohol intake does not affect warfarin control. Intoxication should be avoided.

Other dosing considerations: There are reports that changing from one brand of warfarin to another or to a generic equivalent may destabilized the dose-response. Formal evaluations suggest this concern is usually unfounded.

Patient Education and Communication: Surveys of warfarin-treated patients find distressing levels of ignorance about the drug. Appropriate education about benefits, hazards and appropriate uses of warfarin, and effective communication about INR results and dose, are essential to good management.

Point of Care (POC) devices allow immediate face-to-face feedback about INR and dose-adjustment, and can be used by patients to self-test and self-adjust their warfarin dose. Drawbacks include limited external quality control and the cost of disposable test cartridges. Randomised comparisons find similar or better dose control than with laboratory based dose adjustment. Education about warfarin plus self-monitoring in patients aged over 65 halved their risk of major bleeding during a six month randomized comparison with usual care (27).

Antidote: Vitamin K1 corrects the warfarin effect.

Response to excessive INR and to warfarin-associated bleeding

Management depends on the presence or absence of bleeding and may require vitamin K1 and clotting factor replacement. Clotting factors should be given only if there is immediate need to reverse warfarin effect.

Vitamin K1: The iv formulation is orally absorbed. Intravenous injection has the quickest and most predictable response but may rarely cause serious (sometimes fatal) anaphylaxis. Oral dosing is usually effective (28), sc vitamin K1 is less reliable (29), and intramuscular injection may cause local bleeding and should be avoided.

Excessive INR without clinically important bleeding: An INR of 3.0–4.0 has little effect on bleeding risk and only needs an earlier appointment. Further increase to ≤ 5 requires a small dose reduction of $\leq 20\%$ after omitting one dose (30). Response above 5–6 depends on INR and intrinsic bleeding risk. Temporarily withholding warfarin plus close monitoring may be enough, but INR takes three to four days to reach safer levels of < 4 after stopping warfarin if INR > 6, and longer when the starting INR > 10; giving vitamin K1 achieves the same result within 24–48 hours (28). The aim is to return INR to within its target range but avoid sub-therapeutic levels that may permit thrombosis and perhaps cause resistance when restarting warfarin. It is also important to seek possible explanations for unexpected fluctuation of the INR.

When there is a need to quickly correct an INR >5 but bleeding risk remains acceptable, then small oral doses of vitamin K1 are usually sufficient and are unlikely to over-correct the prolonged INR. The response by 24 hours depends on the dose of Vitamin K1 and the initial INR (28). Studies have shown that oral doses of 2.5 or 5.0 mg reduce INR to safer levels of 2–5 within 14 hours in 75% people whose starting INR is 8–12 and in 50% of those with a starting INR of >12 (31). The effect of 2 mg orally is similar. An iv dose of 0.5 mg is equivalent to 2.5 mg given orally, but response to 0.5 mg iv is slower and less complete when the baseline INR is very prolonged (> 10) (29).

Guidelines for managing an INR of 5–9 depend on bleeding risk. If this is low, then stop warfarin and closely monitor the INR before restarting warfarin at a reduced dose. If the bleeding risk is high, then give Vitamin K1. All patients with an INR >9 should receive vitamin K1. Clotting factor replacement may be added to vitamin K1 administration if bleeding risk is very high (3; 32). Bleeding risk can be significant when INR is > 5–6. Clotting factor replacement may be added to vitamin K1 if bleeding risk is very high.

Response to bleeding during warfarin therapy: If significant bleeding cannot be controlled by local measures, then stop warfarin, give 5–10 mg of vitamin K1 iv, and correct the co-agulation defect with clotting factor infusion. Warfarin should be restarted only if there is strong reason for ongoing therapy and after bleeding has stopped (3).

Anticoagulant treatment and the need for surgery or invasive procedures (bridging)

When faced with the need for surgery or an invasive procedure during warfarin therapy, first assess thrombosis risk without warfarin (high for prosthetic heart valves, or atrial fibrillation with previous stroke, or soon after VTE; much lower months to years after the most recent VTE), then consider if warfarin can be safely continued (as with most dental work) or devise peri-operative management to minimize the combined risks of bleeding and thrombosis. This should be done with a cardiologist and/or haematologist. Warfarin may continue if bleeding risk is acceptable, aiming for a peri-operative INR of 1.6–2 (or 1.5 for more extensive surgery). Or warfarin may be replaced with iv heparin or sc LMWH for several days. If surgical bleeding risk is very high, then anticoagulants should be stopped for several days unless this is totally contraindicated. Before urgent surgery, warfarin effect can be reversed with vitamin K1 and (if needed) clotting factor infusion, since it takes INR 2–4 days after stopping warfarin (longer in older people) to normalize from a steady state of 2.0–3.0.

REFERENCES

1. Waldo AL, Beccker RC, Tapson VF, Colgan KJ. Hospitalized patients with atrial fribrillation and a high risk of stroke are not being provided with adequate anticoagulation. *Journal of the American College of Cardiology* 2005; **46**(9): 1729–36.

2. Hirsh J, Raschke R. Heparin and Low-Molecular-Weight Heparin. The Seventh ACCP Conference on Antithrombotic and Thrombolytic Therapy. *Chest* 2004; **126**: 188S–203S.

3. Ansell J, Hirsh J, Poller L, Bussey H, Jacobson A, Hylek E. The pharmacology and

management of the vitamin K antagonists. The Seventh ACCP Conference on Antithrombotic and Thrombolytic Therapy. *Chest* 2004; **126**: 204S–233S.

4. Ufer M. Comparative pharmacokinetics of vitamin K antagonists: warfarin, phenprocoumon and acenocoumarol. *Clinical Pharmacokinetics* 2005; **44**: 1227–46.

5. Sconce EA, Khan TI, Wynne HA et al. The impact of CYP2C9 and VKORC1 genetic polymorphism and patient charactreristics upon warfarin dose reuirement: proposal for a new dosing regimen. *Blood* 2005; **106**: 2329–33.

6. Singer DE, Albers GW, Dalen JA, Go AS, Halperin JL, Manning WJ. Antithrombotic therapy in atrial fibrillation. The seventh ACCP conference on antithrombotic and thrombolytic therapy. *Chest* 2004; **126**: 429S–456S.

7. Gage BF, Waterman AD, Shannon W, Boechler M, Rich MW, Radford MJ. Validation of clinical classification schemes for predicting stroke: Results from the National registry of Atrial Fibrillation. *Journal of the American Medical Association* 2001; **285**(22): 2864–70.

8. van Walraven C, Hart RG, Singer DE et al. Oral anticoagulants vs aspirin in nonvalvular atrial fibrillation: an individual patient meta-analysis. *Journal of the American Medical Association* 2002; **288**(19): 2441–8.

9. The ACTIVE Writing Group. Clopidogrel plus aspirin versus orl anticoagulation for atrial fibrillation in the Atrial fibrillation Clopidogrel Trial with Irbesartan for the prevention of Vascular Events (ACTIVE W): a randomised controlled trial. *Lancet* 2006; **367**: 1903–12.

10. Buller HR, Agnelli G, Hull RD, Hyers TM, Prins MH, Raskob GE. Antithrombotic therapy for venous thromboembolic disease. The Seventh ACCP Conference on Antithrombotic and Thrombolytic Therapy. *Chest* 2004; **10**: 401S–428S.

11. Lee AY, Levine MN, Baker RI. Low-molecular-weight heparin vesrsus a coumarin for the prevention of recurrent venous thromboembolism in patients with cance3r. *New England Journal of Medicine* 2003; **349**: 146–53.

12. Levine MN, Raskob G, Beyth RJ, Kearon C, Schulman S. Hemorrhagic complications of anticoagulant treatment. The Seventh ACCP Conference on Antithrombotic and Thrombolytic Therapy. *Chest* 2004; **126**: 287S–310S.

13. Gage BF, Yan Y, Milligan PE et al. Clinical classification for predicting hemarrhage: results from the National Registry of Atrial Fibrillation (NRAF). *American Heart Journal* 2006; **151**: 713–19.

14. Choudhry NK, Anderson GM, Laupacis A, Ross-Degnan D, Normand S-LT, Soumerai SB. Impact of adverse events on prescribing warfarin in patients with atrial fibrillation: matched pair analysis. *British Medical Journal* 2006; **332**: 141–5.

15. Man-Song-Hing M, Gage BF, Montgomery AA et al. Preference-based anticoagulant therapy in atrial fibrillation: implications for clinical decision making. *Medical Decision Making* 2005; **25**: 548–59.

16. Locadia M, Bossuyt PMM, Stalmeier PFM et al. Treatment of venous thromboembolism with vitamin K antagonists: patients' health state valuations and treatment preferences. *Thrombosis and Haemostasis* 2004; **92**: 1336–41.

17. Johnson CE, Lim WK, Workman BS. People aged over 75 in atrial fibrillation on warfarin: the rate of major haemorrhage and stroke in more than 500 patient-years of follow-up. *Journal of the American Geriatric Society* 2005; **53**: 655–9.

18. Man-Song-Hing M, Laupacis A. Anticoagulant-related bleeding in older persons with atrial fibrillation. Physicians' fears often unfounded. *Archives of Internal Medicine* 2003; **163**: 1580–6.

19. Kearon C, Ginsberg JS, Julian JJ et al. Comparison of fixed-dose weight-adjusted unfractionated heparin and low-molecular-weight heparin for acute treatment of venous thromboembolism. *Journal of the American Medical Association* 2006; **296**: 935–42.

20. Harrington RA, Becker RC, Ezekowitz M et al. Antithrombotic therapy for coronary artery disease. The Seventh ACCP Conference on Antithromboyic and Thrombolytic Therapy. *Chest* 2004; **126**: 513S–548S.

21. Geerts WH, Pineo GF, Heit JA et al. Prevention of venous thromboembolism. *Chest* 2004; **126**: 338S–400S.

22. Perret-Guillaume C, Wahl DG. Low dose warfarin in atrial fibrillation leads to more thromboembolic events without reducing major bleeding when compared to adjusted dose-a meta-analysis. *Thrombosis and Haemostasis* 2004; **91**: 394–402.

23. Freedman JE, Adelman B. Pharmacology of heparin and oral anticoagulants. In: Loscalzo J, Schafer AI, eds *Thrombosis and Hemorrhage*. Boston: Blackwell Scientific Publications, 1994: 1155–71.

24. Kovacs MJ, Rodger MA, Anderson DR et al. Comparison of 10-mg and 5-mg warfarin initiation nomograms together with low-molecular-weight heparin for outpatient treatment of venous thromboembolism. A randomized, double-blind, controlled trial. *Annals of Internal Medicine* 2003; **138**: 714–19.

25. Garcia D, Regan S, Crowther M, Hughes RA, Hylek EM. Warfarin maintenance dosing patterns in clinical practice: implications for safer anticoagulaton in the elderly population. *Chest* 2005; **127**: 2049–56.

26. Johnson MA. Influence of vitamin K on anticoagulant therapy depends on vitamin K status and the source and chemical forms of vitamin K. *Nutrition Reviews* 2005; **63**: 91–7.

27. Beyth RJ, Quinn L, Landefeld CS. A multicomponent intervention to prevent major bleeding compications in older patients receiving warfarin. A randomized controlled trial. *Annals of Internal Medicine* 2000; **133**: 687–95.

28. Hanslik T, Prinseau J. The use of Vitamin K in patients on anticoagulant therapy. A practical guide. *American Journal of Cardiovascular Drugs* 2004; **4**: 43–55.

29. DeZee KJ, Shimeall WT, Douglas KM, Shumway NM, O'Malley PG. Treatment of excessive anticoagulation with phytonadione (vitamin K). A meta-analysis. *Archives of Internal Medicine* 2006; **166**: 391–7.

30. Banet GA, Waterman AD, Milligan PE, Gatchel SK, Gage BF. Warfarin dose reduction vs watchful waiting for mild elevations in the International Normalized Ratio. *Chest* 2003; **123**: 499–503.

31. Baker P, Gleghorn A, Tripp T, Paddon K, Eagletin H, Keeling D. Reversal of asymptomatic over-anticoagulation by orally administered vitamin K. *British Journal of Haematology* 2006; **133**: 331–6.

32. Baglin TP, Keeling DM, Watson HG, for the British Committee for Standards in Haematology. Guidelines on oral anticoagulation (warfarin): third edition—2005 update. *British Journal of Haematology* 2005; **132**: 277–85.

17 Haematological disorders

Bryone J. Kuss and Sabria Alhashami

Department of Haematology and Genetic Pathology, Flinders Medical Centre, Flinders University, Adelaide, Australia

INTRODUCTION

Haematological diseases or abnormalities are common among the elderly. Anaemia due to a variety of chronic illnesses or underlying pathology; myelodysplasia and chronic lymphocytic leukaemia are frequent entities seen in private and public pathology laboratories and also general practise. The increasing expectation of a long life with good quality and the changing availability of treatments means that more needs be considered when managing the elderly patient.

Recent studies evaluating the quality of life and outcome in the elderly population have shown that some patients do extremely poorly. However, the group with low risk disease performs far better than expected for this age group as a whole. Overall, outcomes for the elderly population will improve if efforts are made to obtain a diagnosis and to treat the underlying condition, rather than to ignore abnormal haematological parameters until the condition significantly affects quality of life. Most importantly the patient should be well informed and given treatment choices that are appropriate to their philosophy of life and work within the limits of their co-morbidities.

ANAEMIA

Anaemia is a common problem in the elderly with an overall prevalence of 20 % in men and 13.7 % in women in the UK (22, 25). The presence of anaemia contributes significantly to ill health and cardiovascular stress including a greater than chance association with microvascular dementia and increased mortality. It is important to note that when assessing the complete blood picture of a geriatric population, the values for haemoglobin, white cell count and platelet numbers are not significantly altered by age alone and numerical values outside the reference range for an adult population represent underlying pathology. Reduction in overall haematopoiesis within the bone marrow is evident. However this reflects reduced bone marrow reserve and does not affect baseline blood levels in healthy elderly individuals. The ESR is however affected by age and relates to fibrinogen concentration which also increases with age >70 years.

Iron Deficiency

The most common cause of anaemia is iron deficiency, usually signifying blood loss which occurs in 3.5–5.3 % of elderly patients in the UK and USA (22). This classically presents with a microcytic picture but a falling Hb and MCV should alert one to the fact that iron stores may be reduced prior to the development of anaemia. Iron studies will usually confirm the diagnosis of iron deficiency however interpretation of ferritin in the elderly population may be confounded by co-existent inflammatory disease, underlying malignancy or liver disease.

Prescribing for Elderly Patients Edited by Stephen Jackson, Paul Jansen and Arduino Mangoni
© 2009 John Wiley & Sons, Ltd

Investigation

The underlying cause of iron deficiency should be sought and primarily gastrointestinal blood loss should be excluded with faecal human haemoglobin (FHH) testing as a minimum. Lower GI endoscopy is recommended with positive FHH due to the relatively high incidence of colonic carcinoma in this age group (41 % of demonstrated lower GI bleeding in the elderly) which may be treated and cured in early stages. Other causes such as NSAID usage/gastritis, coeliac disease, gastric cancer and intestinal telangiectasia should be considered and investigated appropriately. Endoscopy and biopsy may be required at the outset to exclude coeliac disease or other upper GI causes of anaemia.

Management

Iron replacement should then be initiated using oral therapy wherever possible remembering the high frequency of GI side effects encountered. Where absorption is normal, intramuscular replacement of iron will result in no faster improvement in haemoglobin (Hb) than oral iron therapy using vitamin C. Intravenous replacement has the advantage of a single time-point of replacement of whole iron stores and subsequent to restoration of Hb the ferritin may then be used to monitor for continued blood loss, particularly in the setting of no demonstrable upper or lower GI lesion. The dosage is calculated using the formula taken from Ganzoni (1970). *Schweiz Med Wschr* **100**: 301–619.

Iron dose (mg) = Body Wt (kg) × (Target Hb − Actual Hb in g/L) × 0.24 + Iron Depot (500 mg)
NB: The factor $0.24 = 0.0034 \times 0.07 \times 1000$. Up to 34 kg body weight: target Hb = 130g/L, iron depot = 15 mg/kg body weight. Over 34 kg body weight: targetHb = 150g/L.

Protocol for Iron Administration

100 mg Iron Polymaltose in 2 ml ampoule (FERROSIG®). Total dose to be administered to be aseptically added to 500 ml of sterile Sodium Chloride 0.9 % (up to 2500 mg may be given in 500 ml). Doses <1200 mg may be added to 250 ml of Sodium Chloride 0.9 %.

Premedications should be administered 30–60 minutes before the commencement of the infusion if required due to previous reactions or high risk patient.

Administration and monitoring

- **First 5 ml**:
  - Infuse over 10 minutes (Rate: 20–40 ml/hr)
  - Monitor patient closely (vital signs every 2 minutes)

- **If no reaction**:
  - Increase Rate to 100 ml/hr
  - Measure vital signs every 30 minutes

Adverse effects

- Anaphylactoid reactions can occur especially at the beginning of infusion. If this occurs, stop the infusion immediately. Resuscitation equipment should be available including:
  - Adrenaline 1 in 10 000, 10 ml ampoule
  - Hydrocortisone 250 mg vial
  - Promethazine 50 mg ampoule
- Phlebitis: usually develops within 24–48 hours
- Flushing, sweating, fever, joint pains, nausea and vomiting: if not severe, infusion may be continued +/− analgesia and antihistamines.

Transfusion should be reserved for anaemia resulting in significant cardiovascular signs or symptoms. Guidelines for transfusion when Hb <85 g/L are not as useful in the elderly population and each individual needs to be assessed on their underlying cardiorespiratory tolerance of the anaemia. In a fully active bone marrow, after the first week it is expected that with replacement of iron stores, Hb will rise approximately 10 gm/L/week.

VITAMIN B12 AND FOLIC ACID DEFICIENCIES

Deficiency of these haematinics is frequent in the elderly population for a variety of reasons other than pernicious anaemia and coeliac disease. Included in this is the increasing use of proton pump inhibitors in treatment of oesophageal reflux and gastritis. The chronic use of these drugs leads to a low B12 without the presence of gastric parietal cell or intrinsic factor antibodies as would be expected in pernicious anaemia. Oral replacement with 1000 mcg/d of B12 will however effect satisfactory restoration of levels in most cases. For true pernicious anaemia 1000 mcg should be administered by intramuscular injection initially monthly for approximately three months, then three monthly ever after. Blood levels should be measured particularly in the first six months to establish that replacement is satisfactory.

Folate deficiency is more likely to be due to the high incidence of poor nutritional status in the elderly population as a whole and lowered intake of green leafy vegetables. Folate supplementation in the elderly has been addressed in terms the effects on cognitive function demonstrating a positive outcome (8) but this has not been addressed in terms of its effect on Hb specifically in the elderly. Multiple haematinic deficiencies should raise concerns of both dietary deficiency and malabsorption in the elderly considering late onset coeliac disease as a possible underlying pathology.

THROMBOCYTOPENIA

Thrombocytopenia is defined as a platelet count of less than 150×10^9/L. The severity of the thrombocytopenia has been classified into mild ($<150 \times 10^9$/L), moderate ($<100 \times 10^9$/L) and severe ($<50 \times 10^9$) on clinical grounds. Although bleeding tendency cannot be predicted by platelet count alone serious bleeding risk increases substantially when the count falls below 20×10^9/L. Clearly, the risk of bleeding is increased with co-existent NSAID or aspirin intake.

Presentation

Thrombocytopenia may be found incidentally on routine blood testing or in response to clinical signs and symptoms. The bleeding tends to be mucocutaneous, the commonest findings being purpura, petechiae, ecchymosis and epistaxis which may be exacerbated by the thin fragile skin of senescence. Few patients present with life threatening gastrointestinal or cerebral bleeding.

Aetiology

Thrombocytopenia can be due to one or a combination of the following:

- Reduced production: associated with primary bone marrow disease, e.g. myelodysplasia, leukaemia, aplastic anaemia or secondary to bone marrow fibrosis or infiltration by malignancies. Reversible causes include infections especially viral, vitamin B12 and/or folic acid deficiencies and drugs.
- Increased destruction and/or consumption: commonly immune thrombocytopenic purpura (ITP); disseminated intravascular coagulopathy (DIC) and drugs effects; also includes thrombotic thrombocytopenic purpura (TTP) and heparin induced thrombotic thrombocytopenia (HITT).
- Splenic sequestration: This is characterized by mild to moderate pancytopenia with near normal total body content of platelets.
- Massive transfusion.

Investigation

Thrombocytopenia should be confirmed by performing a blood film to eliminate platelet aggregation. Other significant morphological findings on the blood film include the presence of red cell fragments, seen in microangiopathy, tear drop cells as seen in bone marrow infiltration or fibrosis. The blood film examination will also test for the presence of leukocyte abnormalities as seen in leukaemia, lymphoma and myelodysplasia.

Other investigations should include coagulation profile; liver function and renal function tests; LDH; vitamin B12 and folate levels if there is accompanying macrocytosis and autoimmune screen where appropriate. Imaging studies should be considered individually depending on clinical suspicion. Much can be gained by careful peripheral blood film inspection without the need for bone marrow biopsy. Other specific tests, e.g. HIT screen and viral serology need to be decided according to the clinical context.

Management

This should be based on:

- the immediate risk of bleeding and the need for urgent correction of the thrombocytopenia by platelet transfusion;
- identifying the cause of the thrombocytopenia and then initiating specific treatment where possible.

Patients at highest risk of bleeding are those who:

- have a platelets count of $<10 \times 10^9/L$;
- have concurrent coagulation abnormalities;
- are on drugs affecting platelet function;
- have concurrent infection and fever.

Where thrombocytopenia is mild, other than identifying the cause and determining risks, no treatment may be required. The potential problem of concurrent anti-platelet drugs needs to be considered weighing the overall cardiovascular or cerebrovascular risks, as high risk of bleeding may be considered for platelet transfusion. A bleeding patient with significant thrombocytopenia should receive platelet transfusion until the bleeding stops aiming to keep the platelets count equal or above $50 \times 10^9/L$. Coagulation profile should be corrected if abnormal. If the patient is not bleeding or at high risk for bleeding, then a wait and watch approach is safe until full diagnostic work up for the cause of thrombocytopenia is performed.

The only two contraindications for platelet transfusion would be in the setting of TTP and HITT, since platelet transfusion may worsen the clinical status of the patient. TTP is a rare condition and it is defined clinically by thrombocytopenia, microangiopathy, renal dysfunction and neurological deficit. Treatment should be urgently instituted including intensive plasmapheresis since delays in the treatment can be fatal.

HITT is predominantly associated with the use of unfractionated heparin which must be immediately ceased and other forms of anticoagulation considered.

Acute ITP can be a life threatening event in the elderly with increased risk of intra-cerebral haemorrhage compared with younger age groups. Quinine ingestion needs to be excluded as this is more common in the elderly. Therapy may not be required if thrombocytopenia is mild and transient but platelet levels should be kept above $20 \times 10^9/L$. While transfusion of platelets is not generally effective, it may be justified in intracerebral haemorrhage while waiting for the effect of immunosuppression. ITP is most often managed with steroids alone or in combination with intravenous immunoglobulin (3). However, elderly patients are at higher risk for steroid psychosis, uncontrolled blood glucose levels as well as gastrointestinal ulcers and osteoporosis. The use of proton pump inhibitors is recommended with steroid usage. Other immunosuppressant agents including MabThera (antiCD20 antibody), vincristine, azathioprine, vinblastine and chronic anti-D therapy are also used with variable effect (5). Dapsone in small doses can be effective at maintaining safe platelet levels, the main side effect being mild anaemia from low grade haemolysis. Splenectomy may be considered depending on the patient's fitness for surgery.

The management of the thrombocytopenia which is associated with primary bone marrow disease is discussed below.

MYELODYSPLASTIC SYNDROMES

These are clonal disorders of multi-potential haemopoietic cells. The key pathogenetic features are the ineffective haemopoiesis resulting in cytopenias or dysfunctional cells and the tendency to progress to acute myeloid leukaemia (AML). The frequency and speed with which the MDS progresses to acute leukaemia varies with the different subtypes and the various cytogenetic abnormalities present in the MDS haematopoietic stem cells. These disorders affect mainly the elderly, showing a median age of 69 years with increasing prevalence rising to >20–30 per 100 000 in the over 70 years population. A prior history of chemo and or radiotherapy predisposes to MDS as well as AML and these secondary forms tend to be more aggressive and resistant to therapy.

Classification and Prognostication

There are currently two classification systems, the French- American- British (FAB) and WHO classification. In both, the morphological classification of MDS depends on the percent of leukaemic blasts in the bone marrow or blood, the type and degree of dysplasia and the presence of ringed sideroblasts. For practical purposes the MDS subtypes can be separated into two risk groups: low risk group containing solitary refractory anaemia (RA) and refractory anaemia with ringed sideroblasts. The high risk group contains refractory anaemia with excess blasts (RAEB) and refractory cytopenia with multilineage dysplasia (RC) with or without ringed sideroblasts. Further prognostication can be made using the International Prognostic Scoring System (IPSS) (16) and requires cytogenetic analysis. Overall life expectancy in patients with MDS is reduced compared to age and sex matched controls regardless of disease subtypes.

Additionally there is another group of disorders defined in the WHO classification system which presents predominantly in the elderly. These disorders have been defined as myelodysplastic/myeloproliferative disorders and the most common of these is chronic myelomonocytic leukaemia (CMML). Clonal cytogenetics is found in 20–40 % of CMML and survival varies from 1–100 months.

Clinical findings

The patients may be asymptomatic and diagnosed on incidental full blood count and morphology. Some may have anaemia related symptoms and signs. Few will present with bleeding or infection but most will progress to these problems in time. Hepatomegaly is seen in 5 % and splenomegaly in 10 % at presentation. In CMML patients with high monocytosis, the incidence of hepatosplenomegaly is up to 50 %. Those with severe leucopenia and thrombocytopenia at presentation are likely to have higher risk disease categories.

Laboratory investigations

- Full blood and reticulocyte counts which may show isolated or combined cytopenia. Monocytosis may be present.
- Blood film examination is crucial to demonstrate the morphological abnormalities seen in either one or all the lineages. Leukaemic blasts may also be seen and may herald progression to acute leukaemia.
- Estimations of vitamin B12, serum folate and ferritin levels are recommended.
- Bone marrow examination, if performed should include a trephine biopsy and cytogenetic analysis. In those selected patients, the trephine may identify a subtype of hypoplastic MDS which can respond to immunosuppression, although this is rare. Cytogenetic analysis is critical for accurate prognostication and management (14).

Management

Supportive care

Both good and poor risk groups in whom poor clinical status does not allow more active treatment are candidates for supportive therapy. The principles of this involves transfusion of cell products to correct cytopenia, rapid response to infection with appropriate antibiotic or antifungal therapy and appropriate home supports to maintain quality of life. (4)

The major side effect of red blood cell (RBC) transfusion is iron overload. The need for iron chelation has been addressed in these patients. However, in many patients it has not been practical for several reasons. Firstly continuous subcutaneous deferoxamine is not tolerated or acceptable for elderly patients. Secondly life expectancy of these patients is reduced and therefore cost benefit analysis of chelation has not been positive (16).

The advent of oral iron chelation has changed this. Currently the recommendations for iron chelation are as follows: receipt of 20–30 RBC transfusions; ferritin level >1000–1500 µg/L; low or intermediate risk patients with survival >1 year or higher risk patients if undergoing curative therapy (transplantation) (2). Prospective studies on overall survival and quality of life are awaited.

Pro-active Therapy

Therapeutic options in MDS particularly the higher risk subtypes have increased in recent years. While standard chemotherapeutic approaches are generally not associated with increased survival, newer agents whose mechanism of action is either demethylation or immunomodulatory/microenvironment modification have resulted in favourable outcomes. In the USA, three new agents have been approved for the treatment of MDS. These include: 5-azacytidine, lenalidomide and 5-aza-2-deoxycytidine (decitabine). Decitabine is a hypomethylating agent. The net effect is reactivation of epigenetically repressed genes such as tumour suppressor genes and others that may trigger cell differentiation and improve outcome in MDS (18). The usefulness of these agents is under clinical investigation.

Chronic myelomonocytic leukaemia may be indolent for many years and hydroxyurea is considered when there is progressive increase in the white cell count. Etoposide is also used but without an increased survival advantage.

Growth Factors in Refractory Anaemia

Routine use of granulocyte colony stimulating factor (GCSF) and/or prophylactic antibiotics or anti-fungal agents for neutropenia is not in general use. However, severe sepsis should be treated as per the local protocols for management of febrile neutropenia with broad spectrum antibiotics and consider the use GCSF to maintain the neutrophil count $>1.0 \times 10^9$/L. Studies have examined the use of EPO +/- GCSF and while there is a reduction in the overall use of blood products in a percentage of patients and some improvement in quality of life estimates these studies are yet to show a benefit to long term outcome.

ACUTE LEUKAEMIA

Acute leukaemia is a clonal proliferation of cells derived from the bone marrow. It may be of lymphoid or myeloid origin. Acute myeloid leukaemia is the commonest leukaemia in adults with increasing frequency with increased age (median age 64 years). Although 27 % of patients in leukaemia trials are over 65 years of age, patients above 65 years of age comprise 63 % of all leukaemia cases (SWOG report). Although acute lymphoblastic leukaemia is commoner in children, there is a late peak above the age of 80 years. Management of acute leukaemia rests with haematologists and palliative care physicians most commonly.

The prevalence of poor risk cytogenetic abnormalities and secondary AML that has evolved from myelodysplasia is higher in the elderly than in the young. Elderly patients tolerate intensive chemotherapy less well than the young adult and even with intensive chemotherapy the chance of achieving remission is lower in the elderly. Conversely the risk of early relapse is higher even after achieving complete remission. Allogeneic bone marrow transplantation is not recommended. (20)

Poor prognostic features include advanced age, co-morbidities, infection, bleeding, chromosomal abnormalities and high blasts count. Patient with preceding MDS, MPD and cytotoxic therapy have long been known to have inferior response to therapy and survival compared with those with de novo AML. The poor outcome is probably due to the fact that elderly patients tend to have multi-lineage dysplasia, antecedent haematological diseases, prognostically unfavourable karyotypes, multi drug resistance, impairment of major organs, high frequency of age associated alteration in pharmacokinetics of anti-cancer agents and reduced capacity of the haemopoietic system to tolerate the chemotherapy.

Management

For most elderly patients aggressive chemotherapy does not improve outcome. (24) Supportive care therefore is an important aspect of the management, since most of these patients are very ill at presentation (24, 25). Supportive care may take one of several forms. Firstly, similar to the management of patients with myelodysplasia and cytopenia; transfusion of blood products is required in an effort to maintain outpatient care and quality of life for as long as possible. Secondly: the use of hydroxyurea to control high white cell counts when platelet levels are not life threatening ($>50 \times 10^9$/L). Thirdly: end stage or comfort-care where the leukaemia is advanced or rapidly progressive is usually best achieved as an inpatient. Bleeding is a major problem with marked thrombocytopenia. Patients who are neutropenic and have fever should be evaluated for infection and should be covered with broad spectrum antibiotics as per the local protocol for febrile neutropenia. Opiate analgesia may be required to control bone aches. The median survival of acute leukaemia managed in this fashion is 6 weeks and patients need to be aware of this and make provision for their soon to be realised mortality.

There are several instances where chemotherapy improves long term survival in patients with no major co-morbidities these are predominantly patients with favourable cytogenetics (*Brit J Haem* 2001; **115**: 25–33). In particular t(15; 17)—APML: acute promyelocytic leukaemia which results in the formation of a fusion protein (PML/RARα) that arrests the differentiation of myeloid cells.

All-Trans-retinoic acid (ATRA) can bind to this fusion protein and overcome the arrest, allowing the blasts to differentiate and is effective when used with anthracyclines. APML should be diagnosed and treated early to prevent death from disseminated intravascular coagulopathy (DIC). Overall relapse free survival approaches 75 % of patients, elderly patients also respond favourably. Additionally arsenic trioxide is recommended in relapsed disease with suggestions of its earlier use in the elderly (26).

Where active treatment is to be entertained the major issues become hydration to maintain good urinary output, especially in the case with high blasts count, since those patients are at risk of leucostasis and tumor lysis syndrome. Hyperuricemia which should be treated with allopurinol, usually at 300 mg daily adjusted in presence of renal dysfunction. Fluid overload should not be overlooked in these patients and judicious use of diuretics in combination with hydration may be required. Cyto-reduction by leucopheresis may be required in the event of high blast count and when there is clinical evidence of leucostasis. Lower dose regimens and newer agents are being tried in elderly patients with good prognosis AML (21, 29). However, this is not the path that most elderly acute leukaemic patients will chose, even if given a choice.

LYMPHOPROLIFERATIVE CONDITIONS

Introduction

The most common lymphoproliferative conditions are B cell disorders: chronic lymphocytic leukaemia (CLL) and non Hodgkin lymphoma (NHL). The overall incidence of non-Hodgkin's lymphoma (NHL) has been rising during the past few decades. The increase has been largely confined to two age groups: men 24 to 54 years of age and individuals above 65 years of age. Whereas the increase in NHL among younger men is likely the result of the acquired immunodeficiency syndrome (AIDS) reasons for the increase among older persons remain unclear. In view of the higher occurrence of NHL in the elderly, clinicians who treat this population must be familiar with all aspect of the disease from clinical and pathological standpoints. Treatment is once again tempered by the existence of co-morbidities in this age group.

Furthermore, older patients typically have alteration in drug handling, which modify the pharmacokinetics of therapeutic treatment. Decreases in glomerular filtration rate and tubular reabsorption delay drug excretion and because of decreased liver function, the metabolism of certain drugs such as cyclophosphamide and anthracycline might be altered. Haematopoietic reserve capacity might also be altered, and myelotoxicity has been shown to increase with standard doses.

Chronic Lymphocytic Leukaemia

Chronic lymphocytic leukaemia (CLL) is the most common leukaemia in adults and with a median age at presentation of 70 years. It displays heterogeneity in both biology and clinical outcome with an overall survival of about 48 % at five years and 28 % at ten years. Differences in clinical course and outcome has prompted enquiry into prognostic indicators. Current accepted and widely used clinical markers include lymphocyte doubling time, serum lactate dehydrogenase and β2-microglobulin all of which denote the leukaemic cell kinetics. The later development of fludarabine resistance which is associated with TP53 gene deletion: a tumour suppressor gene, has a particularly poor outcome.

As with MDS, cytogenetic and FISH analysis is playing an increasingly important role with particular reference to 17p or TP53 deletions and mutations; trisomy 12; 11q (ATM gene deletions) and 13q14 which has a good prognosis (19). Revision of the guidelines for diagnosis and therapy of CLL have recently occurred in an attempt to clarify the use of prognostic markers (9).

Diagnosis

Lymphocyte count $>10 \times 10^9$/L although lower counts can be relevant with the appropriate immunophenotype:

- CD19 CD5 positive;
- Surface Ig expression weak expression;
- CD23, 20, 22, 79a weak expression;
- Cyclin D1, FMC7 and CD10 negative.

Patients usually present in an early stage (http://www.cancer.gov/cancertopics/pdq/treatment/CLL/HealthProfessional/page2). They are often asymptomatic and are referred due to the incidental diagnosis of CLL on routine blood tests. Bone marrow involvement occurs early in the disease. Lymphadenopathy and hepatosplenomegaly are variably present at presentation.

Management

The mainstay of treatment in the elderly with early disease is wait and watch. Many may not require treatment for a decade if at all and their overall survival may not be affected. Recurrent infection may become a problem due to immune paresis and hypo-gammaglobulinaemia and regular infusions of gamma-globulins have been shown improve infection rates. If the tempo of the disease declares itself to be more rapid, i.e. a lymphocyte doubling time <12 months or the advent of "B symptoms" with night sweats, fevers, anorexia or significant weight loss then treatment will help disease and symptom control in most patients. A meta-analysis of randomized trials showed no survival benefit for immediate versus delayed therapy for patients with early stage disease, nor for the use of anthracycline containing regimens over a single-agent alkylator for advanced stage disease. The management of CLL beyond the initial assessment and the watch and wait period is chiefly the domain of physicians with an interest in CLL.

Treatment is largely chemotherapeutic with a role for radiotherapy to troublesome peripheral nodes in selected cases. Systemic therapy consists one of the following approaches.

- Alkylating agents:
  - Chlorambucil as a single agent or with prednisolone in cases of auto immune cytopenias
  - Combination chemotherapy: Cyclophosphamide, vincristine and prednisolone.

- Bendamustine—studies from early usage in East Germany
- Purine analogues:
  - Fludarabine +/− cyclophosphamide
  - Cladribine
- Antisense agent: BCL2 antisense—ongoing clinical trials
- Monoclonal antibodies: alone or in combination with above agents
  - antiCD20 (MabThera/Rituximab)
  - antiCD52 (alemtuzumab/CamPath) (Faderl 2003)
  - antiCD23 (lumiluximab)—currently in clinical trials.

In essence, the advent of purine analogues has taken the complete remission rates in CLL from 0–5% in the chlorambucil era to 20–30% with single agent fludarabine then 35% by the use of any number of fludarabine-cyclophosphamide combinations (Rai 2000) to >50% when chemo-immunotherapy is used (28). As yet, as shown by a Cochrane review, 2006, this has not translated to an increase in overall survival, particularly for the elderly group. However, active research and clinical trials are increasing our understanding of CLL biology.

Non Hodgkin Lymphoma

This is best considered pathologically as low, intermediate and high grade lymphoma using pathological appearances, immunophenotype and cytogenetics or molecular analysis to further grade the tumour biology. Low grade lymphoma is increasing in frequency in the elderly. Similar to CLL, treatments have been considered to be palliative and therefore the wait and watch approach has been widely used. However, the advent of antiCD20 antibody MabThera (Rituximab) revised this concept. This agent relies on the expression of CD20 on the surface of B lymphocytes and binding of the CD20 antibodies leads to an apoptotic or sometimes lytic cell death. Used in combination with chemotherapy these actions have resulted in marked increase in complete remissions and prolonged relapse free survivals. Use of MabThera in maintenance therapy approaches has prolonged these remissions further. Long term outcomes of these studies are awaited but disease free survivals are significantly different at four years.

Diagnosis

The usual presentation is one of painless adenopathy by the patient or adenopathy found on routine clinical examination. The patient may be otherwise symptomless in low grade disease. The rapidity of the disease depends on the pathological grade and like CLL progression can vary from years to weeks. CT imaging is performed to fully evaluate the extent of adenopathy. Bone marrow aspirate and trephine may be required to assess extent of marrow involvement and the surrounding normal marrow. Co-existent myelodysplasia is not uncommon in the elderly. PET scans are used to assess the extent of higher grade disease and are an important tool in follow up.

Management

Principles are similar to CLL: watch and wait for follicular low grade NHL. Combination chemotherapy with RCVP—cyclophosphamide, vincristine and prednisolone are a common first line therapy in association with rituximab (anti-CD20) particularly when anthracyclines cannot be used due to poor baseline cardiac function. RCHOP—rituximab, cyclophosphamide, doxorubicin, vincristine and prednisolone has been shown to be highly effective in both low grade and high grade NHL (6). European studies have pioneered the use of CHOP and RCHOP as active regimens in the over 60 age group with excellent outcomes (7) Maintenance rituximab appears to improve long term survival even if used in the original regimen in low grade lymphoma (27).

Peripheral blood stem cell transplant is used in situations of relapse after a re-induction regimen of choice. Obviously this is restricted to the age group biologically below the age of 70 years. However, each patient needs to be assessed on the basis of co-morbidities and likely risk of this procedure. Other salvage regimens are used depending on fitness of the patient including bone marrow reserve (30). These are administered in specialist units and the choices available to elderly patients are more restricted than with a younger cohort.

MULTIPLE MYELOMA

Like CLL the incidence of monoclonal and polyclonal gammopathies increases with age. The finding of a monoclonal immunoglobulin does not however equate to a malignancy. Both monoclonal gammopathy of uncertain significance (MGUS) and smouldering myeloma occur in the elderly and neither may require treatment. Of importance is a thorough screening examination and investigations which include biochemical assays for creatinine, globulins and calcium, complete blood picture, immunoglobulin profile as well as serum electrophoresis to identify the monoclonal subtype, urinary protein electrophoresis and quantification of Bence Jones Protein, SFLC analysis, skeletal survey, and consideration of MRI examination if there is concern about vertebral involvement with myelomatous deposits. Bone marrow biopsy is also necessary for diagnosis but if all other parameters point to MGUS rather than myeloma, this may be delayed and may never become necessary in the elderly patient. As most myelomas are secretory, progress may be monitored by peripheral blood paraprotein quantification and symptoms, non secretory myeloma may be monitored by serum free light chain assay.

Bone disease should be treated with bisphosphonates either an oral weekly preparation or monthly intravenous form. Of note is the infrequent but devastating side effect of the bisphosphonate family, osteonecrosis of the jaw. This is most commonly seen in the elderly, associated with tooth decay and in increasing frequency with the strength of the bisphosphonate (residronate, olendronate, pamidronate, zolendronate). Although it may be reversible if occurring with the oral preparations, it should be considered permanent. However, these agents have made an enormous impact in controlling the serious bone disease previously a hallmark of myeloma.

The mainstays of therapy have changed and even for the elderly some of the newer drugs may be appropriate. Melphalan and prednisolone/dexamethasone is a useful first treatment option. The combination of +/− cyclophosphamide thalidomide and dexamethasone are probably the treatment of choice in this age group being mindful of the increased side effects of high dose steroids in the elderly and of the neuropathy accompanying thalidomide use. Beyond these agents, the newer agents of Velcade (Bortezomib—proteosome inhibitor) and Revlimid (Lenalidomide—immune modulatory and anti-angiogenic) are making substantial impact on disease behaviour and are available on or off clinical trial. High dose melphalan autologous transplant is not generally applicable to the elderly unless biologically younger with few co-morbidities.

KEY POINTS

- Haematological parameters in the elderly outside the reference ranges are due to underlying pathology which should be diagnosed and treated.
- Diagnosis and appropriate treatment results in superior outcomes in the elderly.
- New agents and approaches to treat malignancy (NHL and myeloma) are applicable to the elderly with excellent disease control and should be considered at diagnosis.
- Cytogenetic analysis in leukaemia may identify treatable disease.
- Supportive therapy may provide the best quality of life for the elderly patient with acute leukaemia.

REFERENCES

1. Atallah E, Kantarjian H et al. The role of decitabine in the treatment of myelodysplastic syndromes *Expert Opinion on Pharmacotherapy* 2007; **8**(1): 65–73.
2. Balducci L. Transfusion independence in patients with myelodysplastic syndromes: impact

on outcomes and quality of life. *Cancer* 2006; **106**(10): 2087–94.

3. Borst F, Keuning J, van Hulsteijn H, Sinnige H, Vreugdenhil G. High-dose dexamethasone as a first- and second-line treatment of idiopathic thrombocytopenic purpura in adults. *Ann Haematol* 2004; **83**(12): 764–8.

4. Bowen DT. Treatment strategies and issues in low/intermediate-1-risk myelodysplastic syndrome (MDS) patients *Seminars in Oncology* 2005; **32**(4 Suppl 5): S16–S23.

5. Braendstrup P, Bjerrum O, Nielsen O, et al. Rituximab chimeric anti-CD20 monoclonal antibody treatment for adult refractory idiopathic thrombocytopenic purpura. *Am J Haematol* 2005; **78**(4): 275–80.

6. Cheung M, Haynes A, Meyer R, et al. (2007) Rituximab in lymphoma: a systematic review and consensus practice guideline from Cancer Care Ontario *Cancer Treat Rev* **33**(2): 161–76.

7. Coiffier B, Lepage E, Briere J, et al. CHOP chemotherapy plus rituximab compared with CHOP alone in elderly patients with diffuse large-B-cell lymphoma *N Engl J Med* 2002; **346**(4): 235–42.

8. Durga J, van Boxtel MP et al. Effect of 3-year folic acid supplementation on cognitive function in older adults in the FACIT trial: a randomised, double blind, controlled trial.[see comment] *Lancet* 2007; **369**(9557): 208–16.

9. Eichhorst B, Hallek M. Revision of the guidelines for diagnosis and therapy of chronic lymphocytic leukaemia (CLL) *Best Pract Res Clin Haematol* 2007; **20**(3): 469–77.

10. Estey E. Acute myeloid leukemia and myelodysplastic syndromes in older patients *Journal of Clinical Oncology* 2007; **25**(14): 1908–15.

11. Estey E, Dohner H. Acute myeloid leukaemia. [see comment]. *Lancet* 2006; **368**(9550): 1894–907.

12. Faderl S, Thomas D, O'Brien S, et al. Experience with alemtuzumab plus rituximab in patients with relapsed and refractory lymphoid malignancies *Blood Rev* 2003; **101**(9): 3413–5.

13. Feugier P, Van Hoof A, Sebban C, et al. Long-term results of the R-CHOP study in the treatment of elderly patients with diffuse large B-cell lymphoma: a study by the Groupe d'Etude des Lymphomes de l'Adulte *J Clin Pathol* 2005; **23**(18): 4117–26.

14. Galili N, Cerny J, Raza A Current treatment options: Impact of cytogenetics on the course

of myelodysplasia *Curr Treat Options Oncol Epub*, 2007.

15. Goss TF, Szende A et al. Cost effectiveness of lenalidomide in the treatment of transfusion-dependent myelodysplastic syndromes in the United States *Cancer Control* 2006; **13** (Suppl): 17–25.

16. Greenberg PL. Myelodysplastic syndromes: iron overload consequences and current chelating therapies *Journal of the National Comprehensive Cancer Network* 2006; **4**(1): 91–6.

17. Holyoake TL, Stott D, McKay PJ, et al. Use of plasma ferritin concentration to diagnose iron deficiency in elderly patients *J Clin Pathol* 1993; **46**: 857–60.

18. Kantarjian HM, O'Brien S et al. Update of the decitabine experience in higher risk myelodysplastic syndrome and analysis of prognostic factors associated with outcome *Cancer* 2007; **109**(2): 265–73.

19. Kay N, Rai K, O'Brien S. Chronic lymphocytic leukaemia: current and emerging treatment approaches *Clin Adv Haematol Oncol* 2006; **4**(11(Suppl 22)): 1–12.

20. Kiss T, Sabry W, Lazarus H, Lipton J. Blood and marrow transplantation in elderly acute myeloid leukaemia patients—older certainly is not better *Bone Marrow Transplant* 2007; **40**(5): 405–16.

21. Manoharan A, Reynolds J et al. Flexible low-intensity combination chemotherapy for elderly patients with acute myeloid leukaemia: a multicentre, phase II study *Drugs and Aging* 2007; **24**(6): 481–8.

22. Mukhopadhyay D and Mohanaruban K. Iron deficiency anaemia in older people: investigation, management and treatment.[see comment]. *Age and Ageing* 2002; **31**(2): 87–91.

23. Rai K, Peterson B, Appelbaum, et al. Fludarabine compared with chlorambucil as primary therapy for chronic lymphocytic leukaemia *N Engl J Med* 2000; **343**(24): 1750–7.

24. Rodrigues CA., Chauffaille ML et al. Acute myeloid leukemia in elderly patients: experience of a single center *Brazilian Journal of Medical and Biological Research* 2003; **36**(6): 703–8.

25. Steensma DP, and Tefferi A. Anemia in the elderly: how should we define it, when does it matter, and what can be done? *Mayo Clinic Proceedings* 2007; **82**(8): 958–66.

26. Tsimberidou AM, Kantarjian H et al. Optimizing treatment for elderly patients with acute promyelocytic leukemia: is it time to replace

chemotherapy with all-trans retinoic acid and ar-senic trioxide? *Leukemia and Lymphoma* 2006; **47**(11): 2282–8.

27. van Oers M, Klasa R, Marcus R, et al. Ritux-imab maintenance improves clinical outcome of relapsed/resistant follicular non-Hodgkin lym-phoma in patients both with and without ritux-imab during induction: results of a prospective randomised phase 3 intergroup trial *Blood* 2006; **108**(10): 3295–301.

28. Wierda W, O'Brien S, Wen S, Faderl S, et al. Chemoimmunotherapy with fludarabine, cyclophosphamide, and rituximab for relapsed and refractory chronic lymphocytic leukaemia *J Clin Oncol* 2005; **23**(18): 4070–8.

29. Yamauchi T, Negoro E et al. Combined low-dose cytarabine, melphalan and mitox-antrone for older patients with acute myeloid leukemia or high-risk myelodysplastic syn-drome *Anticancer Research* 2007; **27**(4C): 2635–9.

30. Zinzani PL. Salvage chemotherapy in follicular non-Hodgkin lymphoma: focus on tolerability *Clin Lymphoma Myeloma* 2006; **7**(2): 115–24.

18 COPD and asthma in the elderly

Martin Connolly[1] and Tina L. Davies[2]

[1]*Department of Geriatric Medicine, North Shore Hospital, Auckland, New Zealand*
[2]*Newcastle University, Newcastle, UK*

Chronic respiratory disorders such as chronic obstructive pulmonary disease (COPD) and asthma are increasing in prevalence in older people, in whom there are high levels of morbidity and mortality. In the near future demographic changes will result in a further substantial increase of chronic obstructive airway disorders with huge socio-economic consequences. COPD and asthma are two distinct chronic respiratory disorders sharing one chronic functional feature of airflow limitation. Correctly diagnosing and treating these diseases in older people has proved more difficult than in younger patients because of the potential for presenting with concomitant diseases, and the similarities among diseases. Despite their similarities, it is important not to misdiagnose asthma as COPD because asthma has a different natural history different treatment, and a better prognosis. Awareness of COPD and asthma in the UK has recently been increased by the publication of two separate national guidelines (1, 2).

RISK FACTORS AND TRIGGERS

In older people, as in other age groups, cigarette smoking is by far the most important risk factor for COPD. Childhood respiratory disease and exposure to occupational dusts and chemicals, and indoor and outdoor air pollutants have also been associated with COPD in this age group. Risk factors for COPD interact amongst themselves in a synergistic way (Figure 18.1).

Compared to young asthmatics, the prevalence of allergic asthma in elderly patients is considerably lower. Moreover, the sensitivity of both immediate skin testing and IgE levels decreases with age, reducing the negative predictive value of these tests.

Asthma triggers in elderly subjects are similar to those in younger patients; they include viral infections, environmental allergens or irritants, emotional triggers and adverse drug effects. Viral infection, chronic sinusitis and gastroesophageal reflux disease appear to play a larger role in the initial presentation and exacerbation of asthma in older people.

The potential for drugs to trigger or worsen asthma is greater in elderly patients because these patients are likely to be on multiple medications for other conditions, in particular heart disease (Table 18.1). For instance, aspirin and other anti-inflammatory medications used to treat arthritis and other pain, beta-blockers for hypertension and heart disease, and beta-blocker eye drops used to treat glaucoma are all known to potentially cause or worsen bronchoconstriction. Symptoms with a new medication might be as subtle as a new cough, or more obvious, such as decreased exercise tolerance, wheezing or shortness of breath.

Prescribing for Elderly Patients   Edited by Stephen Jackson, Paul Jansen and Arduino Mangoni
© 2009 John Wiley & Sons, Ltd

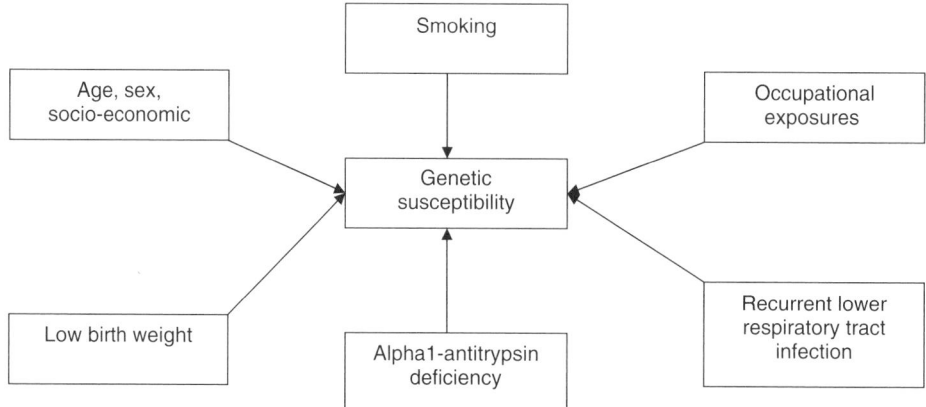

Figure 18.1. Interaction of risk factors for COPD, modified from (1) National Institute for Clinical Excellence. *Thorax* 2004; **59** (Supplement 1):i1–i232

PRESENTATION AND DIAGNOSIS

The diagnoses of COPD and asthma are clinical judgements based on a combination of history, physical examination and confirmation of the presence of airflow obstruction by spirometry. Table 18.2 describes definitions for COPD and asthma.

NICE suggested (1) that COPD should be considered in any individual over the age of 35 years who has a risk factor (generally a significant smoking history) and one or more of the following:

- Breathlessness on exertion.
- Chronic cough.
- Chronic sputum production.
- Frequent winter bronchitis.
- Wheeze.

Physical examination is important but rarely diagnostic in COPD as a normal physical examination is common in early disease. Signs of airflow limitation are rarely present until significant impairment of lung function has occurred.

The presenting symptoms of asthma in an elderly person are similar to those in the younger adult. To avoid misdiagnosis BTS/SIGN guideline advised that people with asthma may suffer from a variety of symptoms, none of which is specific for asthma:

- Wheeze.
- Shortness of breath.

- Chest tightness.
- Cough.

The hallmark of asthma is that these symptoms tend to be:

- Variable.
- Intermittent.
- Worse at night.
- Provoked by triggers including exercise.

However *all* the above features are less common in asthma in older people, and clinically asthma in an elderly person often presents in a similar fashion to COPD.

Physical examination is normal in younger asthmatics outside acute episodes. However, during an exacerbation the patient will often have wheeze and reduced lung function, either reduced peak flow or an obstructive pattern on spirometry. In elderly asthmatics physical examination and/or spirometry may reveal evidence of small airways obstruction between acute episodes.

OBJECTIVE TESTS

COPD produces a decrease in peak expiratory flow (PEF) and forced expiratory volume in one second (FEV1). Spirometry, as opposed to PEF monitoring, is particularly helpful in assessing progress in elderly patients with greatly compromised lung function because PEF measurements can be relatively well preserved in older

Table 18.1. Medications with increased potential for adverse effects and interactions in the elderly patient with asthma

Medication	Co-morbid conditions for which drug is prescribed	Adverse effect	Comment
Beta-blocker	Hypertension Heart Disease Tremor Glaucoma	Worsening Asthma Bronchospasm Decreased response to bronchodilator	Avoid where possible; when must be used, use a highly beta-selective drug
Non steroidal anti-inflammatory drugs	Arthritis Musculoskeletal diseases	Worsening asthma Bronchospasm	Not all elderly with asthma have non-tolerance of NSAIDs, but are best avoided if possible
Non-potassium-sparing diuretics	Hypertension Congestive heart failure	Worsening cardiac function/ dysrhythmias due to hypokalemia	Additive effect with anti asthma medications that also produce potassium loss (steroids, beta-agonist); elderly also more likely to be receiving drugs (e.g., digitalis) where hypokalemia is of increased concern
Certain non-sedating antihistamines (terfenadine and astemizole)	Allergic rhinitis	Worsening cardiac function/ventricular arrhythmias due to prolonged QT interval	
Cholinergic agents	Urinary retention Glaucoma	Bronchospasm Bronchorrhea	Some over-the-counter asthma medications contain ephedrine, which could aggravate urinary retention, glaucoma
ACE inhibitors	Heart failure Hypertension	Precipitation of cough	

Table 18.2. Definitions of COPD and asthma

COPD	Asthma
'characterised by airflow obstruction. The airflow obstruction is usually progressive, not fully reversible and does not change markedly over several months' (1)	'a chronic inflammatory disorder of the airways.... In susceptible individuals, inflammatory symptoms are usually associated with widespread but variable airflow obstruction and an increase in airway response to a variety of stimuli. Obstruction is often reversible, either spontaneously or with treatment' (3)

Table 18.3. Severity of airflow obstruction in COPD according to post bronchodilator FEV1 as a percentage of the predicted value, modified from (1)

Severity of airflow obstruction	Post bronchodilator FEV1
Mild	50–80 % predicted
Moderate	30–49 % predicted
Severe	<30 % predicted

people with COPD in the presence of greatly reduced spirometric values. Simple spirometry is easy and quick, but requires expensive equipment and training. Poorly performed spirometry can lead to misdiagnosis or a missed diagnosis. Spirometry is useful in confirming the diagnosis of COPD, as well as giving a measure of the severity of airflow obstruction (Table 18.3).

Variability of PEF and FEV1, either spontaneously over time or in response to therapy is a characteristic feature of asthma (Table 18.4). Sequential measurement of PEF may be useful in the diagnosis of asthma. In asthma, ideally both PEF and FEV1 should be measured and are normal if the measurement is made between episodes of bronchoconstriction (though this is less likely in the elderly).

Table 18.5 summarizes the history, physical examination and laboratory findings, and response to beta$_2$-agonist therapy of COPD and asthma, in older people.

DIFFERENTIAL DIAGNOSES

The differential diagnosis of episodic chest symptoms in the elderly increases as cardiovascular disease and other forms of chronic lung disease become more prevalent. In addition the co-existence of COPD or asthma with other chronic cardiovascular or lung diseases may complicate the diagnosis.

Distinguishing between asthma and COPD may also be difficult as the clinical presentations of these diseases overlap. Elderly asthmatic patients often have incomplete reversibility of their airflow obstruction. A trial of corticosteroids may be necessary to establish that there is reversible airflow obstruction.

MANAGEMENT OF COPD AND ASTHMA

In order to effectively manage COPD and asthma, a partnership needs to be established between the physician, the patient and the patient's family. The components of management include identification and control of factors contributing to severity, objective monitoring of the disease and pharmacological therapy.

Both COPD and asthma are classified by severity, and treatment is stepped up or stepped down as needed, according to guidelines, Figures 18.2 (1) and 18.3 (2) respectively. A stepwise approach aims to abolish symptoms as soon as possible. Patients should start treatment at the stage most appropriate to the initial severity of their disease. The aim is to achieve early control and to maintain control by stepping up treatment as necessary and considering stepping down control when control is good.

Long-term management strategies for COPD and asthma in the elderly must take into consideration the greater likelihood of co-existing conditions and diseases. The drugs used to treat COPD and asthma, and potential adverse reactions are given in Tables 18.6 and 18.7. The

Table 18.4. Diagnosis of asthma using spirometry, based on (2)

>20 % diurnal variation on ≥3 days in a week for 2 weeks on the PEF diary
Or FEV1 ≥15 % or 200 ml increase after short acting $\beta_2$agonist (e.g. salbutamol 400 µg by pMDI + spacer or 2.5 mg by nebuliser)
Or FEV1 ≥15 % or 200 ml increase after trial of steroid tablets (30 mg prednisolone/day for 14 days)
Or decrease after six minutes of exercise (running)
Histamine or methacholine challenge in difficult cases

Table 18.5. Comparison of differences between COPD and asthma in history, physical examination, laboratory findings and response to beta$_2$-agonist therapy, in older people

Characteristic	Asthma	COPD
History		
Episodic wheeze	Sometimes	Less common; may occur with exacerbations
Nocturnal dyspnoea or Cough	Common (episodic)	Less common but often troublesome in severe disease
Cough with phlegm	Common, especially in those who smoke	Characteristic of chronic bronchitis
Other allergic symptoms (rhinitis, conjunctivitis)	Uncommon	Uncommon
Smoking history	Uncommon	Almost always associated
Past history of asthma	Common	Uncommon
Family history of allergy	Moderately common	Uncommon
Physical Examination		
Wheeze	Common	Common after forced expiration or cough
Laboratory Findings		
Pulmonary function	Similar to COPD	Similar to asthma
Chest x-ray	Often normal; may show hyperinflation	Normal in mild (even moderate) disease ↓vessels, focal hyperaeration (emphysema) markings (chronic bronchitis)
Eosinophilia	Uncommon	Uncommon
Positive skin tests	Uncommon	Uncommon
Total serum IgE	Usually normal	Usually normal
Response to Therapy		
FEV 1 response to beta$_2$-agonist	FEV1 improves with symptom relief	Little/no change in FEV1 (but often symptom relief)

differences between therapeutic approaches between COPD and asthma are summarized in Table 18.8.

Based on the guideline established by BTS/SIGN (2), patients with asthma should start treatment at the step most appropriate to the initial severity of their disease. The aim is to achieve early control and to maintain control by stepping up treatment as necessary and stepping down when control is good.

Step 1: Prescribe an inhaled short-acting beta$_2$-agonist as a short-term reliever therapy for all patients with symptomatic asthma.

Step 2: All patients on high usage of inhaled short-acting beta$_2$-agonists should have their asthma management

initially reviewed. Inhaled steroids as a preventer medication should be considered in patients with:

• exacerbations of asthma in the last two years;
• using inhaled beta$_2$-agonists three times a week or more;
• are symptomatic three times a week or more, or waking one night a week.

The guideline recommends a daily starting dose of inhaled steroids of 400 mcg per day (refers to beclomethasone given via a MDI). Inhaled steroids are best given twice daily, though where compliance is poor a double dose may be given once daily and is almost as effective (e.g. a patient with dementia who has once daily carer input).

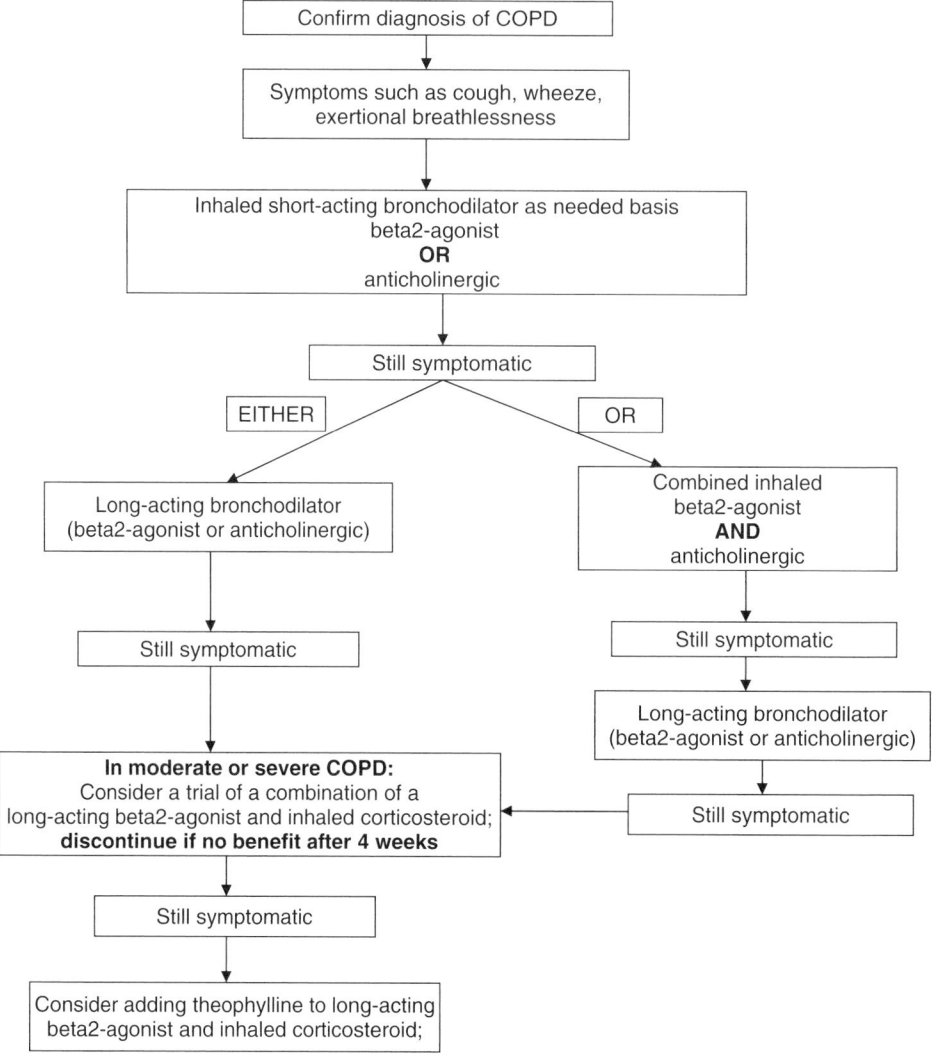

- Long-acting bronchodilators should also be used in patients who have two or more exacerbations per year

- The choice of drug(s) should take into account the patient's response to a trial of the drug, the drug's side effects, patient preference and cost

Figure 18.2. Stepwise approach to drug therapy for breathlessness and exercise limitation in chronic stable COPD, modified from (1) National Institute for Clinical Excellence. *Thorax* 2004; **59** (Supplement 1):i1–i232

Step 3: Check compliance, inhaler technique and eliminate trigger factors before changing therapy. The guideline recommends the following:

- Carry out a trial of other treatments before increasing the inhaled steroid dose above 800 mcg/day

in adults as many patients will benefit more from add-on therapy than from increasing inhaled steroids.

- If an add-on therapy is required, an inhaled long-acting beta$_2$-agonist is advised.

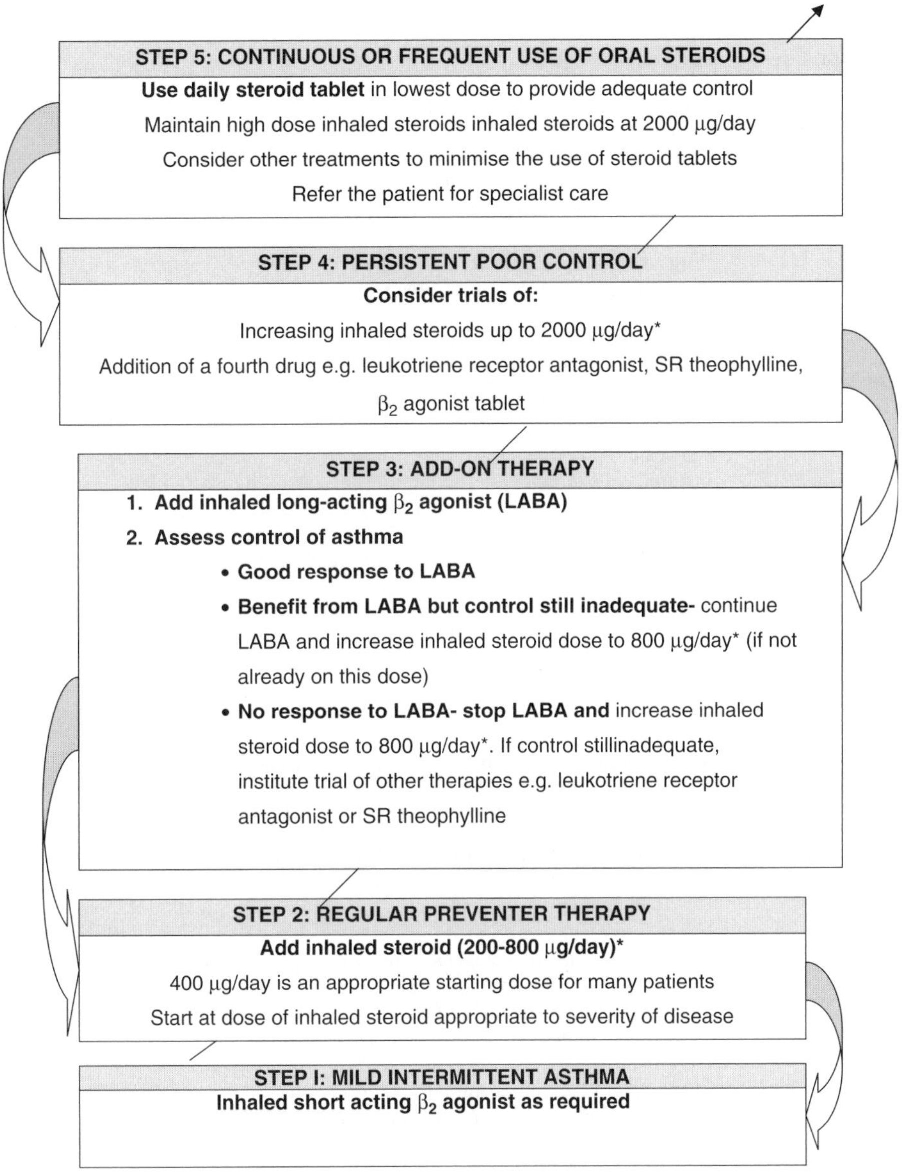

STEP 5: CONTINUOUS OR FREQUENT USE OF ORAL STEROIDS

Use daily steroid tablet in lowest dose to provide adequate control

Maintain high dose inhaled steroids inhaled steroids at 2000 µg/day

Consider other treatments to minimise the use of steroid tablets

Refer the patient for specialist care

STEP 4: PERSISTENT POOR CONTROL

Consider trials of:

Increasing inhaled steroids up to 2000 µg/day*

Addition of a fourth drug e.g. leukotriene receptor antagonist, SR theophylline,

β_2 agonist tablet

STEP 3: ADD-ON THERAPY

1. **Add inhaled long-acting β_2 agonist (LABA)**

2. **Assess control of asthma**

   - **Good response to LABA**
   - **Benefit from LABA but control still inadequate-** continue LABA and increase inhaled steroid dose to 800 µg/day* (if not already on this dose)
   - **No response to LABA- stop LABA and** increase inhaled steroid dose to 800 µg/day*. If control stillinadequate, institute trial of other therapies e.g. leukotriene receptor antagonist or SR theophylline

STEP 2: REGULAR PREVENTER THERAPY

Add inhaled steroid (200-800 µg/day)*

400 µg/day is an appropriate starting dose for many patients

Start at dose of inhaled steroid appropriate to severity of disease

STEP I: MILD INTERMITTENT ASTHMA

Inhaled short acting β_2 agonist as required

*All doses of inhaled steroids in this section refer to beclomethasone (BDP) given via a metered dose inhaler (MDI).

Figure 18.3. Stepwise management of chronic asthma in adults, taken from (2)

- If asthma control remains sub-optimal after the addition of an inhaled long-acting beta$_2$-agonist then the dose of inhaled steroids should be increased to 800 mcg/day.
- If control is still inadequate the guideline recommends a sequential trial of add-on therapy, i.e. leukotriene receptor antagonists, theophyllines, slow release beta$_2$-agonist tablets. However, there are no current trials available regarding the use of leukotriene antagonists in older people.
- The use short-acting anticholinergics is not recommended.

Table 18.6. Bronchodilator drugs used in obstructive airways diseases and potential adverse effects

Bronchodilator drugs	Potential adverse effect
Short-acting beta$_2$-agonist	Myocardial ischaemia due to increased myocardial oxygen consumption and mild increase in hypoxemia Complex ventricular arrhythmia due to myocardial irritability Cardiac arrhythmias and muscle weakness related to hypokalemia Hypotension or hypertension Tremor With excessive use, bronchodilator effect and airway hyperresponsiveness related to downregulation of beta receptors
Long-acting beta$_2$-agonist	Same as for short-acting beta$_2$-agonist
Theophylline	Cardiac arrhythmias; effect is related to increased catecholamine release and is additive with beta$_2$-agonists Anorexia, nausea and vomiting from central (brain) effects Insomnia, seizures related to central nervous system stimulant Cardiac arrhythmia due to inotropic and chronotropic effects Serum levels increased by heart failure, liver disease, beta-blocker therapy, selected H$_2$-blocker therapy, quinolone therapy, macrolide therapy, ketoconazole therapy
Anticholinergics	Dry mouth Acute angle glaucoma from mist of the nebulised drug

Table 18.7. Anti-inflammatory drugs used in obstructive airways diseases and potential adverse effects

Anti-inflammatory drugs	Potential adverse effects
Oral corticosteroids	High blood pressure, oedema, congestive heart failure due to sodium retention Hypokalemia, alkalosis, and resulting arrhythmias due potassium and hydrogen excretion Worsening diabetes mellitus, cataracts, polyuria with dehydration due to elevated blood glucose Thinning of the skin, reduced muscle mass with myopathy and osteoporosis Hypoadrenalism due to decreased ACTH Cataracts Altered cognitive function, depression Joint effusions and articular pain with corticosteroid withdrawal Osteoporosis due to decreased calcium absorption Glaucoma due to decreased absorption of aqueous humour Aggravation of existing peptic ulcer disease
High dose inhaled corticosteroids	Oral thrush Laryngeal myopathy Effects on ACTH secretion with hypoadrenalism Effects on calcium absorption with acceleration of osteoporosis Development of cataracts
Sodium cromoglycate	No significant adverse effect known
Nedocromil	• No significant adverse effect known

Table 18.8. Differences in therapeutic approaches to asthma and COPD

Drug	Asthma	COPD
Beta$_2$-agonist		
Aerosol	Excellent response	Slight to moderate response
Long Acting	May be useful	Useful
Oral	Rarely needed	Rarely needed
Ipratropium	Sometimes useful, egg, in smokers	Excellent response in many patients
Theophylline	Sometimes useful	Often useful, particularly if patient cannot use aerosols or as an add-on therapy
Corticosteroids		
Intravenous	Essential for severe exacerbations	Recommended in severe exacerbations
Oral	Essential for severe asthma attack	Recommended in acute exacerbations
Aerosol	Essential if regular beta$_2$-agonist aerosol is used	Reduces exacerbation rate and rate of deterioration of quality of life
Cromoglycate/ nedocromil	Useful in specific cases e.g. exercise-induced asthma	Value not established; unlikely to be useful in most cases unless asthmatic component is pronounced
Antibiotics	Needed if evidence of infection	Needed for infectious exacerbations
Mucolytics	Value not established	Indicated patients with difficulty expectorating sticky sputum
Long-term oxygen therapy (LTOT)	Rarely needed	Often needed in severe cases Particularly indicated as LTOT in chronic hypoxia

Step 4: If control remains inadequate on 800 mcg daily of an inhaled steroid plus a long-acting beta$_2$-agonist, the guideline recommends the following interventions:

- Increase inhaled steroids to 2000 mcg/day.
- Add-on theophylline.
- Add-on slow release beta$_2$-agonist tablets, though caution needs to be used.
- Add-on leukotriene receptor antagonists.

If a trial of an add-on treatment is ineffective, the guideline advises to stop the drug (or in the case of increased dose of inhaled steroid, reduce to the original dose).

For Step 5, patients on long-term steroid tablets (e.g. longer than three months) or requiring frequent courses of steroid tablets (e.g. three to four per year) are at risk of systemic side-effects of corticosteroids (Table 18.7). The guideline advises that patients receiving prednisolone for over three months should be prescribed a long-acting bisphosphonate.

The aim of treatment is to control the asthma using the lowest possible dose of steroids or if possible, to stop long-term steroid tablets completely.

There is a role for a trial of treatment with long-acting beta$_2$-agonists, leukotriene receptor antagonists, and theophyllines for about six weeks. They should be stopped if no improvement in steroid dose, symptoms or lung function is detected.

Immunosuppressants (methotrexate, cyclosporin and oral gold) may be given as a three month trial, once other drug treatments have proved unsuccessful. The guideline recommends that the risks and benefits of these potentially toxic drugs should be discussed with the patient and their side-effects carefully monitored. Treatment should be in a centre with experience of using these medicines.

Stepping down therapy once asthma is controlled is recommended, but often not implemented leaving some patients over-treated. The guideline advises:

- Regular review of patients as treatment is stepped down.

- Patients should be maintained at the lowest possible dose of inhaled steroid.
- Reduction in inhaled steroid dose should be slow, decreasing the dose by approximately 25–50 % every three months, dependent on symptoms.

ACUTE ASTHMA

The BTS/SIGN guideline recommends the following (2):

- Patients should be referred to hospital if they have any features of acute severe or life threatening asthma (Table 18.9).
- Patients should be admitted to hospital if they have any features of a near fatal attack (Table 18.9).
- Patients should be admitted to hospital if they have any features of an acute severe attack persisting after initial treatment (Table 18.9).
- Patients whose peak flow is greater than 75 % best or predicted one hour after initial treatment may be discharged from A&E, unless they have other criteria, when admission may be appropriate.

Treatment of acute asthma, according to the SIGN/BTS guideline is summarized in Table 18.10 (2).

The BTS/SIGN guideline does not suggest an age limit for asthmatics who require referral to the intensive care unit (ICU) (2). Indications for admission to ICU or a high dependency unit included those patients requiring ventilatory support and those with severe acute or life threatening asthma who are failing to respond to therapy as evidence by:

- deteriorating PEFR;
- persisting or worsening hypoxia;
- hypercapnea;
- arterial blood gas analysis showing fall in pH or rising H^+ concentration;
- exhaustion, feeble respiration.
- Drowsiness, confusion;
- coma or respiratory arrest.

Not all patients admitted to ICU need ventilation, but those with worsening hypoxia or hypercapnea, drowsiness or unconsciousness and those who have had a respiratory arrest require intermittent positive pressure ventilation. Intubation in such patients is very difficult and should ideally be performed by an anaesthetist or ICU consultant.

Hypercapneic respiratory failure developing during the evolution of an acute asthmatic episode is regarded as an indication for urgent admission to the ICU. It is unlikely that non invasive ventilation (NIV) would ever replace intubation in these very unstable patients. Future studies might usefully examine its role in the gradually tiring patient, but at present this treatment cannot be recommended outside randomized controlled trials.

MANAGEMENT OF EXACERBATIONS OF COPD

NICE defined an exacerbation of COPD as 'a sustained worsening of the patient's symptoms from their usual stable state which is beyond

Table 18.9. Features of near fatal, life threatening and acute severe asthma attacks

Near fatal asthma	• Raised P_aCO_2 and/or requiring mechanical ventilation with raised inflation pressure
Life threatening asthma	• Silent chest, cyanosis or feeble respiratory effort
	• Exhaustion, confusion or coma
	• Bradycardia or hypotension
	• PEFR <30 % of best or predicted
	• Blood gas markers: P_aCO_2 > 6 kPa, P_aO_2 < 8 kPa and pH < 7.35
Acute severe asthma	• Inability to complete sentences in one breath
	• Respiratory rate >25 breaths/min
	• Tachycardia >110 beats/min
	• PEFR<50 % best or predicted

Table 18.10. Treatment of acute asthma, according to BTS/SIGN Guideline (2)

	Recommendations
Oxygen	• In hospital, ambulance and primary care, nebulised beta$_2$-agonist bronchodilators should be driven by oxygen. • Outside hospital, high dose beta$_2$-agonist bronchodilators may be delivered via large volume spacers or nebulisers. • Whilst supplemental oxygen is recommended, its absence should not prevent nebulised therapy being given if indicated.
Beta$_2$-agonist bronchodilators	• Use high dose inhaled beta$_2$-agonists as first line agents in acute asthma and administer as early as possible • Nebulisers should be driven by oxygen • Intravenous beta$_2$-agonists should be reserved for those patients in whom inhaled therapy cannot be used reliably.
Corticosteroids	• Give steroid tablets in adequate doses (prednisolone 40 to 50 mg daily) in all cases of acute asthma • Continue prednisolone 40 to 50 mg daily for at least five days or until recovery.
ipratropium bromide	• Nebulised ipratropium bromide (0.5 mg 4–6 hourly) should be added to beta$_2$-agonist treatment for patients with acute severe or life threatening asthma or those with a poor initial response to beta$_2$-agonist therapy

Magnesium	• Consider giving a single dose of IV magnesium sulphate for patients with:
	  • acute severe asthma who have not had a good initial response to inhaled bronchodilator therapy
	  • life threatening or near fatal asthma.
	  IV magnesium sulphate (1.2 to 2 g IV infusion over 20 minutes) should only be used following consultation with senior medical staff

Antibiotics	• Routine prescription of antibiotics is not indicated for acute asthma
Heliox	• Not recommended
Leukotriene receptor antagonists	• Not recommended
Intravenous fluids	• When appropriate
Potassium supplements	• Correct if potassium level if low

normal day-to-day variations, and is acute in onset' (1). This change in symptoms often requires a change in treatment based on the guidelines established by NICE (1). Frequent exacerbations accelerate lung function decline and lead to worsening quality of life and prognosis.

The common symptoms of an exacerbation include:

• increasing breathlessness;
• cough;
• increased sputum production;
• increased sputum purulence.

Decisions about whether the patient requires hospital admission can be complex and may not be based solely on medical grounds, particularly in the elderly. NICE advises that specific factors

(Table 18.11) should be used to assess the need to treat patients in hospital.

The treatment of exacerbations should follow a stepwise approach to therapy, with consideration of patient characteristics, co-morbidities, failure of initial treatment, and the severity of the exacerbation itself.

Increased breathlessness should be treated with increased doses of a bronchodilator. In the community, patients can use more doses of their usual inhaler, take their treatment regularly rather than as needed, or an additional bronchodilator can be added. In the hospital setting nebulised therapy may be required. If the patient is hypercapneic, nebulisers should be driven with air <u>not</u> oxygen. If oxygen is needed at the same time, it can be delivered via nasal cannulae to avoid giving too high

Table 18.11. Factors to consider when deciding where to manage patient with exacerbation of COPD, modified from (1)

Factor	Favour for treatment at home	Favour for treatment in hospital
Able to cope at home	Yes	No
Breathlessness	Mild	Severe
General condition	Good	Poor/deteriorating
Level of activity	Good	Poor/confined to bed
Cyanosis	No	Yes
Level of consciousness	Normal	Impaired
Already receiving LTOT[+]	No	Yes
Social circumstances	Good	Living alone/not coping
Acute confusion	No	Yes
Rapid rate of onset	No	Yes
Significant co-morbidity*	No	Yes
$S_aO_2 < 90\%$[†]	No	Yes
Changes on the chest radiograph	No	Present
Arterial pH level	$\geqslant 7.35$	< 7.35
Arterial P_aO_2[‡]	$\geqslant 7\,kPa$	$< 7\,kPa$

*Particularly cardiac disease and insulin-dependent diabetes.
[+]LTOT long-term oxygen therapy.
[†]S_aO_2 oxygen saturation of arterial blood.
[‡]P_aO_2 partial pressure of oxygen in arterial blood.

a flow rate of oxygen. The need for a nebuliser during an exacerbation does not mean that the patient requires nebulised therapy in the long term. This needs to be explained to the patient and their relatives. Patients should be changed back to their normal inhalers as soon as possible.

Antibiotics are administered according to the NICE guideline in exacerbations of COPD. This has a proven evidence base. In the community, antibiotics are prescribed if the sputum is purulent and the choice of antibiotic should follow local bacterial resistance patterns. An aminopenicillin, tetracycline or macrolide usually provide adequate cover and sputum cultures are not usually necessary. Hospitalized patients need to have a sputum culture taken to subsequently check the appropriateness of their antibiotic therapy. Antibiotics are required if the sputum is purulent, or if there are clinical signs of pneumonia or consolidation on the chest radiograph.

NICE recommends oral corticosteroids if the exacerbation is associated with marked breathlessness, sufficient to interfere with daily activity. All hospitalized patients with an exacerbation should be treated with oral corticosteroids to improve lung function and shorten hospital stay. A seven to 14 day course of prednisolone 30 mg daily is sufficient and no additional benefit is seen with prolonged courses.

An exacerbation can precipitate or worsen respiratory failure. Drowsiness or confusion, cyanosis and worsening ankle oedema are common presenting symptoms. NICE advises that arterial blood gases are needed to confirm the diagnosis. In the hospital setting, oxygen saturations must be monitored. The aim of supplementary oxygen therapy is to maintain adequate oxygenation (oxygen saturations greater than 90 %) without precipitating respiratory acidosis or worsening hypercapnea.

NIV is the treatment of choice for persistent hypercapnea and respiratory acidosis (pH less than 7.35) during acute exacerbations despite optimal medical therapy. A recent study has shown that elderly patients with acute exacerbations of COPD and persistent respiratory acidosis not only tolerate but benefit from NIV (4). It is vital that a decision about what to do if NIV failure is reached is agreed and documented before therapy is started. For some patients, admission to intensive care and invasive ventilation will be an option.

Following successful hospital treatment of severe exacerbation, optimisation of medical treatment and prompt outpatient follow-up is essential as the one year mortality rate after hospital discharge is 25–40 % (up to half of which occurs in the first three months).

MANAGEMENT OF STABLE COPD

The stepwise approach to drug therapy for breathlessness and exercise limitation in chronic stable COPD according to NICE is summarized in Figure 18.1 (1) and drugs used listed in Table 18.8.

NICE recommends that

- Short-acting bronchodilators, as necessary, should be the initial empirical treatment for the relief of breathlessness and exercise limitation.
- Patients who remain symptomatic on monotherapy should have their inhaled treatment increased to include long-acting bronchodilators or combined therapy with a short-acting beta$_2$-agonist and a short-acting anticholinergic.
- Long-acting bronchodilators should be used in patients who remain symptomatic despite treatment with short-acting bronchodilators because these drugs appear to have additional benefits over combinations of short-acting drugs.
- Long-acting bronchodilators should also be used in patients who have two or more exacerbations per year.
- Inhaled corticosteroids should be added to long-acting bronchodilators to decrease exacerbation frequency in patients with an FEV1 less than or equal to 50 % predicted who have had two or more exacerbations requiring treatment with antibiotics or oral corticosteroids in a 12-month period.

Theophylline

The guideline recommends the use of theophyllines (slow release preparations) only after a trial of short-acting bronchodilators and long-acting bronchodilators, or in patients who are unable to use inhaled therapy. This is because theophyllines require monitoring of blood plasma levels and there is a high risk of drug interactions, particularly in the elderly.

Oral Corticosteroids

Maintenance use of oral corticosteroid therapy in COPD is *not* recommended by NICE. However, it is acknowledged that some patients with advanced COPD may require maintenance oral corticosteroids when these cannot be withdrawn following an exacerbation. In these cases, the dose of oral corticosteroids should be kept as low as possible.

Oxygen

Recommendations for long-term oxygen therapy (LTOT) by NICE are summarized in Table 18.12.

LTOT prolongs life in chronically hypoxic COPD sufferers. The guideline also advises that assessment for LTOT should be considered in patients with moderate airflow obstruction (FEV1 30–49 % predicted).

The assessment of patients for LTOT should comprise the measurement of arterial blood gasses on two occasions at least three weeks apart in patients who have a confident diagnosis of COPD, who are receiving optimum medical management and whose COPD is stable.

NIV

Adequately treated patients with chronic hypercapneic ventilatory failure who have required assisted ventilation (whether invasive or non-invasive) during an exacerbation or who are hypercapneic or acidotic on LTOT should be referred to a specialist centre for consideration of long-term NIV.

CONCLUSION

COPD and asthma continue to be significant heath care problems in older people in the UK. These conditions pose many clinical challenges, particularly in the elderly. These include diagnosing the disease correctly, deciding the correct treatment options and following

Table 18.12. Indications for long term oxygen therapy, modified from (1) National Institute for Clinical Excellence

General indications

FEV1 is below 1.5 litres
AND
Non smoker
AND
PaO_2 is less than 7.3kPa
OR
PaO_2 7.3 to 8kPa in the presence of:

polycythaemia,
OR
pulmonary hypertension
OR
peripheral oedema

Special situations

If the patient is normoxaemic (PaO_2 was greater than 7.3 kPa) at rest but desaturates on exercise.

established guidelines, and considering concomitant medications in treating the older patients with concurrent disease. Only through increased understanding of their similarities and differences can there be progress in simplifying the differential diagnosis of these two disease entities.

KEY POINTS

- Common conditions.
- Significant morbidity and mortality.
- Often missed or misdiagnosed.
- Avoid triggers and STOP SMOKING.
- Research is needed to evaluate the effectiveness and safety of current and new therapies in the older population.

LEARNING RESOURCES

Asthma UK http://www.asthma.org.uk
Breathe Easy British Lung Foundation Support Group http://www.lunguk.org/support-groups.asp
British Lung foundation http://www.lunguk.org
British Thoracic Society http://www.brit-thoracic.org.uk
European Respiratory Society http://www.ernet.org

General Practice Airways Group http://www.gpiag.org
Global Initiative for Asthma http://www.ginasthma.com
National Institute for Clinical Excellence http://www.nice.org.uk
Scottish Intercollegiate Guidelines Network http://www.sign.org.uk

GUIDELINES

National Institute for Clinical Excellence. Chronic Obstructive Pulmonary Disease. National clinical guideline on management of chronic obstructive pulmonary disease in adults in primary and secondary care. *Thorax* 2004; **59** (Supplement 1): i1-i232.

The British Thoracic Society and Scottish Intercollegiate Guidelines Network. British Guideline on the Management of Asthma. *Thorax* 2003; **58** (Supplement 1): 1–94.

GINA (Global Initiative for Asthma). Global strategy for asthma management and prevention. National Institutes of Health Publication No. 02–3659. Management segment: Chapter 7. January 2005. Available at: http://www.ginasthma.com/ download. Accessed February 28, 2006.

Celli BR, MacNee W, Agusti A, et al. Standards for the diagnosis and treatment of patients with COPD: a summary of the ATS/ERS position paper. *European Respiratory Journal*. 2004; **23**: 932–46.

Pauwels R, Buist A, Calverly P, et al. Global strategy for the diagnosis, management, and prevention of chronic obstructive lung disease. NHLBI/WHO Global Initiative for Chronic Obstructive Lung Disease (GOLD) Workshop summary. *American Journal of Respiratory Critical Care Medicine*. 2001; **163**: 1256–76.

REFERENCES

1. National Institute for Clinical Excellence. Chronic Obstructive Pulmonary Disease. National clinical guideline on management of chronic obstructive pulmonary disease in adults in primary and secondary care. *Thorax*. 2004; **59** (Supplement 1): i1–i232.

2. The British Thoracic Society, Scottish Intercollegiate Guidelines Network. British Guideline on the Management of Asthma. *Thorax*. 2003; **58** (Supplement 1): 1–94.

3. National Heart Lung and Blood Institute, National Institutes of Health. International consensus report on the diagnosis and treatment of asthma. *European Respiratory Journal*. 1992; **5**: 601–41.

4. Balami J, Packham S, Gosney M. Non-invasive ventilation (NIV) for respiratory failure due to acute exacerbations of chronic obstructive pulmonary disease (COPD) in older patients. *Age & Ageing*. 2006; **35**: 75–8.

19 Pneumonia in the elderly

Peter A. Frith[1] and Karin S. Nyfort-Hansen[2]

[1] Southern Adelaide Health Service and Repatriation General Hospital, Adelaide, Australia
[2] Pharmacy Department, Repatriation General Hospital, Adelaide, Australia

INTRODUCTION

Pneumonia is inflammation of the lung parenchyma (alveoli and bronchioli) resulting from bacterial, viral and other organisms or immunological insults. Both community acquired (CAP) and hospital acquired (HAP) pneumonia increase in prevalence (and danger) with advancing age and the presence of chronic disease. This review will concentrate particularly on CAP, its causes, assessment, impact and treatment in older patients. Since increasing numbers of the elderly reside in long-term care facilities (LTCF), where CAP is generally more severe, we have contrasted CAP in LTCF with CAP in home-based individuals. Further, elderly people are at increased risk of aspiration events, and treatment options for aspiration pneumonia are included. The American Thoracic Society (ATS) and Infectious Diseases Society of America (IDSA) have included management of CAP contracted in LTCF in Guidelines for HAP.

EPIDEMIOLOGY

The incidence of CAP overall is estimated between 8 and 15 per 1000 persons per year (UpToDate v13.3, 2005). Around 20 % require hospitalization (1), of whom up to a third need treatment in Intensive Care (IC) areas (2, 3). Mortality is not uncommon, especially in people who require IC management, and is reported as high as 50 % in some series (3). In a recent Spanish study the incidence of CAP increased sharply in older adults, especially males – in people aged over 75 years the incidence was 10 per 10000 person-years. There were also some differences in causative organisms (more viruses and *Chlamydophila spp*) (4).

In LTCF residents the incidence of CAP is much higher – 33 per 1000 residents required hospitalization (5) – and 90 % of deaths from CAP are seen in the over-65 age group. CAP is the leading cause of morbidity, hospitalisation and mortality in elderly LTCF residents (5, 6, 12). It is the sixth leading cause of death in the USA and fourth in Japan (8).

CAP consumes health resources mainly through hospitalization, and there is mounting evidence that these costs can realistically be reduced by treating patients who do not need hospitalization in the community (9, 10). It therefore has societal implications to ensure patients are accurately assessed.

AETIOLOGY AND PATHOGENESIS

Organisms reach the lower respiratory tract by inhalation from ambient air or from the oral

Prescribing for Elderly Patients Edited by Stephen Jackson, Paul Jansen and Arduino Mangoni
© 2009 John Wiley & Sons, Ltd

cavity (much less commonly via the blood-stream). Impaired oral hygiene and poor gag reflex are especially important in LTCF residents and the elderly, leading to inhalation of mouth or gastric commensal organisms. Sub-optimal immune defences compound the problems (7).

Influenza, respiratory syncytial virus and parainfluenza are common viral causes of CAP, and account for up to 30 % of CAP cases (11). Bacterial CAP is more common, however. The major bacterial pathogens are *Streptococcus pneumoniae, Mycoplasma pneumoniae, Legionella spp, Chlamydophila pneumoniae* and *Haemophilus influenzae*. The most common micro-organisms for HAP, on the other hand, are aerobic gram negative bacilli *(Escherichia coli, Klebsiella pneumoniae, Enterobacter spp, Pseudomonas aeruginosa, Acinetobacter spp)* and gram positive cocci *(Streptococcus spp, Staphylococcus aureus* including MRSA). The spectrum in CAP occurring in LTCF patients has been found to be similar (12). In immunocompromised patients viruses and fungi are also important causes of HAP.

In a recent large study of 1511 consecutive patients admitted with CAP, 40 % had demonstrable bacterial pathogens, and 13 % of these had mixed pathogens. The most frequent combination involved *S. pneumoniae* with *H. infuenzae*, and mixed CAP was more severe than CAP with a single organism (13).

Older people are at increased risk of CAP or HAP for a variety of reasons that are especially prevalent in the elderly and LTCF residents. Poor oral hygiene, impaired swallowing, gastric hypoacidity, repeated aspiration, use of sedatives, impaired nutrition, immobility, and chronic diseases (especially Diabetes mellitus and Chronic Obstructive Pulmonary Disease) are the most important pre-disposing factors in the elderly (12, 14). Other medications are also more prevalent in the elderly, and these may contribute further to the increased risk of CAP – such as acid-suppressive agents (15). Use of HMG-CoA reductase inhibitors ("statins") may be protective (16), though the evidence for this is disputed (17). Multi-drug resistant pathogens are emerging as important considerations in this population (18).

SYMPTOMS AND SIGNS

Cough is the most usual symptom, and this is usually productive of purulent, muco-purulent or haemo-purulent sputum; chills and fever are also often seen. Pleuritic chest pain occurs in a third. Malaise, nausea and vomiting are also common. Classical symptoms, however, are poorly predictive of pneumonia in general practice, and the best symptom model in 246 patients (mean age 52 years) included dry cough, diarrhoea, and temperature $\geq 38\,°C$. This model plus C-reactive protein ≥ 50 or ESR ≥ 40 had high predictive value. C-reactive protein below $20\,mg/L$ in combination with only one symptom (including fever $\geq 38\,°C$) predicts a low risk of pneumonia and therefore safety in avoiding antibiotic use (19).

Symptoms are less obvious in older patients, and develop more slowly than in younger individuals. Delirium, confusion and falls are often the first manifestation (20). Among elderly residents of LTCF with CAP, a third have no fever (21). Mortality in this group is as high as 44 % (22), and the survivors often fail to recover their former functional status (23).

Because the symptom profile lacks sensitivity, especially in the elderly, combinations of clinical signs (such as fever, tachycardia, and pulmonary crackles) have been evaluated, but none has been found to have sensitivity more than 50 % (24). At least half have tachycardia and increased respiratory rates. Indeed, increased respiratory rate is more sensitive than most other signs in the elderly. Pulmonary crackles are common, albeit sometimes faint and in unusual regions, and frank signs of consolidation are found in about one-third.

DIAGNOSIS

The "gold standard" for confirming pneumonia is the plain chest x-ray, where alveolar infiltrates, patchy interstitial changes, consolidation and air bronchograms are most common. In CAP these are often lobar or lobular in distribution, though diffuse and less distinct opacities may be seen ("bronchopneumonia"). In early stages, especially if the patient is dehydrated, infiltrates may only emerge after rehydration (25). A prospective cohort study of 192 patients (age 56.8 ± 17.6 years) with a GP diagnosis of suspected pneumonia were referred for confirmatory chest x-ray – no abnormalities were seen in 98 patients (52 %), and the chest x-ray changed the probability rating of pneumonia in 53 % of patients, and management plans were changed after chest x-ray in 69 % (26).

A microbiological diagnosis is an ideal goal, but early empirical therapy should not be delayed while awaiting results. In any case, positive identification seldom exceeds 20 %. In HAP, however, it may be more important to identify causative organisms so potential sources of infection can be identified, cross-infection can be minimized, and antibiotic resistance patterns can be documented. Blood cultures, sputum cultures, and deeper respiratory specimens can all be used, although none has high sensitivity. Gram stains are even less sensitive.

PATIENT ASSESSMENT

Over recent years large studies have been done to rate the severity of CAP, the need for hospitalisation, and the risk of death. Fatal outcome from CAP is most often associated with the following: afebrile, bedridden, swallowing disorder, immunosuppressed (major features in the elderly), respiratory rate over 30, creatinine above 1.4 mg/dL, involvement of three or more lobes on chest X-ray, rapid progression of chest X-ray infiltrates, and APACHE score ≥ 22 (27, 28). Scoring systems using these data have been used to predict 30-day mortality in LTCF residents with CAP (29). Patients admitted with CAP who also have COPD need ICU care more frequently and have significantly greater mortality at 30 and 90 days than those without COPD (30). Increasing age, male sex, prior heart failure, stroke or dementia and use of anti-depressant medications or benzodiazepines are significant risk factors for complications or death (31). Diabetes is not an independent risk factor for case fatality in CAP (32).

The Pneumonia Severity Index (PSI – Table 19.1. includes 20 criteria, which were derived from a study of a cohort of 14 199 patients with CAP (33). It has been shown to allow better targeting of care (34), especially in identifying those at lowest risk. The BTS criteria (35) aimed to identify high risk patients, and were subsequently modified to include confusion (36) and other (37) criteria (BTS-CURB). A recent study of 696 consecutive patients validated several prediction formulae against the PSI for predicting both Intensive Care admission and death (38). The BTS-CURB and the American Thoracic Society (ATS) (3) rules were simple to use and reliable. The "gold standard" – the PSI – is rather difficult to use (Table 19.1), although it is amenable to computerisation (39). Alternatively it can be replaced in routine clinical practice by the BTS-CURB index (Table 19.2). Rating need for critical care and likelihood of death can be easily measured by the modified ATS criteria (Table 19.3)

Home management versus hospital care of mild to moderate CAP has been examined in a randomized controlled trial in New Zealand (40), in part validating the CURB-65 scoring system (41). Patients with CURB-65 scores 0 to 2 were considered suitable for management in the community and randomized. There were similar outcomes in home-care as in hospital-care patients, but patients preferred community treatment. Use of the risk predictions is more problematic in LTCF patients, but mortality rates may not be worse if patients stay in the LTCF for their treatment compared to hospital transfer (42), providing appropriate care resources are available. While the PSI was designed to distinguish patients with CAP who would be suitable for home treatment, it has been found very useful for stratifying likelihood of mortality (Table 19.1). However the value of the PSI in determining the best site for care may be limited as it does not include some important social factors (43).

In conclusion, it has proven useful to stratify the severity of CAP to predict who can successfully be cured without hospitalisation, and to predict risk of mortality and the urgency and

Table 19.1. Pneumonia Severity Index (PSI)

Patient characteristics		Points
Demographics	Age (males)	Age (yrs)
	Age (females)	Age − 10 (yrs)
	LTCF resident	+10
Comorbidities	Neoplastic disease	+30
	Liver disease	+20
	Chronic heart failure	+10
	Cerebrovascular disease	+10
	Renal disease	+10
Physical examination findings	Altered mental status	+20
	Pulse rate >124 bpm	+10
	Respiratory rate >29 bpm	+20
	Systolic blood pressure <90 mmHg	+20
	Temperature <35°C or >39.9°C	+15
Laboratory findings	Haematocrit <30%	+30
	pH <7.35	+30
	Urea >10 mmol/L	+20
	Sodium <130 mmol/L	+20
	Glucose >13.9 mmol/L	+10
	pO2 <60 mmHg	+10
	Pleural effusion	+10
Total point score represents the PSU Risk Score		

Likelihood of Mortality with Pneumonia Severity Index categories

PSI risk class	Points assigned	30-day mortality (%)
I		0.1
II	≤70	0.6
III	71–90	0.9
IV	91–130	9.3
V	>130	27.0

Table 19.2. CURB-65 Criteria for CAP Severity

C	Confusion	
U	Urea >7mm/L	
R	Respiratory rate ≥30/min	1 point for each
B	BP systolic <90mm Hg	
	Diastolic ≤ 60mm Hg	
65	65 years of age or above	

Score	CURB-65 Risk Group	30-day mortality (5%)
0 to 1	1	1.5
2	2	9.2
3 to 5	3	22

intensiveness of supportive therapy. PSI is the best-validated tool, though complex (Table 19.1). The CURB-65 (Table 19.2) is a more simple alternative measure with good performance characteristics. Severity of pneumonia can also be effectively predicted by the modified ATS criteria (Table 19.3).

THERAPY

Choice of antibiotic for CAP depends largely on local antibiotic sensitivity patterns, especially for *Streptococcus pneumoniae*, although clinical failure with beta-lactams (e.g. penicillin) has not been reported. On

Table 19.3. Modified ATS Criteria for CAP Severity

Minor Criteria	Systolic BP < 90 mmHg
	$\geq$ 2 lobes involved
	PaO$_2$/Fi O$_2$ < 250
Major Criteria	Mechanical ventilation required
	Septic shock present

Severe pneumonia present if two minor or one major criteria are present
−sensitivity 69%, specificity 98%, PPV 87%, NPV 94%

the other hand, mortality is lower when a beta-lactam is combined with another antibiotic (especially macrolide or tetracycline); North American guidelines recommend use of fluoroquinolones. One Australian guideline applicable to empirical therapy in non-tropical areas is shown (Table 19.4).

Parenteral (IV) therapy should only be necessary for patients unable to swallow or absorb oral preparations. This approach would be suitable for most other bacterial causes of CAP, but immuno-incompetence, unusual origin of CAP, "atypical pneumonia", and likely aspiration would warrant a less empirical approach with more specific drugs. Since aspiration is not uncommon in the elderly, especially LTNC residents (28), antibiotic choice in this setting should provide anaerobic cover (Table 19.5).

Patients with moderate to severe CAP (eg PSI grades III to V or CURB-65 grades 2 to 5) should be treated in a hospital environment. Those with severe pneumonia should be considered early for ICU management, including supportive measures (eg IV fluids, assisted ventilation). While there is as yet no consensus on the role of glucocorticosteroids (GCS), a preliminary randomized trial suggests that by controlling the inflammatory reaction with GCS does improve outcome in patients with severe CAP (44).

IMPORTANT CONSIDERATIONS FOR DRUG USAGE

The primary role of antibiotics is to decrease bacterial load and allow the balance of host defences to be restored in favour of cure. If bacterial proliferation is allowed to proceed – by incorrect, ineffective or delayed antibiotics,

or because of late presentation or impaired immune defences – cure cannot occur, and death may ensue. Many of these characteristics are found in older individuals, as indicated above. Patients with severe CAP due to *Streptococcus pneumoniae* that is sensitive to penicillin can still die despite all bacteria being eliminated. Further, antibiotic therapy appears not to affect clinical outcome in many people with "atypical" CAP (e.g. due to *Mycoplasma pneumoniae* and *Chlamydophilia pneumoniae*) (46). These findings can be used to underline the importance of maintaining a high index of suspicion of CAP in the elderly who have rapid respiration rate, confusion and hypotension, or fever, then to implement effective safe antibiotic therapy as soon as possible. **A delay in initiating antibiotics by more than 4 hours is associated with higher death rates** (48).

Which antibiotic to use? The antibiotics in Tables 19.4 and 19.5 are generally well-tolerated by the elderly. Doxycycline should be avoided in patients with swallowing disorders due to a risk of oesophagitis, and for the same reason doxycycline should not be administered at bedtime. Patients prescribed a macrolide (erythromycin, azithromycin, clarithromycin, roxithromycin) who are also taking warfarin require close INR monitoring. Of the macrolides azithromycin has the least potential for interaction with warfarin or other drugs. These macrolides may also be associated with unpredictable reversible hearing loss or tinnitus in some patients. Due to age-related decline in renal function gentamicin doses require adjustment in all elderly patients in order to minimize nephro- or oto-toxicity. Trough gentamicin concentrations <0.5 mg/L are recommended if therapy continues beyond

Table 19.4. Empirical choice of early antibiotics for Pneumonia in the elderly (non-tropical Australia)*

PSI Class	First line therapy	Alternatives
I and II	Oral amoxicillin 1Gm 8-hourly for 7 days If intending to treat for Mycoplasma pneumoniae or Chlamydia pneumoniae add: Oral doxycycline 200 mg stat then 100 mg daily for 5 days OR Oral clarithromycin 250 mg 12-hourly for 7 days OR Oral roxithromycin 300 mg daily for 5 days	IF PENICILLIN HYPERSENSITIVITY: Oral cefuroxime 500 mg 12-hourly for 7 days. IF IMMEDIATE PENICILLIN HYPERSENSITIVITY: Oral moxifloxacin 400 mg daily for 7 days
III and IV	IV benzylpenicillin 1.2Gm 6-hourly OR IV amoxy/ampicillin 1 G 6-hourly till clinical stability, THEN oral amoxicillin 1 G 8-hourly for total 7 days PLUS EITHER Oral doxycycline 100 mg 12-hourly for 7 days OR Oral clarithromycin 500 mg 12-hourly for 7 days OR roxithromycin 300 mg daily for 5 days. IF GRAM NEG organisms in sputum or blood: ADD gentamicin OR substitute ceftriaxone or cefotaxime for benzylpenicillin or amoxy/ampicillin. IF ASPIRATION possible: IV metronidazole 500 mg b.d. added if aspiration and for nursing-home residents.	IF PENICILLIN HYPERSENSITIVITY: IV ceftriaxone 1Gm daily OR IV cefotaxime 1 G 8-hourly till clinical stability. THEN oral as above. IF IMMEDIATE PENICILLIN HYPERSENSITIVITY: Oral/IV moxifloxacin as above (if Immediate Penicillin Hypersensitivity).
V	IV azithromycin 500 mg daily OR IV erythromycin 0.5 to 1Gm 6-hourly PLUS EITHER IV ceftriaxone 1Gm daily OR IV cefotaxime 1 G 8-hourly OR COMBINATION of IV benzylpenicillin 1.2Gm 4-hourly PLUS IV gentamicin 4 to 6 mg/kg/day (adjust dose to renal function).	IF IMMEDIATE PENICILLIN HYPERSENSITIVITY: IV moxifloxacin 400 mg daily.

*from Therapeutic Guidelines. *Antibiotic*. Version 13, 2006 Melbourne : Therapeutic Guidelines Ltd, pp. 206–8 (http://www.etg.hcn.net.au/).

Table 19.5. Empirical antibiotic therapy for aspiration pneumonia*

First line therapy	Alternatives
benzylpenicillin 1.2 g IV 6-hourly	In patients with immediate penicillin hypersensitivity:
PLUS	
metronidazole 500 mg IV 12-hourly or 400 mg orally 12-hourly	clindamycin 450 mg IV or orally 8-hourly
	OR
If Gram-negative pneumonia is suspected (e.g. in alcoholic patients) use:	lincomycin 600 mg IV 8-hourly
metronidazole 500 mg IV 12-hourly or 400 mg orally 12-hourly	Switch to oral therapy after there has been significant improvement and patient is able to tolerate oral medication: clindamycin 450 mg orally 8-hourly
PLUS EITHER	
ceftriaxone 1 g IV daily or	
cefotaxime 1 g IV 8-hourly	
OR (as a single agent)	
piperacillin+tazobactam 4/0.5 g IV 8-hourly or	
ticarcillin+clavulanate 3/0.1 g IV 6-hourly	
Switch to oral therapy after there has been significant improvement and patient is able to tolerate oral medication:	
amoxycillin+clavulanate 875/125 mg orally 12-hourly	

*from Therapeutic Guidelines. *Antibiotic*. Version 13, 2006 Melbourne : Therapeutic Guidelines Ltd, pp. 206–8 (http://www.etg.hcn.net.au/).

one dose. Moxifloxacin and clarithromycin may prolong the QTc interval and should therefore be avoided in patients who have known prolongation of QTc or are also taking amiodarone, sotalol, tricyclic antidepressants or antipsychotics.

Although early antibiotic use is of critical importance, **duration of antibiotic therapy** is not widely agreed. Guidelines suggest seven to 21 days (42, 49, 50), but adherence to guidelines is at best variable (39, 51, 52). A recent study in adult patients with mild-moderate CAP concluded that in a subgroup who showed a good early response, three days of treatment with IV amoxycillin was as effective as a total of eight days of IV and oral therapy (53). Attempts have been made to develop markers that might be used as "stopping rules". Clinical markers, though, are unreliable, and culture results are not useful. Biomarkers therefore are attractive, especially those that can be measured in peripheral blood and are reflective of cytokine expression or mediators. A particularly promising chemical is procalcitonin, which is high in

bacterial infections (52), and its measurement to guide therapy has been shown to reduce antibiotic prescriptions yet optimize recovery (55). Furthermore, persistently high levels are associated with poor outcome (56) and decreasing levels with favourable outcome (57). In the first randomised controlled trial of reducing duration of antibiotics (55) a median duration of five days was achieved (from a median of 12 days). Procalcitonin has proven better than C-reactive protein (CRP) both to guide initiation of antibiotics and to indicate when antibiotics can be withdrawn (58). Until external validation of these findings in larger multicentre trials, this remains for the present a very promising marker.

Response to therapy should be monitored by simple clinical indicators, notably respiratory rate, heart rate, blood pressure (if shocked), temperature and gas exchange (pulse oximetry or arterial blood gas analysis). Improvements in radiology lag behind clinical resolution, so chest X-ray cannot be relied upon for early evidence of improvement. The duration of hospital stay is dictated by (a) the stabilization of clinical parameters and (b) recovery of functional status. Once heart rate has stabilised below 100 beats/min, systolic blood pressure above 90 mmHg, respiratory rate below 24 breaths/min, temperature below 37.2 °C and oxygen saturation above 90 %, discharge can be considered as long as home supports and functional status are satisfactory. It is advisable to follow up older people with pneumonia with a chest X-ray about 6 to 12 weeks later to monitor full resolution. Failure to resolve suggests recurrent aspiration events, antibiotic resistance or development of complications like lung abscess or empyema, but the possibility of obstructive pneumopathy due to lung cancer should also be considered. If recovery takes place, two-year mortality thereafter may still be as high as 32 %, higher mortality being associated with severe comorbid conditions (relative rise 9.4), but not with age (45). Elderly residents of LTCF admitted to hospitals had higher mortality rates (around 58 % at one year) (46). Functional status in one study was the chief determinant of survival (22).

Despite these objective findings, **recovery** of overall health status can be prolonged. In 102 patients with moderate-to-severe CAP followed for 18 months post-CAP, respiratory symptoms disappeared within two weeks. Health-related quality of life took longer and had certainly returned to pre-CAP levels at six months. Any residual symptoms or health status impairments could be attributed entirely to age or comorbid conditions (59).

PREVENTION

Pneumococcal vaccination reduces severity of infection in the elderly, though without influencing the incidence (60–63). In a community cohort of 11241 in Spain, slightly under half of whom had been vaccinated and slightly over half had not, there were important reductions of death risk from CAP (hazard ratio 0.28; 95 % CI:0.09-0.83). All-cause mortality was also less in the vaccinated group (HR-0.67;

95 % CI:0.54-0.83) (60). On these grounds alone a good case can therefore be made for pneumococcal vaccination in people over the age of 65 years as well as people with impaired immunocompetence. Further details can be found in the vaccination schedule for Australia (64), which recommends an initial vaccination at age 65 with a single booster five years later. Both are provided free to those over age 65.

REFERENCES

1. Oosterheert J, Bonten MJM, Hak E, Schneider MM, Hoepelman AI. Severe community-acquired pneumonia: What's in a name? *Curr Opin Infect Dis* 2003; **16**: 153–9.
2. Moine P, Vercken J-B, Chevret S, Chastang C, Gajdrs P. Severe community-acquired pneumonia: etiology, epidemiology and prognosis factors. *Chest* 1994; **105**: 1487–95.
3. Ewig S, Ruiz M, Mensa J, Marcos MA, Martinez JA, Arancibia F, et al. Severe community-acquired pneumonia. Assessment of severity criteria. *Am J Respir Crit Care Med* 1998; **158**: 1102–8.
4. Guttierrez F, Masia M, Mirete C, Soldan B, et al. The influence of age and gender on the population-based incidence of community-acquired pneumonia caused by different microbial pathogens. *J Infect* 2006; **53**: 166–74.
5. Marrie TJ. Pneumonia in the long-term-care facility. *Infect Control Hosp Epidemiol* 2002; **23**: 159–64.
6. van der Steen JT, Ooms ME, Mehr DR, van der Wal G, Ribbe MW. Severe dementia and adverse outcomes of nursing home-acquired pneumonia: evidence for mediation by functional and pathophysiological decline. *J Am Geriatr Soc* 2002; **50**: 439–48.
7. Yoneyama T, Yoshida M, Ohrui T, Mukaiyama H, Okamoto H, Hoshiba K, et al. Oral care reduces pneumonia in older patients in nursing homes. *J Am Geriatr Soc* 2002; **50**: 430–3.
8. Japanese Respiratory Society. Definition of pneumonia. *Respirology* 2006; **11**: 582.
9. Fine MJ, Pratt HM, Obrosky DS, et al. Relation between length of hospital stay and costs of care for patients with community-acquired pneumonia. *Am J Med* 2000; **109**: 378–85.
10. Bartolomé M, Almirall J, Morera J, Pera G, et al. A population-based study of the costs of

care for community-acquired pneumonia. *Eur Respir J* 2004; **23**: 610–16.

11. deRoux A, Marcos MA, Garcia E, Mensa J, Ewig S, Lode H, Torres A. Viral community-acquired pneumonia in non immuno-compromised adults. *Chest* 2004; **125**: 1343–52.

12. El-Solh AA, Sikka P, Ramadan F, Davies J. Etiology of severe pneumonia in the very elderly. *Am J Respir Crit Care Med* 2001; **163**: 645–51.

13. deRoux A, Ewig S, Marcos MA, Mensa J, Lode H, Torres A. Mild community-acquired pneumonia in hospitalised patients. *Eur Respir J* 2006; **27**: 795–800.

14. Marrie TJ. Community-acquired pneumonia in the elderly. *Clin Infect Dis* 2000; **31**: 1066–78.

15. Laheij RJ, Sturkenboom MC, Hassing RJ, Stricker BH, Jansen JB. Risk of community-acquired pneumonia and use of gastric acid-suppressive drugs. *JAMA* 2004; **292**: 1955–60.

16. Mortensen EM, Restrepo MI, Anzueto A, Pugh J. The effect of prior statin use on 30-day mortality for patients hospitalized with community-acquired pneumonia. *Respir Res* 2005; **6**: 82.

17. Majumdar SR, McAlister FA, Eurich DT, Padwal RS, Marrie TJ. Statins and outcomes in patients admitted to hospital with community acquired pneumonia: population based prospective cohort study. *BMJ* 2006; **333**: 999–.

18. Craven DE. What is healthcare-associated pneumonia, and how should it be treated? *Current Opin Infect Dis* 2006; **19**: 153–60.

19. Hopstaken RM, Muris JW, Knottnerus JA, et al. Contributions of symptoms, signs, erythrocyte sedimentation rate of C-reactive protein to a diagnosis of pneumonia in acute lower respiratory tract infection. *Br J Gen Pract* 2003; **53**: 358–64.

20. Riquelme R, Torres A, El-Ebiary M, Mensa J, Estruch R, et al. Community-acquired pneumonia in the elderly. Clinical and nutritional aspects. *Am J Respir Crit Care Med* 1997; **156**: 1908–14.

21. Muder RR. Pneumonia in residents of long-term care facilities: epidemiology, etiology, management, and prevention. *Am J Med* 1998; **105**: 319–30.

22. Medina-Walpole AM, Katz PR. Nursing home-acquired pneumonia. *J Am Geriatr Soc* 1999; **47**: 1005–15.

23. Fried TR, Gillick MR, Lipsitz LA. Short-term functional outcomes of long-term care residents with pneumonia treated with and without hospital transfer. *J Am Geriatr Soc* 1997; **45**: 302–6.

24. Metlay JP, Fine MJ. Testing strategies in the initial management of patients with community-acquired pneumonia. *Ann Intern Med* 2003; **138**: 109–18.

25. Basi SK, Marrie TJ, Huang JQ, Majumdar SR. Patients admitted to hospital with suspected pneumonia and normal chest radiographs: epidemiology, microbiology, and outcomes. *Am J Med* 2004; **117**: 305–11.

26. Speets AM, Hoes AW, van der Graaf Y, et al. Chest radiography and pneumonia in primary care: diagnostic yield and consequences for patient management. *Eur Respir J* 2006; **28**: 933–8.

27. Riquelme R, Torres A, El-Ebiary M, De La Bellacasa JP, Estruch R, Mensa J, et al. Community-acquired pneumonia in the elderly. A multivariate analysis of risk and prognostic factors. *Am J Respir Crit Care Med* 1996; **154**: 1450–5.

28. Rello J. Rodriguez R, Jubert P, Alvarez B, the Study Group for Severe Community-Acquired Pneumonia. Severe community-acquired pneumonia in the elderly: epidemiology and prognosis. *Clin Infect Dis* 1996; **23**: 723–8.

29. Mehr DR, Binder EF, Kruse RL, Zweig SC, Madsen R, et al. Predicting mortality in nursing home residents with lower respiratory tract infection: the Missouri LRI study. *JAMA* 2001; **286**: 2427–36.

30. Restrepo MI, Mortensen EM, Pugh JA, Anzveto A. COPD is associated with increased mortality in patients with community-acquired pneumonia. *Eur Respir J* 2006; **28**: 346–51.

31. Hak E, Bont J, Hoes AW, Verheij TJM. Prognostic factors for serious morbidity and mortality from community-acquired lower respiratory tract infections among the elderly in primary care. *Family Pract* 2005; **22**: 375–80.

32. Thomsen RW, Hundborg HH, Lervang H-H, Johsen SoP, et al. Diabetes and outcome of community-acquired pneumococcal bacteremia: A 10-year population – based cohort study. *Diabetes Care* 2004; **27**: 70–6.

33. Fine MJ, Auble TE, Yealy DM, Hanusa BH, Weissfeld LA, et al. A prediction rule to identify low-risk patients with community-acquired pneumonia. *N Engl J Med* 1997; **336**: 243–50.

34. Marrie TJ, Lau CY, Wheeler SL, Wong CJ, Vandervoort MK, Feagan BG. A controlled trial of a critical pathway for treatment of

community-acquired pneumonia. *JAMA* 2000; **283**: 749–55.

35. Farr BM, Sloman AJ, Fisch MJ. Predicting death in patients hospitalised for community-acquired pneumonia. *Ann Intern Med* 1991; **115**: 428–36.

36. Neill AM, Martin IR, Weir R, Anderson R, Chereshsky A, et al. Community-acquired pneumonia: aetiology and usefulness of severity criteria on admission. *Thorax* 1996; **51**: 1010–6.

37. Lim WS, Macfarlane JT, Boswell TC, Harrison TG, Rose D, et al. Study of community acquired pneumonia aetiology (SCAPA) in adults admitted to hospital: implications for management guidelines. *Thorax* 2001; **56**: 296–301.

38. Ewig S, deRoux A, Bauer T, Garcia E, Mensa J, et al. Validation of predictive rules and indices of severity for community acquired pneumonia. *Thorax* 2004; **59**: 421–7.

39. Wright AA and Maydom BW. Improving the implementation of community-acquired pneumonia guidelines. *Intern Med J* 2004; **34**: 507–9.

40. Richards DA, Toop LJ, Epton MJ, McGeoch GRB, Town GI, et al. Home management of mild to moderately severe community-acquired pneumonia: a randomised controlled trial. *Med J Aust* 2005; **183**: 235–8.

41. Lim WS, van der Eerden MM, Laing R, Boersma WG, Karalus N, et al. Defining community acquired pneumonia severity on presentation to hospital: an international derivation and validation study. *Thorax* 2003; **58**: 377–82.

42. Naughton BJ, Mylotte JM. Treatment guideline for nursing home-acquired pneumonia based on community practice. *J Am Geriatr Soc* 2000; **48**: 82–8.

43. Goss CH, Rubenfeld GD, Park DR, Sherbin VL, Goodman MS, Root RK. Cost and incidence of social comorbidities in low risk patients with community acquired pneumonia admitted to a public hospital. *Chest* 2003; **124**: 2148–55.

44. Confolonieri M, Urbino R, Potena A, Piattella M, Parigi P, et al. Hydrocortisone infusion for severe community-acquired pneumonia: a preliminary randomized study. *Am J Respir Crit Care Med* 2005; **171**: 242–8.

45. Brancati FL, Chow JW, Wagener MM, Vacarello SJ, Yu VL. Is pneumonia really the old man's friend? Two year prognosis after community-acquired pneumonia. *Lancet* 1993; **342**: 30–3.

46. Marrie TJ, Blanchard W. A comparison of nursing home-acquired pneumonia patients with patients with community-acquired pneumonia and nursing home patients without pneumonia. *J Am Geriatr Soc* 1997; **45**: 50–5.

47. Meehan TP, Fine MJ, Krumholz HM, Scinto JD, et al. Quality of care, process, and outcomes in elderly patients with pneumonia. *JAMA* 1997; **278**: 2080–4.

48. Mandell LA, Bartlett JG, Dowell SF, File TM, Musher DM, Whitney C. Update of practice guidelines for the management of community-acquired pneumonia in immunocompetent adults. *Clin Infect Dis* 2003; **37**: 1405–33.

49. Woodhead M, Blasi F, Ewig S, Huchon G, et al. Guidelines for the management of adult lower respiratory tract infections. *Eur Respir J* 2005; **26**: 1138–80.

50. Aujesky D, Fine MJ. Does guideline adherence for empiric antibiotic therapy reduce mortality community-acquired pneumonia? *Am J Respir Crit Care Med* 2005; **172**: 655–6.

51. Menendez R, Torres A, Zalacain R, Aspa J, et al. Guidelines for the treatment of community-acquired pneumonia: predictors of adherence and outcome. *Am J Respir Crit Care Med* 2005; **172**: 757–62.

52. Muller B, Becker KL, Sehachinger H, Rickenbacher PR, et al. Calcitonin precursors are reliable markers of sepsis in a medical intensive care unit. *Crit Care Med* 2000; **28**: 977–83.

53. el Moussaoui R, de Borgie AJM, van den Broek P, Hustinx WN, et al. Effectiveness of discontinuing antibiotic treatment after three days versus eight days in mild to moderate-severe community acquired pneumonia: randomised, double blind study. *BMJ* 2006; **332**: 1355.

54. Christ-Crain M, Stolz D, Bingisser R, Muller C, et al. Procalcitonin guidance of antibiotic therapy in community-acquired pneumonia. *Am J Respir Crit Care Med* 2006; **174**: 84–93.

55. Harbarth S, Holeckova K, Froidevaux C, Pittet D, et al. Diagnostic value of procalcitonin, interleukin-6, and interleukin-8 in critically ill patients admitted with suspected sepsis. *Am J Respir Crit Care Med* 2001; **164**: 396–402.

56. Becker KL, Nylen ES, White JC, Muller B, Snider RH. Procalcitonin and the calcitonin gene family of peptides in inflammation, infection, and sepsis: a journey from calcitonin back to its precursors. *J Clin Endocrinol Metab* 2004; **89**: 1512–25.

57. Simon L, Gauvin F, Aunre DK, Saint-Louis P, Lacroix J. Serum procalcitonin and C-reactive

protein levels as markers of bacterial infection: a systematic review and meta-analysis. *Clin Infect Dis* 2004; **39**: 206–17.

58. Vila-Corcoles A, Ochoa-Gondor O, Llor C, Hospital I, Rodriguez J, Gomez A). Protective effect of pneumococcal vaccine against death by pneumonia in elderly subjects. *Eur Respir J* 2005: **26**: 1086–91.

59. el Moussaoui R, Opmeer BC, de Borgie CAJM, et al. Long-term symptom recovery and health-related quality of life in patients with mild-to-moderate-severe community-acquired pneumonia. *Chest* 2006; **130**: 1165–72.

60. Dear K, Holden J, Andrews R, Tatham D. Vaccines for preventing pneumococcal infection in adults. *Cochrane Database Syst Rev* 2003; **4**: CD000422–.

61. Mykietiuk A, Carratala J, Domingues A, Manzur A, et al. Effect of prior pneumococcal vaccination on clinical outcome of hospitalized adults with community-acquired pneumococcal pneumonia. *Eur J Clin Microbiol Infect Di* 2006; **25**: 457–62.

62. Fisman DN, Abrutyn E, Spaude KA, Kim A, et al. Prior pneumococcal vaccination is associated with reduced death, complications, and length of stay among hospitalized adults with community-acquired pneumonia. *Clin Infect Dis* 2006; **42**: 1093–1101.

63. Vila-Corcoles A, Ochoa-Gondor O, Llor C, Hospital I, et al. Protective effect of pneumococcal vaccine against death by pneumonia in elderly subjects. *Eur Respir J* 2005; **26**: 1086–91.

64. 64http://www.immunise.health.gov.au /internet/immunise/publishing.nsf/.

20 Therapeutic aspects of pulmonary tuberculosis

Paul Van den Brande

Division of Pulmonology, University Hospital Gasthuisberg, Leuven, Belgium

INTRODUCTION

Tuberculosis (TB) is a disease that has affected the population of the whole world for many thousands of years. Since the introduction of efficient anti-tuberculous medication and control programmes initiated after World War II, an annual decline in the number of TB-cases was observed in Western countries. In the mid 1980s this decline levelled off and an increase in the number of cases was observed. Within the global emergence of TB, there appear to be two different patterns. In low-income countries, TB is related mainly to poverty and the Human Immunodefiency Virus (HIV)-epidemic, but the principal reason is demographic, the world population is increasing most rapidly in the areas of the world where TB is also most prevalent, particularly sub-Saharan Africa and South-East Asia. In high-income countries, TB is related mainly to the impoverishment and marginalization of some risk-groups and to the dismantling of the TB-control programmes, with approximately one third of the new cases found in immigrants from countries with a high TB-prevalence, with one fourth attributed to elderly patients.

In the elderly age group, TB remains an important challenge. The non-specific complaints, the unrewarding physical examination, the atypical roentgenographic findings, the difficulties in interpreting the tuberculin skin test, and the confounding associated diseases often result in a long delay between initial complaints and final diagnosis, in an initial misdiagnosis, and also in the fact that diagnosis may be made only at autopsy. The management of active TB in elderly patients does not differ fundamentally from that in younger patients in terms of the outcome and side effects of treatment. Empiric treatment can perhaps be considered more readily in the elderly patient. When compared to the past, the guidelines have become less reluctant regarding the use of tuberculin skin testing and the treatment of latent tuberculosis infection in elderly persons and the prevention of transmission of tuberculosis in nursing homes.

PATHOGENESIS

TB is caused by Mycobacterium tuberculosis (MTB) and infection generally occurs by inhalation of infected droplets, expelled by coughing, sneezing, or even laughing and singing by patients with sputum-positive TB. The first infection occurs in the best ventilated portions of the lungs. In the alveoli the TB bacillus is ingested by the macrophages and through a cell-mediated immune response, an inflammation is initiated. This tuberculous primo-infection not always evolves to disease. After six to eight weeks the immunologic response is maximal and a resorption of the inflammation takes place together with the

Prescribing for Elderly Patients Edited by Stephen Jackson, Paul Jansen and Arduino Mangoni

deposition of collagen and even calcium, resulting in the formation of a scar. However, TB can develop immediately after the primary infection, which then is called 'progressive primary TB'. Simultaneously with the primary infection, an occult bacillemia occurs with small foci of infection in the apices of the lungs, the surrenals, the brain and the metaphysis of long bones. Essential to the pathogenesis of TB is the fact that in those scar lesions a few TB bacilli can survive in a dormant situation with a very low metabolism. Those dormant bacilli divide only very rarely but sustain the immunologic response as expressed by the positive tuberculin skin test. Long after the primary infection (years to decades), those lesions may reactivate and proceed into TB-disease, which then is called 'post-primary TB' or 'reactivation TB'. Without treatment, TB can heal spontaneously but there is always an incidence of relapse in 2 to 13% per 1000 persons per year, especially in those patients with very extensive fibrotic scar lesions (more than 2 cm diameter) in the apices of the lung. There is general agreement that in an area with a low prevalence of TB, the majority of TB cases in the elderly are due to reactivation TB. This concept is not surprising, since it is accepted that today's elderly patients were infected by MTB at the beginning of the 20th century, a period of high TB-prevalence, and now thus present with reactivation of a remote infection, due to decreased immune resistance with aging. Cavitary TB or phtisis was until the mid 1970s the disease found in approximately 90% of the adult population. The lesions resulted from reactivation from bronchogenic or hematogenic dissemination contracted earlier in life and formed the 'link' between the primary infection and the reactivation, sometimes after a period of several decades. This knowledge remained a 'dogma' until the 1970s–80s, when it was found that a number of patients presented with TB, but in whom the clinical and radiological picture was initially attributed to other diseases, which were much more commonly found in the elderly, i.e. bronchogenic carcinoma, lymphoproliferative

malignancies, systemic disease and other infectious diseases. When ultimately the diagnosis of TB was made after a long delay or even post-mortem, physicians became alert to this problem and those presentations were judged as 'unusual' and/or 'atypical' for this age-group. Taking into account the 'changed view' of the pathogenesis of TB in the elderly, it became clear that a number of elderly subjects developed primary progressive TB even if they were known with a previous TB-infection or even with a history of TB-disease. Although the largest number of cases of TB occurs among community dwelling elderly persons, there is increasing concern about TB in elderly persons living in nursing homes, especially the ease with which the disease can spread in closed environments.

PRESENTATION OF TUBERCULOSIS IN THE ELDERLY

Although approximately 75% of elderly persons with TB present as pulmonary TB, non-pulmonary TB such as miliary TB, pleural TB, lymph node TB, tuberculous meningitis, skeletal and genitourinary TB increase in frequency with advancing age. The clinical presentation can be an atypical and subtle and unexplained weight loss, weakness or change in cognitive status may be the only manifestations of the disease in the elderly. The clinical signs of TB in the elderly are variable and range from total absence of any symptom or mild illness to a fulminate course and even death. The "classic" symptoms of TB such as night sweats and fever are more often seen in the younger age group, whereas non-specific symptoms such as anorexia and weight loss are noted in a higher proportion of the elderly patients. These general symptoms are not unusual in older subjects and do not make the physician readily suspicious of TB; they are often attributed to the ageing process itself, to concomitant chronic illness, or even to mental disorders. More specific pulmonary symptoms such as hemoptysis and purulent expectorations occur equally in both age groups. Chronic cough and dyspnea are noted more often among patients with chronic obstructive pulmonary disease, which is seen more frequently in the older age group. A changing cough pattern is often not recognized by the patient or by the persons surrounding him, i.e., family members and the general practitioner. The radiographic findings of pulmonary TB can be classified into two major categories. 'Usual' are infiltrations (with of without cavitation) in the apicoposterior segments of one or both upper lobes and/or in the apical segments of one or both lower lobes. 'Unusual' findings for adult PTB are characterized by the absence of the above-mentioned abnormalities but the presence of pleural effusion, miliary pattern, anterior and basal infiltrations, lymphadenopathy, or solitary rounded nodules. The radiographic pattern is not different between both age groups: 'usual' apicoposterior lesions are found in more than 70 % of both groups. However, initially a wrong diagnosis is made more often in the elderly, especially when presenting with 'unusual' radiographic findings.

The non-specific complaints, the unrewarding physical examination, the atypical roentgenographic findings and the confounding associated diseases often result in a postponement of diagnosis or even in an initial misdiagnosis.

DIAGNOSIS OF TUBERCULOSIS

The first step in diagnosing TB is to include the disease in the differential diagnosis, followed by demonstration of (or trying to demonstrate) MTB in clinical specimens. A provisional diagnosis of TB can be based on the detection of acid fast bacilli (AFB) in pulmonary and non-pulmonary specimens. More aggressive diagnostic intervention should be considered even in elderly patients, especially as they are not always able to expectorate sputum. Fiberoptic bronchoscopy with bronchial washings and bronchial or peripheral biopsy specimens is feasible, even in frail elderly patients without excessive risk of side effects. The final diagnosis of TB is based on the growth of M. tuberculosis from the specimens, usually in egg-based media (Löwenstein-Jensen) and other solid media (Middlebrook-7H10 and varieties). Fast diagnosis of TB can be achieved by new molecular techniques, especially by the technique of nucleic acid amplification as in the 'polymerase chain reaction' (PCR) or by a transcription-mediated amplification to amplify the RNA. Modern techniques using PCR can detect MTB in less than five hours, with a specificity as high as 99 % at least with a positive staining, but specificity can be uncertain when direct staining is negative even when culture later on is positive. Sensitivities are usually lower, ranging from less than 70 % in smear-negative specimens to more than 90 % in smear-positive specimens.

PCR is approved for use in both smear-positive and smear-negative patients who are suspected of having TB. Newer techniques (ligase chain reaction) with higher sensitivity and specificity rates and kits for Rif LiPA have recently become commercially available and are of additional benefit especially for identifying RMP resistance.

TREATMENT OF TUBERCULOSIS

The recommendations for the treatment of TB in the elderly are in general no different from those in the adult. With the current regimens, the cure rate in Western countries is around 80 %. Although all-cause mortality during therapy can be as high as 21 %, underlying illness and immuno suppression, but not age, are shown to be important predictors of death during treatment. The major challenge for elderly patients is to select a highly effective therapeutic regimen without major adverse reactions. Nevertheless, the guidelines have been adapted recently, due to concern about the emergence of multi-drug resistant TB (MDRTB) and the complex interaction of TB and the HIV-epidemic. The vast majority of TB cases in the elderly in Western countries are probably caused by sensitive strains of MTB. In the elderly, TB mostly is a problem of reactivated TB with an organism that was acquired at the beginning of the 20th century, prior to the availability of effective anti-tuberculous chemotherapy. Exceptions are older patients who were born in a country with a high prevalence of MDRTB, who have not been treated adequately previously, or who have been infected recently by contact with MDRTB.

Principles of anti-tuberculous chemotherapy

Anti-tuberculous chemotherapy is designed to kill as rapidly and as much as possible tubercle bacilli, to minimize the potential for the organisms to develop resistance to the medication and to sterlize the host's tissues. This results in the three principal goals of adequate treatment: (a) to prevent treatment failure thereby rapidly decreasing infectiousness ('one man's cure is several men's prevention'), (b) to prevent resistance and (c) to prevent relapse. In general, accomplishing those goals requires the prescription of multiple potent anti-tuberculous drugs taken for a sufficiently long period, which can be translated into three rules.

The first rule is to start with potent bactericidal drugs. In this regard, isoniazid (INH) is followed by rifampicin (RMP), streptomycin (SM) and ethambutol (EMB), whilest pyrazinamide (PZ) shows only very weak bactericidal activity. Those drugs with potent early bactericidal activity also reduce the risk of developing resistance within this bacillary population. There is a natural risk of random mutations, with a frequency of about 10^6 for INH and SM, 10^8 for RMP and 10^5 for EMB. Fortunately, the mechanisms of resistance are independent for drugs when given in combination and for that reason, the likelihood of spontaneous resistance to two or more drugs occurring is the product of the probabilities for resistance to each individual agent. So, the cumulative risk for resistance to both INH and RMP is estimated to be 10^{14}. This results in the second rule that at least two initial drugs should be administered in sensitive organisms and more if resistance is suspected. Because the risk of developing monotherapy, a single drug should never be added to an existing regimen. Since the bactericidal activity of PZ is low, PZ should not be used solely with another drug.

With the above-mentioned strategy, the rapidly growing population of bacilli is eliminated quickly, resulting in the clearing of live bacilli from sputum within two months in 80 % of patients. The remaining group of slow multiplying bacilli or intermittently dividing bacilli can be responsible for relapse, if the duration of therapy is inadequate. Therefore sterilizing drugs are needed and the most active drug in this matter is RMP, followed by PZ and in a lesser degree INH and SM. In contrast with PZ, RMP shows sterilizing activity throughout the whole course of therapy. In regimens with RMP, PZ shows additional sterilizing activity only in the first two months of therapy. A large number of investigations have been performed with various numbers of drugs and for various durations, but it is agreed that regimens of less than six months in duration have unacceptable high rates of relapse in patients with smear-positive pulmonary tuberculosis. This results in the third rule for achieving adequate anti-tuberculous treatment, i.e. the administration of drugs for a sufficiently long duration.

Anti-tuberculous drugs

Prescribers have at their disposal five potent first-line tuberculostatics with limited toxicity, of which four have a bactericidal action: INH, RMP, PZ and SM and one with bacteriostatic activity: EMB (Table 20.1). A number of second-line tuberculostatics are less potent and exhibit major toxicity, such as ethionamid, clofazimin, para-aminosalicylic acid, cycloserin and thiacetazon. A number of 'new' products also show activity against MTB: fluoroquinolones (FQ), macrolides, derivatives of RMP such as rifabutin and rifapentin. All of these tuberculostatics have their own properties of absorption, distribution, metabolism, excretion, interaction pattern with other medication, pharmacokinetics, pharmacodynamics and toxicity (Table 20.2). It is not yet fully clear how each tuberculostatic establishes its activity, but at least RMP, AG, FQ and probably also INH and PZ act in a concentration-dependent way. For those drugs, the highest possible dosage is favoured in order to maximize drug

Table 20.1. First-line anti-tuberculous medication and recommended dosage

	Administration 7 days/week	Administration 3 days/week
Isoniazid (INH)	5 mg/kg (300 mg)	15 mg/kg (900 mg)
Rifampicin (RMP)	10 mg/kg (600 mg)	10 mg/kg (600 mg)
Pyrazinamid (PZ)	18.2–26.3 mg/kg* (2 g)	27.3–39.5 mg/kg* (2g)
	2 g for adults $\geq$50 kg#	2.5 g for adults $\geq$50 kg#
Ethambutol (EMB)	14.5–21.1 mg/kg* (1.6 g)	21.8–31.6 mg/kg* (2.4 g)
	15 mg/kg#	30 mg/kg#
Streptomycin (SM)	10 mg/kg° (750 mg)	10 mg/kg° (750 mg)

Figures between brackets indicate maximal dosis
*AmericanThoracic Society guidelines for adults weighing 40–90 kg
°ATS guidelines for persons more than 50 years of age
#British Thoracic Society guidelines

concentration. Since INH and EMB appear to be active against the mycobacterial cell wall, it may be appropriate to ensure that time above the minimal inhibitory concentration is maximized for these agents.

Pharmacodynamics include also the persistence of antimicrobial effect after the drug has been removed, designated as the postantibiotic effect, which has been demonstrated as against MTB for INH, RMP, SM and EMB. This postantibiotic effect is also the reason for the possibility of administering infrequently large doses of antibiotics in the treatment of TB.

INH is a very potent bactericidal agent and acts on both intracellular (macrophages) and extracellular (necrotic tissue) bacilli by inhibiting the synthesis of mycolic acid, an important part of the mycobacterial wall. INH is generally absorbed quickly from the gastro-intestinal tract and reaches its maximal concentration (C_{max}) one to two hours post dose when given on an empty stomach. Antacids, food and especially high-fat meals may delay and reduce the absorption of INH. Since INH is cleared hepatically, dose adjustment is not required in patients with renal impairment. Metabolization in liver occurs through acetylation, which is determined genetically. In fast acetylators the drug has a half-life of one hour and in slow acetylators the drug has a half-life of three hours and especially elderly slow acetylators show higher plasma concentrations. Therefore it was suggested that reduction of INH dosage in older slow acetylators of the drug could prove to be a useful measure in order to prevent side effects without negative effects on the efficacy of regimens, but there seems to be no increased hepatotoxicity in those patients when compared to rapid acetylators. INH increases the plasma concentration of a number of drugs, often used in elderly patients, by inhibiting their metabolism (Table 20.2) and in such cases, it is advisable to decrease their dosage, instead of adjusting INH. The major toxicity of INH is hepatotoxicity, due to its metabolite hydrazine.

Some patients may experience central nervous system and/or peripheral neuropathies and after two weeks of daily treatment, less frequent dose administration may be appropriate. INH interferes with the metabolism of pyridoxine, especially in diabetes mellitus, uremia, malnutrition, alcoholism and in the elderly. Pyridoxine in a dosage of 10 mg daily or 250 mg weekly can be offered to prevent neurotoxicity.

RMP is also a bactericidal agent, acting by inhibiting the RNA-polymerase, necessary for the protein synsthesis of the bacil. It has the unique ability to kill MTB in different conditions, i.e. intracellularly (together with INH but in a lesser degree) and in the persister status, i.e. during their short spurts of metabolic activity. This makes the drug of great importance for the sterilisation of the process and thus for the prevention of relapse. The absorption of RMP is the most variable among the tuberculostatics. C_{max} is reduced and the time to maximal concentration is delayed by high-fat meals, so the drug should be given on an empty stomach, then reaching a C_{max} of 8 to 24 µg/ml, two hours after ingestion of 600 mg. Only a C_{max} of less than 4 µg/ml, as can be observed in malabsorption, requires a dose increase. For

Table 20.2. Potential adverse reactions and interaction patterns of first-line tuberculostatics

Drug	Major adverse reactions	Interaction with other medications
Isoniazid	Asymptomatic increases in hepatic enzymes Hepatitis Peripheral neuropathy Central Nervous System effects	Isoniazid increases concentration of phenytoin, carbamazepine, wafarin, vitamin D, diazepam, disulfiram and phenobarbital Prednisolone decreases level of isoniazid
Rifampicin	Hepatitis Fever Trombocytopenia Flu-like syndrome	Rifampicin lowers concentration of quinidine, methadone, digitalis glycosides, cyclosporin, wafarin, oral contraceptives, disopyramide, mexiletine, metoprolol, propranolol, verapamil, diazepam, oral hypoglycaemic drugs, corticosteroids, theophylline, chloramphenicol, sulfasalazine, dapsone, phenytoin, ketoconazole, protease inhibitors, non-nucleoside reverse transcriptase inhibitors
Pyrazinamide	Gastrointestinal upset Hepatotoxicity Asymptomatic hyperuricemia Arthralgias	Probeniced increases level of pyrazinamide
Ethambutol	Diminished red-green colour discrimination Decreased visual acuity Rash	Aluminium decreases level of ethambutol
Streptomycin	Renal toxicity	
Amikacin	Cochleo-vestibular toxicity	

RMP, a dose-related toxicity is observed and doses above 900 mg and given once or twice daily were associated with higher rates of the flu-like syndrome. It is believed that this is associated with anti-rifampicin antibodies that are built up when the drug is given intermittently. This problem can be avoided by the daily administration of RMP. Less frequent but dangerous side effects of RMP are respiratory distress, hemolytic anemia, purpura with trombocytopenia and renal insufficiency. The most common side effect of RMP is hepatotoxicity, especially in the combination with INH and PZ and this seems to be more prevalent in older patients. Since RMP is predominantly is cleared by the liver, dose adjustment is not necessary in patients with renal impairment. The half-life is about two hours. RMP is a strong inducer of hepatic microsomial enzymes and leads to decreased plasma concentrations of drugs (Table 20.2). It is suggested that the dosage of those medications be adjusted instead of RMP. Because of its interaction with

inhibitors of proteases, rifabutin is preferred in cases of HIV-infection.

PZ only works in an acid environment as a bactericidal agent, yet to a lesser degree than INH. Its action is through its conversion by the enzyme pyrazinamidase of M. tuberculosis into pyrazinoic acid, thereby lowering the pH in the macrophages and killing the intracellular bacilli, which makes PZ so important in the initial phase of the treatment when combined with rifampin.

PZ is reliably absorbed from the gastro- intestinal tract and one to two hours post dose reaches a C_{max} of 20 to 40 µg/ml after a 25 mg/kg daily dose and of 40 to 60 µg/ml after a 50 mg/kg biweekly dose. Since PZ inhibits renal tubular secretion of uric acid, increased levels of uric acid are often observed, but mostly without arthritis. PZ penetrates the intact meninges and is therefore a very useful drug in the treatment of tuberculous meningitis. The concomitant administration of PZ and RMP lowers the AUC of RMP and increases its clearance, but it is not clear whether this effect therefore requires adaptation of dosage.

EMB is a bacteriostatic agent in a dose of 15 mg/kg and is bactericidal in doses of 25 mg/kg. It influences the RNA-synthesis of the tubercle bacillus and inhibits mycolic acid. Since EMB is responsable for retrobulbar neuritis with disturbances in colour vision, its bactericidal dose is only used during the first two months of treatment since a longer duration of higher doses increases the risk of ocular side effects, especially in elderly patients. EMB is well absorbed from the gut and is excreted unchanged in the urine, making the agent a useful drug for patients with liver disease, but requiring dosage modification in patients with renal insufficiency. The half-life is about four hours.

Aminoglycosides (AG), such as SM and amikacin, block the synthesis of ribosomal RNA. The drugs are bactericidal in aerobic circumstances, but their use is limited to extra-cellular multiplying mycobacteria. AG are not absorbed from the gastrointestinal tract and thus require parenteral administration. The activity of AG relies on a high C_{max}/MIC ratio and peak concentrations occur within one hour of an intramuscular administration, but the drug persists in the serum for 12 to 24 hours. AG do exhibit a post-antibiotic effect, which makes the effect of the drug persist and makes a once daily dosing of AG feasible. AG are not protein bounded or metabolized and the renal excretion therefore follows closely creatinine clearance. In persons with normal renal function, the plasma half-life is about two hours but increases steadily with reduced renal function from nine hours with creatinine clearance of 35 ml/min to 18 with creatinine clearance of 18 ml/min. AG are reabsorbed and accumulate in the renal tubules, reducing glomerular filtration and causing tubular necrosis and resulting in increase of the half-life. Nephrotoxicity is mostly reversible. AG affect the vestibular and cochlear branch of the eighth cranial nerve and this phenomenon is often irreversible. Ototoxicity is related to serum levels at the end-of-dose period, which should not exceed 10 mg/l of amikacin. Serum concentration monitoring is recommended in the elderly, a trough level be drawing 30 min before the next dose. A pre-treatment audiogram is also advisable for documenting ototoxicity. Because of their side effects, which are not significantly different between the most important agents in their class, AG are not the preferred tuberculostatics for elderly patients. When necessary, amikacin is preferred over SM since it has no cross-resistance to SM, although it offers no benefit in terms of mode of administration and side effects. The risk of nephrotoxicity and ototoxicity is increased when administering cisplatin or methotrexate.

Fluoroquinolones (FQ) are potent bactericidal agents, inhibiting the DNA-gyrase involved in supercoiling the DNA of the bacillus, resulting in impaired DNA replication and protein synthesis. The later generation FQ, such as gatifloxacin and moxifloxacin are the most potent and seem to induce the least likely resistance. Moxifloxacin exhibits an early bactericidal activity comparable to that of INH. FQ are currently approved by the WHO as second-line agents for the treatment of MDRTB, but those drugs are potential first-line agents. With more FQ experience, more serious adverse effects have become apparent: tendon rupture, especially in elderly patients with concomitant corticosteroid use, QT prolongation in the case of sparfloxacin with concomitant use of cisapride, amiodarone, sotalol and other agents known to prolong the QT interval. Photosensitivity, renal dysfunction, anaphylactoid reactions, gastrointestinal intolerance and hepatitis can occur especially when given together with PZ. Central nervous system effects such as dizziness, insomnia, headache, acute psychosis are rare but occur especially when administered together with nonsteroidal anti-inflammatory drugs, and are dose dependent and reversible. The drugs are well absorbed unless given together with antacids, are less bounded to albumin and are eliminated renally and by transintestinal secretion. The half-life varies from one hour to > 4 hours. Ciprofloxacin interacts with theophylline, resulting potentially in adverse theophylline reactions.

In the group of macrolides, claritromycin and azytromycin have shown considerable activity against M. tuberculosis, although in second line, but show activity especially against the M. avium-intracellulare complex. Claritromycin and azytromycin achieve very high intracellular concentrations (e.g. in the macrophages). These drugs cause frequently upper gastrointestinal side effects, such as nausea and vomiting. They are eliminated by hepatic metabolism and biliary excretion and may therefore interact with other drugs (e.g. astemizole and terenadine). Serum half-life varies from one hour to > 12 hours.

The use of anti-tuberculous agents in the elderly is not fundamentally different from that in younger adults, although there are some changes in the pharmacokinetics of the drugs in the elderly because of alterations in absorption, distribution, protein binding and elimination with age.

Anti-tuberculous regimens

Taking into account the above-mentioned essential rules for prevention of treatment failure, relapse and development of resistance,

the 'two-phase concept' of anti-tuberculous therapy is generally accepted, consisting of a two month 'initial' (intensive, bactericidal) phase with INH, RMP and PZ followed by a four month 'continuation' (consolidation, sterilizing) phase with INH and RMP (Table 20.3). In the bactericidal phase, the vast majority of bacilli are killed, reducing symptoms, risk of transmission and emergence of resistance) and in the sterilizing phase, the few remaining persisters are eradicated, reducing the risk of relapse. Addition of EMB or SM in the initial phase does not change the outcome if the bacilli are sensitive to INH and RMP, i.e. if there is less than 4 % of primary resistance to INH in the community, if the patient was not treated previously with anti-tuberculous medication, if the patient has not come from a country with a high prevalence of MDRB or has no known exposure to a drug resistant case. Nevertheless, from the beginning of the 1990s, the generally accepted regimen has included initially four drugs (INH, RMP, PZ and EMB), which can be adapted when the pattern of sensitivity of the strain is known. Although few trials have

Table 20.3. WHO recommendations for treatment of tuberculosis

Patients	Treatment	
	Initial phase	Continuation phase
New cases of smear-positive pulmonary tuberculosis Severe extra-pulmonary tuberculosis Severe smear-negative pulmonary tuberculosis Severe concomitant HIV disease	2(H7R7Z7E7) or 2(H7R7Z7S7) 2(H3R3Z3E3) or 2(H3R3Z3S3)	4(H7R7) or 6(H7E7) 4(H3R3)
Previously treated smear-positive pulmonary tuberculosis Relapse Treatment failure Failure after default	2(H7R7Z7E7S7)/1(H7R7Z7E7) 2(H3R3Z3E3S3)/1(H3R3Z3E3)	5(H7R7E7) 5(H3R3E3)
New cases of smear-negative pulmonary tuberculosis Less severe forms of extrapulmonary tuberculosis	2(H7R7Z7E7) 2(H3R3Z3E3)	4(H7R7) or 6(H7E7) 4(H3R3)

Figure before brackets refers to the number of months of treatment
Figures after letters refers to the number of doses per week
H = isoniazid; R = rifampicin; Z = pyrazinamide; E = ethambutol; S = streptomycin

been carried out in patients with non pulmonary tuberculosis, it is generally suggested that the six-month regimens recommended for PTB can be used in most cases of non pulmonary TB. The successful treatment of tuberculous meningitis depends on the concentration achieved in the cerebrospinal fluid and in this regard, INH and PZ penetrate well whereas RMP, EMB and SM only achieve adequate concentrations in the early stages of treatment when the meninges are inflamed. In cerebrospinal TB, a regimen of 12 months is mostly recommended, which has to be prolonged to 18 months if PZ is omitted or cannot be tolerated.Since corticosteroids can ameliorate the inflammatory manifestations in patients with severe overwhelming disease and also in some forms of extra-pulmonary TB, the adjunctive treatment with corticosteroids appears to be protective, reducing mortality in pericarditis and decreasing neurological sequelae in meningitis.

Non-adherence to the anti-tuberculous regimens is well known to be the most common cause of treatment failure, relapse and the development of drug resistance. With the current regimens, even in a compliant patient and with a susceptible organism, there is less than a 5 % risk that the patient will fail to improve during therapy or relapse after completing therapy (5 % is the accepted limit of risk by the WHO). However, about one third of the patients (up to 50 %) is not compliant with the therapy (especially in some risk groups such as homeless people and intravenous drug users), increasing the risk of relapse and the emergence of resistant germs as well as the need for longer treatment regimens and a longer duration to convert to negative culture.

One of the possible reasons for failure is drug malabsorption, even in the non-HIV infected patient. In those cases, therapeutic drug monitoring can eliminate drug malabsorption as a possible cause, but can also be effective in guiding therapy even if they exceed the so-called 'maximum' doses. Success of treatment increases with short-course regimens, in hospitalized patients or when the medication is delivered under supervision, the latter is called 'Directly Observed Therapy' (DOT). Although

there is no information on DOT in elderly patients, the DOT strategy can be of value for the community-dwelling elderly. These patients often take a lot of drugs for other health problems, with the risk of confusion between the different drugs; or they cease the intake of the tuberculostatics because of intolerance or because they feel better after a few weeks of treatment, subsequently ignoring the necessity for further treatment.

Treatment of MDRTB is generally disappointing and often requires more than five anti-tuberculous agents, with an increased risk of toxicity. In a group of patients receiving DOT, 18 % experienced non-compliance with DOT, which was closely associated with alcoholism and homelessness and also with a 10-fold increase of poor outcome from treatment. Nevertheless, MDRT can be treated successfully, but requires a great deal of effort from both patients and carers, and the costs may be higher than is affordable in resource-poor countries.

It was suggested that administration of therapy on an intermittent basis, as opposed to classical daily dosing, could facilitate the supervision of therapy and improve outcome. During in vitro studies, it was noted that exposure of tubercle bacilli to drugs was followed by a long period of post antibiotic effect, lasting as long as four days without loss of activity. A series of clinical trials showed that intermittent regimens were as effective as daily regimens without increasing toxicity, resulting in a currently accepted regimen of treating TB.

Initiation of anti-tuberculosis treatment

Patients suspected of having TB should give appropriate specimens for AFB smear (for pulmonary TB preferentially three) and culture and for susceptibility testing. Rapid amplification tests can also confirm diagnosis. Based on this information and on epidemiological information, clinical and radiographic features, the likelihood of TB can be estimated and therapy can be initiated.

Initiation of therapy should not be delayed because of negative AFB smears, especially in life-threatening situations, such as military tuberculosis. In elderly patients with clinically suspected pulmonary TB, that was smear-negative but later on culture-positive, empiric treatment with INH, RMP and EMB was shown to be effective with a cure rate of 90 % and acceptable toxicity (severe hepatotoxicity necessitating withdrawal of one or more tuberculostatics in 9.7 %). This treatment modality, however, is limited to countries with a low primary INH-resistance but the addition of EMB in stead of PZ avoids potential increased hepatotoxicity of PZ and risk of monotherapy.

It is recommended that all patients with TB to be tested for HIV infection and patients at risk for hepatitis be tested for hepatitis B and C. Measurements of liver and renal function tests, as well as platelet count is advised in every elderly patient, as well as testing for visual acuity and colour vision when EMB is used.

Follow-up during treatment

Patients who still have positive cultures after four months of treatment should be considered to be failures and should be managed accordingly. In those circumstances in which the risk of treatment failure is judged to be higher than normal, therapeutic drug monitoring could be an appropriate measure in order to ensure correct serum drug concentrations. Therapeutic monitoring, however, is not the standard of care, the more so since it was found that the risk of recurrence was not related to serum levels of tuberculosis drugs, HIV-status or even to age.

In addition to the microbiological evaluations, it is essential that patients have clinical evaluation for compliance to therapy and detection of possible adverse advents.Occurrence of any major side effect (rash, fever, hepatitis or gastro-intestinal upset, necessitating modification or discontinuation of medication) was associated with the female sex and with age over 60 years, and the drug most likely responsible for hepatitis or rash during therapy appeared to be PZ. Special attention is needed for the development of hepatotoxicity since drug-induced hepatitis can be caused by INH, RMP and PZ. It seems reasonable that in elderly patients other options should be possible:

RMP, PZ and EMB for six months, thereby avoiding INH; INH and RMP for nine months with EMB supplementation until INH and RMP susceptibility is verified, thereby avoiding PZ; RMP and EMB for 12 months with use of a FQ for the first two months in patients with severe liver disease. For example, in elderly patients with PTB treated with INH, RMP and EMB, elevated levels of liver function tests were observed in one third of the patients, whereas it was the case in only one fifth of the younger group; furthermore, there was no higher incidence of major hepatotoxicity in the elderly group. CDC define hepatitis as a serum AST level equal or greater than three times the upper limit of normal in the presence of symptoms or greater than or equal to five times the upper limit of normal in the absence of symptoms. It appears to be unnecessary to monitor liver or renal function or platelet count for patients being treated with first line drugs, unless there were abnormalities at baseline. Further investigation should be initiated promptly if abnormalities are detected when asking for complaints or detected by clinical examination. However, it is not clear whether this can be extrapolated to the elderly patients, taking into account the increased risk of hepatotoxicity especially when dealing with co-morbidities and interactions with other drugs that might act synergistically so as to produce an increased likelihood of drug-induced hepatitis. If drug-induced hepatitis is diagnosed, the following could be done: (1) discontinue INH, RMP and PZ; (2) discontinue any other medication that may cause hepatic injury; (3) question the patient about the use of other hepatotoxic agents and alcohol intake; (4) rule out hepatitis A, B and C or other aetiology of hepatitis; (5) wait until liver function has normalized; (6) reintroduce INH at 50 mg and daily increase with 50 to 100 mg up to 300 mg daily; (7) restart RMP at 50 mg with daily increase of 50 mg up to 150 mg and then with an increase of 150 mg every two days up to 600 mg; and (8) eliminate the offending hepatotoxic agent if found. It is also possible to start treatment with two new anti-tuberculosis medications with no major hepatotoxic properties, such as EMB, amikacin or a FQ.

TREATMENT OF LATENT TUBERCULOSIS INFECTION

In addition to the detection and treatment of active TB, screening and treatment of groups with 'latent tuberculosis infection' (LTBI) is needed. In most people infection with M. tuberculosis is contained by host defences, especially cytokines, leaving the infection latent but with the potential to develop into active TB at any time after the immune system being altered. This particular ability of MTB to infect a patient and to remain latent for many years before reactivation is indeed the key obstacle to the control and elimination of tuberculosis, since patients with reactivation of remote infection become sources of new infections. It is obviously clear and evident that elderly subjects represent a very important group when considering treatment of LTBI. Elderly patients belong to almost all of the above-mentioned risk groups for different reasons, the most important being the depressed immunological status due to concomitant diseases or medication and the fact they are the largest reservoir since they were infected at the beginning of the 20th century, and are thus prone to reactivation TB. A recent example is the use of TNF-α blockers in the treatment of rheumatoid arthritis. Since TNF-α provides protection against reactivation by containment of M. tuberculosis in the formation of granulomas, it is suggested that patients, intended to be treated with TNF-α blockers, should have a TST and be treated for LTBI if appropriate. The tuberculin skin test can be used for identification of those infected persons and criteria for cut-off will depend on the epidemiological features in the different population group being tested, influenced by the likelihood of being infected with M. tuberculosis and the risk of developing the active disease when infected.

For treatment of LTBI, most generally, a daily dosage of 300 mg of INH is recommended for six or preferably nine months and in HIV-infected persons 12 months is mostly advised, although in the latter group the optimal duration is not clear yet. However, other strategies of single agents or in combination and of different duration are currently available (Table 20.4). RMP (600 mg per day) alone for six months or in combination with EMB for three or four months can be offered to subjects with INH intolerance or to contacts of an INH-resistant strain.

In cases of recent infection with MDRTB and no active disease, treatment should include at least two and preferably three drugs chosen on the knowledge of the drug susceptibility pattern of the index case. If the drug susceptibility pattern is not known then the administration of ofloxacin or ciprofloxacin with PZ has been suggested or the combination of EMB and PZ, although increased hepatoxicity can be expected.

When residing in a nursing home, elderly subjects become infected more easily than the younger staff-members from a (mostly undisclosed) infectious case of TB. It was shown that using INH in elderly subjects with a TST conversion, a protective rate of 98.4 % was calculated in preventing the development of clinical TB, without increased risk for hepatitis (4.4 %) resulting in a ratio of benefit of 1.6 for women and 3.4 for men. The former recommendation of treating LTBI only in persons under the age of 35 years was thus abandoned because the benefits of treatment outweighed risk of adverse events and there is no age limit

Table 20.4. Recommended regimens for the treatment of latent tuberculosis infection

Drugs	Duration of treatment in months	Dose	
		Daily	Twice weekly
Isoniazid	6–9	5 mg/kg (300 mg)	15 mg/kg (900 mg)
Rifampicin and pyrazinamide	3	10 mg/kg (600 mg) and 5 mg/kg (300 mg)	10 mg/kg (600 mg) and 15 mg/kg (900 mg)
Rifampicin	4	10 mg/kg (600 mg)	

for initiation of treatment of LTBI. Nevertheless, there still appears to be reluctance to use INH in the treatment of LTBI due probably to many of non-rational reasons such as private preferences, asymptomatic liver enzyme level elevation and the fear of INH-induced hepatitis, thus leading to under utilization of therapy especially in older persons. In general, known active hepatitis and end-stage liver disease are relative but not absolute contraindications of treatment of LTBI with INH or PZ. Clinical monitoring for unexplained anorexia, nausea, vomiting, icterus, rash, fatigue, weakness, fever, abdominal tenderness or darkened urine should be employed in all patients. It is not generally accepted that routine baseline laboratory measurement of serum alanine aminotransferase or aspartate aminotransferase or bilirubin should be performed for all patients. However, in HIV-infected persons and in persons with hepatitis B and C, alcoholic hepatitis and liver cirrhosis, baseline laboratory investigation followed by monthly monitoring is advised. Furthermore, all those patients should be educated in recognizing these non-specific symptoms and in seeking counsel from the treating physician.

KEY POINTS

- As TB is receding in Western countries amongst the indigenous population, this may lead to a decrease in vigilance and expertise with regard to the problem of TB in the elderly.
- Diagnosis is often difficult because of the non-specificity of the complaints, clinical findings and radiological patterns and therefore attempts should be made to obtain as soon as possible a diagnosis in order to avoid postponement of therapy.
- Treatment does not essentially differ from that in the younger age groups.
- The outcome of treatment can be compromised because of the frailty of the elderly

patient, the presence of concomitant diseases and concurrent medication.
- Ask on a monthly basis for complaints suggestive of drug toxicity, provide further investigation if necessary and adjust medication.

REFERENCES

1. American Thoracic Society. Diagnostic standards and classification of tuberculosis in adults and children. *Am J Respir Crit Care Med* 2000; **161**: 1376–95.
2. American Thoracic Society/Centers for Disease Control and Prevention/Infectious Diseases Society of America: treatment of tuberculosis. *Am J Respir Crit Care Med* 2003; **167**: 603–62.
3. American Thoracic Society. Targeted tuberculin testing and treatment of latent tuberculosis infection. *Am J Respir Crit Care Med* 2000; **161**: S221–S247.
4. Blumberg HM, Leonard MK, Jasmer RM. Update on the treatment of tuberculosis and latent tuberculosis infection. *JAMA* 2005; **293**: 2776–84.
5. Douglas JG, McLeod M-J. Pharmacokinetic factors in the modern drug treatment of tuberculosis. *Clin Pharmacokinet* 1999; **37**: 127–46.
6. Frieden TR, Sterling TR, Munsiff SS, Watt CJ, Dye C. Tuberculosis. *Lancet* 2003; **362**: 887–99.
7. Horsburgh CR Jr, Feldman S, Ridzon R. Practice guidelines for the treatment of tuberculosis. *Clin Infect Dis* 2000; **31**: 633–9.
8. Iseman MD. *A Clinician's Guide to Tuberculosis*. Lippincott Williams and Wilkins, Philadelphia, 2000.
9. Joint Tuberculosis Committee of the British Thoracic Society. Chemotherapy and management of tuberculosis in the United Kingdom: recommendations 1998. *Thorax* 1998; **53**: 536–48.
10. Joint Tuberculosis Committee of the British Thoracic Society. Control and prevention of tuberculosis in the United Kingdom: code of practice 2000. *Thorax* 2000; **55**: 887–901.
11. Migliori GB, Raviglione MC, Schaberg T, Davies PD, Zellweger JP, Grzemska M, Mihaescu T, Clancy L, Casali L. Tuberculosis

management in Europe. Task Force of the European Respiratory Society (ERS), the World Health Organisation (WHO) and the International Union against Tuberculosis and Lung Disease (IUATLD) Europe Region. *Eur Respir J* 1999; **14**: 978–92.

12. Van den Brande P. Revised guidelines for the diagnosis and control of tuberculosis. Impact on management in the elderly. *Drugs Aging* 2005; **22**: 663–86.

13. Zevallos M, Justman JE. Tuberculosis in the elderly. *Clin Geriatr Med* 2003; **19**: 121–38.

21 Interstitial lung disease in the elderly

Jeffrey Bowden

Department of Medicine, Flinders Medical Centre, Adelaide, Australia

INTRODUCTION

The treatment of interstitial lung disease (ILD) is complex, due to the difficulty in achieving a specific diagnosis, the limited efficacy of many treatments, and the difficulty in assessing response. Moreover there is a large array of causes, many with confusing nomenclature and these disorders are uncommon, difficult to diagnose in their early stages and response to treatment in many cases is poor (1, 2). Of particular concern is the potential toxicity of many treatments in the elderly.

Given the paucity of well designed clinical trials of treatment of ILD and lack of consensus on treatment, decisions with regard therapy are difficult (3). Moreover, some 60 % or more of patients with established fibrosis will not gain benefit form corticosteroid or cytotoxic treatment. In the elderly, lung transplantation is not an option for treatment of pulmonary fibrosis with refractory respiratory failure. Nonetheless, it would appear that selected patients may receive substantive benefit from therapy and a large number of patients may benefit from supportive therapies.

Critical to management of interstitial lung disease is knowledge of the classification of these disorders, given the substantive variations in prognosis and response to treatment between groups. It is important to recognize that the histological appearance of interstitial lung disease represents common patterns of injury in the lung and multiple etiologies may have similar histological appearances.

In this chapter a brief outline of presentation and assessment of ILD will be provided, followed by a summary of drugs used in ILD and options for treatment of the more common forms of ILD.

PRESENTATION OF INTERSTITIAL LUNG DISEASE

Interstitial lung disease tends to present with insidious onset of breathlessness with progressive reduction in exercise tolerance. Cough is also a common feature of presentation. In view of the gradual onset of breathlessness, patients will present often at a late stage of disease with significant fibrosis already established. The breathlessness is due to a number of factors including reduced compliance of the lungs (increased stiffness), which results in increased work of breathing, and impaired gas exchange, particularly with exercise when red blood cell transit times through the pulmonary circulation are reduced (see Table 21.1).

The history at presentation is particularly important in identifying inhaled agents that may contribute to ILD such as mineral dusts (e.g. asbestos and silica) organic materials (e.g. in farmer's lung) and drugs which may also contribute to its development (4). It is also important to identify connective tissue disorders including

Prescribing for Elderly Patients   Edited by Stephen Jackson, Paul Jansen and Arduino Mangoni
© 2009 John Wiley & Sons, Ltd

Table 21.1. Aetiology of interstitial lung disease

Common Causes
- Environmental
  - –Organic, inhaled allergens: eg farmers lung
  - –Inorganic: eg asbestos, silica (coal)
- Drugs
  - –Amiodarone
  - –Nitrofurantoin
  - –Cytotoxic agents, including methotrexate and bleomycin
  - –Others (see Camus et al., 4)
- Autoimmune
  - –Usual interstitial pneumonitis
  - –Non-specific interstitial pneumonitis
  - –Sarcoidosis
  - –Secondary to connective tissue disorders (eg rheumatoid arthritis, scleroderma, Sjogren's syndrome, systemic lupus erythematosus)

Uncommon Causes
- Tobacco associated
  - –Respiratory Bronchiolitis/Interstitial Lung Disease
  - –Desquamative Interstitial Pneumonitis
- Malignancy
  - –Lymphangitis carcinomatosis
  - –Bronchoalveolar cell carcinoma
- Pulmonary Haemorrhage
- Infection
  - –Viral pneumonitis
  - –Miliary Tuberculosis
- ARDS (Adult Respiratory Distress Syndrome)
  - –Diffuse alveolar damage

rheumatoid arthritis, systemic lupus erythematosus and scleroderma which may be associated with ILD. Occasionally the onset of interstitial lung disease may predate systemic manifestations of these disorders (see Table 21.2) (5).

A variety of classifications of interstitial lung disease have been proposed (1). Interstitial lung disease itself is a general term which identifies diseases affecting predominantly the lung parenchyma and helps to distinguish these forms of disease from those affecting which predominantly affect airways, e.g. asthma and COPD. In the early stages of interstitial lung disease inflammatory changes affecting alveoli and bronchi are prominent, whereas in later stages fibrosis and thickening of alveoli may be prominent. These disorders may also be referred to in histopathological terms as interstitial pneumonitis with acute interstitial pneumonitis representing an idiopathic form of "diffuse alveolar damage" which is the pathological equivalent of

"adult respiratory distress syndrome". Various forms of chronic interstitial pneumonitis (also known as cryptogenic fibrosing alveolitis and idiopathic pulmonary fibrosis) have been divided into usual interstitial pneumonitis (UIP) and non-specific interstitial pneumonia (1, 6).

Whereas NSIP may have significant fibrosis, it is usually uniform, and fibroblastic foci and honeycombing, if present, are rare. The temporal uniformity is different from the pattern seen in UIP. Nonetheless, end-stage or fibrotic NSIP can be difficult to distinguish radiologically or pathologically from UIP. Even amongst expert histopathologists, there is significant inter-observer variability. Unlike patients with UIP, most patients with nonspecific or non-classifiable interstitial pneumonia have a good prognosis with a five-year mortality rate estimated at 10 to 15 %. Moreover, NSIP will frequently show improvement with corticosteroid treatment. In contrast, UIP is defined

Table 21.2. Assessment of ILD

Assessment	Feature	Comment
History	Respiratory Symptoms	Progressive exertional breathlessness & dry cough
	Occupational	
	Medication	Exclude connective tissue disease
	Environment	
Examination	Tachypnea	
	Reduced chest expansion	
	Bibasilar end-inspiratory dry crackles	
	Clubbing	Common in idiopathic fibrosis, rare in sarcoid
	Pulmonary hypertension & cor pulmonale	May be seen in advanced ILD
	Primary feature of scleroderma/CREST	
Imaging	Chest X-ray	May underestimate severity of ILD
	High resolution CT	Critical to evaluation
	Tc-DTPA clearance lung scan	Limited use
Pulmonary Function Testing	Spirometry	Spirometry does not correlate well with histopathology in ILD
	Lung Volumes	
	Resting & exercise gas exchange, including 6 minute walk test	Same measures monitor disease & treatment response
		Resting & exercise gas exchange establish degree of physiologic impairment
		Cardiopulmonary exercise testing may identify early physiological change
Serology	Fungal and avian precipitins	
	Rheumatoid Factor	
	ENA	
	ANA	
	ACE	
Biopsy	Transbronchial	Limited value
	Video Assisted Thoracoscopy	May be required if clinical features and HRCT are non-diagnostic
	Open Lung Biopsy	

by heterogenous fibrosis with fibroblastic foci and honeycombing, has a poor prognosis and is relatively refractory to corticosteroid therapy.

High resolution CT (HRCT) scanning has contributed significantly to the evaluation of patients with interstitial lung disease (8). The characteristic radiographic features of the idiopathic interstitial pneumonias on HRCT scans are well described and are summarized briefly in Table 21.3. It is often possible to achieve a diagnosis by combining clinical history and examination, serological assessment, and HRCT findings without resorting to lung biopsy. Nonetheless if features of the history are atypical or HRCT findings are non-diagnostic or incongruent with other findings, then biopsy may be required.

PARTICULAR PROBLEMS IN THE ELDERLY

Interstitial lung disease is more prevalent in the elderly with over two thirds of patients with idiopathic pulmonary fibrosis over the age of 60 (1). Diagnosis is potentially more difficult, as patients may incorrectly attribute symptoms of dyspnoea due to aging. Clinicians may also be reluctant to undertake lung biopsy in the elderly. Treatment is also limited in that lung transplantation is not an option in most patients over 60 and certainly in all patients over 65. Moreover there are well justified concerns that treatment may have an increased risk of side effects, with significant toxicity in the elderly.

Table 21.3. Forms of interstitial lung disease

Disease	Pathological features	Radiological features	Distribution	Prognosis
Acute interstitial pneumonia	Early stage; hyaline membranes, interstitial oedema Late stage; inflammatory infiltrate, uniform changes	Ground glass attenuation +/− patchy consolidation		Variable, depending on severity
Usual interstitial pneumonia	Fibroblastic foci Temporal and topographic heterogeneity of fibrosis Relatively little inflammatory infiltrate	Fibrotic change, honey-combing traction bronchiectasis	Basal and sub-pleural predilection	Poor
Non-specific interstitial pneumonia	Uniform disease Interstitial inflammatory infiltrate or fibrotic change Absence of hyaline membranes and honey-combing	Ground-glass attenuation, usually symmetrical and bilateral Absence of honey-combing		Generally good, but depends also on associated systemic illness
Lymphocytic interstitial pneumonia	Diffuse or patchy lymphocytic interstitial infiltrate	Ground glass opacity Nodules		Depends on associated systemic illness and possible development of lymphoma
Desquamative interstitial pneumonia	Confluent sheets of macrophages in alveoli	Ground glass opacity, with fibrotic change in 50% of cases	Lower lobe predominance	Good with smoking cessation
Hypersensitivity pneumonitis	Lymphocytic infiltrate Poorly formed granuloma	Ground glass attenuation or profuse micro-nodules	Upper lobe predominance	Good with avoidance of antigen
Sarcoidosis	Epithelioid non-caseating granuloma Patchy fibrotic change Variable lymphocytic infiltrate	Nodular, reticular and ground glass opacities, +/− lymph node enlargement	Predilection for broncho-vascular and lymphatic channels Sub-pleural nodules	Generally good
Bronchiolitis obliterans organising pneumonia	Pulmonary architecture maintained Intra-alveolar and bronchiolar plugs of proliferative fibrous tissue No micro-organisms	Subpleural or peri-bronchovascular consolidation Patchy ground glass attenuation		Good with steroid treatment

GENERAL COMMENTS WITH REGARD TO THERAPY

Treatment of ILD is broadly based on the use of immunosuppressive drugs and to a lesser extent antifibrotic agents (2). The treatment is in many cases unsatisfactory and a key aspect of therapy is the ability to recognize when therapy is ineffective and the need to avoid the extended use of potentially toxic agents.

ASSESSING THE RESPONSE TO THERAPY

A favorable response to glucocorticoid therapy is defined by a decrease in symptoms, (especially dyspnoea, cough, hemoptysis, chest pain, or fatigue), a reduction or clearing of radiological abnormalities and physiological improvement.

Significant physiologic improvement is identified by; a 10 to 15 % or greater increase in FVC or TLC, a 20 % or greater increase in DLCO, or an improvement in gas exchange (a 4 mmHg or greater increase in the arterial PO2 or a decline of 4 mmHg or more in the alveolar-arterial oxygen gradient at rest or during exercise).

Stable lung function or exercise capacity over three to six months may also be considered a positive response to therapy. Nonetheless, subjective improvement can occur without objective change and therefore should not be the sole factor in determining whether to continue treatment. Failure to respond to therapy (or a relapse) is often defined as; a fall of 10 % or more in FVC or TLC, worsening of radiographic opacities, particularly with development of cavities, honeycombing, or signs of pulmonary hypertension, or decline in arterial blood gases.

DRUGS USED IN ILD

Corticosteroids

Many forms of lung disease are treated with corticosteroids. Previous recommendations with regard the use of corticosteroids have recommended high doses (up to 1 mg/kg of prednisone or prednisolone) to avoid failing to identify a steroid responsive condition. Nonetheless the optimal dose of steroids remains to be determined and chronic treatment with high doses is likely to produce serious side effects in the elderly. Such effects include osteoporosis, myopathy, and steroid induced diabetes mellitus. Although it remains difficult to predict whether specific side effects will occur in a given patient, in general, complications of therapy are more likely to occur with longer durations of treatment and with higher doses of corticosteroids. Moreover, patients with latent tuberculosis have a risk of reactivation with chronic corticosteroid therapy. In patients from areas of moderate risk of tuberculosis, treated with chronic moderate dose of steroid treatment, consideration should be given to screening for tuberculosis with skin testing and to giving isoniazid prophylaxis.

Cytotoxic and Antifibrotic Agents—several cytotoxic drugs have been used in treating interstitial lung disease including azathioprine, cyclophosphamide and methotrexate. These drugs have been used both as single treatment, and in those who have failed to respond to steroids or who require high doses of steroids, in combination with steroids as steroid sparing agents.

Azathioprine

Mechanism of action—Azathioprine, a purine analog, is converted to mercaptopurine, which inhibits synthesis of RNA and DNA, suppressing both cellular and humoral immunity.

Adverse effects—Azathioprine commonly causes fatigue and gastrointestinal symptoms, including nausea, vomiting, and diarrhea. Severe hepatitis is rare although abnormal liver function tests are not uncommon. As with any cytotoxic agent anemia and neutropenia may occur. There is an increased risk of malignancy associated with prolonged use in renal transplant recipients. Azathioprine unlike cyclophosphamide does not cause bladder injury.

Cyclophosphamide—Cyclophosphamide is an alkylating agent which is metabolized to active metabolites which cross-link DNA strands and impair cell replication, particularly in lymphocytes. It is most often used as a second-line drug in patients whose condition is deteriorating despite corticosteroid and aza-thioprine therapy.

Adverse effects—Reductions in all blood cell lines may be seen and require dose adjustment. The WBC count should be monitored monthly and cyclophosphamide dose adjusted to maintain WBC counts between $4-7 \times 10^9$/L. As with most immunosuppressive therapies, patients on cyclophosphamide are at increased risk of infection. Other toxicities include hemorrhagic cystitis, fatigue, stomatitis, nausea, diarrhea, hepatotoxicity (rarely), and carcinoma of the bladder, particularly with prolonged use. Cystitis may in part be avoided by encouraging high fluid intake: i.e. >2 litres/water per day.

Methotrexate

Methotrexate (MTX), an antimetabolite with both immunosuppressive and anti-inflammatory properties, is an analog of folic acid that inhibits the enzyme dihydrofolate reductase. Its immunosuppressive properties can probably be attributed to inhibition of replication and function of T and possibly B lymphocytes.

Adverse effects—A major side effects of methotrexate is hepatic fibrosis (the risk being dose dependent, occurring in up to 10 % of cases with total dose >5 gms). Uncommonly interstitial pneumonitis may occur, often with insidious onset. Liver function tests and WBC count should be monitored monthly to assess for toxicity in patients of methotrexate. After 24 months or one gm of therapy, liver biopsy should be considered. Other toxicities include bone marrow suppression, nausea, alopecia, and skin rash.

TREATMENT FOR SPECIFIC FORMS OF LUNG DISEASE

Idiopathic pulmonary fibrosis (usual interstitial pneumonitis)

Current treatments for IPF are based on expert opinion and on clinical trials showing limited efficacy. The most recent Cochrane reviews suggest that for patients with IPF/UIP there is no evidence that either corticosteroid or non-corticosteroid therapy plays a role in modifying the course of the disease (9, 10). However, there is little good quality information regarding the efficacy of agents in IPF(UIP) (3). In the absence of definitive clinical trials there are a variety of opinions with regard the optimal treatment of UIP (11) with some clinicians suggesting that no treatment is appropriate and others suggesting that azathioprine and low-dose corticosteroids have become a "standard of care" for IPF. In general, if a trial of immunosuppressive therapy is used, the patient must be carefully monitored for side effects and at least three to six months allowed to assess response to therapy.

Treatment with corticosteroids alone is currently not favoured in the treatment of UIP, particularly as a substantial percentage of patients will not respond to corticosteroid therapy and there is no demonstrated survival advantage for patients treated with corticosteroids alone (2, 12).

Chronic progressive disease—when used in conjunction with azathioprine the typical starting dose of prednisolone is 0.5 mg/kg per day given as a single daily oral dose, ideal body weight. This dose is continued for approximately 8 weeks, at which time the patient is reevaluated. If the patient's condition is felt to be stable or improved, the dose is tapered to 0.4 mg/kg per day and then 0.3 mg/kg per day one month later. If the patient continues to remain stable or improved, the dose is progressively reduced over months four through six to 10 mg per day. This dose is maintained for as long as the treatment appears indicated (13).

Acute or rapidly progressive disease–Pulse therapy with methylprednisolone 1 gm/day for 5 days may rarely be of benefit (14).

Intermittent pulse therapy—Intermittent pulse therapy has also been used, especially in patients with severe and aggressive disease (14) This regimen consists of the administration of intravenous methylprednisolone 2 g once a week) plus oral prednisone (0.25 mg/kg per day); however, this approach has not clearly been shown to improve the lung disease.

Azathioprine—Azathioprine and low-dose corticosteroids have become a "standard of care" for IPF (13).

Dosage and administration—A dose of up to 2 to 3 mg/kg per day given orally as a single dose. Dosing should begin at 25 to 50 mg/day and increase gradually, by 25 mg increments, every seven to 14 days, monitoring white blood cell counts (WBC, to ensure that neutropenia does not develop) until the maximum tolerated dose is reached (not exceeding 150 mg/day).

Cyclophosphamide, in combination with corticosteroids has shown marginal benefit.

Dosage and administration—Oral cyclophosphamide is usually administered at 2 mg/kg per day in one dose. The starting dose is 25 to 50 mg/day; and the dose is increased by 25 mg increments every seven to 14 days, aiming to reduce and maintain the WBC count between 4000 and 7000/µL. WBC count should be measured twice weekly for the first six to 12 weeks and then at least monthly thereafter. A maximum dose no higher than 150 mg/day is recommended, even if the WBC count remains above 7000/µL.

Intravenous therapy—in patients with rapidly progressive disease, intravenous cyclophosphamide therapy has been used, 2 mg/kg ideal body weight over 30 to 60 minutes, once daily for three to five days. Following this treatment, oral daily therapy is initiated as detailed above.

Methotrexate published experience with methotrexate for the treatment of interstitial lung disease is very limited. Case reports have described patients with IPF associated with connective tissue disease who have responded favorably to methotrexate.

Methotrexate may be administered orally or intramuscularly. Initial dosing is 7.5 mg once weekly, increasing by 2.5 mg per week at two to four weekly intervals to a maximum dose of 15 mg per week.

In a patient with IPF treated with methotrexate, it may be difficult to distinguish pulmonary drug toxicity from progression of the underlying disease and detailed assessment may be required. Other toxicities include bone marrow suppression, nausea, alopecia, and skin rash.

Other agents

Acetylcysteine—Acetylcysteine may delay progression of pulmonary impairment when used in conjunction with immunosuppressive therapy. It is generally well tolerated although may cause nausea and vomiting and, rarely, rash and fever. Acetylcysteine is a precursor of glutathione, an antioxidant, and potentially restores depleted glutathione levels in the lung.

Dosage and administration—The dose of acetylcysteine for the treatment of IPF is 600 mg administered as effervescent tablets orally three times per day (1800 mg/day).

Sarcoidosis

Sarcoidosis is a multisystem granulomatous disorder of unknown aetiology manifested by non-caseating infiltration. The granulomas may occur in any organ, with the most commonly affected sites being the lungs, lymph nodes, skin, eyes, and liver. Although affected patients may present with a wide variety of signs and symptoms, the patient with pulmonary sarcoidosis most commonly presents without symptoms but with an abnormal chest roentgenogram obtained for an unrelated purpose. When symptomatic, the patient most commonly presents with dyspnoea with or without exertion, nonproductive cough, or nonspecific chest pain. Spontaneous resolution of the disease is common, but progressive and disabling organ failure can occur in up to 10 % of patients.

The current therapy of sarcoidosis is aimed at suppressing the inflammatory response, reducing the burden of granulomas, and preventing the development of fibrosis. Because of their ability to attenuate the inflammatory response, glucocorticoids are thought to be capable of halting or slowing the progression of the pulmonary parenchymal fibrosis that can develop in sarcoidosis. As a result, glucocorticoids have been the most commonly used agents for the treatment of pulmonary sarcoidosis. Based on the current evidence, their use in this setting is justified for relief of symptoms and for control of disabling systemic involvement. In many cases treatment may not be required if symptoms are mild or remitting. Indications for treatment include progressive pulmonary impairment, hypercalcaemia, severe disfiguring skin disease, cardiac or occular disease.

Protocol for use of glucorticoids—The optimal dose of glucocorticoids is not known, so that choosing a dose requires balancing the risk of adverse effects with the likelihood of response. Theoretically, one wishes to choose the lowest dose necessary to obtain optimal benefit in those patients who have the potential for glucocorticoid responsiveness.

Therapy is initiated with moderate to high doses of oral prednisolone. This is followed by a gradual reduction to the lowest effective dose, aiming for a total duration of therapy between six and 12 months (12). The usual starting dose is 0.5–0.7 mg per kg of ideal body weight (usually 30 to 60 mg). After four to six weeks, if improvement is observed the dose should be reduced (by 5 to 10 mg every four to eight weeks) down to 0.25 to 0.5 mg/kg (usually 15 to 30 mg/day).

If the condition improves or stabilizes, the dose may be further reduced until a maintenance dose is reached (approximately 0.25 mg/kg of ideal body weight or less per day, usually 10 to 15 mg daily and continued for at least six to eight months, in view of risk of relapse, (occurring in about 60 % of patients). A short course of an increased dose may be required for relapse (increases of 10 to 20 mg above the maintenance dose given for two to four weeks). For patients who are stable on low dose corticosteroids over 6 months medications can be ceased, i.e. total duration of therapy is six to 12 months. Few patients may require lifelong low dose therapy (0.25 mg/kg alternate days). If there is no relapse after 12 months further relapse is rare.

Inhaled glucocorticoids may be of limited benefit in patients with sarcoidosis although have relatively little effect in improving lung function. Treatment may be appropriate in cases of coexistent asthma, which may coexist in up to 30 % of cases of symptomatic sarcoidosis. In those patients with sarcoidosis with only pulmonary disease and requiring long term low dose steroids, inhaled corticosteroids may be of benefit and a trial of medication could be considered. Budesonide (800 mcg twice daily) would be recommended.

Methotrexate—Whereas experience with MTX for sarcoidosis is limited, several case reports and small series suggest that it can be effective in patients with pulmonary and extrapulmonary disease. The proportion of patients who might benefit from MTX is probably in the range of 40 to 60 %.

Dosage and administration—orally or intramuscularly. Initially 7.5 mg oral weekly, increasing by increments of 2.5 mg every two weeks, until a dose of 10 to 15 mg per week is achieved. A trial of methotrexate therapy should last at least four to six months to allow adequate assessment of effectiveness.

Liver function tests and the white blood cell count should be monitored monthly to assess for toxicity. Liver biopsy should be considered after 18 months of treatment.

Cyclophosphamide—cyclophosphamide has been used rarely as a glucocorticoid-sparing agent in the treatment of sarcoidosis. It is most often given as a "second-line" drug in patients whose condition is deteriorating despite glucocorticoid therapy.

Dosage and administration—Dose is as used for treatment of UIP.

Azathioprine—Azathioprine is another agent that has been used as second line therapy for sarcoidosis]. It has been suggested that azathioprine is best used as a steroid-sparing agent rather than as a single drug for treatment of pulmonary sarcoidosis.

Dosage and administration—Dose is as used for treatment of UIP.

Bronchiolitis obliterans organizing pneumonia

BOOP may occur following intercurrent infection or may be associated with auto-immune disorders. This disorder is highly responsive to steroids and in the majority of cases a limited course only is required. Nonetheless, in a small number of cases chronic corticosteroid therapy may be required, particularly after relapse or in association with connective tissue disorders (12).

Non-specific interstitial pneumonia

Most patients with nonspecific or nonclassifiable interstitial pneumonia have a good prognosis and show improvement after treatment with corticosteroids although those with severe disease, a poor response to treatment or side effects from corticosteroids may also require treatment with cytotoxic therapy to minimize corticosteroid dosing (12). Initial treatment protocols should be as described above for sarcoidosis.

Lymphocytic interstitial pneumonitis

LIP most likely represents a spectrum of disorders including autoimmune processes (given its association with diseases such as pernicious anemia, rheumatoid arthritis, systemic lupus erythematosus, Sjögren's syndrome, chronic active hepatitis, and biliary cirrhosis) and neoplastic disorders (16). When associated with a dysproteinemia or autoimmune process, LIP may predate the establishment of lymphoma.

Corticosteroid therapy alone or in combination with other agents has been used to treat symptomatic patients with LIP, although its efficacy has not been established in a controlled trial. However, some patients have responded to this treatment, while others may spontaneously remit. The initial corticosteroid dose regime is as outlined for sarcoidosis.

Desquamative interstitial pneumonitis

Represents an uncommon form of interstitial lung disease typically associated with tobacco smoking and possessing a more benign prognosis than UIP with a mean survival of 12.2 years, as compared to 5.6 years in usual interstitial pneumonia (17, 18). Smoking cessation is critical in initial management and if the disease fails to ameliorate treatment with corticosteroids is appropriate, using a protocol as listed for treatment of NSIP.

Asbestosis

There is currently no specific treatment for asbestosis. There have been no studies of patients with asbestosis using anti-inflammatory or immunosuppressive agents such as steroids or cytotoxic therapy showing substantive benefit. Thus, management of patients with asbestosis should focus on prevention of further asbestos exposure, in addition to other supportive measures outlined below.

Silicosis

There is no proven specific therapy for any form of silicosis. Corticosteroid therapy has been shown to produce a small improvement in lung function in patients with chronic disease and may have benefit in accelerated and acute silicosis (15). Nonetheless, no large, randomized, double-blinded, prospective clinical trials have demonstrated an impact of steroid therapy on the long-term clinical outcome of silicosis. Symptomatic therapy should include treatment of airflow obstruction with bronchodilators, aggressive management of respiratory tract infection with antibiotics, and supportive measures as listed below.

Hypersensitivity pneumonitis

Although antigen avoidance forms the basis of treatment of hypersensitivity pneumonitis, in severe or refractory cases or where antigen avoidance can not be undertaken corticosteroid therapy may be required. Antigen avoidance may be particularly difficult in cases of occupational exposure for financial reasons, or in bird fancier's lung where patients may be reluctant to give up their birds, or where a specific antigen can not be identified. Nonetheless, in mild to moderate cases of farmer's lung modifications of the work environment, rather than leaving employment, may be sufficient to arrest progress.

Corticosteroids accelerate recovery from farmer's lung and bird fancier's lung, particularly in severely affected patients; however, they do not appear to change the long-term outcome (19). Treatment with steroids is therefore appropriate in severely ill patients. Generally a dose of 0.5–1.0 mg per kilogram of ideal body weight of prednisolone may be given once daily. This dose could be given over two weeks and then tapered over two to four weeks. Maintenance steroids should not be seen as a substitute for reducing exposure to the offending antigen, although may be indicated where the antigen can not be identified or removed form the environment. Inhaled steroids may be of benefit in treatment of this disorder although evidence of efficacy is lacking.

General supportive therapies

Ambulatory oxygen therapy may provide symptomatic benefit although has not been demonstrated to improve long term survival or quality of life (20). Opiates, (e.g. morphine 10 mg slow release once daily), may be of benefit in treating dyspnoea associated with interstitial lung disease although have the potential to cause respiratory depression in higher doses. General measures to maintain respiratory health and prevent decline include smoking cessation, pulmonary rehabilitation, maintaining optimum nutrition, prompt treatment of intercurrent respiratory infections and vaccination for pneumococcal infection and influenza.

KEY POINTS

- Interstitial lung disease represents a heterogeneous group of disorders with variable prognosis and response to therapy.
- Diagnosis is usually achieved through a combination of history, examination, serological markers, HRCT and in some cases lung biopsy, and hence requires close consultation between physicians, radiologists and pathologists.
- As treatments are of uncertain efficacy and possess potential side effects, any trial of treatment requires close monitoring and demonstration of therapeutic benefit to justify continuation.
- Although corticosteroids remain the mainstay of therapy, many forms of interstitial lung disease are relatively refractory to treatment and if a trial of corticosteroids is undertaken treatment steroids should not be continued in the absence of objective measures of improvement.

- Where corticosteroids are effective, treatment should be undertaken with the minimum effective dose and with measures to minimize complications, particularly osteoporosis.
- Ongoing use of immunosuppressive therapies in the elderly requires close monitoring.

LINKS

http://www.nlm.nih.gov/medlineplus/pulmonaryfibrosis.html
Useful NIH site providing information for patients about aetiology and nature of pulmonary fibrosis.

http://www.lungusa.org/interstitiallungdisease
what Patient information site provided by the American Lung Association.

http://www.thoracic.org/sections/publications/statements/pages/respiratory-disease-adults/idio02.html
Provides web access to ATS/ERS 2001 Consensus statement on Classification of Pulmonary Fibrosis.

http://www.brit-thoracic.org.uk/Portals/0/Clinical%20Information/DPLD/Guidelines/Parenchymaltext.pdf
Provides web access to 1999 British Thoracic Guidelines, due to be updated in mid 2008.

REFERENCES

1. American Thoracic Society (ATS) and the European Respiratory Society (ERS), Idiopathic pulmonary fibrosis: diagnosis and treatment: international consensus statement. *Am J Respir Crit Care Med* 2000; **161**: 646–64.
2. King Jr TE, Clinical advances in the diagnosis and therapy of the interstitial lung diseases. *Am J Respir Crit Care Med* 2005; **172**: 268–79.
3. Raghu, G. Pulmonary Fibrosis: treatment options in pursuit of evidence-based approaches. *Eur Respir J* 2006; **28**: 463–5.
4. Camus PH. Foucher P. Bonniaud PH. Ask K. Drug-induced infiltrative lung disease. *Eur Respir J - Supplement*. 2001; **32**: 93s–100s.

5. Tzelepis G. E, Toya S. P, and Moutsopoulos H. M. Occult connective tissue diseases mimicking idiopathic interstitial pneumonias. *Eur Respir J* 2008; **31**: 11–20.

6. Daniil ZD; Gilchrist FC; Nicholson AG; Hansell DM; Harris J; Colby TV; du Bois RM A histologic pattern of nonspecific interstitial pneumonia is associated with a better prognosis than usual interstitial pneumonia in patients with cryptogenic fibrosing alveolitis. *Am J Respir Crit Care Med* 1999; **160**: 899–905.

7. Raghu G; Depaso WJ; Cain K; Hammar SP; Wetzel CE; Dreis DF; Hutchinson J; Pardee NE; Winterbauer RH Azathioprine combined with prednisone in the treatment of idiopathic pulmonary fibrosis: a prospective double-blind, randomized, placebo-controlled clinical trial. *Am Rev Respir Dis* 1991; **144**: 291–6.

8. Gotway, Michael B 1; Freemer, Michelle M 2; King, Talmadge E Jr Challenges in pulmonary fibrosis 1: Use of high resolution CT scanning of the lung for the evaluation of patients with idiopathic interstitial pneumonias *Thorax* 2007; **62**: 546–53.

9. Davies HR, Richeldi L, Walters EH. Immunomodulatory agents for idiopathic pulmonary fibrosis. *Cochrane Database of Systematic Reviews* 2003, Issue 2. Art. No: CD003134.

10. Richeldi L, Davies HR, Ferrara G, Franco F. Corticosteroids for idiopathic pulmonary fibrosis. *Cochrane Database of Systematic Reviews* 2003, Issue 3. Art. No: CD002880.

11. Collard HR, Loyd JE, King Jr TE, Lancaster LH, Current diagnosis and management of idiopathic pulmonary fibrosis: A survey of academic physicians. *Respir Med* 2007; **101**: 2011–16.

12. Danoff SK, Terry PB, and Horton MR. A clinicians guide to the diagnosis and treatment of interstitial lung diseases. *South Med J* 2007; **100**: 570–87.

13. Demedts M; Behr J; Buhl R; Costabel U; Dekhuijzen R; Jansen HM; MacNee W; Thomeer M; Wallaert B; Laurent F; Nicholson AG; Verbeken EK; Verschakelen J; Flower CD; Capron F; Petruzzelli S; De Vuyst P; van den Bosch JM; Rodriguez-Becerra E; Corvasce G; Lankhorst I; Sardina M; Montanari M, High-dose acetylcysteine in idiopathic pulmonary fibrosis. *N Engl J Med* 2005; **353**: 2229–42.

14. Keogh BA; Bernardo J; Hunninghake GW; Line BR; Price DL; Crystal RG Effect of intermittent high dose parenteral corticosteroids on the alveolitis of idiopathic pulmonary fibrosis. *Am Rev Respir Dis* 1983; **127**: 18–22.

15. Sharma SK; Pande JN; Verma K Effect of prednisolone treatment in chronic silicosis. *Am Rev Respir Dis* 1991; **143**: 814–21.

16. Strimlan CV; Rosenow EC 3d; Weiland LH; Brown LR Lymphocytic interstitial pneumonitis. Review of 13 cases. *Ann Intern Med* 1978; **88**: 616–21.

17. Carrington CB; Gaensler EA; Coutu RE; FitzGerald MX; Gupta RG Natural history and treated course of usual and desquamative interstitial pneumonia. *N Engl J Med* 1978; **298**: 801–9.

18. Moon, J, du Bois, RM, Colby, TV. Clinical significance of respiratory bronchiolitis on open lung biopsy and its relationship to smoking related interstitial lung disease. *Thorax* 1999; **54**: 1009.

19. Kokkarinen JI; Tukiainen HO; Terho EO Effect of corticosteroid treatment on the recovery of pulmonary function in farmer's lung. *Am Rev Respir Dis* 1992; **145**: 3–5.

20. Crockett AJ, Cranston JM, Antic N. Domiciliary oxygen for interstitial lung disease. *Cochrane Database of Systematic Reviews* 2001, Issue 3. Art. No: CD002883.

22 Lung Cancer in the elderly

Jeffrey Bowden

Department of Medicine, Flinders Medical Centre, Adelaide, Australia

INTRODUCTION

Lung cancer occurs most frequently in those over the age of 65 with up to 40 percent of patients older than 70 at diagnosis (1). Consequently, many of those presenting with lung cancer will have co-morbid illness, particularly cardiovascular, respiratory and renal disease, and age related decline in physiological function. These factors are particularly important in determining fitness for treatment for lung cancer and will impact on both the ability to undertake surgery and on the use of chemotherapy in lung cancer. Moreover, cognitive impairment and social isolation may have a major impact on the ability of the elderly to respond to potential complications of cytotoxic chemotherapy and should be taken into account in deciding on whether an individual patient is suitable for treatment.

Importantly though, chronological age alone should not be the principal determinant of therapy. Surveys of clinical practice have shown that relatively few elderly patients with advanced non-small cell lung cancer (NSCLC) are treated with cytotoxic chemotherapy, presumably due to concerns regarding efficacy, tolerability and toxicity (1). Although few studies have specifically examined outcomes of treatment with cytotoxic chemotherapy in the elderly, subgroup analysis of elderly patients included in large clinical trials have demonstrated benefits of treatment in the elderly comparable

to those of younger patients. Overall these results suggest that elderly patients with carcinoma of the lung with good performance status may derive significant benefit from chemotherapy and should be offered such treatment (2).

In this chapter the rationale and protocols for treatment of lung cancer, including small cell and non-small cell lung cancer and mesothelioma will be briefly outlined. The protocols provide a general guide to treatment and cannot substitute for the opinion of an experienced oncologist but should assist in selecting and monitoring treatment in elderly patients.

AETIOLOGY

In developed nations, tobacco smoking is the most common cause of lung cancer with up to 90 % of cases in males and 80 % in females directly attributable to smoking (3). Nonetheless, a small but significant proportion of cases may occur in non-smokers and may have a different molecular biological basis, and response to therapy, particularly in Asian females and in those with adenocarcinoma. It is anticipated that lung cancer will remain prevalent in western societies, given current smoking rates and that it will increase in developing nations associated with the uptake in tobacco use and the promotion of tobacco products in these countries (4).

Prescribing for Elderly Patients   Edited by Stephen Jackson, Paul Jansen and Arduino Mangoni
© 2009 John Wiley & Sons, Ltd

SYMPTOMS AND SIGNS

Patients may present with respiratory symptoms, systemic symptoms or those of metastatic disease. Moreover, in 10 % of cases the carcinoma may be detected in asymptomatic patients with imaging undertaken for an unrelated problem. Respiratory symptoms are the most common cause of presentation (cough, haemoptysis, chest pain or dyspnoea) and are present in 85 % of those diagnosed with lung cancer (4). Nearly two thirds of patients will present with locally advanced or metastatic disease.

DIAGNOSIS AND STAGING

Optimal treatment of lung cancer depends upon accurate histological diagnosis, accurate staging and assessment of co-morbid illness.

Histological subtypes of carcinoma of the lung may be divided into small cell carcinoma and non-small cell carcinoma, the latter of which includes adenocarcinoma, squamous cell carcinoma and large cell carcinoma. The staging system of non-small lung cancer is based upon a TNM system with stages from 1–4 (see Table 22.1, (5)). Simply stated, stage 1 is intrapulmonary disease; stage 2 is intrapulmonary disease with intrapulmonary nodal metastases; stage 3 refers to disease spread to the mediastinum or with pleural effusion and stage 4 represents metastatic disease. Optimal treatment for stage 1 or 2 would be surgical resection (6); for stage 3A a number of treatment options are available for treatment, pneumonectomy with adjuvant chemotherapy or combined chemotherapy and radiotherapy (7); for stage 4 disease chemotherapy may be of survival benefit and improvement of symptom

Table 22.1. International staging system for lung cancer, 1997 revision

Primary tumor (T)
- T1: A tumor that is 3 cm or smaller in greatest dimension, is surrounded by lung or visceral pleura, and is without bronchoscopic evidence of invasion more proximal than the lobar bronchus (i.e., not in the main bronchus).
- T2: A tumor with any of the following features of size or extent:
  - Larger than 3 cm in greatest dimension
  - Involves the main bronchus and is 2 cm or larger distal to the carina
  - Invades the visceral pleura
  - Associated with atelectasis or obstructive pneumonitis that extends to the hilar region but does not involve the entire lung
- T3: A tumor of any size that directly invades any of the following: chest wall (including superior sulcus tumors), diaphragm, mediastinal pleura, parietal pericardium; or, tumor in the main bronchus less than 2 cm distal to the carina but without involvement of the carina; or, associated atelectasis or obstructive pneumonitis of the entire lung
- T4: A tumor of any size that invades any of the following: mediastinum, heart, great vessels, trachea, esophagus, vertebral body, carina; or, separate tumor nodules in the same lobe; or, tumor with a malignant pleural effusion.

Regional lymph nodes (N)
- N0: No regional lymph node metastasis
- N1: Metastasis to ipsilateral peribronchial and/or ipsilateral hilar lymph nodes, and intrapulmonary nodes including involvement by direct extension of the primary tumor
- N2: Metastasis to ipsilateral mediastinal and/or subcarinal lymph node(s)
- N3: Metastasis to contralateral mediastinal, contralateral hilar, ipsilateral or contralateral scalene, or supraclavicular lymph node(s)

Distant metastasis (M)
- M0: No distant metastasis
- M1: Distant metastasis present. [Note: M1 includes separate tumor nodule(s) in a different lobe (ipsilateral or contralateral).]

AJCC Stage Groupings Stage IA (T1, N0, M0) Stage IB (T2, N0, M0) Stage IIA (T1, N1, M0) Stage IIB (T2, N1, M0) Stage IIIA (T1, N2, M0) (T3, N0, M0) (T2, N2, M0) (T3, N1, M0) (T3, N2, M0) Stage IIIB (Any T, N3, M0) (T4, any N, M0) Stage IV (Any T, any N, M1)

Table 22.2. Ecog performance status*

Grade	ECOG
0	Fully active, able to carry on all pre-disease performance without restriction
1	Restricted in physically strenuous activity but ambulatory and able to carry out work of a light or sedentary nature, e.g., light house work, office work
2	Ambulatory and capable of all self-care but unable to carry out any work activities. Up and about more than 50% of waking hours
3	Capable of only limited self-care, confined to bed or chair more than 50% of waking hours
4	Completely disabled. Cannot carry on any self-care. Totally confined to bed or chair
5	Dead

*see (8).

control. In addition to anatomical staging it is also important to assess performance status (see Table 22.2, (8)) as this assists in determining overall fitness and the appropriateness of chemotherapy. Generally chemotherapy would not be recommended for patients with an ECOG performance status of >2.

GOALS OF THERAPY

For adjuvant treatment (chemotherapy given after surgical resection) of stage 2 and 3 disease, 5-year survival is improved, with potentially a small number of patients being cured (disease free after five years). The magnitude of improved survival is 5–10%. For treatment of locally advanced disease, the combination of chemotherapy and radiotherapy may result in cure in a small number of cases (up to 20%) and a significant improvement in survival in others. In treating metastatic disease, a modest improvement in survival may be seen, with an increase in median survival of one to two months (9). In addition, such patients may derive an improvement in cancer-related symptoms and overall quality of life. An additional benefit demonstrated in clinical trials (not specifically dealing with the elderly) is of cost savings when comparing overall treatment costs in patients with good performance status treated with chemotherapy versus best supportive care.

Although haematological toxicity is particularly common in older patients, it remains difficult to predict bone marrow reserve in individual subjects. In considering chemotherapy in the elderly it is important that the patient and their family or carers are well informed of the potential benefits and potential complications of treatment. It is particularly important that consideration be given as to how they may respond to problems of chemotherapy, that ability to use the telephone, ability to use public transport and ability to take medication reliably, and that they be informed of the risk of neutropaenia and sepsis and that they be given clear written instructions as to how to respond to such an episode.

CHEMOTHERAPEUTIC AGENTS

Platinum compounds

Platinum compounds exert a cytotoxic effect by forming adducts with DNA and subsequent cross-linking of strands thereby inhibiting transcription and replication (10). They have been shown to be of benefit in combination with other drugs in improving survival when given as adjuvant chemotherapy, in chemo-radiotherapy and in treating metastatic disease. The two main formulations are cisplatin and carboplatin (a third platinum compound, oxaliplatin, is not routinely used in lung cancer treatment). A major concern with the use of cisplatin is the risk of nephrotoxicity and this drug should not be given to patients with GFR less than 40 ml/min. This drug requires fluid loading at the time of administration. These drugs are highly emetogenic and require aggressive therapy to diminish nausea and vomiting ((11) and Table 22.10).

Carboplatin may be better tolerated, but likewise has potential for renal impairment. Both agents have the potential for haematological toxicity with the risk of thrombocytopaenia being greater with cisplatin. The dose of cisplatin is based on calculated body surface area, assuming satisfactory renal function. The dose of carboplatin is based on creatinine clearance with a predicted serum concentration × time (area under the curve, AUC) of 5 or 6. For example, for an AUC of 5, the dose in mg is derived from the following formula: Dose = AUC(GFR + 25)

It is strongly recommended that patients to receive platinum based compounds should have GFR estimated with a nuclear scan, as calculations based on serum creatinine alone may overestimate GFR. As these drugs are renally excreted, toxicity may be potentiated by the use of nephrotoxic agents (eg aminoglycosides) or diuretics.

Gemcitabine

Gemcitabine is a nucleoside analogue which is active in treating small cell and non-small cell carcinoma. Major toxicity is related to myelosuppression, although non-haematologic toxicity with transient flu-like symptoms including fever, headache, myalgia and asthenia are common (12). Rarely, use of gemcitabine may be associated with pulmonary toxicity with the risk of development of an acute respiratory distress type syndrome.

Vinca alkaloids (Vincristine, Vindesine, Vinblastine, Vinorelbine)

Vinorelbine, vinblastine and vindesine are vinca alkaloids which exert their effect principally by interacting with tubulin and disrupting microtubule function particularly the microtubule apparatus involved in cell division (12). Neurotoxicity is particularly associated with vincristine, although may occur infrequently with other vinca alkaloids. Myelosuppression may occur with any of these agents and neutropenia may be dose limiting for vinblastine, vindesine and vinorelbine.

Taxanes (Paclitaxel and Docetaxel)

Taxanes exert their effect by binding to microtubules at sites different to those of vinca alkaloids, thereby stabilizing the microtubule network and inhibiting reorganisation which is essential for cellular functions in mitosis and interphase (12). The major toxicity of taxanes is myelotoxicity. Hypersensitivity reactions including dyspnoea, bronchospasm, urticaria, hypotension and chest pain are common if no prophylaxis is given, and require pre-treatment with corticosteroids and antihistamines.

TREATMENT PROTOCOLS FOR NSCLC

Stage 1

Surgical resection is recommended as primary treatment for Stage 1 carcinoma. For patients unfit for surgery, radiotherapy is of benefit, and may offer long term survival in a small number of cases. Chemotherapy is not recommended as primary treatment for Stage 1 disease. Currently, adjuvant chemotherapy is not indicated following complete resection of stage 1 carcinoma as there is insufficient benefit for stage 1 disease, (which carries a relatively good prognosis), to justify its use in this group of patients (13).

Stage 2, Adjuvant chemotherapy

Surgical resection is similarly recommended as primary treatment of Stage 2 carcinoma, However, survival post resection may be improved by the use of adjuvant chemotherapy. At least five randomized control trials have demonstrated benefit for the use of chemotherapy, with a relative improvement of survival of about 5–10 % (13). Several treatment protocols have been recommended, although the best results have been achieved with a combination of cisplatin and vinorelbine (see Table 22.3). This regime would require satisfactory renal function (GFR >50 ml/min), particularly if given in the elderly.

Stage 3A, Adjuvant chemotherapy or Chemo-radiotherapy

Where ipsilateral mediastinal nodal involvement is identified during the process of staging for NSCLC, the optimal treatment would be concurrent chemotherapy and radiotherapy. A variety of protocols are available for such treatment although the standard of care is cisplatin and etoposide (see Table 22.4). Where surgical resection has been undertaken, and metastatic spread identified on pathological examination of resected mediastinal nodes, adjuvant chemotherapy is also recommended (7).

Table 22.3. Adjuvant chemotherapy protocols

Drug	Dosing	Frequency	Duration	Precautions	Side effects
Vinorelbine	25 mg/m2 day 1 and 8	3 weekly	4 Cycles	Monitor for haematological toxicity and renal imparment,	Fatigue, Anorexia, Alopecia, Diarrhoea, Nausea, Vomiting, Constipation, Infection, Febrile neutropenia,
Cisplatin	80 mg/m2 day 1*			Monitor for nephrotoxicity, otoxicity, hypo-magnesaemia, hypocalcaemia and ensure adequate hydration.	Hearing loss, Sensory neuropathy, Motor neuropathy, Dyspnoea, Thrombocytopenia
Paclitaxel	200 mg/m2 day 1	3 weeks	Haematological toxicity	Reduce paclitaxel if hepatic impairment or neuropathy	Hypersensitivity reactions, Neuropathy, anorexia, fatigue
Carboplatin	AUC 6 on day 1		Nephrotoxicity,	Renal impairment, Neutropenia Thrombocytope-nia,	Hearing loss, Sensory neuropathy, Motor neuropathy, Dyspneoa,

*the original protocol used doses of 100 mg/m2 Day1 or split 50 mg/m2 day 1 and 8.

Stages 3B and 4, Chemotherapy

Cytotoxic chemotherapy produces improvement in survival and quality of life when compared with best supportive care in patients with good performance status (ECOG performance status of 0–2) with advanced NSCLC. There is some debate as to the optimal combination of treatment for elderly patients with metastatic disease, and no single regime is appropriate for all patients. For patients with good performance status, no co-morbidities and good renal function a combination of platinum based therapy and a second agent may be used, provided that patients are carefully monitored for toxicity (see Table 22.5). For those patients at risk of chemotherapy related complications, treatment with a single agent, such as docetaxel, vinorelbine or gemcitabine, may be most appropriate (1) (see Table 22.6). There are conflicting data with regard the benefit of two non-platinum containing cytotoxic compounds over a single agent (eg vinorelbine versus vinorelbine plus gemcytabine) in treating elderly patients and

Table 22.4. Chemotherapy for combined therapy (chemo-radiotherapy) for stage 3A and 3B disease

Drugs	Dosing	Frequency	Duration	Comments
Cisplatin	50 mg/m^2 by IV infusion Days 1, 8, 29, and 36	Single course, concurrent with radiotherapy	36 days	Reduce dose if GFR < 60 ml/ min and do not use if GFR < 40 ml/min
Etoposide	50 mg/m^2 by IV infusion Days 1 to 5 and 29 to 33			Modify if haematological toxicity Consider dose reduction of etoposide if hepatic impairment

Table 22.5. 1st line therapy for advanced disease: combination therapy

Drug	Dosage	Treatment cycle	Side effects	Dose modification required
Docetaxel	75 mg/m2 day 1	3 weeks	Haematological toxicity Nephrotoxicity,	Reduce docetaxel if hepatic impairment Renal impairment, Neutropenia
Cisplatin	75 mg/m2 day 1		Ototoxicity, Peripheral neuropathy	Thrombocytopenia, Neuropathy
Docetaxel	75 mg/m2 day 1	3 weeks	Haematological toxicity	Reduce docetaxel if hepatic impairment
Carboplatin	AUC 5 on day 1		Nephrotoxicity,	Renal impairment, Neutropenia Thrombocytopenia,
Gemcitabine	1000 - 1250 mg/m2 on days 1, 8	3 weeks	Haematological toxicity	Renal impairment Hepatic impairment Neutropenia
Cisplatin	80 mg/m2 day 8		Nephrotoxicity, Ototoxicity, Peripheral neuropathy	Thrombocytopenia Neuropathy
Gemcitabine	1000 - 1250 mg/m2 on days 1, 8	3 weeks	Haematological toxicity	Renal impairment Hepatic impairment Neutropenia
Carboplatin	AUC 5 on day 8		Nephrotoxicity,	Thrombocytopenia Neuropathy
Vinorelbine	25 mg/m2 Days 1, 8	3 weekly	Haematological toxicity	Renal impairment Hepatic impairment Neutropenia
Cisplatin	80 mg/m2 day 1		Nephrotoxicity, Ototoxicity, Peripheral neuropathy	Thrombocytopenia
Paclitaxel	200 mg/m2 day 1	3 weeks	Haematological toxicity	Reduce paclitaxel if hepatic impairment or neuropathy
Carboplatin	AUC 6 on day 1		Nephrotoxicity,	Renal impairment, Neutropenia Thrombocytopenia,

combinations of non-platinum compounds could not be routinely recommended at this time (14).

Similarly a variety of "doublet" protocols are available, including combinations of platinum based compounds and newer cytotoxic agents including vinorelbine, gemcitabine and taxanes. In general, combination chemotherapy has yielded better response rates and improves survival, although carries with it an increased risk of toxicity. In the elderly, single agent chemotherapy is likely to give less toxicity and only slightly inferior response rates to double agent chemotherapy. Currently there is no role for using three cytotoxic agents in the treatment of lung cancer.

In patients who have failed to respond or have relapsed after first line therapy, second line treatment with docetaxal or pemetrexed may offer a small survival advantage (15) (see Table 22.7).

NON CYTOTOXIC AGENTS: EGFR INHIBITORS

Selective inhibitors of EGFR linked tyrosine kinase have been investigated in the treatment of non-small cell carcinoma of the lung, and are currently indicated for locally advanced or metastatic NSCLC after failure of prior chemotherapy or in patients not amenable to

Table 22.6. Single agent therapy for advanced NSCLC

Drug	Dosage	Treatment cycle	Max No of cycles	Side effects	Dose adjustments
Docetaxel[†]	60–75 mg/m2 Day 1	3 weeks	4	Anaemia, Neutropenia Thrombocytopenia, Pulmonary toxicity, Fatigue, Fever	Haematological Liver impairment
Pemetrexed	500 mg/m2 Day 1*	3 weeks	Benefit beyond 4 cycles is unproven	Neutropenia, anemia, fatigue, nausea, diarrhea, stomatitis, rash	Renal impairment Neurotoxicity
Gemcitabine	1000 mg/m^2 by IV infusion Day 1, 8 and 15	4 weeks	4	Anaemia, Neutropenia Thrombocytopenia, Nausea and vomiting, Diarrhoea, Fatigue, Fever	If CrCl < 30 consider reduction Delay if haematological Toxicity
Vinorelbine	IV 25–30 mg/ m2 days 1 and 8 Oral 60 mg/m2 days 1, 8, 15	3 weeks	Depending on response and toxicity	Anaemia, Neutropenia Nausea and vomiting Diarrhoea Mucositis Fatigue Fever, Constipation, Peripheral neurotoxicity	Delay if haematological toxicity Reduce if hepatic insufficiency

[†]Pretreatment with dexamethasone 8 mg orally the morning of chemotherapy is recommended. Docetaxel administered at a dose of 33.3–40 mg/m2 (for six weeks on an eight-week cycle or for three weeks on a four-week cycle) may be considered in patients at high risk of hematologic toxicity or with a previous history of febrile neutropenia using the three-weekly docetaxel schedule. Ontario guidelines
*Should be administered with vitamin supplements: oral folic acid 350–1000 mcg daily and intramuscular vitamin B12 1000 mcg every nine weeks, beginning between one to two weeks before, and continuing until three weeks after chemotherapy

Table 22.7. 2nd line therapy for advanced NSCLC

Drug	Dosage	Treatment cycle	Side effects	Dose adjustments
Docetaxel	75 mg/m2 Day 1	3 weeks	Haematological toxicity Myalgia Hypersensitivity reactions	Neutropenia Thrombocytopenia
Docetaxel	35 mg/m2 Day 1, 8, 15	4 weeks*	Haematological toxicity Myalgia Hypersensitivity reactions	Neutropenia Thrombocytopenia
Pemetrexed[†]	500 mg/m2 Day 1	3 weeks	Haematological toxicity, fatigue, mucositis	Neutropenia Thrombocytopenia Renal impairment Neuropathy

*Docetaxel administered at a dose of 33.3–40 mg/m2 weekly (for six weeks on an eight-week cycle or for three weeks on a four-week cycle) may be considered in patients at high risk of hematologic toxicity or with a previous history of febrile neutropenia using the three-weekly docetaxel schedule. (Ontario guidelines)
[†]Should be administered with vitamin supplements: oral folic acid 350–1,000 mcg daily and intramuscular vitamin B12 1,000 mcg every nine weeks, beginning between one to two weeks before, and continuing until three weeks after chemotherapy

cytotoxic chemotherapy (16). These agents should only be continued in cases of tumour regression or stable disease or where cancer related symptoms continue to improve. These agents are particularly effective in patients of East Asian background and to a lesser extent non-smokers with lung malignancy.

Dosing: Erlotinib 150 mg orally daily, Gefitinib 250 mg orally daily. Side effects: diarrhoea and skin rash are commonly encountered with these agents and if severe may require discontinuation of the drug. Interstitial lung disease has been identified in some populations treated with these medications (primarily Japanese).

TREATMENT OF SMALL CELL CARCINOMA

Small cell carcinoma accounts for 10–20 % of cases of primary lung cancer. Staging of small cell carcinoma is divided into limited and extensive disease. Limited stage disease is confined to the thorax and can be encompassed

within a radiotherapy field, whereas extensive disease represents clinically or radiologically detectable disease outside the thorax (17, 18). The median survival without treatment for extensive disease is very poor (less than two months) whereas that of limited disease is around eight months. Survival in both groups is substantively improved with chemotherapy. For extensive stage disease treatment is usually chemotherapy alone whereas limited stage disease is treated with chemotherapy, local radiotherapy and prophylactic cranial irradiation. Chemotherapy protocols are listed in Table 22.8.

TREATMENT OF MESOTHELIOMA

A number of chemotherapy regimes used in the treatment of malignant mesothelioma have shown improvements in survival, symptoms and quality of life, although none is curative. Response rates for combination chemotherapy range from 20–40 % with improvement in

Table 22.8. Chemotherapy for small cell carcinoma

Drugs	Dosage	Treatment cycle	Max No of cycles	Side effects	Dose adjustments
Carboplatin Etoposide	5 AUC by IV infusion D1 100 mg/m^2 by IV infusion per day on D1-3	4 weeks	6	Haematological toxicity, Nephrotoxicity, Ototoxicity, Peripheral neuropathy	Renal impairment, Neutropenia Thrombocytopenia, Neuropathy
Cisplatin Etoposide (if concurrent radiotherapy)	60 mg/m^2 by IV infusion D1 120 mg/m^2 by IV infusion per day on D1-3	3 weeks	6	Haematological toxicity, Nephrotoxicity, Ototoxicity, Peripheral neuropathy	Renal impairment, Neutropenia Thrombocytopenia, Neuropathy
Cisplatin Etoposide	80 mg/m^2 by IV infusion D1 100 mg/m^2 by IV infusion per day on D1-3	3 weeks	6	Haematological toxicity, Nephrotoxicity, Ototoxicity, Peripheral neuropathy	Renal impairment, Neutropenia Thrombocytopenia, Neuropathy
Cyclophosphamide Adriamycin Vincristine	1000 mg/m2 40–50 mg/m2 1 mg/m2 Day 1	3 weeks	6	Haematological toxicity, Peripheral neuropathy	Neutropenia Thrombocytopenia, Neuropathy

Table 22.9. Chemotherapy protocols for treatment of mesothelioma*

Drug	Dosage	Frequency	Duration	Side effects	Comments
Pemetrexed	500 mg/m2, day 1	3 weeks	4-6 cycles until maximum clinical benefit, No evidence for treating beyond 6 cycles.	Haematological toxicity	Delay until recovery to ANC >1.5 × 10^9/L and platelets >100 × 10^9/L.
Cisplatin	75 mg/m^2 by IV infusion Day 1				Consider treating at 75 % of total dose in the presence of any significant grade 3 or 4 event.
Pemetrexed	500 mg/m2, day 1	3 weeks	4-6 cycles until maximum clinical benefit, No evidence for treating beyond 6 cycles.		Carboplatin is contraindicated if CrCl < 20 ml/min Pemetrexed dose to be delayed if CrCl < 45 ml/min.
Carboplatin	5 AUC by IV infusion day 1				Full dose to be given if CrCl > 45 ml/min Treatment should be delayed if neutropenia

*Protocols using gemcitabine and platinum compounds, and also single agent vinorelbine have also shown efficacy and may be considered as alternatives (see Tables 22.5 and 22.6).

survival. The best efficacy has been shown with the use of the multi-targeted agent pemetrexed, combined with either cisplatin or carboplatin (see Table 22.9), although combinations of platinum compounds and gemcytabine, and single agent vinorelbine (as per lung cancer protocols in Tables 22.5 and 22.6) have also shown efficacy.

ANTI-EMETIC THERAPY

For chemotherapy regimes of high emetogenic potential a combination of three drugs as pre-treatment is recommended (5-hydroxytryptamine-3 (5-HT3) serotonin receptor antagonist, dexamethasone, and aprepitant) (11). For patients receiving chemotherapy of moderate emetic risk, a two-drug combination is recommended (5-HT3 receptor serotonin antagonist and dexamethasone). Moreover in patients receiving cisplatin, dexamethasone and aprepitant are recommended to be given on days 2 and 3 to prevent delayed emesis (see Table 22.10).

KEY POINTS

- Lung cancer is common in the elderly and will remain common.
- Most patients present with advanced disease.
- For early stage disease, surgery is the treatment of choice.
- For locally advanced and metastatic disease, chemotherapy may improve symptoms, quality of life and overall survival.
- Chronological age alone should not be the determinant of therapy, and should not preclude patients from potentially curative surgery, nor from aggressive therapies such as radiotherapy or chemotherapy.
- In selected older patients with good performance status, chemotherapy gives outcomes similar to that seen in younger patients and older patients should be offered such treatments.

Table 22.10. Risk of emesis with cytotoxic chemotherapy and anti-emetic agents (based on ASCO guidelines, (11))

Drug	Emesis potential	Recommended initial anti-emesis protocol
Cisplatin Cyclophosphamide <1500 mg/m2	High	5 HT3 Receptor antagonist Dexamethasone (12 mg) Aprepitant (125 mg)
Carboplatin Cyclophosphamide <1500 mg/m2 Doxorubicin Irinotecan	Moderate	5 HT3 Receptor antagonist Dexamethasone (12 mg)
Paclitaxel Docetaxel Mitoxantrone Topotecan Etoposide Pemetrexed Mitomycin Gemcitabine	Low	Dexamethasone (12 mg), single dose
Vinblastine Vincristine Vinorelbine	Minimal	As needed: Dexamethasone 8 mg, single dose
Bevacizumab		Metoclopramide 10 mg orally 4 hourly prn

- Prevention by smoking cessation is the best method to reduce the burden of illness.

GUIDELINES

https://www.treatment.cancerinstitute.org.au/
Excellent summary of commonly used chemotherapy protocols, including toxicities and advice on dose modification.

http://www.nice.org.uk/Nice
Guidelines, good summary of evidence base but don't deal specifically with the elderly.

http://www.nhmrc.gov.au/publications/synopses/cp97syn.htm
Detailed summary similar to NICE

http://www.chestjournal.org/content/123/1_suppl/
Supplement to Chest outlining ACCP evidence based guidelines for diagnosis and management of Lung Cancer, updated September 2007.

http://www.cancercare.on.ca/index_lung
Cancerguidelines.htm Excellent summary of Canadian guidelines for Lung Cancer management, including chemotherapy protocols.

http://www.sign.ac.uk/guidelines/published/index.html.

http://www.cancer.gov/cancertopics/types/lung.

REFERENCES

1. Gridelli C, A. M., Ardizzoni A, Balducci L, De Marinis F, Kelly K, Le Chevalier T, Manegold C, Perrone F, Rosell R, Shepherd F, De Petris L, Di Maio M, Langer C. Treatment of advanced non-small-cell lung cancer in the elderly: results of an international expert panel. *American Society of Clinical Oncology* 2005; **23**: 3125–37.

2. Maione, P, Perrone, F, Gallo, C, et al. Pretreatment quality of life and functional status assessment significantly predict survival of elderly patients with advanced non–small-cell lung cancer receiving chemotherapy: a prognostic analysis of the multicenter Italian lung cancer in the elderly study. *J Clin Oncol* 2005; **23**: 6865–72.

3. Alberg AJ, Ford JG and Samet JM. Epidemiology of Lung Cancer ACCP Evidence-Based Clinical Practice Guidelines. *Chest* 2007; **132**: 29S–55S.

4. Skuladottir H and Olsen JH, Epidemiology of Lung Cancer *Eur Respir Mon* 2001; **17**: 1–12.

5. Mountain CF, Revisions in the International System for Staging Lung Cancer. *Chest* 1997; **111**: 1710–7.

6. Cerfolio RJ and Bryant AS, Survival and Outcomes of Pulmonary Resection for Non-Small Cell Lung Cancer in the Elderly: A Nested Case-Control Study *Ann Thorac Surg* 2006; **82**: 424–30.

7. Robinson LA, Ruckdeschel JC, Wagner H and Stevens CW Treatment of Non-small cell lung cancer-Stage IIIA; ACCP Evidence-Based Clinical Practice Guidelines. *Chest* 2007; **132**: 243S–265S.

8. Oken, M.M., Creech, R.H., Tormey, D.C., Horton, J., Davis, T.E., McFadden, E.T., Carbone, P.P.: Toxicity And Response Criteria Of The Eastern Cooperative Oncology Group. *Am J Clin Oncol*, 1982; **5**: 649–55.

9. Stewart LA, Pignon JP. Chemotherapy in non-small-cell lung cancer: a meta-analysis using updated data on individual patients from 52 randomized clinical trials. *Br Med J* 1995; **311**: 899–909.

10. Devita VT, Hellman S and Rosenberg SA. *Cancer. Principles and Practice of Oncology* Lippincott Williams and Wilkins, Philadelphia 2005.

11. Kris MG, Hesketh PJ, Somerfield MR, et al. American Society of Clinical Oncology guideline for antiemetics in oncology: update 2006. *J Clin Oncol* 2006; **24**: 2932–47.

12. Tsao AS New Chemotherapeutic agents in Lung Cancer pp 315–333 in *Lung Cancer* ed Roth JA, Cox JD and Hong, WK Blackwell, Oxford 2008.

13. Alam N, Darling G, Shepherd FA, et al. Postoperative chemotherapy in non-small cell lung cancer: a systematic review. *Ann Thoracic Surg* 2006; **81**: 1926–36.

14. Langer CJ, M. J., Bernardo P, Kugler JW, Bonomi P, Cella D, Johnson DH. Cisplatin-based therapy for elderly patients with advanced non-small-cell lung cancer: implications of Eastern Cooperative Oncology Group 5592, a randomized trial. *J Natl Cancer Inst* 2002; **94**: 173–81.

15. Weiss GJ, Langer C, Rosell R, Hanna N, et al. Elderly patients benefit from second-line cytotoxic chemotherapy: a subset analysis of a randomized phase III trial of pemetrexed compared with docetaxel in patients with previously treated advanced non-small-cell lung cancer. *J Clin Oncol*. 2006; **24**: 4405–11.

16. Molina JR, Adjei AA, Jett JR. Advances in Chemotherapy of Non-small Cell Lung Cancer. *Chest*. 2006; **130**: 1211–9.

17. Rossi A, Maione P, Colantuoni G, Guerriero C, Ferrara C, Del Gaizo F, Nicolella D, Gridelli C. Treatment of small cell lung cancer in the elderly. *The Oncologist* 2005; **10**: 399–411.

18. Cooper S, Spiro S.G. Small cell lung cancer: treatment review. *Respirology* 2006; **11**: 241–48.

23 Nutritional disorders and the older person

Robert K. Penhall and Renuka Visvanathan

Department of Geriatric and Rehabilitation Medicine, Royal Adelaide Hospital, Adelaide, Australia

INTRODUCTION

There is no one gold standard that defines malnutrition but what is poorly understood is that it should not only include under-nutrition but also include over- nutrition (obesity). Obesity is an emerging public health issue in older people and is briefly discussed here. The Body Mass Index (BMI) is often used to classify older people as over-weight or obese but the use of waist-to-hip ratio may be more appropriate as it is really visceral adiposity that is of interest. The BMI measures not only fat mass but also lean mass, total body water and bone mass. The mere advice to lose weight may result in detrimental loss of lean mass. Physical activity accompanying dietary advice may result in an appropriate loss of fat mass and preservation of lean mass.

Sadly, under-nutrition in the older person is often missed and a greater portion of this chapter is devoted to this topic for this reason. Under-nutrition in older people is associated with a myriad of poor health outcomes. Both physiological (sarcopenia and the anorexia of ageing) and non-physiological factors are associated with under-nutrition in the older person. Screening should occur to identify those at risk and several screening tools exist: the Mini Nutritional Assessment, the Malnutrition Universal Screening Tool and the Rapid Screen. Assessment of the nutritional status of those at risk should be confirmed by the dietitian, the subjective global assessment or the standardized nutritional assessment. Management should begin with attention to the management of non-physiological factors. Non-pharmacological strategies may include enhancement of taste, nutrient content and quantity. In under-nourished older people, protein and energy supplementation may result in weight gain and reduce mortality risk. Orexigenic and anabolic agents are associated with adverse effects and the evidence supporting their use is weak.

OBESITY AND THE OLDER PERSON

Obesity is on the rise. The Body Mass Index (BMI) has been used extensively to define overweight and obesity and the WHO categorization of $25-29.9\,\text{kg/m}^2$ for overweight and obese $\geq 30\,\text{kg/m}^2$ is often used (1). The Australian experience is confirmed by Australian Bureau of Statistics (2001) data demonstrating that the percentage of obese or overweight people in the community is increasing for all age groups, particularly over the last 15 years (2). The increase was greatest in the 65–74 age group increasing from 45% in 1995 to 56% in 2001 (2). Similarly, in Europe, obesity is said to already be at pandemic levels with one

Prescribing for Elderly Patients Edited by Stephen Jackson, Paul Jansen and Arduino Mangoni
© 2009 John Wiley & Sons, Ltd

fifth of its total population obese (3). Managing adiposity is recognized as an important public health issue. Increased visceral adiposity is associated with the metabolic syndrome. Obesity in its own right in older people may result in osteoarthritis and its ensuing disability (4).

Weight loss has been associated with increased mortality. For example, in one study of 1749 community dwelling Mexican American older (age 65+) adults, weight loss of 5 % or more of body weight was associated with increased (Hazard Ratio 1.35 [95 % CI 1.06–1.70]) mortality risk compared to no change in weight or weight gain of 5 % of body weight (Hazard Ratio 0.78 [95 % CI 0.58–1.05]) after controlling for baseline demographics, waist circumference and BMI (5). Interestingly in one study, men who lost weight as a result of personal choice had a reduced risk of mortality whilst those who lost weight because they were asked to do so by their physicians or those who lost weight intentionally due to ill health had an increased risk of dying (6).

In people older than 70 years, it is not clear if an increased BMI is associated with an increased risk of mortality. The study by Flegal et. al. looking at data and risk from the combined National Health and Nutrition Examination Survey (NHANES) data sets over

a 6 to 20 year follow–up showed that the increased mortality risk was mainly seen with body mass index (BMI) $<18.5\,kg/m^2$ in people aged 70 years and older (Figure 23.1) (7). A very recent meta-analysis concluded that in older people (>65 years), BMI in the overweight range ($25\text{--}29.9\,kg/m^2$) was not associated with an increased risk of mortality (RR 1.00 [95 % CI 0.97–1.03]) compared to the normal weight range (WHO classification). Mortality risk was only very slightly increased for BMI in the obese category (RR 1.10 [95 % CI 1.06–1.13] (8)). Therefore, the sole use of BMI to assess mortality risk is inappropriate in the older person. Should the intention for assessment be to assess circulatory mortality risk, then the waist-to-hip ratio may be more appropriate. An increasing waist-to-hip ratio in older non-smoking men and women (≥75 years) has been shown to be associated with increasing risk of circulatory mortality (9). This would be in keeping with the evidence that abdominal adiposity is an important risk factor for circulatory mortality (8). The weight of a person is the combination of at least four components and consists of bone plus muscle plus fat plus water. The possibility of significant variations in each of the components of this collective is rarely

BMI Level	Relative Risk (95% Confidence Interval) by Age Category		
	25-59 y	60-69 y	≥70 y
Overall			
<18.5	1.38 (0.82-2.32)	2.30 (1.70-3.13)	1.69 (1.38-2.07)
<18.5 to <25	1.00	1.00	1.00
25 to <30	0.83 (0.65-1.06)	0.93 (0.80-1.13)	0.91 (0.83-1.01)
30 to <30	1.20 (0.84-1.72)	1.13 (0.89-1.42)	1.03 (0.91-1.17)
>35	1.83 (1.27-2.62)	1.63 (1.16-2.30)	1.17 (0.94-1.47)
Never-Smokers Only			
<18.5	1.25 (0.29-5.49)	2.97 (1.17-7.54)	1.50 (1.11-2.02)
18.5 to <25	1.00	1.00	1.00
25 to <30	0.66 (0.38-1.16)	0.81 (0.56-1.16)	0.90 (0.79-1.04)
30 to <30	0.77 (0.46-1.28)	1.21 (0.83-1.77)	1.13 (0.96-1.31)
>35	1.25 (0.76-2.06)	2.30 (1.47-3.59)	1.12 (0.87-1.45)

Abbreviations BMI, body mass index (increased as weight in kilograms divided by the square of height in meters): NHANES, National Health and Nutrition Examination Survey

Reproduced with permission from Flegal et al JAMA 2005[7]

Figure 23.1. Relative risks by age group and BMI level from the combined NHANES I,II and III Data set. Reproduced from Flegal et al. Excess deaths associated with underweight, overweight, and obesity. *JAMA* 2005; **293**: 1861–1867. Copyright © 2005, the American Medical Association

considered. Consequently a possible flaw is the notion that the use of BMI to define overweight and obesity is accurate and is directly measuring fat levels.

The next issue becomes whether weight can be lost safely. Water decreases initially when attempts are made to lose weight. Additionally adiposity decreases with weight loss too (10). Unfortunately bone mass also decreases with weight loss. This was confirmed by a study conducted by Ensrud who looked at 1342 men aged 65 and over from two centres, who were participating in the Osteoporotic Fractures in Men Study (11). The essential exclusion criteria were men with a history of bilateral hip replacement and those who were unable to walk without assistance from another person. They were followed for an average of 1.8 years to determine the amount of weight change and any change in bone mineral density. Figure 23.2 shows the mean annualized percentage change in total hip bone mineral density (BMD) by category of percent weight change and intention to lose weight. BMD was lost as weight was lost whether intentional or not. The same pattern was also seen in overweight people with BMI $>30 \, \text{kg/m}^2$ when weight was lost. Therefore,

older men who lose weight have increased rates of hip bone loss. Weight bearing exercise is known to be of benefit in the preservation of bone mass (12).

The final component of weight to consider is muscle. With increasing age, if weight is maintained, there is a loss of 1.5 kg of fat free mass per decade (13). The recommended dietary intake of protein for older people may be inadequate to maintain muscle mass. A 14 week study by Campbell provided 10 older men with a diet containing 0.8 g/kg/day of protein (current recommended dietary intake) (14). By week 14, mid-thigh muscle area was decreased by 1.7 +/− 0.6 cm^2 (p = .019) when compared with week 2. Therefore, a simple recommendation of reducing oral intake would most likely result in a further reduction in dietary protein intake and so muscle loss. Including all age groups, a meta-regression revealed that diets where protein intake was greater than 1.05 g/kg/day were associated with an additional retention of fat free mass versus diets containing less than 1.05 g/kg/day and this retention increased when the diets were longer than 12 weeks[10]. Diets consisting of ≤35 % carbohydrate resulted in a greater loss of lean

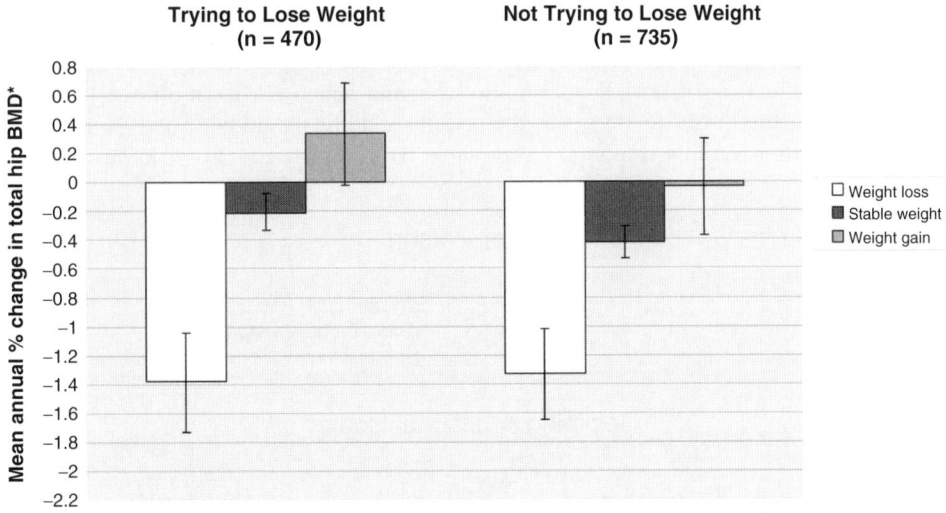

* Adjusted for age; health status; physical level; smoking status; alcohol use; total calcium intake; history of one or more select medical conditions including stroke, diabetes, hyperthyroidism, hypothyroidism, Parkinson;s disease, coronary heart disease; congestive heart failure, chronic obstructive lung disease, and non-skin cancer, body mass index; lean mass; leg power; and total hip bone density.

Figure 23.2. Bone mineral density change with weight loss. Reproduced with permission of The Endocrine Society from Ensrud et al., *J Clin Endocrinol Metab* **2005; 90**: 1998–2004

mass than diets containing $>41.4\%$ carbohydrate and this loss increased when the duration of the diet was more than 12 weeks (10). Low carbohydrate diets are associated with significantly greater fat free mass loss than high carbohydrate diets and an increase in protein intake is required to mitigate this loss somewhat. Exercise may also be of some benefit in ensuring maintenance of muscle or fat free mass. In a small study of 27 obese elderly people randomized to a control group and a treatment group which underwent an exercise programme and behavioural therapy for weight loss, compared to the control group, fat mass reduced (8.4% lost) without a significant reduction in fat free mass in the treatment group (15). The safety and effectiveness of weight reduction medications in older people need evaluation and so cannot be recommended for use in older people (16).

NUTRITIONAL FRAILTY

What is frailty? There are many definitions but that provided by Rockwood is perhaps the most clinically understandable (17). Frailty is "a vulnerable state of health, arising from the complex interaction of medical and social problems, resulting in a decreased ability to respond to stress, and associated with a decline in functional performance".

Under-nutrition contributes to frailty in the older person. Nutritional frailty (Figure 23.3) is the disability that occurs in old age due to rapid, unintentional loss of body weight and sarcopenia (18). The term 'Anorexia of Ageing' refers to the physiological decline in energy intake and appetite that occurs with progressive ageing (19, 20). This reduction in energy intake often exceeds the decrease in energy expenditure that occurs with normal physiological ageing, so body weight is unintentionally lost (21). When body weight decreases in older people, lean body tissue is thought to be lost disproportionately (sarcopenia) (21, 22). A complex interaction exists between unintentional weight loss, sarcopenia and the numerous health, physical, social and psychological insults that occur with increasing age, and this in turn can result in increasing physical frailty and its undesirable outcomes which include nursing home placement, falls, malnutrition, immobilization and increased dependency and eventually death (18, 23).

UNDER-NUTRITION IN OLDER PEOPLE

This is an area that has been consistently overlooked. To date, the percentage of older underweight Australians is still not known through the Australian census data and this may be complicated somewhat by the debate as to what the actual BMI cut-off for underweight in the elderly should be. There is a suggestion that BMIs between $20-22 \, \text{kg/m}^2$ should be

The Older Person

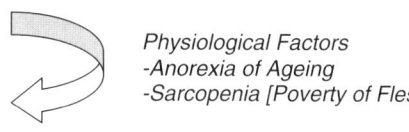

Physiological Factors
-Anorexia of Ageing
-Sarcopenia [Poverty of Flesh]

Declining Nutritional Health

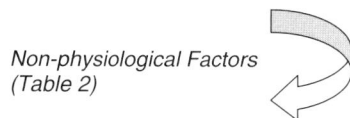

Non-physiological Factors
(Table 2)

Nutritional Frailty

Figure 23.3. The spiral of decline to nutritional frailty

the lower cut-off, there being differences with different ethnic groups and gender, but more evidence is required (24, 25). This notion of a higher BMI cut-off point is also supported by the results of a large prospective study of 1 million adults where the lowest death rates from all causes were at BMIs between 23.5 and 24.9 for men and 22.0 and 23.4 for women (26). Relative risks were not significantly increased for the range of BMIs between 22.0 and 26.4 in men and 20.5 and 24.9 in women in that study.

In three recent Australian studies 20 % of acute hospital inpatients, 30 % of sub-acute hospital inpatients and 5 % of community dwelling domiciliary care recipients were malnourished as defined by the Mini Nutritional Assessment (MNA) (27–29) (Figure 23.4). The respective figures for being at-risk of malnourishment were 30 %, 45 % and 40 % This gives a combined rate of under-nutrition (malnutrition and risk of malnutrition) at greater than 40 % in older people in the three different settings—particularly 50 % in the acute care hospital, 75 % in the sub-acute hospital and 45 % in the community.

Under-nutrition is associated with poor health (Table 23.1). However, it may be difficult to determine which comes first - under-nutrition or poor health. For example, poor health may lead to reduced oral intake and poor nutritional health as seen in many hospitalized patients. Nutritional status often deteriorates after admission to an acute hospital when there can be inadequate intake of food for days at a time (30). In one study from Scotland,

Table 23.1. Adverse effects of under-nutrition. Reproduced from *Am J Med* 2006; 119:1019–1026. Copyright © 2006, Elsevier

The adverse effects

- increased mortality
- frequent and prolonged hospitalisation
- institutionalization (i.e. being placed in nursing homes)
- increased falls and hip fractures
- increased post-operative complications
- delayed wound healing
- immune impairment and increased infections
- development of pressure sores
- increased health care costs
- increased health care utilization
- reduced quality of life.
- cognitive impairment
- anemia

40 % of patients admitted to an acute hospital were under-nourished and 75 % of those that were under-nourished had lost weight during the hospital stay when reassessed at discharge (31). In contrast to this, poor nutritional health could also lead to poor health and disability. For example, an older person with reduced oral intake and poor nutritional health would experience unintentional weight loss and lose muscle mass and develop sarcopenia (18). This would put them at risk of falls and hip fracture (32). Should a hip fracture occur, this could lead to reduced mobility, increased frailty, institutionalization or death- Nutritional Frailty (32, 33). In a prospective study of patients admitted to 5 tertiary centres with serious medical illnesses, BMI below or equal to the

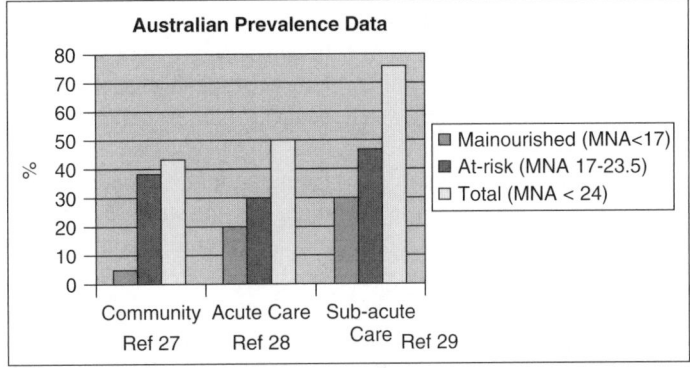

Figure 23.4. How common is under-nutrition in older people?

Table 23.2. Factors associated of under-nutrition in older people (35). Reproduced from *Nutrition* 2000; 16:983–995. Copyright © 2000, Elsevier

Physiological Factors	Social Factors	Emotional and Cognitive Factors
Reduced Taste	poverty	Alcoholism
Reduced Appetite	inability to shop	Depression
Early Satiety	inability to prepare and cook meals	Bereavement
Sarcopenia	inability to feed oneself	Cognitive Impairment
Cachexia	living alone	Abnormal Food Restriction (cholesterol phobia)
Medical Factors	social isolation	
Acute and Chronic Illness	failure of meal services or institutions	
Medications (Table 21.3)	to cater to ethnic food preferences	
Poor Dentition	lack of staff at institutions	
Impaired Vision		

15th percentile was associated with increased risk of mortality (Risk Ratio 1.23; $P < 0.01$) when compared to the reference 15th to 85th percentile (34). Many factors have been shown to be associated with the poor nutritional health of older people and can be viewed as risk factors (Table 23.2).

SCREENING AND ASSESSMENT OF UNDER-NUTRITION

In the acute hospital setting, usually at the time of major illness, nutrition has been the one area of acute care that has been side-stepped at the time it is most needed. Over the first two weeks of hospital stay, parameters of nutrition decrease in many patients (36). It has been an area rarely acknowledged by doctors and infrequently specifically treated in the hospital setting (37).

Assessment of nutrition provides an opportunity for holistic care. Evaluation and management should encompass all aspects of care. The pathological causes of weight loss and poor nutrition need a diagnostic evaluation because appropriate intervention can help. Social factors such as poverty, isolation, and lack of services can be addressed. Psychological (cognitive) problems such as dementia, depression and alcoholism can be screened for. Poor dentition, taste and smell are frequently not recognized, and medication review is essential. Factors in Tables 23.2 and 23.3 that can be addressed should be managed in all patients to avoid the risk of developing poor nutritional health (i.e.

prevention). Where these risk factors exist but there is a need not to alter management for medical reasons, then monitoring of nutritional health is required to ensure that under-nutrition does not develop.

The first step for the practitioner is to have a high index of suspicion for the contribution of protein-calorie malnutrition and its contribution to the presenting state. This requires acceptance of its importance and its possible contribution to the clinical picture. There are some specific signs of protein-calorie malnutrition (Table 23.4). These features may be difficult to recognize, if not thought of or looked for, amongst the signs and drama of the presenting illness.

At a bare minimum, screening for under-nutrition should occur routinely in clinical practice. Screening should occur before assessment. When risk is confirmed, the presence of disease should be confirmed using assessment tools or skilled clinicians (described later). There are many screening tools and frequently a lot of time is spent arguing as to which tool is the best. However, given that mostly screening does not occur, it is the opinion of the authors that perhaps it is best to use the tool that is best suited for individual clinical practice rather than arguing about the strengths and weaknesses of individual screening tools. Any form of screening would be better than nothing. Below, several screening tools are described.

The Mini Nutritional Assessment is an easily administered, valid (in the elderly) and widely used screening tool that can be performed

Table 23.3. Frequently used classes of medications (and some examples) and the frequency of reported adverse effects that may detrimentally affect nutritional health

Medication Class	Reported Adverse Effects (http://www.rxlist.com)
	—the % below is those reported in subjects taking medication. Some of the same symptoms were also reported in the placebo arm sometimes to the same extent but this is not described below. Therefore, not always is the symptom conclusively attributable to the medication.
Non Steroidal Anti-Inflammatory Drugs	
Indomethacin	Nausea, vomiting, dyspepsia, abdominal pain, diarrhoea, constipation-(all >1%), anorexia (<1%)
Cardiac Medications	
Digoxin	Dose dependent- anorexia, nausea, vomiting—almost 25% of adverse events
Diltiazem (calcium channel blocker)	Nausea, anorexia, constipation, diarrhoea, dry mouth, altered taste (all<2%)
Atenolol (beta-blocker)	Depression (<2%), fatigue (3–6%), tiredness (up to 26%), nausea (3%)
Perindopril (angiotensin converting enzyme inhibitor)	Dyspepsia (<2%), abdominal pain (2.7%), vomiting (1.5%), somnolence (1.3%)
Spironolactone (potassium sparing diuretic)	Gastric bleeding, gastric ulceration, gastritis, nausea and vomiting (% not stated)
Frusemide (loop diuretic)	Pancreatitis, nausea, vomiting, diarrhoea, constipation, gastric irritation (% not stated)
Simvastatin (HMG-CoA reductase inhibitor)	Constipation (2.3%), dyspepsia (1.1%), abdominal Pain (3.2%)
Antibiotics (examples)	
Augmentin	Diarrhoea (2.5%), vomiting (1.4%)
Cephalexin	Dyspepsia, gastritis, nausea, vomiting and diarrhoea have been reported
Trimethoprim	Nausea, vomiting and glossitis have been reported
Opioids	
Oxycodone	Nausea, vomiting, sedation
Bladder Agents	
Ditropan	Dry mouth (61%), constipation (13%), nausea (9%), somnolence (12%)
Anti-Parkinsonian Medication	
Sinemet (carbidopa-levodopa)	Dry mouth, taste alteration, diarrhoea, duodenal ulceration, constipation, dyspepsia, somnolence
Diabetic Medications	
Metformin (biguanide)	Diarrhoea (53%), nausea and vomiting (26%), taste disorder (2–5%).
Glipizide (sulphonylurea)	Nausea and diarrhoea (1.5%), constipation (1%), gastralgia (1%), drowsiness (2%)
Bisphosphonates	
Risedronate	Abdominal pain (9.4%), nausea (10.7%), diarrhoea (9.6%), gastritis (2.3%)
Benzodiazepines	
Temazepam	Nausea (3.1%), drowsiness (9.1%), diarrhoea (1.7%), abdominal discomfort (1.5%)
Cognitive Agents	
Donepezil (acteylcholinesterase inhibitor)	Anorexia, nausea, diarrhoea, vomiting-up to 5%
Memantine (NMDA receptor antagonist)	Constipation (3%), vomiting (2%), somnolence (2%)
Anti-depressants	
Sertraline (selective serotonin reuptake inhibitor)	Dry mouth (14%), diarrhoea (20%), nausea, anorexia (6%),
Amitriptyline (tricyclic)	Constipation, dry mouth, nausea, anorexia, vomiting, dysgeusia.

This list is not exhaustive but is merely there to illustrate that side-effects are reported frequently with medication use and it may interfere with oral intake and contribute to under-nutrition

Table 23.4. Clinical presentation of protein-calorie malnutrition in the older person; Features associated with poor nutritional health

- wasting of fat and muscle
- generalized weakness
- dry skin
- flaking dermatitis
- thin hair, easily removed
- peripheral oedema
- abdominal distension
- hepatomegaly
- parotid enlargement
- transverse lines on nails
- hyperpigmented plaques over areas of trauma

in about 10 minutes that does not need biochemical testing or nutritional training (38, 39). It comprises anthropometic measures (weight, height and weight loss), a global assessment (of six questions relating to lifestyle, medication and mobility), a dietary assessment (of eight questions dealing with number of meals, food and fluid intake, and autonomy of feeding) and a subjective assessment (of self-perception of health and nutrition).

The Malnutrition Universal Screening Tool (MUST) is widely used in the United Kingdom and has been shown to have a good agreement with the Subjective Global Assesment (40). An overall risk of malnutrition is assessed by totalling scores for a low BMI, weight loss, the presence of acute illness and the likelihood of experienced reduced oral intake of more than five days. Management guidelines for those classified as medium or high risk by the tool also exist.

A low BMI and weight loss are known to contribute greatly towards mortality and morbidity in older people and are the two most important contributors to a low MNA score so a simple assessment incorporating those two variables could also possibly function as a quick measure of under-nutrition. Our study has shown that the Rapid Screen, consisting of one or both of BMI $<22\,\mathrm{kg/m^2}$ and reported weight loss of greater than 7.5 % in the preceding three months, was as effective as the above two tools in that all indicated those malnourished and those with poor discharge outcomes (28). In this paper, it was recommended that

when resources permit, the MNA might be the screening instrument of choice. When resources are more limited, the Rapid Screen is a simple yet effective tool.

There is no one accepted gold standard for the diagnosis of under-nutrition in older people. In most instances, the accepted gold standard is confirmation of poor nutritional health by trained specialist (dieticians). However, in clinical practice, there may be logistical barriers to obtaining a diagnosis by a skilled dietician. In such instances, the use of assessment tools may be of benefit.

The subjective global assessment (SGA) is a widely used clinical tool for the assessment of nutritional status (41). It requires the clinician to identify in the history the following: the presence of gastrointestinal symptoms, weight loss, functional dysfunction and illness and a change in dietary intake. Physical examination is required to determine loss of subcutaneous fat and muscle and the presence of oedema and ascites. A water test is also administered to assess swallowing but there is no need for laboratory investigations. From here, the patient is classified as well-nourished, moderately malnourished or severely malnourished. Compared to the Standardized Nutritional Assessment (see below), there is more subjectivity with the SGA but it has been shown that with training there is a good inter-observer reliability (kappa = 0.78; P = 0.001) (41).

The Standardised Nutritional Assessment (SNA) was devised based on the usual clinical practices of the dietitians working in a sub-acute facility in South Australia and may be of some benefit in some settings (28). The criteria assessed include total lymphocyte count, serum albumen level, total cholesterol concentration, number of risk factors (from nausea, vomiting, diarrhoea, constipation, difficulty chewing or swallowing, history of gastro-intestinal disease), percentage of unintentional weight loss over three months (which is subjective) and BMI. There are cut-off values for normal, borderline and under-nourished and a scoring system allows allocation to normal, mild or moderate-severe under-nourished groups.

THE MANAGEMENT OF THE UNDER-NOURISHED OLDER PERSON

Non-pharmacological Managment

When under-nutrition is confirmed, then ideally advice should be sought from a dietician specifically with regards to enhancing nutrient content and taste (flavour enhancement) or the use of nutritional supplements (either snacks or energy drinks). Dietary advice can also be based on published guidelines (Table 23.5). Another useful source of dietary advice is at http://www.MyPyramid.gov which actually helps a person choose the foods and amounts that are right for that individual. It is a website created by the Centre for Nutrition Policy and Promotion, an organization of the United States Department of Agriculture. My Pyramid Plan is based on the information provided about an individual and the average needs for that person's age, gender and physical activity level. The results indicate the amounts one should eat from five food groups daily, namely grains, vegetables, fruits, milk, meat and beans. It provides specific advice for daily intake for that person with the crucial link being the amount of physical activity. When dysphagia is present, the speech therapist may need to require some

Table 23.5. Dietary guidelines for older Australians-National Health and Medical Research Council (http://www.nhmrc.health.gov.au)

1. enjoy a wide variety of nutritious foods
2. keep active to maintain muscle strength and body weight
3. eat at least three meals every day
4. care for your food: prepare and store it correctly
5. eat plenty of vegetables (including legumes) and fruit
6. eat plenty of cereals, breads and pastas
7. eat a diet low in saturated fat
8. drink adequate amounts of water and/or other fluids
9. if you drink alcohol, limit your intake
10. choose foods low in salt and use salt sparingly
11. include foods high in calcium
12. use added sugars in moderation

food modification and the dietician may need to make specific recommendations with this in view. Adequate hydration is always important.

Treating clinicians should counsel patients and their families making them aware of the need for good nutrition to avert ill health. When possible, families should play a role by either providing financial assistance, preparing food or eating with the older person. Meals on Wheels may be of benefit in settings where food may need to be prepared for the client but clinicians should be aware that this is a supplementary service and can not meet the total dietary needs of older people. Older people should be encouraged to eat in the company of others. The help of an occupational therapist may be of benefit in settings where devices to assist feeding may be required. Where community service providers are involved and care packages exist, then services could be tailored to assist with shopping and meal preparation ensuring that nutritious food is prepared in the usual way the older person would have made it.

Patients in nursing homes are vulnerable and in addition to the above, consideration can be given to encouraging family to assist with feeding when there are resource constraints (i.e. lack of staff). Providing feeding assistance, enhancing nutrition quality and content, promoting socialization and enhancing comfort are likely to improve nutritional health. In a recent Danish study, when family-style dining which included the right ambiance in the dining hall, a member of staff eating with residents at a table and residents being able to choose their meal, was compared to the control group who chose their food 2 weeks before, had their medications dispensed during meals and had a choice of either eating in their room or to assigned seats, residents in the intervention arm maintained body weight and energy intake while both decreased in the control group (42, 43). Liberalizing diets as opposed to the prescription of restrictive diets is also more likely to enhance quality of life and food intake in long term care residents (44). Similarly, smaller but energy enhanced food has been shown to result in increased energy intake in comparison to standard meals (45).

Prescribed or Pharmacological Management

The routine prescription of protein and energy supplementation (commercial sip feeds) to all older people cannot be recommended. However, protein and energy supplementation has been shown to reduce mortality (OR 0.66 95 % CI 0.49–0.90) in malnourished hospitalized patients (46). Also, protein and energy supplementation in at-risk older people may result in some weight gain and reduction in mortality risk but has not been shown conclusively to be of benefit in reducing length of hospitalization or improving physical function and clinical outcomes (47).

Unfortunately for proponents of vitamins or anti-oxidant supplements, there is no compelling evidence that non-specific micro-nutrient supplementation really works. There is some suggestion that one multi-vitamin daily may be of benefit in older people (>65 years old) when used for more than 6 months but further trials are required to confirm this (48). Over-supplementation may result in adverse effects from vitamin overdose or excessive anti-oxidant activity. Perhaps the most useful public health action in this area is to consider vitamin D supplementation for older men and women who are deficient (with calcium), given the high prevalence of osteoporosis in the community (49).

The use of orexigenic agents and anabolic agents cannot be recommended due to adverse effects and a lack of evidence supporting benefits in older people. It can be debated that it may play a role in the terminal phases of malnutrition or cachexia. The use of mergestrol acetate for periods less than 3 months has been reported to be of benefit but it is associated with the development of adrenal insufficiency and deep vein thrombosis (50–52). Cannabinoids have been used to stimulate appetite in AIDS-related cachexia (53). It has been suggested that dronabinol which is a cannabinoid may be useful in stimulating appetite in older people with severe malnutrition which may be terminal (50). It can be associated with adverse effects such as sedation, tachycardia, hypotension and seizures (product information). Mirtazapine, an anti-depressant, has been shown to be associated with weight gain and when patients are depressed, it may be used in preference preferably at night (54). Growth hormone has been shown to have some beneficial effects on lean mass but is associated with adverse effects such as the development of diabetes, gynaecomastia and athralgia (55). A very recent randomized controlled trial in elderly subjects showed that neither dehydroepiandrosterone (in men and women) or bioavailable testosterone (in men only) supplementation was associated with benefits in body composition, quality of life or physical performance (56).

Very often in older patients with advanced dementia, the dilemma about the need for percutaneous enteral gastrostomy (PEG) feeding arises. In some ways, advanced directives by patients earlier in the disease process are required to provide guidance in management decisions. But where there is no directive, then often families need to weigh the pros and cons of treatment with clinicians. The goal of any treatment regimen should include an aim to improve quality of life and not merely prolong life. It is known that the majority of older people with PEG placement do not survive beyond one year (57). At least five cohort studies in nursing home residents have shown no benefits to survival with PEG feeding. (57) Only one cohort study in a group of patients with amyotrophic lateral sclerosis showed a survival benefit (57). Therefore, in some patients where there is the potential to improve functional health and quality of life there may be a role for PEG feeding. However, in many cases, failure to eat or thrive is due to the patient entering into the terminal phase of an illness (e.g. advanced dementia) (58). In such cases, the recommendation for PEG feeding may actually reduce quality of life. In many cases, the institution of PEG feeding is associated with denial of oral intake and it could be argued that this impacts significantly on quality of life as being able to taste food is one of life's pleasures. A qualitative study of PEG fed adults and their carers revealed that oral intake of food and fluid was missed (59). While the practice is frowned upon in some countries, the use of physical restraints to prevent the older person from pulling the PEG out is likely to have a detrimental effect on quality of life (60). There is also some evidence that PEG feeding is associated with an increased risk of pressure ulcer formation (60). PEG feeding has not been shown to maintain skin integrity, prevent malnutrition and reduce aspiration risk (60). Therefore, in such cases, a realistic discussion with regards to the evidence and likely discomforts should occur with the family to enable them to make an informed decision. From the evidence, PEG feeding is more detrimental than of benefit to patients with advanced dementia but cultural and religious beliefs should also be taken into consideration (60).

MONITORING AND CHANGE

With any management plan, monitoring for improvement or adverse effects is essential. If benefits or adverse effects are seen, there is a need to reassess, re-evaluate and institute a change to the management plan.

CONCLUSION

Attention to nutritional health in the older person is important. Malnutrition (over- and under-nutrition) is a clinical challenge that requires early intervention because of poor outcomes but especially because it can respond well to corrective measures, that may be simple, but potentially life saving. Obesity is associated with ill health and disability. Weight loss programmes should be individually tailored and preservation of muscle mass is essential. This is an emerging area of research interest. Elderly people losing weight is a common clinical problem that may herald numerous medical and psychosocial disorders. It must not be overlooked. After careful history, thorough physical examination and judicious laboratory investigations, a clinician can accurately identify most patients/clients who have a physical cause for weight loss. That weight loss and the associated under-nutrition might required the identification of and dealing with multiple contributing

factors like so many other scenarios in geriatric medicine.

REFERENCES

1. WHO. Obesity: *Preventing and Managing the Global Epidemic*. Report of a WHO Consultation on Obesitt. Geneva 1998.
2. Statistics AB. Health Risk Factors, Australia, 2001: 4812.0. Available at: http://www.abs.gov.au/Ausstats/abs@.nsf/0e5fa1cc95cd093c4a2568110007852b/b8b08eafca9de7b3ca256dfc0083adf0!OpenDocument.
3. Groves T. Pandemic obesity in Europe. *BMJ* 2006; **333**: 1081.
4. Kopelman P. Health risks associated with overweight and obesity. *Obes Rev* 2007; **8** Suppl 1: 13–17.
5. Amador LF, Al Snih S, Markides KS et al. Weight change and mortality among older Mexican Americans. *Aging Clin Exp Res* 2006; **18**: 196–204.
6. Wannamethee SG, Shaper AG, Lennon L. Reasons for intentional weight loss, unintentional weight loss, and mortality in older men. *Arch Intern Med* 2005; **165**: 1035–40.
7. Flegal KM, Graubard BI, Williamson DF et al. Excess deaths associated with underweight, overweight, and obesity. *JAMA* 2005; **293**: 1861–7.
8. Janssen I, Mark AE. Elevated body mass index and mortality risk in the elderly. *Obes Rev* 2007; **8**: 41–59.
9. Price GM, Uauy R, Breeze E et al. Weight, shape and mortality risk in older persons: elevated waist-hip ratio, not high body mass index, is asociated with a greater risk of death. *Am J Clin Nutr* 2006; **84**: 449–60.
10. Krieger JW, Sitren HS, Daniels MJ et al. Effects of variation in protein and carbohydrate intake on body mass and composition during energy restriction: a meta-regression 1. *Am J Clin Nutr* 2006; **83**: 260–74.
11. Ensrud KE, Fullman RL, Barrett-Connor E et al. Voluntary weight reduction in older men increases hip bone loss: the osteoporotic fractures in men study. *J Clin Endocrinol Metab* 2005; **90**: 1998–2004.
12. Kemmler W, Lauber D, Weineck J et al. Benefits of 2 years of intense exercise on bone density, physical fitness, and blood lipids in early postmenopausal osteopenic women: results of the Erlangen Fitness Osteoporosis Prevention

Study (EFOPS). *Arch Intern Med* 2004; **164**: 1084–91.

13. Forbes GB. Longitudinal changes in adult fat-free mass: influence of body weight. *Am J Clin Nutr* 1999; **70**: 1025–31.

14. Campbell WW, Trappe TA, Wolfe RR et al. The recommended dietary allowance for protein may not be adequate for older people to maintain skeletal muscle. *J Gerontol A Biol Sci Med Sci* 2001; **56**: M373–380.

15. Villareal DT, Banks M, Sinacore DR et al. Effect of weight loss and exercise on frailty in obese older adults. *Arch Intern Med* 2006; **166**: 860–6.

16. Ioannides-Demos LL, Proietto J, Tonkin AM et al. Safety of drug therapies used for weight loss and treatment of obesity. *Drug Saf* 2006; **29**: 277–302.

17. Rockwood K, Fox RA, Stolee P et al. Frailty in elderly people: an evolving concept. *CMAJ* 1994; **150**: 489–95.

18. Bales CW, Ritchie CS. Sarcopenia, weight loss, and nutritional frailty in the elderly. *Annu Rev Nutr* 2002; **22**: 309–23.

19. Wurtman JJ, Lieberman H, Tsay R et al. Calorie and nutrient intakes of elderly and young subjects measured under identical conditions. *J Gerontol* 1988; **43**: B174–80.

20. Morley JE. Anorexia of aging: physiologic and pathologic. *Am J Clin Nutr* 1997; **66**: 760–73.

21. Forbes GB, Reina JC. Adult lean body mass declines with age: some longitudinal observations. *Metabolism* 1970; **19**: 653–63.

22. Chapman IM. Endocrinology of anorexia of ageing. *Best Pract Res Clin Endocrinol Metab* 2004; **18**: 437–52.

23. de Jong N. Nutrition and senescence: healthy aging for all in the new millennium? *Nutrition* 2000; **16**: 537–41.

24. Committee on Diet and Health, Food and Nutrition Board, Comission on Life Sciences et al. *Implications for reducing chronic disease risk*. Washington DC: National Academy Press, 1989.

25. Deurenberg P, Deurenberg-Yap M, Guricci S. Asians are different from Caucasians and from each other in their body mass index/body fat per cent relationship. *Obes Rev* 2002; **3**: 141–6.

26. Calle EE, Thun MJ, Petrelli JM et al. Body-mass index and mortality in a prospective cohort of U.S. adults. *N Engl J Med* 1999; **341**: 1097–1105.

27. Visvanathan R, Macintosh C, Callary M et al. The nutritional status of 250 older Australian recipients of domiciliary care services and its association with outcomes at 12 months. *J Am Geriatr Soc* 2003; **51**: 1007–11.

28. Visvanathan R, Penhall R, Chapman I. Nutritional screening of older people in a sub-acute care facility in Australia and its relation to discharge outcomes. *Age Ageing* 2004; **33**: 260–5.

29. Barone L, Milosavljevic M, Gazibarich B. Assessing the older person: is the MNA a more appropriate nutritional assessment tool than the SGA? *J Nutr Health Aging* 2003; **7**: 13–17.

30. Sullivan DH, Sun S, Walls RC. Protein-energy undernutrition among elderly hospitalized patients: a prospective study. *JAMA* 1999; **281**: 2013–19.

31. Williams CM, Driver LT, Lumbers M. Nutrition in the older hospital patient. *J Roy Soc Health* 1990; **110**: 41–2, 44.

32. Baumgartner RN, Waters DL, Gallagher D et al. Predictors of skeletal muscle mass in elderly men and women. *Mech Ageing Dev* 1999; **107**: 123–36.

33. Rolland Y, Kim MJ, Gammack JK et al. Office management of weight loss in older persons. *Am J Med* 2006; **119**: 1019–26.

34. Galanos AN, Pieper CF, Kussin PS et al. Relationship of body mass index to subsequent mortality among seriously ill hospitalized patients. SUPPORT Investigators. The Study to Understand Prognoses and Preferences for Outcome and Risks of Treatments. *Crit Care Med* 1997; **25**: 1962–8.

35. MacIntosh C, Morley JE, Chapman IM. The anorexia of aging. *Nutrition* 2000; **16**: 983–95.

36. Omran ML, Morley JE. Assessment of protein energy malnutrition in older persons, Part II: Laboratory evaluation. *Nutrition* 2000; **16**: 131–40.

37. McWhirter JP, Pennington CR. Incidence and recognition of malnutrition in hospital. *BMJ* 1994; **308**: 945–8.

38. Guigoz Y, Vellas B, Garry P. *Mini Nutritional Assessment: a practical assessment tool for grading the nutritional state of elderly patients*. Paris: Serdi Publishing Company, 1994.

39. Guigoz Y, Vellas B, Garry PJ. Assessing the nutritional status of the elderly: The Mini Nutritional Assessment as part of the geriatric evaluation. *Nutr Rev* 1996; **54**: S59–65.

40. Stratton RJ, Hackston A, Longmore D et al. Malnutrition in hospital outpatients and inpatients: prevalence, concurrent validity and ease of use of the 'malnutrition universal screening

tool' ('MUST') for adults. *Br J Nutr* 2004; **92**: 799–808.

41. Detsky AS, McLaughlin JR, Baker JP et al. What is subjective global assessment of nutritional status? *JPEN J Parenter Enteral Nutr* 1987; **11**: 8–13.

42. Nijs KA, de Graaf C, Kok FJ et al. Effect of family style mealtimes on quality of life, physical performance, and body weight of nursing home residents: cluster randomised controlled trial. *BMJ* 2006; **332**: 1180–4.

43. Nijs KA, de Graaf C, Siebelink E et al. Effect of family-style meals on energy intake and risk of malnutrition in dutch nursing home residents: a randomized controlled trial. *J Gerontol A Biol Sci Med Sci* 2006; **61**: 935–42.

44. Womack P, Breeding C. Position of the American Dietetic Association: liberalized diets for older adults in long-term care. *J Am Diet Assoc* 1998; **98**: 201–4.

45. Lorefalt B, Wissing U, Unosson M. Smaller but energy and protein-enriched meals improve energy and nutrient intakes in elderly patients. *J Nutr Health Aging* 2005; **9**: 243–7.

46. Milne AC, Avenell A, Potter J. Meta-analysis: protein and energy supplementation in older people. *Ann Intern Med* 2006; **144**: 37–48.

47. Milne AC, Potter J, Avenell A. Protein and energy supplementation in elderly people at risk from malnutrition. *Cochrane Database Syst Rev* 2005; CD003288.

48. Stephen AI, Avenell A. A systematic review of multivitamin and multimineral supplementation for infection. *J Hum Nutr Diet* 2006; **19**: 179–90.

49. Avenell A, Gillespie WJ, Gillespie LD et al. Vitamin D and vitamin D analogues for preventing fractures associated with involutional and post-menopausal osteoporosis. *Cochrane Database Syst Rev* 2005; CD000227.

50. Morley JE. Orexigenic and anabolic agents. *Clin Geriatr Med* 2002; **18**: 853–66.

51. Chidakel AR, Zweig SB, Schlosser JR et al. High prevalence of adrenal suppression during acute illness in hospitalized patients receiving megestrol acetate. *J Endocrinol Invest* 2006; **29**: 136–40.

52. Marshall LL. Megestrol acetate therapy in geriatric patients: case reviews and associated deep vein thrombosis. *Consult Pharm* 2003; **18**: 764–73.

53. Walsh D, Nelson KA, Mahmoud FA. Established and potential therapeutic applications of cannabinoids in oncology. *Support Care Cancer* 2003; **11**: 137–43.

54. Laimer M, Kramer-Reinstadler K, Rauchenzauner M et al. Effect of mirtazapine treatment on body composition and metabolism. *J Clin Psychiatry* 2006; **67**: 421–4.

55. Liu H, Bravata DM, Olkin I et al. Systematic review: the safety and efficacy of growth hormone in the healthy elderly. *Ann Intern Med* 2007; **146**: 104–15.

56. Nair KS, Rizza RA, O'Brien P et al. DHEA in elderly women and DHEA or testosterone in elderly men. *N Engl J Med* 2006; **355**: 1647–59.

57. Mitchell SL, Tetroe JM. Survival after percutaneous endoscopic gastrostomy placement in older persons. *J Gerontol A Biol Sci Med Sci* 2000; **55**: M735–9.

58. Galicia-Castillo M. The PEG dilemma: feeding tubes are not the answer in advanced dementia. *Geriatrics* 2006; **61**: 12–13.

59. Brotherton A, Abbott J, Aggett P. The impact of percutaneous endoscopic gastrostomy feeding upon daily life in adults. *J Hum Nutr Diet* 2006; **19**: 355–67.

60. Cervo FA, Bryan L, Farber S. To PEG or not to PEG: a review of evidence for placing feeding tubes in advanced dementia and the decision-making process. *Geriatrics* 2006; **61**: 30–5.

24 Mouth and dental disorders

Cees de Baat[1] and Isaac van der Waal[2]

[1]Department of Oral Function and Prosthetic Dentistry, Radboud University Medical Centre Nijmegen, Nijmegen,The Netherlands
[2]Department of Oral and Maxillofacial Surgery/Oral Pathology, Vrije Universiteit Medical Center, Amsterdam, The Netherlands

INTRODUCTION

Elderly people's quality of life can be affected by their oral status. For instance, edentulous elderly people wearing complete dentures have decreased chewing ability which may lead to loss of confidence and isolation from other people. Therefore, maintaining good oral health and delivering good quality oral health care to elderly people appear to be prerequisites for successful ageing.

Oral tissues undergo gradual changes in morphology and physiology during ageing. These changes may predispose the involved tissues to pathologic conditions. The occurrence and progress of most oral disorders in the elderly are the result of an interaction between degenerative age changes and pathologic conditions. Although very few oral disorders are characteristic of the elderly, many pathologic conditions are seen more frequently in old age. This chapter focuses on pathologic oral conditions that occur in the elderly which may be treated with medicines.

PERIODONTAL DISEASE

Introduction

Periodontal disease (gingivitis and periodontitis) refers to inflammatory processes in the tissues surrounding the teeth in response to bacterial accumulations in dento-gingival plaque. Dento-gingival plaque is divided into supra- and subgingival plaque. In dentate older individuals, periodontal disease is one of the most prevalent chronic conditions. The periodontal health of frail and functionally dependent elderly people is extremely poor because they are usually dependent on others for the daily removal of dento-gingival plaque. The enhanced severity of periodontal disease is related to the length of time the periodontal tissues have been exposed to dento-gingival bacterial plaque, reflecting the individual's cumulative periodontal history.

Aetiology

Supragingival plaque is dominated by facultative *Streptococcus* and *Actinomyces* species, whereas subgingival plaque harbours an anaerobic gram-negative flora which has been associated with periodontitis.

If left untreated, the dento-gingival plaque will become calcified, forming dental calculus, which is difficult to remove. Any medical condition which affects host antibacterial defence mechanisms, such as diabetes, immunodeficiency, neutrophil disorders, hyposalivation and smoking will predispose to periodontal disease.

Prescribing for Elderly Patients   Edited by Stephen Jackson, Paul Jansen and Arduino Mangoni
© 2009 John Wiley & Sons, Ltd

Symptoms and signs

The early stages of periodontal disease are easily overlooked or ignored because of lack of serious complaints. Eventually, the inflammatory process may result in loss of periodontal tissues and deepened periodontal pockets and, in advanced cases, of tooth mobility and finally tooth loss.

Diagnosis

A clinical examination is carried out in order to assess colour, shape, consistency and contour of the attached gingiva, the marginal gingiva, and the gingival papillae. Plaque deposits, gingival bleeding and pocket depths can be assessed on probing. Probing pocket depths is the backbone of evaluation.

Therapy

A standard treatment approach consists of the combination of increase of the patient's daily oral self care, and regular professional treatment to remove newly formed deposits and calculus. Also in elderly people, periodontal disease can be treated successfully and the prognosis is generally good. Professional mechanical treatment may not eliminate all pathogens because they reside in sites inaccessible for dental instruments. Anti-microbial agents, delivered either locally into the periodontal pocket or systemically, enhance the effect of mechanical treatment. If daily oral self care is compromised, for instance in institutionalized elderly people, mouth rinses or sprays containing 0.2 % or 0.12 % chlorhexidine used daily are very effective in plaque removal. Long-term use is only limited because of its teeth staining side effect. In general, there is no role for systemic antibiotics.

References

Loesche WJ, Grossman NS. Periodontal disease as a specific, albeit chronic, infection: diagnosis and treatment. *Clin Microbiol Rev* 2001; **14**: 727–52.

Ogawa H, Yoshihara A, Hirotomi T, Ando Y, Miyazaki H. Risk factors for periodontal disease progression among elderly people. *J Clin Periodontol* 2002; **29**: 592–7.

DENTAL CARIES

Introduction

Dental caries is the result of gradual loss of calcium and phosphate from the hard tooth tissues. Many dentate older people have coronal and root caries.

Aetiology

Dental caries develops as a result of multiple acid attacks on the tooth surface produced by bacteria in dento-gingival plaque. Intermittent changes in acidity level give rise to demineralization and remineralization at the interface of tooth surface and dento-gingival plaque. The metabolic activities in the plaque may be modified by changes in dietary habits and salivary flow rate.

Symptoms and signs

The enamel surface from which calcium and phosphates are constantly dissolved and redeposited during the active phases of caries, appears clinically dull. As mineral is lost, the enamel becomes more porous. Finally, a clinically detectable cavity in enamel and dentin will result.

Diagnosis

Dental caries can be diagnosed by visual and tactile clinical signs including changes of contour and color and cavitation and by intra-oral radiographs.

Therapy

Restorative dental treatment is the treatment of choice. In order to prevent and control the disease an antimicrobial approach must be considered in order to achieve a shift from an ecologically unfavourable dento-gingival plaque to an ecologically stable biofilm. Fluoride is effective in reducing caries. Products can be either self applied or delivered by a professional. Brushing teeth twice daily with a fluoride toothpaste is the cornerstone of preventing and controlling dental caries. Additional fluoride may be delivered as an adjunct to those considered being at high caries risk, such as dependent elderly people. Fluoride gels, varnishes and tablets may be beneficial, whereas fluoride mouth rinses are not. If daily oral self care is compromised, chlorhexidine is the most effective anti-plaque agent. Mouth rinses or sprays containing 0.2 % or 0.12 % chlorhexidine used daily are very effective in plaque removal.

References

Arneberg P, Hossain ANMN, Jokstad A. Fluoride tablet programs in healthy elderly subjects: distribution of fluoride in saliva and plaque with tablets in different sites. *Acta Odontol Scand* 2005; **63**: 65–72.

Davies RM. The rational use of oral care products in the elderly. *Clin Oral Invest* 2004; **8**: 2–5.

ODONTOGENIC INFECTIONS

Introduction

Odontogenic infections are caused mainly by the destruction of enamel, dentine and periodontal tissues. Common odontogenic infections are pulpitis, apical periodontitis, localised abscess, periodontal abscess, pericoronitis and subperiostal or submucosal abscess.

Untreated odontogenic infections may involve the surrounding cellular adipose tissues. This involvement is called cellulitis. Distant spread can occur by means of the bloodstream or the lymphatic system.

Aetiology

When a carious lesion or a traumatic injury contaminates the dental pulp, pulpitis will follow which results ultimately in pulpnecrosis. Untreated necrosis may lead to apical periodontitis, a perapical granuloma, a periapical or radicular cyst and occasionally to abscess formation or extension into the surrounding soft tissues. In rare cases, periostitis and osteomyelitis of the jaw may occur. If periodontal disease progresses gram-negative anaerobes predominate and an acute periodontal abscess may occur. Pericoronitis around an erupting or partially erupted tooth occurs when bacterial plaque and food debris accumulate beneath the mucosal flap covering the partial erupted tooth.

Symptoms and signs

In case of apical periodontitis, following pulpitis, the involved tooth is usually painful. Pain may be exacerbated by temperature changes and the tooth may be tender to percussion and shows increased mobility. A localized, subperiostal or submucosal abscess may form with fever and illness. Left untreated, the abscess may rupture or, less commonly, progress to cellulitis.

Inflammatory edema, pain, local tenderness, a bad taste caused by pus oozing from beneath the mucosal flap, and regional lympadenopathy are common symptoms of pericoronitis. Cellulitis and trismus may occur, especially if a wisdom tooth is involved. In case of cellulitis, regional lymphadenopathy is common and fever may be present. The infection may spread into the major fascial spaces of the head and the neck. Attendant serious risks are airway obstruction, orbital infections, sinus cavernous thrombosis, cerebral abscess and mediastinitis.

Diagnosis

The provisional diagnosis of odontogenic infections is based on clinical signs and symptoms. Panoramic and intraoral radiographs are helpful diagnostic tools.

Therapy

Management consists primarily of dental or surgical treatment, such as incision and drainage. Antibiotics are of no additional benefit, unless immunocompromised conditions occur or serious complications, such as fever and cellulitis. Pain should be managed with appropriate analgetics such as paracetamol and nonsteroidal anti-inflammatory drugs (NSAIDs). A direct incision of an apical or periodontal abscess may release pus.

Localized forms of cellulitis should be managed with dental treatment. If serious spreading occurs and/or dental treatment is delayed, anti-streptococcal oral antibiotics, such as penicillin in a dosage of 500 mg three times daily are indicated.

References

Matthews DC, Sutherland S, Basrani B. Emergency management of acute apical abcesses in the permanent dentition: A systematic review of the literature. *J Can Dent Assoc* 2003; **69**: 660.

Storoe W, Haug RH, Lillich TT. The changing face of odontogenic infections. *J Oral Maxillofac Surg* 2001: **59**: 739–48.

ALVEOLAR OSTEITIS

Introduction

Alveolar osteitis is an inflammatory complication occurring after tooth extraction. The local inflammation inside and around the tooth alveolus is accompanied by disintegration of the intra-alveolar blood clot.

Occurrence has been reported in 0.5–5 % of all tooth extractions. Alveolar osteitis occurs 10 times more often after removal of impacted mandibular wisdom teeth as compared to other tooth extractions.

Aetiology

This complication is most frequently associated with difficult or traumatic tooth extraction. Contributing factors are increased age, smoking, and most importantly alveolar hypovascularity and focal fibrinolytic activity.

Symptoms and signs

Severe pain and occasionally oral malodour on the second or third day after the tooth extraction are the typical clinical manifestations. After an extraction in the lateral parts of the mandible, pain may irradiate to the homolateral ear.

Diagnosis

The disorder is clinically recognizable by the existence of an empty alveolus after tooth extraction without a blood clot, exposed bony alveolar walls, separation of gingival borders, and sometimes sequestration.

Therapy

Therapy concentrates primarily on daily alveolus irrigation with a saline solution using a needleless syringe. Intra-alveolar dressings with eugenol, lidocaine or 0.12 % chlorhexidine may be beneficial. Without or with treatment, the complication may last for 10 to 15 days. The best treatment is prevention by avoiding surgical trauma, in high risks occasions supported by topical application of 0.12 % chlorhexidine, tetracycline, lincomycine, clindamycin, metronidazole or tinidazole.

References

Torres-Lagares D, Serrera-Figallo MA, Romero-Ruìz MM, Infante-Cossìo P, Garcìa-Calderón M, Gutiérrez-Pérez JL. Update on dry socket: A review of the literature. *Med Oral Patol Oral Cir Bucal* 2005; **10**: 77–85.

XEROSTOMIA AND HYPOSALIVATION

Introduction

Xerostomia is the subjective sensation of dry mouth and is not necessarily related to hyposalivation. Xerostomia affects 14–40 % of all adult people and up to 65 % of institutionalized elderly people. Objective hyposalivation or decreased salivary flow rate and alterations in salivary composition may cause a sensation of dry mouth and a disturbance of oral homeostasis. When salivary volume is reduced significantly, patients are at increased risk for periodontal disease, dental caries, odontogenic infections, alveolar osteitis and fungal mucosal oral infections.

Three pairs of major salivary glands are responsible for 90 % of salivary secretion. Saliva provides a fluid environment for lubrication of the oral cavity to aid in speech, swallowing, the digestive process and cleansing the oral tissues. In addition, saliva possesses acid buffering, antimicrobial and antifungal properties. The biofilm of salivary mucins on the teeth and mucosal surfaces is believed to protect these oral structures from wear. As salivary glands age, salivary producing cells decrease in number and are replaced by adipose and fibrotic tissues. Its total impact on the salivary output is argued, since the glands compensate for cell loss.

Aetiology

Hyposalivation may be caused by salivary gland disease, dehydration, salivary gland destruction associated with head and neck irradiation, autoimmune diseases, poorly controlled diabetes, hormonal disorders and neurological disorders. The most common cause in elderly people is use of medication. Many anticholinergic medications may cause xerostomia and hyposalivation.

Symptoms and signs

Patients with xerostomia often report dry and sticky sensation in the mouth and stringy or foamy saliva. The appearance of the oral mucosa is thin, pale and cracked. Problems are encountered with chewing, swallowing, tasting and speaking. Halitosis and burning sensations are common characteristics.

Diagnosis

Assessing the entire oral cavity is critical in the diagnosis of hyposalivation, palpating the glands, stimulating saliva from the ducts, observing the glands ducts openings, the viscosity of the saliva, dryness of the lips and the lubricity of the mucosa. The diagnostic tools are measuring resting and stimulated salivary flow rates, sialometry, contrast sialography, sequential salivary gland scintigraphy, ultrasonography and labial salivary gland biopsy.

Therapy

Simple methods to counter xerostomia are sipping water frequently, using chewing gum or acidic substances, sucking sweets, and using artificial saliva. Many moistening agents and saliva substitutes are available, manufactured in spray or gel forms.

Pilocarpine hydrochloride 5–10 mg administered three to four times daily, is a cholinergic drug capable of stimulating the salivary glands. Cevimeline hydrochloride 30 mg three times daily may also be beneficial.

References

Cassolato SF, Turnbull RS. Xerostomia: clinical aspects and treatment. *Gerodontology* 2003; **20**: 64–77.

Götrick B, Åkerman S, Torstenson R, Tobin G. Oral pilocarpine for treatment of opioid-induced oral dryness in healthy adults. *J Dent Res* 2004; **5**: 393–7.

CANDIDIASIS

Introduction

Oral candidiasis is a common opportunistic infection caused by an overgrowth of *Candida* species, the commonest being *Candida albicans*. The infection is probably under diagnosed in the elderly, particularly in those wearing dentures. The incidence has been reported to be 30 %–45 % of healthy adults, 50 %–65 % of people wearing removable dentures and 65 %–88 % of residents of long-term care facilities. The different types of candidiasis are pseudomembranous candidiasis, chronic hyperplastic candidiasis, median rhomboid glossitis, and especially in elderly people angular cheilitis and denture stomatitis.

Aetiology

Candida is a normal commensal in the oral cavity, generally not causing signs or symptoms in healthy people. Predisposing factors for overgrowth of *Candida* are old age, hyposalivation, removable dentures, antibiotics, immunosuppressiva, using steroid aerosol inhalers, smoking, diabetes, Cushing's syndrome, HIV-infection and vitamine B deficiency.

Symptoms and signs

Pseudomembranous candidiasis consists of extensive white pseudomembranes of desquamated epithelial cells, fibrin, and fungal hyphae. The membrane can usually be scraped off to expose an underlying erythematous mucosa.

Chronic hyperplastic candidiasis occurs on the buccal mucosa or lateral border of the tongue as speckled or homogenous white lesions. There is an association with smoking. Median rhomboid glossitis is a chronic symmetrical area of atrophic filiform papillae on the tongue anterior to the circumvallate papillae.

Diagnosis

The diagnosis is usually made on clinical findings, ruling out other diagnoses and the response to antifungal treatment and may be confirmed by culture testing.

Therapy

The infection can effectively be managed by oral hygiene measures and local application of nystatin or amphotericin-B as an oral rinse. Systemic medications are clotrimazole and fluconazole, 10 mg administered four to five times daily over 10 days. If therapy is not successful, culture and sensitivity testing is recommended. For those with removable dentures a referral to a dentist for improving the denture fit might be necessary.

References

Akpan A, Morgan R. Oral candidiasis. *Postgrad Med J* 2002; **78**: 455–9.

ANGULAR CHEILITIS

Introduction

Angular cheilitis is characterized by ulcerated fissures or cracks at the outside corners of the mouth.

Aetiology

The predisposing factor is wrinkled and macerated epithelium at the commissures of the mouth. Saliva tends to collect in the commissures, which may become secondarily infected by micro-organisms, particularly *Candida albicans*. Many cases of wrinkled and macerated commissures are due to overclosure of the mandible, such as occurs in edentulous patients with improper vertical facial dimension.

Riboflavin deficiency with a superimposed fungal or bacterial infection is also suggested as aetiologic factor.

Symptoms and signs

The subjective complaints are a burning sensation and pain at the corners of the mouth. Fissures and cracks tend to bleed and to form a superficial exudative crust. The lesions show a tendency for spontaneous remission. Subsequent exacerbation is common and the lesions disappear completely only rarely.

Diagnosis

Infected, wrinkled and macerated commissures of the mouth can be diagnosed clinically and may be confirmed by culture testing.

Therapy

Over closure of the mandible in edentulous patients should be corrected by increasing the vertical dimension of the dentures. The infection at the mouth corners can be treated by antifungal steroid creams and ointments. Riboflavin deficiency can be cured by administration of vitamin B complex.

References

Grimoud AM, Lodter JP, Marty N, et al. Improved oral hygiene and Candida species colonization level in geriatric patients. *Oral Dis* 2005; **11**: 163–9.

DENTURE STOMATITIS

Introduction

Denture stomatitis is characterized by localized chronic erythema of tissues covered by removable dentures, particularly the hard palate and the maxillary residual alveolar ridge. Reported prevalence rates are up to 65 % of denture wearers.

Aetiology

Denture stomatitis is induced by colonization of *Candida* and subsequent dental plaque formation on denture materials, specifically in poorly fitting dentures. Rarely, hypersensitivity to denture base materials is cited as an aetiological factor.

Symptoms and signs

Symptoms are rare. A mild burning sensation is sometimes reported and, very rarely, dysphagia.

Diagnosis

Provisional diagnosis is based on clinical signs. Swabs or saline mouth rinses may be taken for culturing *Candida*.

Therapy

As poorly fitting dentures and *Candida* are the causative factors, therapy includes denture fit improvement and topical or systemic anti-fungal medications. Daily cleaning of the denture is a prerequisite in the elimination of dental plaque formation. Topical anti-fungal agents are nystatin, amphotericin-B and hexetidine. Fluconazole and itraconazole are available for systemic anti-fungal treatment. To avoid side effects, duration of therapy with anti-fungal mouth rinses should not be more than two weeks. Applying denture hygiene and keeping dentures in hexetidine during the night may prevent recurrence of denture stomatitis.

References

Koray M, Ak G, Kurklu E, Issever H, Tanyeri H, Kulekci G, Guc U. Fluconazole and/or hexatidine for management of oral candidiasis associated with denture-induced stomatitis. *Oral Dis* 2005; **11**: 309–13.

Wilson J. The aetiology, diagnosis and management of denture stomatitis. *Br Dent J* 1998; **185**: 380–4.

BURNING MOUTH SYNDROME

Introduction

Burning mouth syndrome is a chronic oral pain condition characterized by an unexplained, usually persistent, burning sensation in the mouth in which the oral mucosa looks normal. Reported prevalence rates in general populations vary from 1 %–15 %. Burning mouth predominantly affects women with an increased prevalence with age and following menopause.

Aetiology

The cause of an oral burning sensation is unknown. A wide range of aetiologic factors has been suggested, such as hyposalivation, allergic reactions, iron and vitamine B_{12} deficiency, menopause, diabetes and psychogenic factors. Recently, the syndrome was suggested as being a neuropathy related to free radical production.

Symptoms and signs

The predominant feature is the symptom of burning pain or discomfort which can be localized to the tongue and/or the lips, the hard palate, the edentulous alveolar ridge or be more widespread and involve the whole oral cavity. It is bilateral in almost all cases. Complaints of altered taste and dry mouth are reported frequently. Many patients show evidence of headache, tinnitus, anxiety, depression, personality disorders, other psychiatric features or an increased tendency for somatization.

Diagnosis

Standard clinical examination of the oral cavity identifies no abnormalities. There are no clinically useful investigations. The diagnosis is usually made after symptoms are reported over more than six months. Burning mouth syndrome as a diagnosis should only be used when a definite cause has not been found.

Therapy

Primarily, any possible irritating factor, such as a sharp tooth, dental restoration material, unclean denture, mouth rinse or acid drink, tobacco or oral medication, should be considered for removal. Reduction of symptoms may be achieved by cognitive therapy and the use of SSRI antidepressants. Recently, it has been indicated that the natural antioxidant alpha-lipoic acid is beneficial in at least some of the patients with complaints of burning mouth.

References

Femiano F, Scully C. Burning mouth syndrome (BMS): double blind controlled study of alpha-lipoic acid (thioctic acid) therapy. *J Oral Pathol Med* 2002; **31**: 267–9.

Zakrzewska JM, Forssell H, Glenny A-M. Interventions for the treatment of burning mouth syndrome: a systematic review. *J Orofac Pain* 2003; **17**: 293–300.

RECURRENT APHTHOUS STOMATITIS

Introduction

Recurrent aphthous stomatitis is one of the most common oral mucosal pathologic conditions, characterized by either single or multiple shallow, painful ulcers which most often affect the non-keratinized oral mucosa. Some 15 %–20 % of the population is reported to be affected by the condition. Three distinct forms of the condition are recognized, namely minor, major and herpetiform. The minor form affects about 80 % of all aphthous patients. Herpetiform aphthous ulcers are the least common form, occurring more often in women and at an older age.

Aetiology

Aphthous ulcerations are of unknown origin. Numerous possible aetiological factors have been suggested, such as heredity, bacterial infection, viral infection, trauma, hormones (menstruation, postmenopausal), immunologic factors, haematinic deficiencies (iron, foliate, vitamine B1, B2, B6, B12), food hypersensitivity (gluten) and stress factors. Some investigators have documented a negative association between occurrence of aphthous ulcers and tobacco use.

The majority of subjects who have recurrent aphthous ulceration tend to be otherwise healthy without signs of systemic disease. Major aphthous ulcers are classified as autoimmune and may originate from an antibody response. They are common in patients with Behçet's disease. Episodes of aphthous ulcers have been observed in coeliac disease, Crohn's disease, patients with cyclic neutropenia and HIV-infected patients.

Symptoms and signs

For 24–48 hours preceding the development of a minor aphthous ulcer, subjects may experience a pricking or burning sensation in the mucosa. In this prodromal stage, erythema of the surrounding mucosa may be observed or it may be appearing normal. Within one or two days an oval or round ulcer with a grey-white centre and erythematous halo develops. Typically the ulcers are less than 1 cm in diameter and less than five occur at one time. These ulcers are self-limiting and require seven to 14 days to heal without scarring. Major aphthous ulcers are similar in appearance, but larger and deeper, and are frequently healing with scarring. Herpetiform aphthous ulcers are distinguished by numerous small punctuate shallow vesicles of irregular shape.

Diagnosis

The minor and herpetic form are characterized by single, shallow, non-indurated ulcers no greater than 5 mm in diameter, regular in outline, and surrounded by an erythematous halo. Major aphthous ulcers are more painful and persist longer.

Therapy

Owing to the unpredictable course of the disease, the primary goals are to control the pain of the ulcer, promote ulcer healing and prevent recurrence.

A multitude of topical agents are available for symptomatic relief including glucocorticoids, antibiotics, local anaesthetics, antihistamines, NSAID, enzymatic preparations, gammaglobulines, immunosuppressants and tissue adhesive 2-octyl cyanoacrylate. Of the topical agents available, amlexanox is the most intensively studied. If this anti-inflammatory and anti-allergic medication is administered in the prodromal stage, it prevents progression to ulcer development and reduces symptoms if an ulcer does develop. The problem with topical agents in the mouth is establishing effective drug delivery, since every substance will inevitably be rubbed or rinsed away. This problem is addressed by compounding a topical agent with a mucosal adherent.

Chlorhexidine and triclosan mouth rinses and gels reduce the incidence, duration and severity of recurrent minor aphthous ulcerations. The mechanism of action is unclear but may relate to a reduction in contamination of ulcers by oral bacteria. Tetracycline hydrochlorite has been found reducing pain and ulcer duration. A 250 mg capsule dissolved in 180 ml water can be used as a three-minute rinse four times daily for three to five days. Rapid pain control and healing has been suggested to be promoted by saturated potassium nitrate and dimethyl isosorbide in an aequous hydroxyethyl cellulose gel.

An experimental dentifrice containing many compounds reduced days with ulcers by more than 50 % in half of the patients.

Pentoxifylline 400 mg three times daily for one month reduced the number of episodes for up to nine months after therapy, without side effects.

The therapies recommended for persistent major ulcers with considerable tissue destruction are topical and systemic antibiotics, topical steroids and combinations of prednisone and azathioprine. Major ulcers which can not be controlled by topical steroids may be treated by thalidomide, two or four times daily 50 mg over two months. Attention must be paid to the possible serious side effects.

References

Coli P, Jontell M, Hakeberg M. The effect of a dentifrice in the prevention of recurrent aphthous stomatitis. *Oral Health Prev Dent* 2004; **2**: 133–41.

Natah SS, Konttinen YT, Enattah NS, Ashammakhi N, Sharkey KA, Häyrinen-Immonen R. Recurrent aphthous ulcers today: a review of the growing knowledge. *Int J Oral Maxillofac Surg* 2004; **33**: 221–34.

Pizarro A, Herranz P, Navarro A, Casado M. Recurrent aphthous stomatitis: treatment with pentoxifylline. *Acta Derm Venereol* 1996; **76**: 79–80.

RECURRENT HERPES SIMPLEX

Introduction

Labial herpes is a common secondary or recurrent viral disease. In a less common manifestation, the lesions occur inside the mouth on the hard palate and the gingiva. Approximately 20 %–40 % of the population will experience labial or peri-oral outbreaks of vesicular herpetic lesions. The frequency of outbreaks varies from rare episodes every five to 10 years in some persons, to monthly or even more frequent outbreaks in a small proportion of persons.

Aetiology

Herpes simplex virus is a common human pathogen with two serotypes. Type 1 most commonly affects the oral cavity. The virus is transmitted by direct contact and can enter a broken mucosal surface. After the primary infection, often presenting as acute gingivo-stomatitis, herpes simplex virus type 1 remains latent in the trigeminal ganglion and may be reactivated by stress, fever, upper respiratory tract infections, ultraviolet light, trauma, menstruation, and immune incompetence.

Symptoms and signs

Secondary herpes simplex comprises a prodromal phase of tingling and/or burning and erythema, followed by an extra-oral painful vesicle involving the lips or nares. In some cases, it may recur as multiple shallow, punctuate oral ulcers, followed by formation of multiple vesicles and ulceration. Finally, there is crusting and healing over eight to 21 days. Active virus is present throughout the vesicular stage.

Diagnosis

Provisional diagnosis is based on clinical signs and symptoms. Viral culture by swab specimens provides confirmation of the disease.

Therapy

Episodic or prophylactic treatment with anti-viral agents is the current standard therapy. Although nucleoside anti-viral agents, including aciclovir, valaciclovir and penciclovir, can be effective, most have toxicity or side effects, and can promote viral resistance. Recently, it was demonstrated that swallowing zinc sulphate granules dissolved in a glass of water twice daily, each day during the months of February, March, September, and October reduced both the number of episodes and the time to recovery.

References

Femiano F, Gombos F, Scully C. Recurrent herpes labialis: a pilot study of the efficacy of zinc therapy. *J Oral Pathol Med* 2005; **34**: 423–5.

Spruance SL, Kriesel JD. Treatment of herpes simplex labialis. *Herpes* 2000; **9**(3): 64–9.

ORAL LICHEN PLANUS

Introduction

Oral lichen planus is an immunologically based, chronic, inflammatory, muco-cutaneous disorder. Molecular alterations related to cell cycle control, such as growth, maturation, proliferation and apoptosis, may produce an epithelial substrate which favours evolution to malignancy. Malignant transformation has been reported for 0.4%–3.7% of cases. Oral lichen planus is estimated to affect about 0.5%–4% of the general population, with a predilection for the late fourth through sixth decades of life. There is a slight female predilection.

Aetiology

A likely aetiological scenario suggests extrinsic antigens, altered self-antigens or superantigens being taken up by Langerhans cells located within the epithelium. Herpes viruses, such as Herpes simplex 1 virus, Epstein-Barr virus, Cytomegalovirus and Herpes virus 6 have been implicated in oral lichen planus. Virtually any restorative material or dental prosthesis is capable of inducing a lichenoid response.

Symptoms and signs

Lesions tend to be symmetrical and bilateral. The most commonly involved site is the buccal mucosa. Other sites of occurrence are the tongue, lips, floor of the mouth, palate and gingiva. Gingival cases, about 10%, present as desquamative gingivitis, characterized by the presence of painful, red, atrophic or denuded attached gingiva.

Lesions can be classified as reticular, atrophic or erosive. The reticular form occurs most frequently and is characterized by keratotic lines, arranged in a lacy pattern (striae), plaques or papules.

Pain is most commonly associated with the erosive form and is aggravated by agents such as spiced food and alcohol. Purely reticular oral lichen planus is usually asymptomatic. Erosive presentations have much greater old patient predominance than reticular and atrophic forms. Malignant transformation is extremely rare.

Diagnosis

In order to confirm the preliminary clinical diagnosis, a biopsy may be considered. The histological features consist of (hyper)keratinization of the surface, loss of basal cells, and the presence of a clearly defined band-like subepithelial lymphocytic infiltrate with a clearly defined lower border.

Therapy

To validate a reticular lichenoid reaction to any material, the suspected cause should be removed. Subsequent lesion resolution should be observed.

Treatment of mild erosive lichen planus usually consists of topical steroids. Commonly used steroids include triamcinolone acetonide 0.1%, betamethasone valerate 0.1%, fluocinonide 0.05%, fluocinolone acetonide 0.15%, dexamethasone 0.5 mg/mL and clobetasol propionate 0.05 %. Persistant local erosive lesions may be managed adequately by local injection of up to 0.4 mL of triamcinolone acetonide 10 mg/mL. As a systemic steroid a maximum 10-day daily morning dose of 40–80 mg prednisone may be prescribed. Promising results in the treatment of erosive oral lichen planus using pimecrolimus 1 % have been described recently.

References

Lodi G, Scully C, Carrozzo M, Griffiths M, Sugerman PB, Thongprasom K. Current controversies in oral lichen planus: Report of an international consensus meeting. Part I Viral infections and ethiopathogenesis. *Oral Surg Oral Med Oral Pathol Oral Radiol Endod* 2005; **100**: 40–51.

Lodi G, Scully C, Carrozzo M, Griffiths M, Sugerman PB, Thongprasom K. Current controversies in oral lichen planus: Report of an international consensus meeting. Part II Clinical management and malignant transformation. *Oral Surg Oral Med Oral Pathol Oral Radiol Endod* 2005; **100**: 164–78.

Swift JC, Rees TD, Plemons JM, Hallmon WW, Wright JC. The effectiveness of 1 % pimecrolimus cream in the treatment of oral erosive lichen planus. *J Periodontol* 2005; **76**: 627–35.

25 Swallowing disorders and medication in the elderly

Eddy Dejaeger

Department of Geriatrics, University Hospital Leuven, Belgium

INTRODUCTION

Swallowing disorders can be quite common in the elderly (1). The reasons are obvious and multiple. First of all, one must take into account the occurrence of pathology associated with deglutition disorders such as a stroke, Parkinson's disease and other neurological conditions.

Secondly, people with serious medical problems are now more likely to survive the acute moment but are prone to develop deglutition problems (e.g. post radiotherapy or post invasive surgery in the pharyngo-laryngeal region).

Finally, there is the aging process by itself. Although this doesn't necessarily cause deglutition problems, it certainly decreases the functional reserve of the patient thereby leading to difficulties in acute situations.

The elderly often take many different medications and this not only leads to possible interaction but we should also bear in mind that the elderly persons have to swallow all those pills.

The epidemiology of dysphagia is not yet thoroughly explored. A study in different medical institutions revealed dysphagia to be present in 12–20 % of patients hospitalized on general medical wards, in nursing homes the incidence was much higher (up to 50 %) (2).

The prevalence of subjective dysphagia in community residents aged over 87 was found to be 16 % (3).

To fully understand the possible problems it is worthwhile to linger shortly with the description of a normal deglutition.

NORMAL DEGLUTITION

Swallowing is a complex mechanism which requires the intricate coordination of several cranial nerves and a very large number of muscles in the face, mouth, pharynx and oesophagus.

It is helpful to divide dysphagia into two types: oropharyngeal and oesophageal. Dysphagia secondary to a lesion above or proximal to the oesophagus is called oropharyngeal dysphagia. This symptom is often characterized as a transfer problem, meaning that the patient has trouble transferring the food from the mouth into the pharynx and oesophagus. Patients with oesophageal dysphagia have difficulty transporting food down the oesophagus once the bolus has been transferred successfully through the pharynx.

For the management of patients with aspiration, the moment of aspiration in relation to the pharyngeal stage of deglutition (before, during or after deglutition) appears to be a crucial element.

The act of swallowing can be subdivided into four stages: oral preparation, oral stage, pharyngeal stage and the oesophageal stage. Oral preparation involves the coordination of lip closure, rotary and lateral motion of the jaw,

Prescribing for Elderly Patients   Edited by Stephen Jackson, Paul Jansen and Arduino Mangoni
© 2009 John Wiley & Sons, Ltd

buccal tone, rotary and lateral motion of the tongue and anterior bulging of the soft palate. The purpose of this stage is to break food down to a consistency appropriate for swallowing and to mix it with saliva. The oral stage starts when the tongue moves upward and backward, contacting the palate in a sequential squeezing or rolling action, propelling the bolus ahead of it into the pharynx. When the complex tongue and bolus reaches a trigger zone, the pharyngeal stage is initiated. The exact localization of this trigger zone is not clearly defined and may not be identical in all subjects. The anterior faucial or palatoglossal arch is probably the main trigger zone, but other places such as the tonsils, the soft palate, the base of the tongue and the adjacent region of the oropharynx can predominate in eliciting the pharyngeal stage. During this stage five very important actions occur, some closely related to each other:

1. Velopharyngeal closure prevents reflux into the nose.
2. Closure of the larynx prevents aspiration in the airways.
3. The pharynx generates a peristaltic contraction.
4. Elevation and anterior movement of the larynx brings it out of the path of the bolus.
5. The upper oesophageal sphincter (UOS) opens. The UOS is a very complicated structure which functions in order to control the passage of material retrograde from the oesophagus into the oropharyngeal cavity as well as the passage of material antegrade into the oesophagus. On manometry the UOS is identified as a high-pressure zone at the juncture of the proximal oesophagus and the hypopharynx. Most studies have indicated that the cricopharyngeus muscle is the predominant muscle in this sphincter zone although this remains a matter of controversy. Motor neurons residing in the nucleus ambiguous in the medulla oblongata provide a continuous stimulation of the UOS and allow it to maintain a constant tone. When the muscle is electrically quiescent, residual pressure in the UOS likely results from passive elastic forces of the muscle and surrounding tissues. Opening of the UOS is not simply a matter of cessation of electrical activity in the UOS. Three additional factors play a role. The first is an active anterior traction on the UOS resulting from the contraction of the muscles that pulls the hyoid bone and laryngeal structures anteriorly. Secondly, the UOS lumen is pushed open by the bolus itself. Thirdly, the intrinsic compliance of the UOS and its attachments will affect the ability of distracting and distending forces so as to increase the luminal diameter of the UOS.

Different studies have shown that manometric relaxation and anterior hyoid traction on the larynx invariably preceded UOS opening. The movement of the larynx and the opening of the UOS are intimately related.

The closure of the larynx is an important component in the protection of the airways against aspiration. The true vocal cords contract and this contraction propagates upwards. This action of the larynx is a crucial protective step and is supported by its up- and forward movement. The epiglottis offers some protection but its contribution is inessential.

The role of the pharynx musculature seems to be threefold: maintenance of an adequate tone and the creation of a rigid chamber, a shortening of the pharynx to engulf the bolus and a clearing function to eliminate the bolus tail or residual bolus. The oesophageal stage includes the passage of the bolus through the oesophagus to the stomach.

CHANGES WITH AGE

There are no significant changes in the oral preparatory phase but bad dentures may lead to the ingestion of only soft food. The oral phase remains untouched but during the pharyngeal phase some changes occur such as a delayed triggering of the swallowing reflex, a decreased pharyngeal sensibility and a decreased upper oesophageal sphincter opening.

As far as the oesophagus is concerned, normal ageing is accompanied by a reduction of secondary peristalsis, in some cases a complete disappearance of peristaltic contractions, an increased proportion of simultaneous contractions and a decrease of the amplitude and of the propagation speed of the oesophageal contractions.

With age there is also an increase of functional oesophageal disorders (e.g. diffuse spasms) of pathologic gastro-oesophageal reflux and of the frequency of oesophageal tumours.

AETIOLOGY OF DEGLUTITION DISORDERS

A wide variety of pathologies can cause deglutition disorders in the elderly.

We can discern three major groups.

Neurological and neuromuscular diseases

Examples: stroke is by far the most frequent cause of dysphagia in the elderly. Parkinson's disease, amyothrophic lateral sclerosis, motor endplate disease, dementia, muscular dystrophies.

Local causes

Examples: Zenker's diverticulum, Local surgery and/or radiotherapy, cervical spine disease.

Motility disorders

Examples: idiopathic achalasia of the upper oesophageal sphincter, gastro-oesophageal reflux disease, systemic disease.

Moreover, we should be aware that there may be several factors which may aggravate an existing problem such as bad dentures, xerostomia, deterioration of the general mobility and loss of autonomy.

Elderly persons are therefore the most likely individuals to acquire dysphagia.

SYMPTOMS AND SIGNS

Swallowing problems can manifest themselves with different aspects.

Dysphagia has already been mentioned.

Other symptoms may be regurgitation, coughing or choking during or after intake of liquid or food, prolonged oral preparation with food, odynophagia (i.e. pain on swallowing) sensation of food sticking in the throat or sternal region, heartburn. This is not an exhaustive list and one should always remain alert to a deglutition problem when a patient has an unexplained weight loss or is showing repeated incidents of upper respiratory infections with or without a clear diagnosis of aspiration pneumonia.

DIAGNOSIS

Following a clinical observation and examination a radiological and/or an endoscopic exploration may be indicated.

A fibre endoscopic evaluation of swallowing (FEES) has several advantages (e.g. no need for transportation of the patient, repeated investigations possible...) although radiology, a modified barium swallow or a videofluoroscopy remains the method of choice while allowing for examination of the deglutition in all its aspects. However, one should consider both investigations as being complementary.

The combination of videofluoroscopy and solid state manometry (manofluoroscopy) has advantages when the problems are situated during the pharyngeal phase.

THERAPY

Apart from specific medication which is only available in rare instances as, for example, in myasthenia gravis other approaches have to be followed.

Of course changes in diet textures may be indicated or exercises be performed under the supervision of a speech language pathologist.

One discerns compensatory and rehabilitative measures. The former deal with the symptoms without altering the pathophysiology of swallowing and can be taken in all patients as little or no cooperation is needed (e.g. positioning of the head, changing the sensory input). The latter, however, interfere with the physiology of swallowing (e.g. swallow manoeuvres such as the Mendelsohn manoeuvre) and here full cooperation is required. Other possibilities are a vocal fold medialization or surgery (e.g. a myotomy of the upper oesophageal sphincter, diverticulopexy of a Zenker's diverticulum).

Of course, caregivers dealing with this kind of patient should be instructed as to how to assist them at mealtimes and they also should be able to perform the Heimlich manoeuvre.

DEGLUTITION DISORDERS AND MEDICATION

Medication can either improve or worsen the symptoms of dysphagia (4–6). Therefore it is important not only to understand the pathophysiology of swallowing but also to be aware of the effects and adverse effects of the numerous medications used frequently for the elderly.

If a drug is not swallowed properly but remains stuck in the pharyngo-oesophageal region, it will not only be ineffective as far as its working is concerned but, moreover, it could be potentially harmful by inducing a local inflammation. First of all, we will discuss some adverse effects which may intervene with swallowing, and then the focus will lie with a few specific groups of medications followed by the risks of certain medications in persons with a swallowing problem. This provides a link with the final part where the administration route will be dealt with.

Adverse effects

Xerostomia

A significant number of medications lead to dryness of the mouth. The question, however, remains whether xerostomia really leads to an objective deglutition problem. It certainly causes subjective problems.

The most common medication leading to xerostomia are anticholinergic drugs or drug with anticholinergic side-effects.

The use of saliva substitutes may provide some relief, these patients should also be encouraged to take frequent sips of water during and between meals.

Taste impairment

Some medications may cause a loss of taste such as allopurinol, carbamazepine, penicillamine while others such as captopril and lithium may produce a metallic taste. This, however rarely, can mimic a swallowing problem.

Some medications have a bitter taste of their own (e.g. promethazine) which makes crushing rather difficult.

Level of alertness

All drugs which cause sedation or in general a reduction of the alertness level may influence deglutition. As a general rule people who are not fully alert should not receive oral feeding at that moment. There remains a huge problem concerning demented people with a severe loss of autonomy. Due not only to the dementia itself but also to the medication they eventually receive, their swallowing ability may be compromised. Breakfast is usually for them the best meal as at that moment their level of agitation is at its lowest.

Specific medication

Medication which might improve deglutition

These are not numerous and are limited to certain well-defined pathologies.

Myasthenia gravis: these patients typically do well at the beginning of a meal but tire towards the end. Anticholinesterase drugs (e.g. pyridostigmin), when administered in the proper dose, greatly facilitate muscle movement. It is important that these medications be coordinated with feeding schedules so that their maximum benefit is directed toward facilitating the necessary muscle strength for deglutition.

Thyroid disorders: hypothyroid and hyperthyroid disease can cause skeletal muscle dysfunction. In rare cases a deglutition problem may arise which responds well to treatment either with thyroid replacement or to chemical or surgical suppression.

Parkinson's disease: many studies have addressed this issue and the main question is whether L-Dopa or dopamine agonists might improve swallowing. These studies teach us that it is by no means certain that L-Dopa or dopamine agonists will improve existing swallowing problems (7). The deglutition problems are probably the result of a deficit in a non-dopaminergic pathway. The medication should then be given some time (up to one hour) prior to meals. If the patient experiences on/off periods he should take great care to avoid meals during the off periods.

Capsaicin: an ingredient of red peppers which has proved to be beneficial when there is a delay in triggering the pharyngeal phase of swallowing (8).

Botulism toxin: this can be used for treating sialorrhee as well as achalasia of the upper oesophageal sphincter. In the case of sialorrhee the toxin is injected into the submandibular salivary glands under local anaesthesia.

The outcome of the procedure, however, is not always optimal and is in most cases transitory.

For treating achalasia of the upper oesophageal sphincter with botulism toxin, in most cases a general anaesthesia is required and although most patients will benefit this is not always the case.

Medication which may provoke a deglutition problem

Antipsychotics: there are several case reports showing the possible adverse effect of antipsychotics on swallowing. Antipsychotics cause extrapyramidal effects and this may lead to severe oral-pharyngeal dysphagia characterized by reduced chewing ability, tongue pumping, defective tongue movements and reduced base of tongue movement, all resulting in reduced oral control. The pharyngeal phase can also be disturbed with a delay in initiating a swallow, pooling of residue and penetration or aspiration of this residue. Such problems have been described with haloperidol and trifluoperazine.

The only treatment for these swallowing disorders is to reduce exposure to antipsychotics. If this is done the swallowing problems are reversible. Atypical antipsychotics as risperidone and olanzapine, are less likely to cause extrapyramidal syndromes and therefore may be preferable but recently case reports have been publicized showing that these medications are also capable of causing severe but reversible swallowing disorders.

Neuroleptic-induced dysphagia is not reported frequently but it is important to be aware that it exists and may be reversed by stopping the exposure.

Medication that decreases the lower oesophageal sphincter pressure

A considerable number of patients with of GORD (gastro-oesophageal reflux disease) experience dysphagia as a primary symptom. This may be due to the development of strictures but even in the absence of strictures dysphagia may be present. Examining patients with a globus sensation (the feeling that something is stuck in the throat even outside mealtimes), approximately one fourth of them seem to be suffering from GORD. Proton pump inhibitors are the treatment of choice when gastro-oesophageal reflux disease has been diagnosed. However, one has to be aware of the fact that it may take some weeks before the deglutition symptoms start to disappear.

In the presence of GORD caution is needed when prescribing certain medications that decrease the pressure at the level of the lower oesophageal sphincter such as anticholinergic agents, benzodiazepines, certain calcium channel blockers and nitrates. Of course alcohol, caffeine and smoking are better avoided.

Steroids

The prolonged use of steroids may cause a Candida infection of the mouth, pharynx and oesophagus. Such an infection causes odynophagia and should be treated properly with antifungal agents.

Moreover, high-dose steroids, certainly when taken for long duration, cause skeletal muscle wasting. This may lead to pharyngeal dysphagia.

Cytotoxic drugs

Several cytotoxic drugs may cause a stomatitis and/or an oesophagitis thereby leading to severe swallowing problems.

It is important to ensure a proper hygiene of the mouth and to administer a local therapy to alleviate the symptoms.

Patients with swallowing disorders

In patients with known swallowing problems one should consider four issues:

1. Try to avoid some medications which can cause severe local irritation when they get stuck.
2. Give your patient proper advice as to how he should take the medication.
3. Evaluate whether the length of time between doses can be increased.
4. Consider whether there are alternative routes of administration.

Medication which should be avoided if possible

There are quite a few medications which may provoke severe local inflammation when their transport to the stomach is interrupted for whatever reason (9, 10). Therefore a proper technique for swallowing pills is of the utmost importance and we will return to this subject later. Medication that is potentially harmful is iron tablets, NSAIDs, potassium chloride, ascorbic acid, alendronate, aspirin and certain antibiotics such as doxycycline.

How to take medication by mouth

One at a time. Do not take medication just before lying down, instead wait for five to 10 minutes. Accordingly, medication to be swallowed at bedtime in fact means before bedtime.

The patient should be well positioned and alert. Even a bedridden patient should be positioned in an upright position and kept in this position for at least five to 10 minutes after the ingestion.

To begin with a water bolus should be swallowed in order to moisten the mouth, followed by the pill and water and to end another glass of water should be swallowed.

Always consider whether liquid medication is available.

Lengthening of time between doses

It is obvious that we should always try to minimize the number of medications and to consider the use of a once-daily extended release formulation. For certain drugs once weekly dosing regimens exist, e.g. for bisphosphonate medications such as alendronate and risedronate.

Alternative routes of administration

There may be severe difficulties when administering oral medication to patients with swallowing disorders. Quite often this results in crushing or opening of medication and thereby in unlicensed administration. Moreover, enteric-coated or extended release forms can not be crushed without losing their specific pharmacologic properties. Medication mixed with food should always be given immediately after mixing to secure the integrity of the active component.

For some medications a liquid form is available, when switching to a liquid form it is important to check the dose. This is advisable when the patient has trouble swallowing solids but is still capable of swallowing liquids. In such cases an effervescent tablet may be useful and for other medications it might be an option to give an orally disintegrating form (e.g. risperidone, olanzapine).

Particular attention should also be paid to alternative routes, e.g. dermal. This has provided a tremendous advantage for pain therapy where a patch can deliver a stable dose for several days. To start such a prolonged pain therapy, however, we would still recommend the classical approach.

KEY POINTS

- Deglutition disorders are quite frequent in particular subgroups of elderly patients.
- A thorough assessment of the medications and limitation of their numbers is warranted.
- Make sure your patients use the correct technique for taking drugs orally.
- There may be alternative routes of administration.
- Avoid if possible some medications which may interfere with swallowing.

LINKS

American Speech-Language-Hearing Association http://www.asha.org

Dysphagia Resource Center http://www.dysphagia.com

REFERENCES

1. Schindler, JS., Kelly, JH Swallowing disorders in the elderly *Laryngoscope* 2002; **112**(4): 589–602.
2. Groher, ME, Bukatman, R The prevalence of swallowing disorders in two teaching hospitals *Dysphagia* 1986; **1**: 3–6.
3. Bloem, BR, Lagaay, AM, Van Beek, W, Prevalence of subjective dysphagia in community residents aged over 87 *Br Med J* 1990; **300**: 721–2.
4. Feinberg, M, Sonies, BC (ed), The effects of medications on swallowing. In: *Dysphagia: A continuum of care*, Aspen Publishers, Gaithersburg, MD, pp.154–9, 1997.
5. Brandt, N Medication and dysphagia: How do they impact each other? Nutrition in *Clinical Practice* 1999; **14**: S27–S30.
6. Stoschus, B, Allescher, HD Drug-induced dysphagia *Dysphagia* 1993; **8**: 154–9.
7. Hunter, PC, Crameri, J, Austin, S, Woodward, MC, Hughes, AJ 'Response of parkinsonian swallowing dysfunction to dopaminergic stimulation', *Journal of Neurology, Neurosurgery and Psychiatry* 1997; **63**: 579–83.
8. Ebihara, T, Takahashi, H, Ebihara, S, Okazaki, T, Sasaki, T, Watando, A, Nemto, M, Sasaki, H, Capsaicin troche for swallowing dysfunction in elderly people *J Am Geriat Soc* 2005; **53**(5): 824–8.
9. O'Neill, JL Drug-induced esophageal injuries and dysphagia *The annals of Pharmacotherapy* 2003; **37**: 1675–84.
10. Akhtar, AJ Oral medication-induced esophageal injury in elderly patients *Am J Med Sci* 2003; **326**(3): 133–5.

26 Upper gastrointestinal disorders

Geoffrey S. Hebbard

Department of Gastroenterology, The Royal Melbourne Hospital, Victoria, Australia

Upper gastrointestinal disorders are common and a source of considerable morbidity and mortality in the elderly, accounting for a substantial number of hospitalizations and deaths each year. Most disorders of the oesophagus and stomach tend to increase in prevalence and severity with age and often require ongoing prophylactic or suppressive therapy.

GASTROOESOPHAGEAL REFLUX DISEASE

Introduction

The major function of the oesophagus is the transport of ingested food from the pharynx to the stomach, whilst preventing reflux of gastric contents into the oesophagus and upper airway. Hiatus hernia increases in prevalence and severity with age, sphincter function is reduced, along with oesophageal peristalsis and clearance. In addition, medications and co-morbid factors such as reduced saliva production and delayed gastric emptying increase the severity of oesophageal reflux and oesophagitis.

The prevalence of gastrooesophageal reflux disease (GORD) rises with age, as does the severity and proportion of complicated gastrooesophageal reflux disease. This, coupled with a reduction in oesophageal sensation, leads to a reduction in the level of symptoms, later presentations and more severe disease, with a high relapse rate on cessation of therapy

Symptoms and signs

Although symptoms of heartburn and regurgitation are the cardinal symptoms of reflux disease and are relatively specific when present, older patients often do not demonstrate these and commonly present with nonspecific symptoms such as nausea, vomiting, weight loss or anaemia. The presence of features such as a short history, weight loss, dysphagia or haematemesis indicate a low threshold for upper GI endoscopy. Atypical symptoms of reflux disease may include pharyngeal/laryngeal symptoms, cough, recurrent pneumonia and chest pain.

Diagnosis

Upper GI endoscopy is useful to assess the severity of disease and for excluding other conditions, but if the patient is medically unfit and endoscopy would not change management, a therapeutic trial of acid suppression may be a useful alternative.

Therapy

Acid suppression is the mainstay of treatment of GORD, and a healing phase followed by a step-down approach is the most efficient method of treatment, providing the patient with

Prescribing for Elderly Patients   Edited by Stephen Jackson, Paul Jansen and Arduino Mangoni
© 2009 John Wiley & Sons, Ltd

rapid symptom relief and supporting the diagnosis with a therapeutic trial of effective therapy. The level of acid suppression may then be gradually titrated down to the lowest level consistent with adequate control of symptoms and prevention of complications.

Healing phase

All currently available proton pump inhibitors (PPIs) are potent suppressors of gastric acid secretion. There are minor differences between agents in terms of pharmacokinetics and potency (see Table 26.1). H2-receptor antagonists (H2Ras) are suitable for occasional symptoms +/− antacids, but are not appropriate for more severe mucosal disease (Los Angeles grade C and D). There are minor differences in metabolism

and potential drug interactions between PPIs which are unlikely to be of clinical significance in most patients, however patients on warfarin and other drugs metabolized by the CYP 2C19 system should undergo therapeutic monitoring as with the commencement of any new medication.

There is evidence that more severe grades of oesophagitis heal more rapidly with more effective acid suppression and these patients should be commenced on higher initial doses of PPI.

Maintenance treatment

Gastrooesophageal reflux disease should be recognized as a chronic disease; the aims of long-term management are to control symptoms and prevent complications. In mild

Table 26.1. Proton pump inhibitors and H2-receptor antagonists for the treatment of reflux disease in the elderly; for maintenance dose and adverse events see text

Drug	Start dose	Pharmaco-kinetics	Metabolism/elimination	Interactions
omeprazole	20 mg	young adults: t1/2 < 0.7–0.8 hrs elderly : t1/21.6–1.7 hrs	Hepatic CYP 2C19	Potential increase in phenytoin and warfarin concentration
esomeprazole	20–40 mg	young adults: t 1/2 1, 3 hrs elderly : t1/21.7 hrs	Hepatic CYP 2C19	Inhibitor of CYP 2C19
lansoprazole	30 mg	young adults: t1/2 1.4 hrs elderly: ? t1/2 2.2–2.9 hrs	Hepatic, CYP 2C19	Inhibitor of CYP 2C19
pantoprazole	40 mg	young adults: t1/2 1 hr Elderly: t1/2 1, 25 hrs	Hepatic CYP 2C19	
rabeprazole	20 mg	young adults: t1/2 0,9 hrs elderly: t1/2 1.2 hrs	Hepatic CYP 3A4 and 2C19 Are you sure aobut this, I thought it was said to be 'nonenzymatic' by Janssen-Cilag?	
cimetidine	400 mg bid	Young adults: t1/2 2.1 hrs elderly: t1/2 2.6 hrs	renal	Enzyme inhibitor CYP450 many interactions
famotidine	20 mg bid	Young adults: t1/2 3 hrs elderly: t1/2 4–6.7 hrs	renal	
nizatidine	150 mg bid	Young adults: t1/2 1.6 hrs elderly: t1/2 1.9 hrs	renal	
ranitidine	150 mg bid	Young adults: t1/2 2.4 hrs elderly: t1/2 3.2 hrs	renal and hepatic (25%)	Increase of glipizide and theopylline concentrations

disease (no oesophagitis or minor oesophagitis at endoscopy), the level of acid suppression should be titrated down to the lowest level consistent with control of symptoms and maintained at this level. This may be on-demand usage of PPI or H₂RA, but this is less common in the elderly than in younger patients.Mucosal complications such as significant ulceration (LA grade C and D) or stricturing diagnosed at upper GI endoscopy will require regular ongoing maintenance therapy, possibly in addition to endoscopic therapy (e.g. dilation). It is not appropriate to use on demand therapy in this situation. There is no evidence for a role for any currently available prokinetic agent in the management of GORD.

Treatment of extraoesophageal manifestations

Pharyngeal, laryngeal and respiratory symptoms are often nonspecific and may require a prolonged (eight week) course of high dose (bd) therapy to determine whether there has been any response.

Surgery

Laparoscopic fundoplication in expert hands has significantly reduced the morbidity associated with surgery for gastrooesophageal reflux disease. Surgery is not specifically contraindicated by age, but significant medical comorbidity is likely to increase the risks and the alternative of prolonged acid suppression is likely to be safer if control of symptoms and complications is adequate. The major indication for surgery is gastrooesophageal reflux disease that cannot be controlled on high doses of PPIs, for example ongoing reflux/regurgitation of acid or nonacidic gastric contents, especially with evidence of aspiration.

Safety of long-term acid suppression

Considering that H2RAs have been in common use for 30 years, and PPIs for 20 years acid suppression has proven to be a very safe form of therapy. Initial concerns regarding the

development of carcinoid tumors have not been borne out in clinical practice.

Recognized risks include occasional idiosyncratic reactions (interstitial nephritis, hepatitis), diarrhoea, increased susceptibility to orally ingested bacterial pathogens and C difficile colitis, especially in hospitalized patients. The rate of community-acquired pneumonia is increased by a factor of approximately two. Increased risk of osteoporosis and hip fracture have also been recently recognized as long term complications.

Helicobacter pylori and gastrooesophageal reflux disease

There is little evidence that the infection with Helicobacter pylori worsens reflux disease, indeed in some patients it may be protective. Concerns relating to a possible interaction between Helicobacter pylori and potent acid suppression in increasing progression of intestinal metaplasia are of more relevance to younger patients. Certainly treating H pylori infection cannot be expected to improve symptoms of reflux disease and these issues should be managed separately

Risk of malignancy

Gastrooesophageal reflux disease and particularly Barrett's oesophagus, which is closely associated with reflux disease, are risk factors for the development of oesophageal adenocarcinoma. Although the incidence of this has increased dramatically over the past three decades and is highest in older age groups, the absolute risks of developing oesophageal adenocarcinoma remain low, even in patients with Barrett's oesophagus (approx 1/50 lifetime risk), and the vast majority of patients with Barrett's oesophagus die of other causes. There is weak evidence that higher levels of acid suppression reduce the risk of oesophageal adenocarcinoma, however there does appear to be a reduction in the risk of oesophageal adenocarcinoma in patients taking low dose aspirin. These issues are currently being examined in ongoing trials. Conventional management of patients with Barrett's oesophagus involves surveillance of the abnormal mucosa at regular intervals, coupled with either local therapy (endoscopic mucosal resection or photodynamic therapy) or oesophagectomy depending on the patient's age and medical condition. As the absolute risks of Barrett's oesophagus are relatively low and many patients have significant comorbidity, this practice should be tailored to the individual patient.

Key Points

- Gastrooesophageal reflux disease is common and more severe in elderly patients.
- Presentation is often nonspecific and upper GI endoscopy is often required to confirm the diagnosis and exclude other conditions.
- The major aims of treatment are to control symptoms and reduce the likelihood of complications.
- Treatment is based on acid suppression, an initial phase of full dose therapy is be followed by step-down therapy to the lowest level of treatment consistent with adequate disease control.
- Treatment should not be ceased or changed to on demand therapy in patients with significant ulceration/structuring.
- Long-term treatment with acid suppression appears to be relatively safe.

OESOPHAGEAL MOTILITY DISORDERS

Apart from gastrooesophageal reflux disease, the most common disorders of oesophageal motor function are ineffective oesophageal peristalsis and diffuse oesophageal spasm. Dysphagia, regurgitation and chest pain which remain undiagnosed despite initial investigation for structural disorders are commonly the result of oesophageal dysmotility

Ineffective oesophageal peristalsis, with absent or weak oesophageal contractions results in poor transit of oesophageal contents, particularly for solids. Diffuse oesophageal spasm involves synchronous, often repetitive and strong contractions of the smooth muscle of the distal oesophagus. These uncoordinated contractions result in holdup of both solids and

liquids, and often intraoesophageal reflux or even regurgitation.

Ineffective oesophageal peristalsis and diffuse oesophageal spasm may be diagnosed on barium swallow or oesophageal manometry (which is the most sensitive investigation).

Initial therapy for oesophageal motility disorders involves dietary modification, with soft foods, chewed well and washed down with liquids. Liquids usually pass well in ineffective peristalsis especially in the upright posture and there is little risk of dehydration or malnutrition with appropriate diet. Prokinetic agents have not been shown to be effective in this condition.

Diffuse oesophageal spasm responds less well to dietary therapy and liquids may be regurgitated. Symptoms may be aggravated or precipitated by acid reflux, and some patients respond to a course of acid suppression with PPI (a therapeutic trial of high dose therapy for four to eight weeks). Alternatively, or in addition to acid suppression, smooth muscle relaxants may be trialed; a sublingual nitrate spray or tablet may relieve intermittent symptoms or be used prophylactically prior to a meal. Long acting nitrates or calcium antagonists may be used prophylactically if symptoms are frequent, but are often associated with postural hypotension. If patients are already on alternative antihypertensive agents, one of these may be substituted, providing a dual therapeutic action. There is a small literature on the effects of Botulinum toxin injected into the oesophageal wall; surgical myotomy of the lower oesophagus has occasionally been used, but has not been adequately evaluated.

Achalasia

Although less common than in young adults, achalasia is seen in older age, however the search for an underlying cause (malignancy) should be more vigorous, with upper GI endoscopy/biopsy and possibly CT scan of the chest/abdomen. The results of balloon dilation or laparoscopic myotomy are similar in the elderly to younger patients and age alone should not be seen as a contraindication to these therapies. Whilst waiting for these, or in patients who are deemed unfit, smooth muscle relaxant drugs may be trialed (as for diffuse oesophageal spasm above), but are often ineffective or associated with unacceptable side effects. Injection of Botulinum toxin into the lower oesophageal sphincter has been evaluated. An injection of 100IU in 4 aliquots into the muscle of the LOS may provide relief, often for months, before retreatment is required and may be of value in patients who are unfit or unwilling to undergo other therapies.

Management of Food Impaction

Food impaction in the oesophagus is a distressing condition, particularly when obstruction is complete and patients cannot swallow saliva. The underlying cause may be obstructive (peptic stricture or malignancy), but not uncommonly no structural abnormality is found and the cause is presumed to be oesophageal spasm. The diagnosis is usually made clinically, with the patient complaining of dysphagia and chest discomfort commencing during a meal and the use of barium makes subsequent endoscopy difficult, and Gastrograffin is problematic if aspirated, so oesophageal contrast radiology should be avoided. The initial management of oesophageal food impaction involves the use of a carbonated beverage (20–50 ml) to distend the oesophagus, stimulating secondary peristalsis and increasing pressure, and smooth muscle relaxants as oesophageal spasm is a contributor in many cases. If unsuccessful, in addition to a further bolus of carbonated beverage, glucagon 1 mg IV with sublingual GTN 600 micrograms may be tried. If the oesophagus cannot be cleared using these interventions, upper GI endoscopy will be required.

NON-CARDIAC CHEST PAIN

When cardiac causes for chest pain have been 'excluded', unexplained chest pain is often ascribed an oesophageal origin. Whilst oesophageal dysfunction can be demonstrated in a proportion of patients, other causes such as chest wall and spinal causes should also be sought as these are frequently overlooked. The presence of 'oesophageal' symptoms such as dysphagia, heartburn and regurgitation supports an oesophageal origin, but are not specific given the underlying high prevalence of these symptoms and endoscopy is often required to exclude severe oesophagitis given the atypical nature of symptoms in the elderly. The most likely treatable causes of non-cardiac chest pain of oesophageal origin are gastrooesophageal reflux disease and diffuse oesophageal spasm, which should be managed as described above. If pains are intermittent, prolonged trials of medication may be required in order to establish the degree of efficacy.

OESOPHAGEAL INFECTIONS

Monilial oesophagitis is common in the elderly, being predisposed to by conditions such as diabetes mellitus and intake of steroid medications. The clinical presentation is nonspecific and may include dysphagia, chest discomfort, nausea or heartburn.

Monilial infection of the pharynx may indicate the presence of oesophageal moniliasis. The diagnosis can be established by endoscopy, which shows a characteristic appearance, and biopsy, however empiric topical treatment of patients at high risk with oral nystatin suspension (swallowed) is also reasonable. Resistant or systemic infections require the use of either orally or systemically administered imidazoles.

Immunosuppression may result in viral infection of the oesophagus, commonly with either HSV or CMV. The presentation is often with odynophagia and the diagnosis is established at upper GI endoscopy with biopsy and specific staining or PCR. Treatment is with intravenous antiviral medication.

PILL-INDUCED OESOPHAGITIS

Many factors present in the elderly make this group particularly prone to medication-induced oesophagitis. This includes a high number of medications, increased prevalence of oesophageal dysmotility and swallowing problems and restrictions on the volume of fluids consumed. A high level of suspicion is required to diagnose medication-induced oesophagitis, which often presents with dysphagia and odynophagia. There may be a long history of milder dysphagia due to underlying oesophageal disease (reflux, webs or ineffective peristalsis). Medications that are particularly likely to cause problems include bisphosphonates, NSAIDs, tetracyclines and slow release potassium preparations. If the diagnosis is suspected clinically, the potentially offending medication should be ceased and the patient observed. If endoscopy is performed, the changes seen are nonspecific but ulceration that is atypical for reflux disease in the presence of a potentially offending medication is suspicious. The treatment is discontinuation of the drug or, if it must be continued, particular attention should be given to the method of administration, with the patient in an upright position and the medication 'washed down' with fluid.

PEPTIC ULCER DISEASE

Introduction

The major risk factors for peptic ulcer disease are NSAID use, Helicobacter pylori infection, previous peptic ulcer disease and age. The presence of comorbidities and the epidemiology of H pylori make this a particular problem in the elderly, who are at greatest risk of death from the complications of peptic ulceration (bleeding and perforation).

Because of the high prevalence of (prescribed and over the counter) usage of low dose aspirin and NSAID, peptic ulcer disease is common in the elderly. The prevalence of gastric ulceration in low dose aspirin users approaches 10 % and in NSAID users up to 30 %, although not all will lead to symptoms or clinical sequelae. Duodenal ulceration, and especially the complication of bleeding duodenal ulcer is also strongly associated with intake of NSAID. Use of enteric coated or rectal preparations does not

substantially reduce risk, however a dose effect is present and different NSAIDs are associated with different levels of risk, with higher doses and longer acting NSAIDs being associated with the greatest risk. COX2 selective NSAIDs are associated with lower gastrointestinal risk, but are contraindicated in patients with risk factors for vascular disease, which effectively excludes many elderly patients. The coprescription of COX2 selective NSAIDS and low dose aspirin negates the gastroprotective effect of the COX2 selective agent. A careful medication history is required to assess for NSAID intake, including specific enquiry regarding low dose aspirin intake, over the counter medications and herbal/alternative medications, some of which may contain NSAIDs.

Most patients with duodenal ulcer and approximately two thirds of patients with gastric ulcer are infected with Helicobacter pylori. The interaction between Helicobacter pylori infection and NSAID intake is synergistic; the combination of Helicobacter pylori infection and use of NSAIDs increases the risk of peptic ulceration by a factor of approximately 60. Helicobacter pylori infection is usually acquired in childhood, mostly related to living conditions and the local prevalence of infection at that time, and thus varies widely with age, socioeconomic group and race, being particularly prevalent in the elderly and in the developing world.

The consequences of Helicobacter pylori infection range from asymptomatic infection with gastritis to complicated peptic ulcer disease and gastric adenocarcinoma. Helicobacter pylori is not a risk factor for gastrooesophageal reflux disease and only a minority of patients with functional dyspepsia have Helicobacter pylori as a contributing factor.

Symptoms and signs

Presentation of peptic ulcer disease in the elderly is often nonspecific, with abdominal pain, nausea or anaemia. Complications such as haemorrhage or perforation present more dramatically, with haematemesis and melaena +/− cardiovascular compromise or an acute abdomen. It is important to recognize that peptic ulcer disease may be asymptomatic until presentation with a major complication, so a high level of suspicion should be maintained and appropriate prophylactic measures instituted (see below).

Complications of peptic ulcer disease include acute upper gastrointestinal bleeding, chronic low-grade bleeding causing iron deficiency anemia, perforation or pyloroduodenal scarring resulting in gastric outlet obstruction. Care should be taken to differentiate benign gastric ulceration from adenocarcinoma, which may present in a similar manner.

Diagnosis

Diagnosis is best made at upper GI endoscopy, which provides a definitive diagnosis, allows biopsy of suspicious lesions, assessment of Helicobacter pylori status and treatment of bleeding lesions. If upper GI endoscopy is unavailable, a barium meal is an alternative, but does not allow histological assessment or diagnosis of H pylori infection.

The production of urease by H pylori provides a convenient diagnostic marker; the presence of urease may be detected in biopsies taken at upper GI endoscopy or on breath testing (^{14}C or ^{13}C depending on local availability). Identification of Helicobacter pylori is more

difficult in patients on PPIs as these suppress Helicobacter pylori, reducing the sensitivity of tests that rely on urease production. Serology is less sensitive overall than urease testing, but is of value in patients on PPI therapy as positivity rates are unaffected by the suppression of Helicobacter pylori.

Therapy

Prophylaxis

Prevention of peptic ulceration should be considered in all patients using low dose aspirin or NSAIDs, however the literature in this area is not yet sufficiently mature to define optimal strategies in terms of efficacy and cost minimization for all patient groups. Concentrating solely on high-risk groups may miss many patients of average risk who develop complicated peptic ulcer disease. Risk factors for peptic ulceration are shown in Figure 26.1, 26.2.

Strategies to minimize the risk of complicated peptic ulceration include optimization of NSAID selection, dose and duration of therapy, use of COX2 selective agents and prophylaxis with gastroprotective agents. These decisions must be made in light of the patient's risk profile, including previous ulcer disease, H pylori

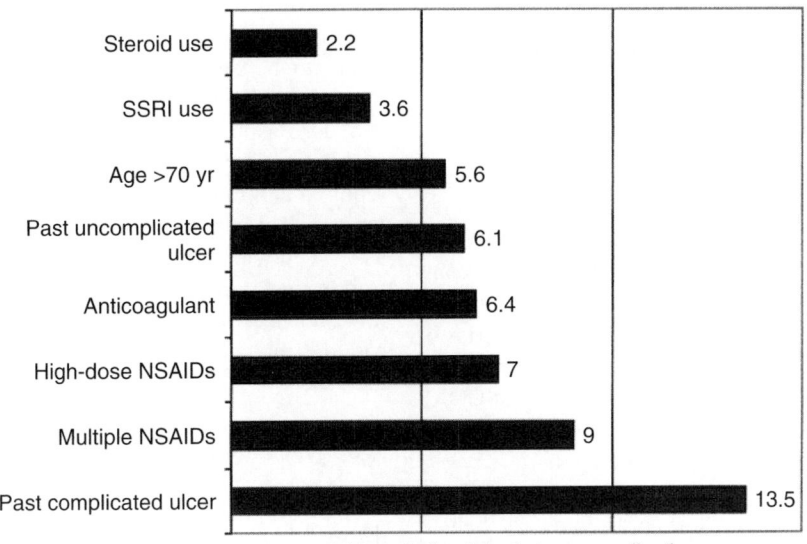

Odds ratio for risk of ulcer complications

SSRI = Selective serotonin reuptake inhibitor.

Figure 26.1. Risk factors for NSAID-induced GI complications. Reproduced from (1)

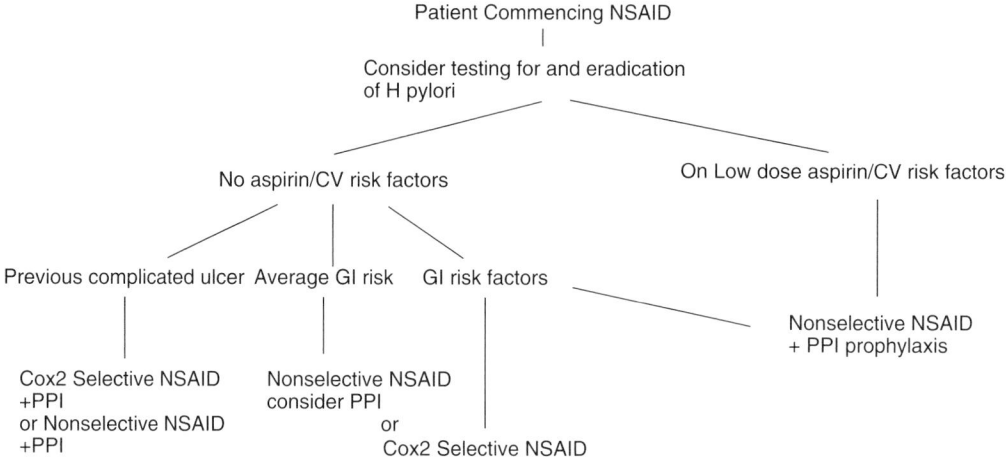

Figure 26.2. Selection of therapy and ulcer prophylaxis in a patient commencing NSAID

status, concomitant conditions/medication and willingness of the patient or a third party to pay for specific drugs.

Average risk patients

The decision to commence a NSAID should only be made once non-drug and simple analgesic options have been exhausted, and a short-acting drug such as indomethacin should be used at the lowest effective dose for the shortest possible period. COX2 selective agents have lower gastrointestinal toxicity than conventional NSAIDs, but are substantially more expensive and increase cardiovascular risk at higher doses. Coprescription of PPI reduces the gastrointestinal toxicity of nonselective NSAIDs, however the benefits of this strategy in average risk patients has not been defined. The issue of whether to test and treat average risk patients for H pylori prior to commencement of NSAID is unclear. Eradication of H pylori would be expected to reduce the risk of ulceration, however the benefit of this strategy in addition or as an alternative to the use of COX2 selective agents has not been defined in patients at average risk for peptic ulceration.

Average risk patients taking low dose aspirin will not gain the same gastrointestinal benefit from the use of COX2 selective NSAIDs the interaction between COX2 selective NSAIDs and aspirin on cardiovascular risk has not been defined and the use of low dose aspirin and nonselective NSAIDs also however substantially increases the risk of gastrointestinal complications, and in the absence of definitive data it seems reasonable to consider ulcer prophylaxis with PPI in average risk patients requiring low dose aspirin in combination with any NSAID, particularly if the patient is H pylori +ve.

High-risk patients

High-risk patients with previous peptic ulcer disease (particularly if complicated) are most likely to benefit from prophylaxis, especially if ongoing risk factors (e.g. H pylori infection, low dose aspirin) are present. COX2 selective agents should be preferred if NSAID therapy is required and the patient has a low cardiovascular risk. The use of clopidogrel is likely to be associated with a lower incidence of upper gastrointestinal ulceration than low dose aspirin, however in patients with previous bleeding ulcer, the rate of rebleeding still appears to be increased.

Prophylaxis regime

Prophylaxis should be undertaken with standard doses of PPI. Misoprostol is also effective in reducing the incidence of ulceration, has a more complicated dosage schedule and is poorly tolerated in some patients.

Established peptic ulceration

The management of established peptic ulceration depends on the mode of presentation, however the principles are to:

- treat complications;
- heal the ulcer;
- identify and treat underlying risk factors;
- reduce the risk of recurrence.

Treatment of complications

Bleeding peptic ulceration should be managed in association with a gastrointestinal physician or surgeon. Resuscitation and early endoscopy with endoscopic therapy to treat bleeding and high-risk lesions with injection and thermal methods have been shown to reduce rates of rebleeding and surgery. Patients should also be treated with intravenous PPI infusion for a period of three days to reduce the risk of rebleeding. The use of tranexamic acid may reduce rebleeding, but is contraindicated in the presence of significant vascular disease.

Ulcer healing

The most important factor in healing of peptic ulcers is acid suppression, with greater degrees of acid suppression resulting in faster rates of healing. Standard doses of PPI therapy are usually sufficient. It is rarely necessary to document duodenal ulcer healing with repeat endoscopy, but this should be considered where the ulcer was large, atypical or complicated, or there are ongoing risk factors such as NSAID use. Gastric ulcers require biopsy and repeat endoscopy to document healing and exclude malignancy, although with the reduction in the incidence of gastric adenocarcinoma the value of this strategy in 'typical' NSAID ulcers is not clear. The duration of therapy should be tailored to the size of the ulcer and is generally between 8 and 12 weeks. NSAID-induced ulcers heal more slowly in the presence of ongoing NSAID intake and larger ulcers take longer to heal than smaller ulcers. The indication for NSAID therapy should be reviewed and the agent ceased if possible.

In uncomplicated duodenal ulcer disease with Helicobacter pylori infection and no ongoing NSAID treatment, a course of treatment for Helicobacter pylori may be sufficient.

Treatment of Helicobacter pylori infection

Treatment for Helicobacter pylori has evolved such that cure rates of 85–90 % are now seen in published trials, however success in the community is probably lower than this because of a lower compliance rate, and side effects remain common, although less that with older regimes. The presence of Helicobacter pylori is not in itself necessarily an indication for treatment, which should be considered in relation to symptoms, overall risks and need for other therapies. The presence of peptic ulcer disease is a strong indication for treatment, however if ongoing acid suppressive therapy will be required in any case (reflux disease/ongoing risk factors) the incremental benefit of Helicobacter pylori eradication may not be large in the elderly. Effective treatment of Helicobacter pylori requires the use of at least three medications: a PPI and two antibiotics. Numerous combinations have been evaluated and success rates are high in patients who are compliant with a full course of treatment. These medications are often available as a combination pack, which makes dispensing and dosing easier. The efficacy of therapy depends on factors such as local antibiotic resistance patterns of Helicobacter pylori and compliance. One example of a seven day regimen with a relatively low rate of side effects and good efficacy is:

- (Es)Omeprazole 20 mg bd, together with
- Clarithromycin 500 mg bd, and
- Amoxicillin 1 g bd.

Patients with penicillin allergy should have metronidazole 400 mg bd substituted for amoxycillin. Patients should be strongly counseled to comply with the therapy, as the first course of treatment is their 'best chance' for eradication.

Confirmation of eradication of Helicobacter pylori following treatment is essential where ulcer disease is present and cessation of PPI therapy is contemplated. Assessment should be carried out at least four weeks after completing eradication therapy or other antibiotic treatment, and after two weeks off PPI (false negatives) Urease breath testing is the most appropriate method as it is noninvasive, however if upper GI endoscopy is planned, urease testing or histopathology may be performed on endoscopic biopsies. In patients who remain on a PPI, histopathology on multiple biopsies from the upper and lower stomach is the most sensitive method of detecting residual infection and culture/antibiotic resistance testing may guide therapy. Serology is not appropriate for the assessment of eradication therapy as the titre of antibody falls only slowly.

Management of failed eradication therapy

Failure of Helicobacter pylori eradication therapy is usually the result of antibiotic resistance or poor compliance (which often results in antibiotic resistance). Repetition of the original course of therapy is only occasionally effective. The management of failed eradication is to use second line therapies, usually PPI with different antibiotics +/− Bismuth subcitrate. A variety of courses have been evaluated, and these patients should be managed in consultation with a practitioner with an interest/expertise in this area.

NSAID intake

The indication for the use of aspirin or NSAIDs should be reviewed and alternatives discussed and trialed.

Key Points

- Age, helicobacter pylori infection and intake of medications commonly used in elderly patients are major risk factors for peptic ulcer disease.
- The first presentation of peptic ulcer disease may be with a major complication such as bleeding or perforation.
- Ulcer risk factors and prophylaxis should be considered in all patients commencing NSAIDs.

- Management involves treatment of complications, healing of the ulcer, identification of risk factors and reducing the likelihood of recurrence.

GASTRITIS

Gastritis indicates inflammation of the gastric mucosa, and may be due to use of drugs such as NSAIDs, Helicobacter pylori infection, autoimmune gastritis or rare causes such as Crohns disease, viral infection, etc. In many cases no specific cause can be identified. Although many symptoms are attributed to 'gastritis' there is little evidence of a causal link except in the case of acute gastritis, for example due to Helicobacter pylori or intake of NSAIDs. Most symptoms attributed to 'gastritis' probably have another cause (reflux disease, peptic ulcer, functional dyspepsia). The treatment of gastritis is the treatment of the underlying cause.

NON-ULCER DYSPEPSIA

Postprandial abdominal discomfort in the absence of peptic ulcer disease or gastro-oesophageal reflux disease is common. Occasionally this symptom is due to other diseases that cause upper abdominal discomfort (gallstones, hepatic disease or musculoskeletal or abdominal wall pain). Functional dyspepsia is a condition which is believed to relate to abnormal perception of visceral stimuli arising in the stomach and upper small intestine. Common symptoms include postprandial discomfort, early satiety, upper abdominal bloating and occasionally nausea, vomiting and weight loss. The differential diagnosis is wide and upper GI endoscopy or barium study is recommended to exclude underlying obstruction or ulceration. A gastric emptying study will differentiate gastroparesis (see separate chapter 27). Depression and anxiety are potent causes of upper GI symptoms and should be actively sought and treated. Management may be difficult and focuses on symptom control. Dietary modification includes avoidance of foods that lead to symptoms, with dietary supplementation as appropriate. A therapeutic trial of acid suppression, antiemetic drugs or prokinetics may be worthwhile, but should not be continued if ineffective. If these measures are ineffective, a trial of a low dose of a tricyclic antidepressant may be helpful.

REFERENCES

1. Anonymous. Prevention of NSAID-induced ulcers in the elderly. *Geriatrics*. 2005 Oct; Suppl: 3–12.
2. Greenwald DA. Aging, the gastrointestinal tract, and risk of acid-related disease. *Am J Med*. 2004 Sep 6; **117** Suppl 5A: 8S–13S.
3. Laine L. Proton pump inhibitor co-therapy with nonsteroidal anti-inflammatory drugs–nice or necessary? *Rev Gastroenterol Disord*. 2004; **4** Suppl 4: S33–41.
4. Johnson DA. Gastroesophageal reflux disease in the elderly–a prevalent and severe disease. *Rev Gastroenterol Disord*. 2004; **4** Suppl 4: S16–24.
5. Johnson DA, Fennerty MB. Heartburn severity underestimates erosive esophagitis severity in elderly patients with gastroesophageal reflux disease. *Gastroenterology*. 2004 Mar; **126**(3): 660–4.
6. Pilotto A. Aging and upper gastrointestinal disorders. *Best Pract Res Clin Gastroenterol*. 2004; **18** Suppl: 73–81.
7. Pilotto A, Franceschi M, Leandro G, Paris F, Cascavilla L, Longo MG, et al. Proton-pump inhibitors reduce the risk of uncomplicated peptic ulcer in elderly either acute or chronic users of aspirin/non-steroidal anti-inflammatory drugs. *Aliment Pharmacol Ther*. 2004 Nov 15; **20**(10): 1091–7.
8. Vergara M, Catalan M, Gisbert JP, Calvet X. Meta-analysis: role of Helicobacter pylori eradication in the prevention of peptic ulcer in NSAID users. *Aliment Pharmacol Ther*. 2005 Jun 15; **21**(12): 1411–8.
9. Williams JL. Gastroesophageal reflux disease in the elderly. *Director*. 2003 Summer; **11**(3): 107–9.

27 Gastric emptying in older patients

Robert J. Fraser

Repatriation General Hospital, Adelaide, Australia

INTRODUCTION

In addition to, and as a result of the effects of disease, the elderly are the greatest consumers in the community of both prescribed and over the counter medication. Many of these impact substantially on gastric emptying (Table 27.1). Furthermore the timing of drug intake in relation to food intake is an important determinant of therapeutic efficacy in the older patient. Hence although gastric emptying per se in healthy older individuals may be relatively normal, disorders of gastric emptying in older patients in general are likely to have a major impact on drug therapy.

Gastric motility can be broadly divided into fasting and postprandial activity and the rate of gastric emptying depends on the properties of the ingested material and the prevailing pattern of gastric motor activity at the time of ingestion (1). Fasting motility is cyclical and characterised by three phases: motor quiescence (phase I), a gradually increasing irregular peristaltic contractile pattern (phase II), and a brief period (3–10 min) of intensive phasic contractions (phase III) which appears to be triggered by peaks in secretion of the neuropeptide motilin It is important to note that non-digestible solids including tablets or capsules are emptied during late phase II or phase III of fasting motility which occurs substantially after meal emptying is complete and food in the gastrointestinal tract may reduce absorption by delaying delivery to the small intestine even in health.

Ingestion of nutrient meals results in a conversion of gastric motility from a fasting to a fed pattern. The proximal stomach (fundus and upper body) relaxes and an irregular pattern of mixing and intermittent propulsive contractions occurs in the antrum. During the postprandial or fed state, nutrient liquids, and digestible solids have different patterns of emptying from the stomach with liquids emptying in a linear fashion, whilst digestible solids are triturated (ground into tiny particles <1 mm in diameter) before emptying occurs (1).

Unlike other areas of the gastrointestinal tract (oesophagus, colon and anal sphincters) where advancing age may be associated with neuro-muscular dysfunctions, both fasting and fed gastric motility (together with gastric secretory function) are usually well preserved into old age (Figure 27.1) (2). Thus although there is some reduction in motor and secretory activity

Table 27.1. Drugs commonly associated with slow gastric emptying

Opiates
Leodopa
Tricyclic antidepressants
Proton pump inhibitors
Sumatriptan
Acarbose
Sildenafil
Somatostatin analogs

Prescribing for Elderly Patients Edited by Stephen Jackson, Paul Jansen and Arduino Mangoni
© 2009 John Wiley & Sons, Ltd

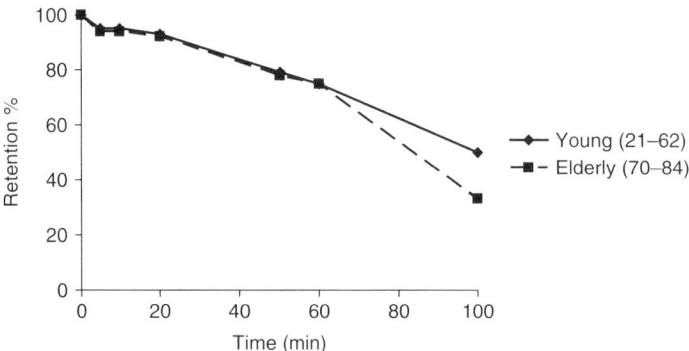

Figure 27.1. Scintigraphic gastric emptying curves showing only minor effects of ageing on emptying of solids (from Horowitz et al ref (2))

of stomach during healthy ageing, this does not usually result in overt symptoms or significantly contribute to altered drug kinetics (3). It has been suggested that delayed gastric emptying may contribute to anorexia of ageing (4) and reduced gastric acid secretion secondary to atrophic gastritis may impair absorption of pH dependent medications (such as ketoconazole) (5). A more common problem however is the impact of various diseases which become more prevalent with increasing age, and adverse effects of both prescribed and over the counter medication.

AETIOLOGY OF DISTURBED GASTRIC MOTOR FUNCTION IN AGEING

Gastric emptying in the healthy elderly patient is only slightly slower than that of young individuals possibly as a result of the autonomic nerve dysfunction seen in with increasing age. The significance of observed changes is unclear but in general the clinical impact of the observed changes probably has a minor impact overall on the gastric absorption of drugs, although loss of gastric acid secretion and vitamin B12 absorption may lead to anaemia.

However, the incidence of diseases such as diabetes mellitus, Parkinson's disease and chronic renal failure which have a major impact on gastric motility increase dramatically with

increasing age. Visceral neuropathy in patients with long-standing diabetes is is associated with gastroparesis in up to 50 % of patients; and acute hyperglycaemia per se also retards emptying (6). Paradoxically, type II diabetes mellitus may also be associated with increased emptying of liquids (7). The unpredictability of gastric emptying in these patients has major implications for glycaemic control. Up to 100 % of patients with Parkinson's disease may have delayed gastric emptying on formal testing (8). Chronic renal failure is also frequently associated with a high incidence of gastroparesis both in patients receiving haemodialysis and those who are not dialysis dependent (9) and lead to malnutrition (10).

SYMPTOMS AND SIGNS

The classic symptoms of delayed gastric emptying are nausea, vomiting and early satiety. These symptoms are sometimes severe enough to cause malabsorption and weight loss. However, slow gastric emptying is often asymptomatic and there is often a poor correlation between the rate of emptying and symptoms even in patients with severe gastroparesis (11). In many patients the clues to problems associated with gastroparesis are more subtle. For example, patients with diabetes mellitus may present with loss of glycaemic control. This may be manifest as either hyperglycaemia or hypoglycaemia due to a mismatch between nutrient absorption and exogenous or endogenous insulin In patients receiving oral drug therapy for Parkinson's disease, erratic absorption of drugs may contribute to fluctuations in symptoms such as the on-off phenomenon.

DIAGNOSIS

Non-specific symptoms such as abdominal pain and bloating are common in the elderly. Anorexia and weight loss are also relatively non-specific. However although gastric emptying rates decline with increasing age, severe symptoms of vomiting and early satiety especially if accompanied by weight loss, should encourage investigation for malignancy or peptic ulcer disease together with assessment for diabetes, depression and a detailed review of medication. Examination findings are also usually non-specific. There may be evidence of weight loss and rarely a succussion splash can be heard.

After exclusion of gastric outlet obstruction, the diagnosis of gastroparesis is best established with a scintigraphic gastric emptying study (1). Ideally both solid and liquid components should be measured and in patients with diabetes mellitus during euglycaemia (12). Stable isotope breath tests may be useful as screening tools in regions where there is expertise in this technique (13). However, breath test techniques whilst less invasive are also less sensitive. Barium studies are too insensitive to be reliable indicators of slow emptying whilst emptying of radio-opaque gastric markers reflects return of the fasting pattern rather than nutrient delivery to the intestine.

THERAPY

Optimal management of glycaemic control is recommended in diabetic patients as hyperglycaemia per se delays gastric emptying (6). Rationalization of drug therapy, such as reduction in opiate use where possible, is logical. Pharmacotherapy with prokinetics such as metoclopramide and domperidone is helpful in a number of patients, although significant side effects in the elderly with metoclopramide are not uncommon. In patients with diabetic or idiopathic gastroparesis the most effective agent for treatment was cisapride (1). However this agent is now unavailable in many countries due to rare but serious cardiac side effects. Low dose (1–3 mg/kg i.v.) erythromycin (a motilin agonist) is useful acutely (14), but oral therapy is less proven. Other agents currently under investigation include non-antibiotic motilin agonists and peripheral opioid receptor antagonists which may have a role in gut dysmotility secondary to opiates. In patients with Parkinson's disease, transdermal delivery of therapy to bypass the stomach may be beneficial.

THERAPY SCHEME OF ADVISED DRUGS FOR GASTROPARESIS

- Metoclopramide (10–20 mg qid);
- Domperidone (10–20 mg tds).

Where the above is unsuccessful consider erythromycin syrup 125 mg po 20 min before meals.

KEY POINTS

- Significant gastroparesis is uncommon in the healthy elderly.
- Slow gastric emptying occurs commonly with disease such as diabetes mellitus, Parkinson's disease and renal failure which have a high incidence in the older age groups. This is frequently asymptomatic but may be associated with alterations in glycaemic control and reduction in control of movement disorders.
- Slow gastric emptying is a consequence of many prescribed medications.
- Drug treatment options are currently limited but include rationalisation or replacement of medication where possible. Tight control of blood sugar concentrations may be beneficial in diabetic patients.

GUIDELINES

http://www.gastrojournal.org/article/
PIIS0016508504016336/fulltext.
   http://ngc.gov/summary/summary.aspx?
ss=15&doc_id=5979&nbr=3938.

EFFECT OF HEALTHY AGEING ON APPETITE REGULATION— ANOREXIA OF AGEING

Introduction

Regulation of food intake to maintain body physiology is a critical function for survival. Maintaining the balance between appetite and satiety mechanisms is highly complex and involves multiple interactions between physiological, psychological and social factors. These include the energy requirements of the organism, the nature and quality of the available food, the setting in which food is presented and nutrients already present in the gut or stored elsewhere within the body. In consequence energy intake at any given time is highly variable. However in the young healthy individual, regulation of food intake is highly controlled with multiple mechanisms in place to ensure that the feeding drive remains intact. One of the characteristics of ageing is the reduction in efficiency of homeostatic mechanisms and it is not surprising that disturbances in weight regulation are well recognised in the elderly (15). Elderly subjects who lose weight due to calorie restriction do not compensate for this by subsequent increase in consumption (16). Weight loss in these patients most markedly affects skeletal muscle mass exacerbating age associated changes in body composition. Such sarcopenia may result in further functional decline.

Aetiology

Weight loss in the elderly may be considered in three broad categories (i) social, (ii) psychological and (iii) medical (16). The mechanisms underlying anorexia are poorly understood, although abnormalities of regulatory pathways

for taste, smell, and sensations such as hunger and satiety such as PYY, CCK and ghrelin, are currently under investigation (17). Animal studies suggest that ageing per se is associated with anorexia and disordered gastrointestinal transit. Even mild slowing of gastric emptying may contribute to anorexia in some older subjects possibly as result of antral distension providing early satiety signals (4). In addition, there are a number of other situations and conditions including social isolation and depression that are characterized by poor appetite and weight loss (Table 27.2). Anorexia and subsequent malnutrition secondary to the effect of medications is an important and often avoidable type of adverse drug reaction. Drugs that are particularly associated with anorexia and weight loss are shown in Table 27.3. In addition many drugs

Table 27.2. Important causes of under-nutrition in older persons (adapted from (17))

Social
Poverty
Isolation, living alone, lack of social supports
Elder abuse
Functional impairment leading to inability to shop
   prepare and cook meals or feed one-self
Institutional factors- failure to cater for ethnic food
   preferences, lack of food choices, other residents
   poor behaviour
Psychological
Depression
Dementia
Bereavement
Paranoia
Phobias- choking, cholesterol
Psychosis
Medical
Cardiac failure
Chronic Obstructive Pulmonary Disease especially
   emphysema
Infection
Alcoholism
Malignancy
Poor Dentition
Rheumatoid arthritis
Gastrointestinal Dysfunction
      Dysphagia- oro-pharyngeal, oesophageal
      Dsypepsia
      Malabsorption
      Vomiting/diarrhoea
Parkinson's disease
Hyperthyroidism
Medications (see below)

Table 27.3. Common drugs causing anorexia in the elderly (adapted from (15))

Digoxin
Amiodarone
Spironolactone
Interferon
Phenothiazines
Topiramate
Tricyclic antidepressant
Selective Serotonin Reuptake Inhibitors
Antibiotics including metronidazole
Iron supplements
Cytotoxic drugs
Colchicine
NSAIDs
Theophylline
Acetyl cholinesterase inhibitors

may also lead to malabsorption (see chapter 28 on large bowel).

Symptoms and signs

Anorexia of ageing resulting in protein calorie malnutrition is associated with protean manifestations. In addition to simple weight loss and loss of body mass, immune deficiency, anaemia, cognitive deficits, poor wound healing and osteopenia are well recognised. Depression may result from as well as contribute to anorexia.

Diagnosis

Historical weight loss is an excellent measure of nutrition deficits. Assessment of protein calorie malnutrition in the elderly by a screening tool such as DETERMINE, SCALES or MNA may also useful 1 (17). Initial investigation of the aetiology of anorexia requires a detailed history with particular emphasis on psychosocial and emotional factors, medication and symptoms suggestive of malabsorption or hypermetabolism. Low albumin concentrations and anaemia are highly predictive of mortality (18).

Therapy

Depression is an important treatable cause of weight loss in the elderly (15). Judicious removal or replacement of medications associated with anorexia may also be important. In undernourished elderly patients, supplements are

beneficial, but there is no evidence of benefit in the healthy older population (17). Sarcopenia is important to take into consideration when calculating drug doses for renally excreted drugs (such as aminoglycosides and enoxiparin) as standard calculations of renal function assume a normal muscle mass and creatinine. Although megestrol, growth hormone and cyproheptadine have all been proposed as possible drugs to treat malnutrition there are currently no convincing data to establish the efficacy of any of these agents (17).

Therapy scheme of advised drugs

See above.

Key points

- Anorexia and weight loss are common in elderly patients.
- Medications may be an important contributor to anorexia.
- Depression is an important treatable cause.
- Low serum creatinine levels associated with sarcopenia may lead to overestimations of renal function when calculating doses for renally cleared drugs.

Guidelines

http:www.mna-elderly.com.

REFERENCES

1. Horowitz M, Dent J. Disordered gastric emptying: mechanical basis, assessment and treatment. *Baillieres's Clinical Gastroenterology*. 1991; **5**: 371–407.
2. Horowitz M et al. Changes in gastric emptying rates with age. *Clin Science*. 1984; **67**: 213–18.
3. O'Mahony D, O'Leary P, EMM Q. Ageing and Intestinal motility. A review of factors that affect intestinal motility in the aged. *Drugs Ageing*. 2002; **19**: 15–27.
4. Clarkston, W et al. Evidence for anorexia of ageing: gastrointestinal transit and hunger in healthy elderly vs young adults. *Am J Physiol*. 1997; **272**: R243–R248.
5. Hurwitz A, et al. Gastric function in the elderly: effects on absorption of ketoconazole. *J Clin Pharmacol* 2003; **43**: 996–1002.

6. Kong M-F, Horowitz M. Gastric emptying in diabetes mellitus. Relationship to blood glucose control. *Clinics in Geriatric Medicine*. 1999; **13**: 321–38.

7. Phillips W, Schwartz J, McMahan C. Rapid gastric emptying in patients with early non-insulin dependent diabetes mellitus. *New Eng J Med* 1991; **324**: 130–1.

8. Goetze O et al. Predictors of gastric emptying in Parkinson's disease. *Neurogastroenterol Motil* 2006; **18**: 369–75.

9. Kao C, Hsu Y, Wang S. Delayed gastric emptying in patients with chronic renal failure. *Nucl Med Commun* 1996; **17**: 164–7.

10. De Schoenmakere G, et al. Relationship between gastric emptying and clinical and biochemical factors in chronic haemodialysis patients. *Nephrol Dial Transplant* 2001; **16**: 1850–5.

11. Samsom M et al. Prevalence of delayed gastric emptying in diabetic patients and relationship to dyspeptic symptoms. *Diabetes Care* 2003; **26**: 3116–22.

12. Fraser R et al. Hyperglycaemia slows gastric emptying in type I diabetes mellitus. *Diabetologia* 1990; **33**: 675–80.

13. Ghoos Y et al. Measurement of gastric emptying rate of solids by means of a carbon-labeled octanoic acid breath test. *Gastroenterology* 1993; **104**: 1640–7.

14. Janssens J et al. Improvement of gastric emptying in diabetic gastroparesis by erythromycin. Preliminary studies. *N Eng J Med* 1990; **322**: 1028–31.

15. Morley J. Anorexia of Ageing: Physiologic and Pathophysiologic. *Am J Clin Nutr* 1997; **66**: 760–3.

16. Roberts S et al. Control of food intake in older men. *JAMA* 1994; **272**: 1601–6.

17. Chapman I. Endocrinology of anorexia of ageing. *Best Practice and Research Clinical Endocrinology and Metabolism* 2004; **18**: 437–52.

18. Miller D, Morley J. Nutritional Epidemiology. *Ann Rev Gerontol Geriatrics* 1995; **15**: 20–53.

28 Lower gastrointestinal disorders

Daniel L. Worthley[1], Graeme P. Young[1,2] and
Robert J. Fraser[2]

[1]*Department of Gastroenterology and Hepatology, Flinders Medical Centre, Adelaide, Australia*
[2]*Repatriation General Hospital, Adelaide, Australia*

MALABSORPTION

Introduction

Effective nutrient absorption requires sufficient intake, digestion, mucosal absorption, and then delivery into the circulation (Figure 28.1). Strictly defined, malabsorption refers to an abnormality of mucosal absorption, most commonly as a consequence of reduced surface area or inflammation. In contrast maldigestion refers to abnormal luminal processing. In reality these processes are frequently intertwined and have common clinical outcomes. In this chapter abnormal nutrient absorption, despite sufficient intake, will be referred to as malabsorption. The exact prevalence of malabsorption in elderly patients is unknown, and the diagnosis, when made, is frequently delayed, because of the often subtle clinical presentation in this group.

Aetiology

Comorbidity and polypharmacy are more relevant to predisposing the aging bowel to malabsorption, than senescence (1). Nevertheless, with advancing age there are physiological changes of the alimentary tract, including impaired gastric acid secretion (2) and a reduction in myenteric plexus neurons (3). In addition, the

capacity of the colon to compensate for more proximal malabsorption may also be impaired. In this chapter we will address several of the specific disease processes that are most clinically relevant in older individuals.

Drug-related malabsorption: Medications may affect the nutrition of elderly patients on multiple levels. Drugs such as digoxin, opiates, and acetylcholinesterase inhibitors may cause nausea and anorexia, whilst methotrexate and non-steroidal anti-inflammatory drugs can cause small intestinal mucosal toxicity. Anticholinergics and opioids can also interfere with alimentary tract motility predisposing to small intestinal bacterial overgrowth (SIBO).

Small intestinal bacterial overgrowth: When the mechanisms that promote the relatively sterile upper gastrointestinal environment, such as small intestinal motility, gastric acid secretion and mucosal immunity, are impaired by drugs (e.g. proton pump inhibitors) or comorbidity (such as diabetes mellitus), bacterial proliferation ($>10^6$ orgs/mL) can result. Bacterial overgrowth in elderly people, however, does not universally cause clinically relevant malabsorption, nor is it necessarily associated with the classical clinical features of bacterial overgrowth, (4) but may present more insidiously with nutritional deficiencies. The pathogenesis of malabsorption in SIBO

Prescribing for Elderly Patients Edited by Stephen Jackson, Paul Jansen and Arduino Mangoni
© 2009 John Wiley & Sons, Ltd

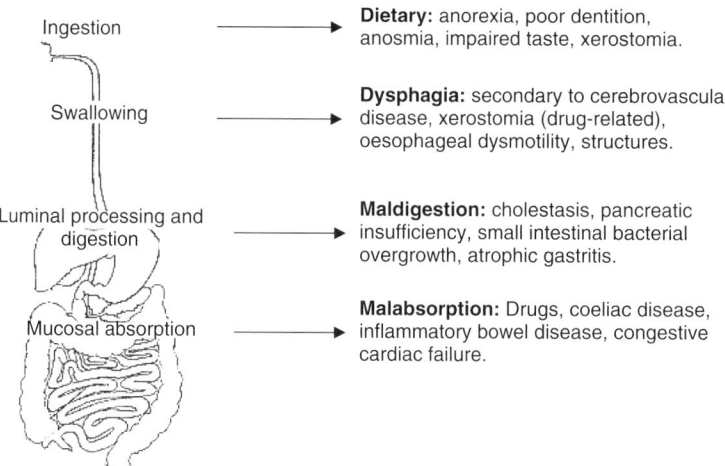

Ingestion → **Dietary:** anorexia, poor dentition, anosmia, impaired taste, xerostomia.

Swallowing → **Dysphagia:** secondary to cerebrovascular disease, xerostomia (drug-related), oesophageal dysmotility, structures.

Luminal processing and digestion → **Maldigestion:** cholestasis, pancreatic insufficiency, small intestinal bacterial overgrowth, atrophic gastritis.

Mucosal absorption → **Malabsorption:** Drugs, coeliac disease, inflammatory bowel disease, congestive cardiac failure.

Figure 28.1. Causes of suboptimal nutrition in elderly people

is multifactorial. Firstly, bacterial proliferation may directly damage enterocytes, blunting intestinal villi and diminishing brush border enzyme activity. Vitamin B_{12} deficiency results from the sequestration of vitamin B_{12} by the enteric bacteria. The bacteria may simultaneously produce folate, thus the individual with SIBO is often replete in folate despite significant vitamin B_{12} deficiency. Steatorrhoea can also occur following bacterial deconjugation of secreted bile salts. When bile salts are deconjugated they form free bile acids that are rapidly reabsorbed in the jejunum, causing a reduction in the luminal concentration of bile salts, and thus impaired micelle formation, critical for fat absorption. This is in contrast to the secretory diarrhoea that may follow terminal ileal disease or resection, when poorly absorbed conjugated bile salts pass into the colon, with consequent fluid and electrolyte secretion from the colonic mucosa.

Coeliac disease: Coeliac disease is sometimes considered a condition of the young. There is, however, a large reservoir of undiagnosed coeliac disease within the elderly population. Several series have shown that up to 25 % of new coeliac disease diagnoses occur in those greater than 60 years of age (5). It should

especially be considered when conditions such as iron deficiency or osteoporosis, accompany other features of malabsorption.

Common co-morbidities that interfere with absorption in elderly people: Comorbidities, common to older age, can influence alimentary tract function. Diabetes mellitus through changes in bowel motility, and predisposition to SIBO, may be important. Heart failure causes venous congestion of the bowel, and major resection of intestine can interfere with absorption (6).

Symptoms and signs

Malabsorption may present with a single complaint or a cluster of symptoms such as diarrhoea, abdominal pain, bloating, weight loss or flatulence. Weight loss despite adequate diet, is a particularly important feature. However, in elderly people the presenting symptoms are often less obvious including lethargy from anaemia or back pain from low-impact osteoporotic fracture. The physical examination of the elderly patient with potential malabsorption should include a full general examination, with particular attention to the patient's weight and height, skin rashes, bruising, nail changes, evidence of heart failure, and neurological examination, particularly of the gait and lower limbs, to assess for signs of B_{12} deficiency.

Diagnosis

Blood tests are valuable and should include complete blood examination and film, routine biochemistry including calcium, albumin, liver function tests, iron studies, glucose, vitamin B_{12} and folate, also INR together with assessment of CRP or ESR if an inflammatory condition is considered. Coeliac disease serology is the first step in investigating coeliac disease and may help triage patients through to upper gastrointestinal endoscopy (7, 8). If the history and examination are suggestive of malabsorption an upper gastrointestinal endoscopy with duodenal biopsy is needed. The next tier of laboratory investigation is directed by symptoms, for example suspicion of SIBO can be tested by the ^{14}C D-xylose breath test. Quantitative or semi-quantitative faecal fat analyses are preferable to the ^{14}C triolein breath test for investigating steatorrhoea, provided it is offered by the local pathology service. Finally, abdominal computed tomography (CT) may be helpful for assessing areas of the bowel beyond the reach of endoscopy, important for Crohn's disease and lymphoma. There is also an evolving role for capsule endoscopy ("pill cam") for diagnosing obscure small intestinal Crohn's disease, particularly when traditional imaging is normal but other features suggest small intestinal inflammation. Investigations should also identify associated problems, for example a dual-energy X-ray absorptiometry scan to assess for osteoporosis.

Therapy

The management of malabsorption in elderly people is directed simultaneously at correcting nutritional deficiencies and specific treatment of the underlying cause. Treatment of coeliac disease involves dietary exclusion of gluten. SIBO associated with problematic symptoms or malabsorption, is usually treated with antibiotics. Amoxicillin, amoxicillin/clavulanate or norfloxacin, prescribed in a seven day course may be effective, albeit that the symptoms can recur after stopping the antibiotic (9). Some patients may only require occasional therapy, whilst those that frequently relapse may benefit from prolonged or cyclical treatment.

Therapy scheme of the advised drugs

Antibiotics, such as those used in SIBO, can be associated with adverse effects particularly diarrhoea, hepatic disturbances, as well as hypersensitivity phenomenon. Hepatitis and cholestatic jaundice associated with amoxicillin/clavulanate preparations have been most frequently reported in elderly males. In elderly patients with a creatinine clearance of $\leq$30 mL/minute, norfloxacin should be reduced from the usual dose of 400 mg twice daily, to 400 mg once daily.

Key Points

- Diagnosis of malabsorption in elderly people is often delayed, because of the subtle and often extra-gastroenterological presentation.
- Elderly people are not predisposed to malabsorption, per se, thus careful consideration is required to identify underlying diseases.
- Drugs and comorbidities are important causes of malabsorption in elderly people.
- The work up of malabsorption should also address the consequences of the identified nutritional deficiencies, such as osteoporosis.
- Treatment of malabsorption requires simultaneous replacement of the identified deficiencies and management of the underlying cause.

Guidelines

British Society of Gastroenterology: tests for malabsorption.

Links

http://www.bsg.org.uk/clinical_prac/guidelines/chronic_diarr.htm.

INFLAMMATORY BOWEL DISEASE

Introduction

Inflammatory bowel disease (IBD) is composed of two major clinical entities, ulcerative colitis (UC) and Crohn's disease (CD), as well as a difficult to categorized subset (approximately 10%) referred to as indeterminate colitis. IBD is frequently diagnosed in young adults. The previously accepted bimodal age presentation of IBD, with a second peak occurring in later decades, has been recently questioned (10). Nevertheless, IBD can occur in all ages, including in elderly patients (10). The incidence of CD and UC in Western countries ranges from 0.7 to 9.8, and 1.5 to 20.3, respectively, per 100 000 person years (10). Pathologically, CD is characterized by patchy inflammation, ranging in severity from subtle aphthous ulcers to deep 'cobble stoning' of the mucosa. CD inflammation may involve all regions of the alimentary tract. In contrast, the inflammation of UC involves the rectum with or without a variable length of continuous, more proximal colitis. In addition, there are two other types of colitis, collagenous and lymphocytic. These present with watery diarrhoea, and occasional weight loss and abdominal pain. These other forms of colitis are characterized by macroscopically normal mucosa, with the diagnosis made on mucosal biopsy, revealing chronic inflammation. These typically affect women in their sixth and seventh decades.

Aetiology

IBD is by definition idiopathic, but results from an interruption in the delicate balance of mucosal immunity, influenced by immunogenetic polymorphisms, luminal bacteria, and environmental factors, such as smoking. Immunosenescence, or impaired immunity with ageing, is characterized by a poorer response to newly encountered antigens (11). These changes also influence the processing of autoantigens, and thus may predispose to autoimmune disease (12). The colonic flora in elderly people is also different to that found in younger individuals and may contribute to the pathogenesis of IBD in elderly patients (13).

Symptoms and signs

The presentation of UC is similar to that for younger patients, typically bloody diarrhoea. In elderly patients the extent of the UC, however, is usually more limited, frequently confined to the distal colorectum (14). Proctitis may be particularly troublesome in elderly patients because it can lead to faecal incontinence. Following the induction of remission the prognosis for elderly patients is more favourable, with fewer recurrent episodes (15). The symptoms attributable to CD usually relate to the chief sites of inflammation. Abdominal pain in the right iliac fossa may indicate ileal disease, haematochezia is common in Crohn's colitis and diarrhoea and weight loss may accompany both. There are several well recognized, although uncommon, extra-intestinal manifestations of IBD, including erythema nodosum, enteropathic spondyloarthropathy and pyoderma gangrenosum.

Diagnosis

The diagnosis requires demonstration of chronic inflammation of the alimentary tract with clinicopathological correlation and exclusion of differential diagnoses. In the acute setting, infectious causes of inflammatory diarrhoea are excluded by clinical course, stool microscopy, culture, and testing for *C. difficile* cytotoxin, particularly when diarrhoea follows antibiotic use. General haematology, CRP and biochemistry are helpful, and may indicate whether this is likely to be an inflammatory process. Plain abdominal radiograph should be performed to exclude colonic dilatation. A CT of the abdomen is helpful when abdominal pain is a prominent presenting symptom. Ultimately, however, diagnosis requires colonoscopy, or often initially flexible sigmoidoscopy, with mucosal biopsies, to assess for chronic inflammatory changes. Anti-*Saccharomyces cerevisiae* antibodies (ASCA), and p-ANCA have a role in better clarifying the nature of indeterminate colitis.

Therapy

The principles of IBD management remain the same for elderly patients, albeit that the effects of the therapy on comorbidities, needs greater consideration. Therapy is multidimensional and the clinician must pay careful attention to both intestinal and extraintestinal consequences of IBD.

Intestinal: Therapy is aimed at managing the acute flare and then maintaining remission. The acute flare of mild to moderate ulcerative colitis, or Crohn's colitis, is often managed by aminosalicylates (5-ASA), such as sulfasalazine. 5-ASA compounds act by inhibiting the products of arachidonic acid metabolism, the chemotaxis of neutrophils as well as inhibiting activation of NF-κB, which is a key regulator of inflammatory gene transcription. The therapeutic effect results from local, rather than systemic effects, thus enemas or suppositories are an attractive option for distal UC. Adverse effects associated with 5-ASA compounds include headache, blood dyscrasias, vomiting, and dyspepsia, which may be slightly more prevalent in the elderly population.

Patients with a moderately severe flare of CD or UC require systemic corticosteroid, either oral prednisolone 50 mg once daily or intravenous hydrocortisone 100 mg every six hours. When Crohn's disease is limited to inflammation of the ileum and ascending colon, oral budesonide 9 mg daily offers an alternative (16). This approach is slightly less effective than other steroid regimens for inducing remission, but has a reduced incidence of steroid adverse effects, (17) related to budesonide's high hepatic extraction (0.9), and thus significant first pass effect.

High dose steroid is usually sufficient to induce remission, albeit that refractory UC may occasionally necessitate intravenous cyclosporine or surgery. Following remission, medications are often required to reduce the frequency and severity of relapses. For mild disease, in which 5-ASA induced remission, 5-ASA compounds are a reasonable first line agent to prevent relapse, particularly in UC. In more severe IBD, however, thioguanines (azathioprine and 6-mercaptopurine, 6-MP) are often necessary to maintain remission, (18, 19) albeit that they take three to four months for their benefits to take full effect. In severe CD, aminosalicylates are no better than placebo for maintaining remission (18). Steroid therapy has no role in maintaining remission. Methotrexate is a second-line option for patients intolerant of the thioguanines.

A number of newer biological agents have emerged for use in IBD. These include monoclonal antibodies such as anti-TNFα, anti-integrins (α4), and anti-IL-2 receptor antibodies, as well as cytokine therapy, for example G-CSF (20). This is a dynamic area, but the biological agent that has received most clinical attention is infliximab, a monoclonal anti-TNFα antibody. This has been used successfully both to induce remission and then as maintenance therapy in CD and UC (21, 22). Infliximab is still expensive and although generally well tolerated is associated with an increased risk of some infections (including reactivation of tuberculosis), and acute infusion reactions. The risk of infusion reactions is increased by the presence of anti-infliximab antibodies that can develop with treatment. These anti-drug antibodies are associated with a shorter duration of response. It is recommended that concomitant immunosuppressive therapy is used with infliximab, in order to reduce the development of these antibodies.

Extra-Intestinal: The extra-intestinal complications of IBD and the consequences of its treatment require careful attention. The careful clinician must remain mindful of the complications of corticosteroid treatment. Nutritional advice from a dietician is important, both in terms of optimizing diet and improving the patient's understanding of how different foods may precipitate symptoms. Monitoring of the bone mineral density is critical, as is the consideration of dietary supplementation with calcium and ergocalciferol, or even treatment with anti-resorptive therapy (i.e. bisphosphonates) in selected cases.

Therapy scheme of the advised drugs

Clinically, the enzyme thiopurine S-methyltransferase (TPMT) has become an important tool in predicting which patients are likely to develop thioguanine related myelosuppression. Azathioprine is a prodrug that is first converted to 6-MP. There are three enzymes that subsequently act on 6-MP (Figure 28.2). Hypoxanthine guanine phosphoribosyltransferase (HG-PRT) initiates the production of 6-thioguanine nucleotides (6-TGNs), which are responsible for both the therapeutic and toxic haematological effects of the drug. The other enzymes xanthine oxidase and TPMT limit the production of 6-TGNs, and consequently reduce toxicity. This explains the agranulocytosis that may accompany concomitant administration of allopurinol (a xanthine oxidase inhibitor) with azathioprine. Approximately 5 % of Caucasians carry a variant TPMT allele, allowing more 6-MP to be metabolized to 6-TGN. TPMT testing is now readily available and worthwhile, particularly in elderly patients, to identify those who require a smaller dose or, more

importantly, those who should avoid thioguanines altogether.

The usual dose for sulfasalazine is 1–2g oral, thrice daily. Azathioprine and 6-MP are prescribed according to weight, with 2–3 mg/kg/day and 1–1.5 mg/kg/day as a guide, respectively. Weekly complete blood examination is required after starting thioguanine therapy (23). In elderly patients with significant renal or hepatic disease, doses of thioguanines should be reduced and careful monitoring undertaken. In addition to blood dyscrasias, thioguanines may also cause pancreatitis and liver function test abnormalities. From the experience of thioguanine use in transplant recipients, there appears to be an increased incidence of both lymphoma and cancers, particularly skin cancer. If there is an association between azathioprine treatment of IBD and malignancy, however, it is likely to be extremely small (24). Nevertheless, it

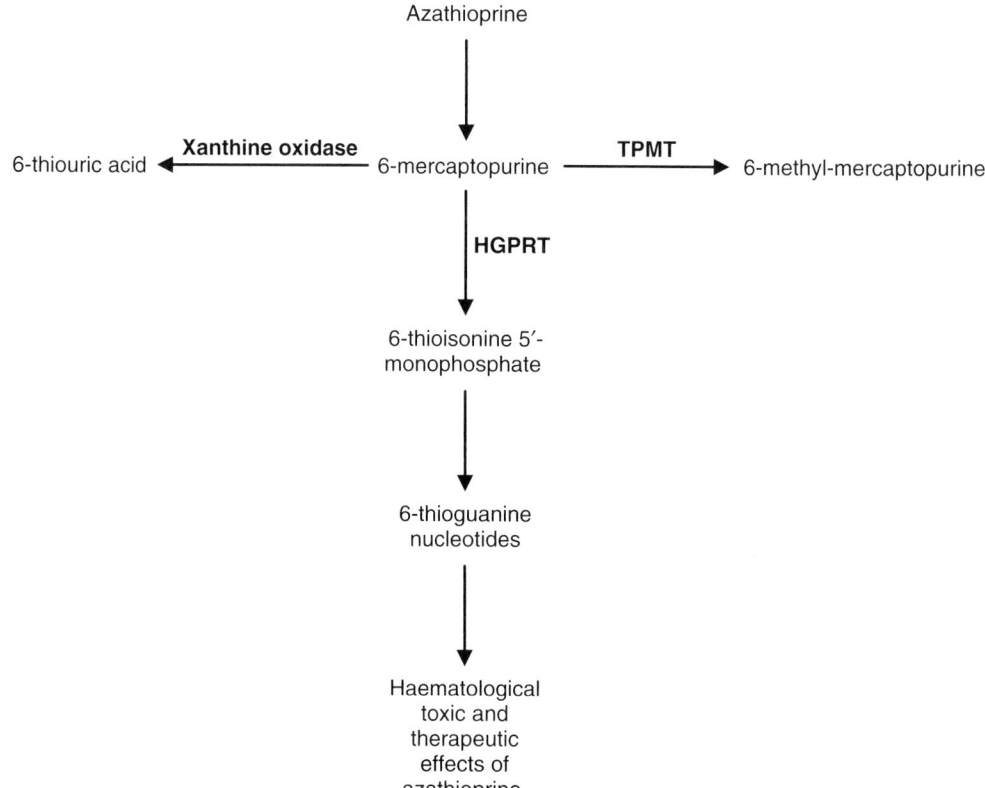

Figure 28.2. Drug metabolism of thioguanines and the role of thiopurine S-methyltransferase

is important for patients on thioguanines to avoid unnecessary sun exposure and use sunscreen.

Key Points

- Inflammatory bowel disease occurs in the elderly population.
- The management of older patients with IBD is similar to the management in younger patients.
- Maintenance therapy with thioguanines is important, both to prevent recurrences, as well as reduce the need for frequent courses of corticosteroid.
- The field of pharmacogenomics can practically assist in deciding on type and dose of maintenance therapy in IBD.
- It is important to screen for extraintestinal complications of IBD in elderly patients, particularly osteoporosis.

Guidelines

British Society of Gastroenterology: Guidelines for the management of inflammatory bowel disease in adults.

European Crohn's and Colitis Organisation Consensus on the management of Crohn's disease.

Links

http://www.bsg.org.uk/clinical_prac/guidelines/mainibd.htm.

DIVERTICULOSIS

Introduction

Diverticulosis refers to herniations of the mucosa and submucosa through the muscular wall of the colon, usually at the point through which the vasa recta penetrates the circular muscle layer (Figure 28.3). The prevalence of diverticulosis increases with age and over half of Westernized populations, greater than 60 years of age have colonic diverticula.

Aetiology

Diverticulosis has been hypothesized to be related to a highly refined diet, low in fibre, which causes exaggerated intracolonic pressures transmitted to the colonic wall and thus diverticula. The pathogenesis may also include changes to the colonic wall microstructure that accompanies aging and alterations in colonic motor function. In Europe, North America and Australia diverticula most

Impaired mural integrity at the point at which the vasa recta penetrates the circular muscle layer, predisposes to diverticula formation.

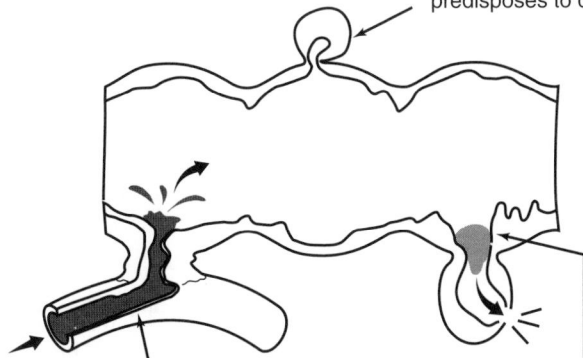

Intimal thickening and medial thinning predisposes the vasa recta to rupture into the diverticula causing haemorrhage.

Obstruction by a faecalith can lead to microperforation and diverticlitis.

Figure 28.3. Schematic representation of colonic diverticula and the chief complications of diverticular haemorrhage and diverticulitis

commonly arise from the sigmoid colon, but in some ethnic groups, particularly from Asia, there is a higher rate of right sided colonic diverticula.

Symptoms and signs

Most patients with uncomplicated diverticulosis are asymptomatic. Some present with abdominal discomfort, bloating and irregular bowel habit, characteristic of irritable bowel syndrome, reflecting the underlying pathogenesis, rather than the diverticulosis. Haemorrhage and inflammation are two potentially serious complications, which often require rapid clinical assessment to exclude alternative causes, and then allow management.

The onset of diverticular haemorrhage is usually abrupt and painless. It may manifest as minor rectal bleeding that scarcely requires medical attention, or it can cause severe haematochezia characterized by hypovolaemic shock. Thus it is important to adequately monitor for clinical signs of shock, particularly heart rate and blood pressure.

Diverticulitis results from colonic microperforation, which leads to peridiverticular inflammation. Uncomplicated diverticulitis can occur in up to 10–25 % of patients with diverticulosis and is often characterized by left lower quadrant discomfort and localized peritonism (25). The inflammation can spread causing generalized sepsis, obstruction, free perforation, abscess or fistula, referred to as complicated diverticulitis. In complicated diverticulitis there may be signs of generalized peritonism, fever, and even septic shock.

Diagnosis

Diagnosis of simple diverticulosis is often made incidentally at colonoscopy, or radiological investigation. In the setting of symptomatic haemorrhage, however, investigation revolves around exclusion of other pathologies, and then specific diagnosis if bleeding persists. When colonic bleeding is massive, it can mimic upper gastrointestinal bleeding, thus upper gastrointestinal endoscopy is usually indicated.

There is an evolving role for emergency colonoscopy, in both the diagnosis and treatment of acute diverticular bleeding (26, 27). It is not routine, however, at many institutions, with the rationale being that the majority of diverticular bleeding settles spontaneously. Investigations should include complete blood examination, coagulation studies and general biochemistry to assist resuscitation and the correction of haemostatic deficiencies. Following exclusion of an upper gastrointestinal source, initial monitoring alone is reasonable. If there is ongoing bleeding, however, then further investigation is required to localize the site of haemorrhage. Urgent colonoscopy, with or without purge preparation, is preferred in some centres (27). If urgent colonoscopy is not available then other choices are angiography, helical CT angiography, and labelled red cell scintigraphy. Advances in enhanced helical CT technology make this the preferred next investigation at our institution, however, diagnostic angiography is a reasonable alternative, with the potential benefit of allowing concurrent therapy. Labelled-red cell scan is rarely sufficient, in isolation, to guide management (27). In patients in whom the bleeding settles, outpatient colonoscopy is usually indicated in order to exclude other colonic pathologies.

The diagnosis of diverticulitis is made on the basis of clinical presentation and often a CT of the abdomen to assess for an abscess. Blood tests reveal a raised white cell count and inflammatory markers, and blood cultures are important when there is fever or peritonitis.

Therapy

Management of diverticulosis itself is frequently aimed at increasing stool bulk through dietary fibre supplements, although the evidence for this is largely observational (28, 29). Some symptoms may in fact be exacerbated by increased fibre. The medical management of diverticulitis involves intravenous fluid resuscitation, restriction of the diet to clear fluids, and broad spectrum antibiotics for seven to 10 days (29). This approach has not, however, been carefully validated by clinical trials (30). Surgery is required only in a minority of patients.

Therapy scheme of the advised drugs

The treatment of diverticulitis will often include gentamicin, which requires careful monitoring when prescribed to an elderly patient, in whom creatinine clearance may be significantly impaired despite normal serum creatinine.

Key Points

- Diverticulosis is common in older individuals.
- Vague abdominal symptoms attributed to diverticulosis may be secondary to other pathology, including irritable bowel syndrome, and should be managed accordingly.
- The management of diverticulitis and diverticular haemorrhage requires simultaneous resuscitation, investigation, and then specific therapy.

MESENTERIC ISCHAEMIA

Introduction

Intestinal ischaemia can cause several different clinical syndromes, depending on the severity of ischaemia and the vascular territory affected. The intestinal arterial supply is provided by branches from the coeliac axis, the superior (SMA) and inferior (IMA) mesenteric arteries (all of which arise from the abdominal aorta), as well as the middle and inferior rectal artery branches from the internal iliac, and internal pudendal arteries, respectively. The coeliac axis provides blood to the stomach, duodenum, pancreas, liver, and spleen. The SMA gives rise to four main branches: the inferior pancreaticoduodenal, the middle and right colic, and the ileocolic arteries, as well as several jejunal and ileal branches. These branches develop into a rich network of arcades, allowing extensive anastomotic communication, and supply the distal duodenum up to and including the proximal two-thirds of the transverse colon (Figure 28.4). The IMA supplies the majority

of the remainder through its left colic, sigmoid branch, and superior rectal arteries, with some assistance in the distal rectum, from branches of the internal iliac. The intestine enjoys a rich collateral circulation, except for the splenic flexure, at the boundary of SMA and IMA territory, which is, therefore, relatively vulnerable to ischaemic insults. Colonic ischaemia is the most common type of mesenteric ischaemia, accounting for one in every 1000 hospital admissions (31).

Aetiology

The aetiology of intestinal ischaemia may be divided into acute, chronic, occlusive or non-occlusive disease, as well as venous infarction. Acute, occlusive mesenteric ischaemia is most often (50%) the consequence of SMA embolus, with cardioembolism a common source. Non-occlusive mesenteric ischaemia, responsible for about 25% of cases, is usually seen with severe splanchnic vasoconstriction in response to stressful stimuli, such as shock, acute pulmonary oedema, or myocardial infarction. Rarely, it may occur during jejunal feeding in the critically ill. Thrombosis of the SMA or superior mesenteric vein, are less common causes of intestinal ischaemia. Chronic stable atherosclerotic plaques within the mesenteric circulation can occasionally cause postprandial abdominal pain, when blood is stolen away from an already compromised circulation, so-called 'intestinal angina'.

Colonic ischaemia is important, particularly in the elderly population. In contrast to small intestinal ischaemia, the main cause of ischaemic colitis is presumed to be regional nonocclusive disease, often arising from a combination of factors such as susceptibility of the splenic flexure to ischaemia, the sensitivity of colonic vasculature to autonomic influence, haemostatic characteristics of the blood, and chronic arterial insufficiency secondary to atherosclerosis or fibromuscular dysplasia.

Symptoms and signs

Acute mesenteric ischaemia presents abruptly, although venous thrombosis may present

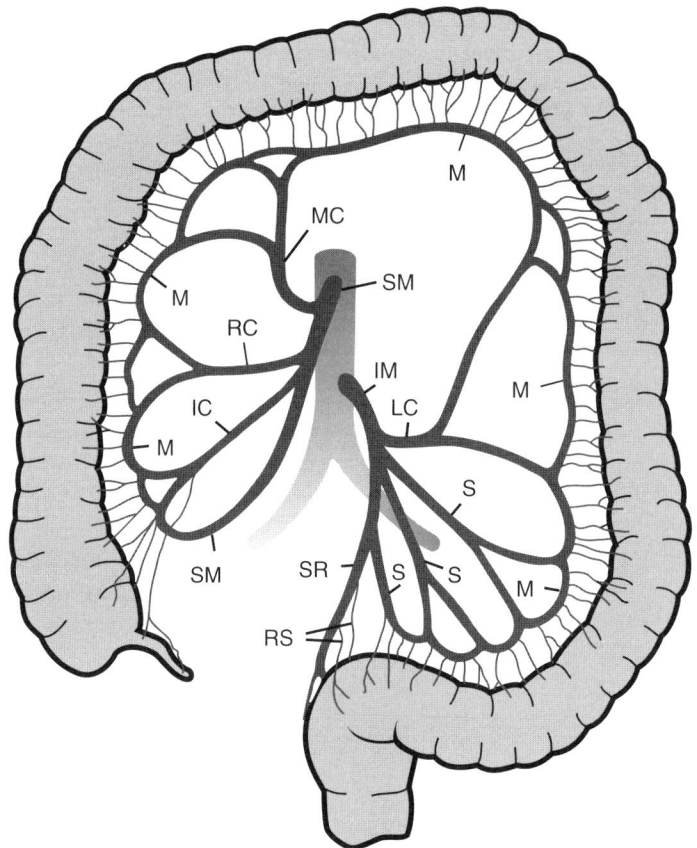

[FN] **D** = duodenum, **SM** = superior mesenteric artery, **MC** = middle colic artery, **RC** = right colic artery, **IC** = ileocolic artery, **M** = marginal artery, **IM** = inferior mesenteric artery, **LC** = left colic artery, **SR** = superior rectal artery, **S** = sigmoid arteries

Figure 28.4. Blood supply of the colon

subacutely, over weeks (32). The chief symptom is abdominal pain, and classically the reported severity of the pain seems more dramatic then the early abdominal examination might suggest. There is often rectal bleeding and abdominal distention. Elderly patients may present with initially vague abdominal symptoms progressing to shock and generalized peritonitis following the loss of intestinal viability. One needs to have a strong clinical suspicion of acute mesenteric ischaemia in elderly patients, particularly in the presence of conditions predisposing to thromboembolism, such as ischemic heart disease, atrial fibrillation, or hypercoagulable states. Colonic ischaemia generally presents in a less dramatic fashion, with mild to moderate left lower quadrant abdominal pain and haematochezia.

Diagnosis

The diagnosis of acute mesenteric ischaemia is suspected on the basis of clinical presentation, along with laboratory indices such as raised white cell count, metabolic acidosis, and elevated lactate. The diagnosis is confirmed, however, by angiography (either CT angiography or interventional selective mesenteric angiography, depending on local expertise), or laparotomy. Colonic ischaemia is ultimately an endoscopic diagnosis. In the absence of peritonitis and a normal abdominal radiograph, it is generally safe to proceed to cautious colonoscopy or at least flexible sigmoidoscopy. During the examination care should be taken to not over inflate the colon and exacerbate the ischaemia. Biopsies may be helpful to exclude other diagnoses. Stool microscopy, culture and analysis for *C. difficile* toxin are also necessary.

Therapy

Acute mesenteric ischaemia is a surgical emergency treated by a combination of radiological and surgical techniques. There is a role for broad spectrum antibiotics once acute mesenteric ischaemia is confirmed, and paparevine is sometimes selectively infused via the angiographic catheter into the mesenteric circulation to relieve secondary vasoconstriction. There may be value of thrombolysis in some cases of SMA embolic occlusion. Medical anticoagulant therapy may be relevant, in the patients who survive a cardioembolic ischaemic episode in order to prevent recurrent events (32).

The therapeutic strategy in colonic ischaemia, is amelioration of exacerbating conditions, particularly hypoxia or hypotension. This involves fluid resuscitation, stopping medications that cause vasoconstriction or hypotension, and optimization of cardiorespiratory function. In addition many centres empirically administer broad spectrum antibiotics, although the evidence base to support this is weak (32).

Therapy scheme of the advised drugs

The medications that may be associated with colonic ischaemia include: antihypertensive agents, diuretics, nonsteroidal anti-inflammatory agents, digoxin, oestrogens, pseudoephedrine, alosetron, the triptans, and psychotropic medications (31). The medical treatment of intestinal ischaemia is largely confined to removing drugs that may exacerbate the problem. Otherwise, the chief management approaches are radiological or surgical intervention, and supportive care.

Key Points

- A strong index of suspicion is required to avoid missing acute mesenteric ischaemia, a potentially life threatening condition.

- The clinical presentation of mesenteric ischaemia includes abdominal pain, tenderness, and haematochezia.
- Colonic ischaemia is the most common type of mesenteric ischaemia, particularly in the elderly population.
- Colonic ischaemia is usually caused by non-occulsive disease, and thus angiography is not indicated.
- The splenic flexure is particularly susceptible to ischaemia because of relatively poor collateralization in this region.

Guidelines

American Gastroenterology Association Institute Guidelines: Technical review on Intestinal Ischemia.

Links

American Gastroenterology Association Institute Guidelines: http://download.journals.elsevierhealth.com/pdfs/journals/0016-5085/PIIS0016508500701831.pdf.

CONSTIPATION

Introduction

Constipation is common in all age groups, but particularly so in older patients. The term constipation is understood differently throughout the community and thus a careful history must be taken to clarify the patient's true symptoms. The clinical research definition for constipation is based on the Rome II criteria (Table 28.1) (33). These criteria describe constipation in terms of bowel motions that are hard, uncomfortable, or infrequent.

Aetiology

Many common conditions predispose to constipation in elderly people. Lifestyle factors may contribute to constipation, including a low residue diet, dehydration and reduced daily activity. Certain diagnoses may be important such as obstructing colonic pathology (e.g. colorectal cancer), constipation predominant

Table 28.1. Rome II criteria for irritable bowel syndrome (33)

The diagnosis requires exclusion of structural and biochemical causes for the symptoms.

At least 12 weeks, which need not be consecutive, in the preceding 12 months of abdominal discomfort or pain that has 2 of 3 features:

1. Relieved with defecation; and/or
2. Onset associated with a change in frequency of stool; and/or
3. Onset associated with a change in form (appearance) of stool.

Symptoms that cumulatively support the diagnosis of IBS:

1. Abnormal stool frequency ("abnormal" may be defined as greater than 3 bowel movements per day or less than 3 bowel movements per week)
2. Abnormal stool form (lumpy/hard or loose/watery stool)
3. Abnormal stool passage (straining, urgency, or feeling of incomplete evacuation)
4. Passage of mucus
5. Bloating or feeling of abdominal distension.

Rome II Criteria for Constipation (33)

At least 12 weeks, which need not be consecutive, in the preceding 12 months of two or more of:

1. Straining in >1/4 defecations
2. Lumpy or hard stools in >1/4 defecations
3. Sensation of incomplete evacuation in >1/4 defecations
4. Sensation of anorectal obstruction/blockade in >1/4 defecations
5. Manual manoeuvres to facilitate >1/4 defecations (e.g. digital evacuation, support of the pelvic floor)
6. <3 defecations/week

Loose stools are not present, and there are insufficient criteria for IBS (see above).

---

irritable bowel syndrome and weakness of defecatory musculature and drugs can impair intestinal motility, for example medications with anticholinergic activity, opiates, calcium channel blockers (particularly verapamil), and iron replacement. Constipation may also be a symptom of extra-gastroenterological disease, including hypercalcaemia and hypothyroidism. Neurological diseases can cause constipation, particularly multiple sclerosis, Parkinson's disease, spinal cord lesions, and autonomic neuropathy. Finally, there are a number of predisposing psychological risk factors, the most important being depression.

Symptoms and signs

It is extremely important to explore what the patient really means by "constipation". Open ended questioning should clarify the duration of the complaint and whether there are any other associated gastroenterological (such as rectal bleeding) or systemic symptoms. In elderly patients, constipation may cause confusion or even spurious diarrhoea and faecal incontinence, as liquid stool seeps around the impacted colonic faeces. It is important to appreciate the time course of the symptoms, and whether this represents an abrupt change, or a chronic problem. A full general examination is required, including a neurological assessment and digital rectal examination to exclude distal malignancy or faecal impaction and assess anal tone. A mental state examination should also be performed.

Diagnosis

Investigating constipation is based on the exclusion of serious pathology and identifying potentially predisposing conditions. Routine blood tests are worthwhile including haemoglobin, erythrocyte sedimentation rate, calcium level and thyroid function tests. The history, examination, routine blood tests, plus or minus a barium enema is usually sufficient to exclude a sinister colonic lesion, particularly in those with chronic constipation. It is important to remember, however, that after 50 years of age there is a sharp increase in the incidence of colorectal cancer, and thus colonoscopy may be needed when there are other factors suggestive of cancer, such as an abrupt onset of constipation, a strong family history, specific symptoms, or abnormal investigations. The role of CT colonography ("virtual colonoscopy") in the diagnostic or screening algorithm for colorectal disease is evolving, but it may be technically difficult in a chronically constipated elderly patient.

Therapy

Once underlying conditions are excluded, the management of constipation is multifactorial. Firstly, support and education is extremely important to reassure the patient that their bowel habit will not make them ill. Diet modification is usually the next step, although the benefits are frequently disappointing. Nevertheless, increasing one's dietary fibre intake to 30 g per day is reasonable advice and may improve some people's symptoms. Unfortunately, an increase of fermentable substrate frequently exacerbates abdominal discomfort and bloating, limiting its effectiveness. Similarly, in addition to poor palatability, unabsorbed sugar preparations such as lactulose and sorbitol, have a relatively limited role in managing chronic constipation. Epsom salts, which are another osmotic laxative, however, are often better tolerated and are amongst the most effective chronic treatments for constipation. Other effective osmotic laxatives, particularly in the initial stages of treatment, are the polyethylene glycol (PEG) based electrolyte solutions. In one randomized comparative study, those that were treated with the PEG-based regimens, had a greater bowel frequency and reported less straining, and passed less flatus, than those randomized to lactulose (34).

Athraquinones, such as senna, are also effective laxatives. These stimulate colonic motor activity and so increase faecal bulk. There is some controversy regarding whether chronic use of this class of laxative impairs long term colonic motility.

Therapy scheme of the advised drugs

A general approach to treatment of constipation is outlined in Figure 28.5. No significant age related dose adjustments are required, although magnesium containing salts should be used with care in elderly patients with renal impairment, due to the risk of hypermagnesaemia.

Key Points

- Constipation is common and understood differently throughout the community.
- The management of constipation involves the exclusion of serious pathology and the identification of any predisposing conditions.
- It is important to stop or reduce, if possible, iatrogenic causes.
- Treatment of constipation includes dietary, psychological and pharmaceutical approaches.
- Epsom salts and PEG-based therapies are effective and well tolerated.

Guidelines

American Gastroenterological Association: Guidelines on constipation.

Links

American Gastroenterological Association: Technical review on constipation. http://download.journals.elsevierhealth.com/pdfs/journals/0016-5085/PIIS0016508500700242.pdf.

American Gastroenterological Association: Guidelines on constipation. http://download.Journals.elsevierhealth.com/pdfs/journals/0016-5085/PIIS0016508500700230.pdf.

DIARRHOEA AND FAECAL INCONTINENCE

Introduction

In Western countries diarrhoea-related mortality and morbidity is considerable in the elderly population (36). Patients often use the term diarrhoea to describe both increased fluidity and frequency of stool. Diarrhoea is strictly defined

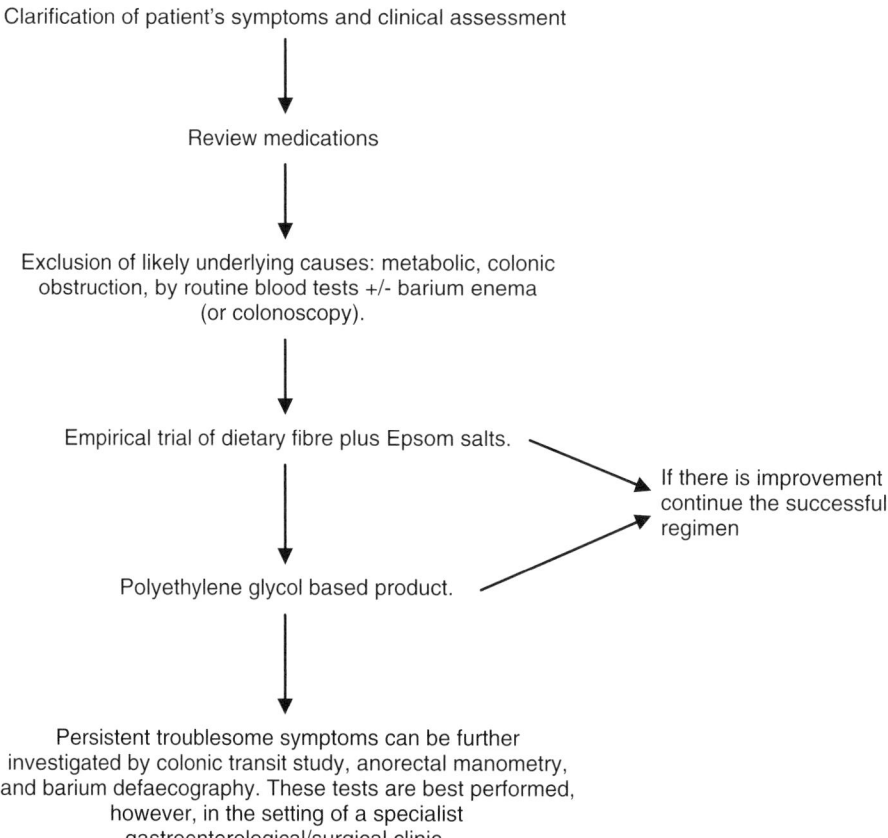

Clarification of patient's symptoms and clinical assessment

Review medications

Exclusion of likely underlying causes: metabolic, colonic obstruction, by routine blood tests +/- barium enema (or colonoscopy).

Empirical trial of dietary fibre plus Epsom salts.

If there is improvement continue the successful regimen

Polyethylene glycol based product.

Persistent troublesome symptoms can be further investigated by colonic transit study, anorectal manometry, and barium defaecography. These tests are best performed, however, in the setting of a specialist gastroenterological/surgical clinic.

Figure 28.5. Management of constipation

as a stool weight greater than 200 g/day or three or more bowel actions per day. Diarrhoea may be either acute (less than two weeks), persistent (between two to four weeks), or chronic (>4 weeks), and in terms of the characteristics of the stool, either inflammatory, watery or fatty. These classifications are helpful when considering the aetiology and thus investigation and treatment.

Faecal incontinence is defined as the failure to perceive, retain and/or evacuate rectal contents at an appropriate time and place, beyond the age of four years. Although faecal incontinence may be a symptom of a significant underlying gastrointestinal disease it is important to consider the possibility of extra-colonic conditions.

Aetiology

A number of factors predispose elderly people to diarrhoea. These include gastric hypochlorhydria (iatrogenic or atrophic gastritis), immunodeficiencies (iatrogenic or comorbidities), recent travel, and prescribed medications, particularly antibiotics. Common causes of diarrhoea in elderly patients are listed in Table 28.2 (37). Simple classification of diarrhoea on the basis of history and stool analysis can help rationalize the diagnostic approach (38).

Watery diarrhoea may be classified as either osmotic or secretory, on the basis of the faecal osmotic gap (Equation 28.1). Osmotic diarrhoea may result from the malabsorption of an ingested solute, such as malabsorption of a

Table 28.2. Causes of chronic diarrhoea in elderly patients (adapted from the British Society of Gastroenterology guidelines) (37)

Colonic
　　Colonic neoplasia
　　Ulcerative and Crohn's colitis
　　Microscopic colitis
　　Bile acid malabsorption
Small bowel
　　Coeliac disease
　　Crohn's disease
　　Mesenteric ischaemia
　　Small intestinal bacterial overgrowth
　　Giardiasis
　　Other small bowel enteropathies (e.g. radiation enteritis, lymphoma, amyloid)
　　Bile acid malabsorption
Pancreatic
　　Chronic pancreatitis
　　Pancreatic carcinoma
Endocrine
　　Hyperthyroidism
　　Diabetes
　　Hormone secreting tumours (VIPoma, gastrinoma, carcinoid)
Other
　　"Surgical" causes (e.g. small bowel resections)
　　Drugs (including intentional and unintentional laxative use)
　　Alcohol
　　Autonomic neuropathy (e.g. secondary to diabetes)
Spurious Diarrhoea
　　Constipation with overflow incontinence.
　　Factitious diarrhoea.

carbohydrate (associated with a low stool pH often <6) or magnesium from laxatives. Secretory diarrhoea results from the malabsorption and/or secretion of luminal electrolytes. Secretory diarrhoea, in contrast to osmotic diarrhoea, does not resolve, or only partially resolves, with fasting. In secretory diarrhoea the osmolality of the stool is accounted for mainly by sodium and potassium salts, and thus the faecal osmotic gap is less than 50 mOsm/kg. In osmotic diarrhoea, however, the diarrhoea is usually driven by an unmeasured solute, often undigested carbohydrate, fats or an osmotic salt from laxative use (e.g. magnesium), thus the faecal osmotic gap

is greater than 50 mOsm/kg. In the case of laxative abuse the faecal osmotic gap is usually greater than 100 mOsm/kg.

$$\text{Faecal Osmotic Gap} = 290 - 2 \times (\text{stool sodium concentration} + \text{stool potassium concentration}) \quad (28.1)$$

In secretory diarrhoea the Faecal Osmotic Gap is <50 mOsm/kg

In osmotic diarrhoea the Faecal Osmotic Gap is >50 mOsm/kg

Inflammatory diarrhoea is caused by mucosal inflammation and is characterized by blood and leukocytes in the stool. Fatty diarrhoea (steatorrhoea) may result from either malabsorption or maldigestion, as is the case in SIBO or pancreatic insufficiency. Stool fat can be measured qualitatively by Sudan stain on a random stool, or by quantitative analysis from a timed collection. Although chronic diarrhoea can be classified according to an underlying chief pathogenic mechanism, in any given patient there are likely to be multiple factors acting concurrently.

In elderly patients faecal incontinence may occur due to comorbidities, e.g. diabetes mellitus, poor mobility and thus difficulty moving to the toilet, anorectal dysfunction following a past insult such as prostatic radiotherapy, surgery, or child birth, or even multiple sclerosis or cord pathology. Faecal incontinence can also be a symptom of rectal prolapse as well as a variety of diarrhoeal diseases. Constipation may cause faecal incontinence through seepage of liquid stool around impacted colonic faeces.

Symptoms and Signs

The presentation of diarrhoea in elderly patients is similar to that seen in any other group, albeit that because of less effective compensatory mechanisms, the individual may be more unwell due to dehydration or electrolyte abnormalities by the time of presentation. Examination should carefully assess the patient's hydration, including heart rate and blood pressure. Signs of systemic inflammation such as temperature should be noted, and an abdominal and general examination should be performed. A full neurological examination and rectal examination (both at rest and on straining) is critical for the patient presenting with faecal incontinence. The elderly patient with faecal impaction and overflow incontinence may present with confusion.

Diagnosis

In chronic diarrhoea, the history and the nature of the stool analysis can help to distinguish whether the diarrhoea is inflammatory, watery (secretory or osmotic) or fatty (i.e. steatorrhoea) (39). A dietary history is important, firstly to determine whether there are any culprit foods, for example dairy produce in lactase deficiency, and secondly to exclude inadvertent use of dietary aperients as are present in many artificially sweetened products.

When osmotic diarrhoea is identified further testing can determine whether there is carbohydrate malabsorption or abuse of laxatives. Laxative abuse may be present in up to one in 20 individuals presenting to gastroenterology clinics with chronic diarrhoea, so this diagnosis should not be lightly dismissed (38). If clinical assessment suggests laxative abuse, there are several tests that can be performed. Firstly, urine or stool water may be tested for anthraquinones, bisacodyl, phenolphthalein, and stool can be analysed for magnesium (normally <45 mmol/L), as well as sulphate and phosphate. Testing of liquid stool for osmolality, is useful if <250 mOsm/kg, which suggests that stool volume is being diluted by another fluid (urine, water). Finally sigmoidoscopy can identify melanosis coli a sign of chronic laxative abuse.

The causes of chronic secretory diarrhoea are numerous. Initial investigation involves exclusion of an enteric infection by stool microscopy and culture. Endoscopy with small bowel biopsy is often required to exclude celiac disease and distal aspirate may be taken for culture to assess for SIBO. Colonoscopy (with ileoscopy) should be performed to exclude inflammatory bowel disease, with random colonic biopsies required to exclude microscopic colitis. For purely secretory diarrhoea, a flexible sigmoidoscopy, rather than colonoscopy, is often sufficient. Abdominal CT may be helpful, followed by consideration of enteroendocrine causes of diarrhoea, particularly hyperthyroidism, with other specific tests only to be considered in the relevant clinical context (39). Investigation of inflammatory diarrhoea involves endoscopy and colonoscopy with biopsies, as does the investigation for steatorrhoea.

Diarrhoea predominant irritable bowel syndrome (IBS) is a common cause of diarrhoea in the elderly population. The working diagnosis for IBS is based on the Rome II criteria (Table 28.1).

The cause of faecal incontinence can often be determined by careful clinical assessment. Nevertheless anorectal manometry and pudendal nerve conduction studies may be helpful to document the neuromuscular pathophysiology. Anorectal ultrasound or MRI is used to better define the regional anatomy, and proctoscopy is helpful to diagnose distal rectal pathologies such as rectal neoplasia, inflammation and rectal prolapse.

Therapy

Therapy should be directed at the underlying cause. Empirical anti-diarrhoeal treatment may be used when no cause is found, or the cause proves resistant to specific therapy (39). Anti-diarrhoeal therapy should not be used, however, in inflammatory colitides, where impairment to colonic motility may promote toxic megacolon. Commonly used agents for diarrhoea include opiates, bile-acid binding resins, and fibre supplements. Drugs such as octreotide are generally only employed in disease specific circumstances, such as the rare hormone-induced secretory diarrhoeas. Some clinicians administer a one off dose of tinidazole 2 g, as empirical treatment for presumed giardiasis, but the clinical utility of this approach is uncertain (39). Anti-diarrhoeal opiates, such as loperamide and diphenoxylate, are effective, relatively safe and preferred because they lack the central activity of other opiates. Cholestyramine may have a role in diarrhoea secondary to bile acid malabsorption. The key issue is whether the diarrhoea is the colonic consequence of bile acid malabsorption (cholestyramine may be effective) or steatorrhoea (cholestyramine may aggravate the diarrhoea). An empirical trial of cholestyramine may be reasonable, but in elderly patients a physician needs to be mindful of the risk of cholestyramine impairing the absorption of concomitantly ingested medications and vitamins.

Therapy scheme of the advised drugs

Cholestyramine may bind other drugs, thus the interval between administration of cholestyramine and other medicaments should be as great as feasible, at least one hour before or four to six hours after cholestyramine.

Key Points

- It is important to clarify the patient's definition of diarrhoea.
- Diarrhoea is strictly defined as a stool weight greater than 200 g/day and/or three or more bowel actions per day.
- On the basis of simple stool testing, diarrhoea may be classified as inflammatory, watery or fatty, which then directs further investigation.
- Anti-diarrhoeal therapy should be directed at the underlying cause, but empirical treatment may be used, if blood is absent from stool analysis, when no cause is found, or the diarrhoea is resistant to specific therapy.
- Faecal incontinence may be a symptom of a gastrointestinal disease, but it is also important to consider the possibility of extra-colonic conditions.

Guidelines

British Society of Gastroenterology: Guidelines for the investigation of chronic diarrhoea.

Links

AGA technical review: http://download.journals .elsevierhealth.com/pdfs/journals/0016-5085/ PIIS0016508599705135.pdf.

British Society of Gastroenterology: Guidelines for the investigation of chronic diarrhea: http://www.bsg.org.uk/clinical_prac/guidelines/ chronic_diarr.htm.

HAEMORRHOIDS

Introduction

Haemorrhoids are extremely common and are in fact normal anatomical structures. They are often asymptomatic but can cause bleeding, pain, pruritus, and prolapse.

Aetiology

Haemorrhoidal disease is often ascribed, in part, to constipation and the resultant straining required to defecate. The pathogenesis, however, is poorly understood, and may relate to ill defined genetic factors (40).

Symptoms and Signs

The presentation in elderly patients is often with fresh red rectal bleeding, either spontaneously on the toilet paper, or on the surface of the stool. The most important issue when an elderly patient presents with haemorrhoidal disease, is whether the symptoms should be ascribed to the haemorrhoids, or if there is some other more serious pathology, such as colorectal cancer. Anal fissures may also cause bleeding, as well as occasionally, severe pain. A palpable mass on rectal examination, suggests rectal neoplasia.

Diagnosis

Careful history and examination is required, including a digital rectal examination. In elderly patients haematochezia should usually prompt colonoscopy, to exclude colorectal neoplasia as the incidence of colorectal cancer is higher. Sigmoidoscopy with barium enema or CT colonography may be a reasonable alternative for more frail patients.

Therapy

Patients are encouraged to adopt a high fibre diet to bulk their stools, and alleviate constipation. This simple measure has been effective in reducing the incidence of bleeding (41). Medical drug treatments, often containing local anaesthetic agents and hydrocortisone, may bring about some symptomatic relief of pain and pruritus. There is no data to suggest, however, that topical medical therapies improve the natural history of the haemorrhoids (40). In fact, high potency corticosteroid creams may be deleterious in the longer term. Improvement of haemorrhoidal pain after using a nitroglycerin ointment has been reported (40), but topical medical therapies remain a short term, symptomatic option. If haemorrhoidal bleeding continues, there should be a careful review of the indications for any prescribed antiplatelet agents, including aspirin and traditional NSAIDs. Most symptomatic second degree (prolapse with defecation, but reduces spontaneously) and third degree (requires manual reduction) haemorrhoids may be treated by outpatient sigmoidoscopic banding. Fourth degree haemorrhoids (irreducible, permanently prolapsed), are usually repaired by surgery.

Therapy scheme of the advised drugs

Initially treat with fibre and symptomatic topical agents, proceed to haemorrhoidal banding if symptoms persist. Surgery is often reserved as a last resort, but may be necessary for the minority that develop complicated haemorrhoidal disease, such as acute incarceration or thrombosis, have large, symptomatic external haemorrhoids, or in whom symptoms persist despite other treatments (40).

Key Points

- Haemorrhoidal bleeding is common, but in elderly patients one cannot assume that haemorrhoids are the cause of haematochezia.
- Medical treatment with high fibre diet softens stool, alleviates constipation, and often improves symptoms.
- Sigmoidoscopic banding or surgery, are reserved for more severe cases.

Guidelines

American Gastroenterological Association Technical Review on the Diagnosis and Treatment of Hemorrhoids. *Gastroenterology* 2004; **126**: 1463–73.

Links

American Gastroenterological Association Technical Review on the Diagnosis and Treatment of Hemorrhoids. http://download.journals.elsevierhealth.com/pdfs/journals/0016-5085/PIIS0016508504003555.pdf.

REFERENCES

1. Hall K, Procter DD, Fisher L, Rose S. American Gastroenterological Association Future Trends Committee Report: Effects of Aging of the Population on Gastroenterology Practice, Education, and Research. *Gastroenterology* 2005; **129**: 1305–38.
2. Jones JIW, Hawkey CJ. Physiology and organ related pathology of the elderly: stomach ulcers. *Best Practice & Research Clinical Gastroenterology* 2002; **15**: 943–61.
3. Hoffman JC, Zeitz M. Small bowel disease in the elderly: diarrhoea and malabsorption. *Best Practice & Research Clinical Gastroenterology* 2002; **16**: 17–36.
4. Saltzman JR, Kowdley KV, Pedrosa MC, Sepe T, Golner B, Perrone G, Russell RM. Bacterial overgrowth without clinical malabsorption in elderly hypochlorhydric subjects. *Gastroenterology* 1994; **106**: 615–23.
5. Freeman H, Lemoyne M, Pare P. Coeliac disease. *Best Practice & Research Clinical Gastroenterology* 2002; **16**: 37–49.
6. Nightingale JM, Lennard-Jones JE, Gertner DJ, Wood SR, Bartram CI. Colonic preservation reduces need for parenteral therapy, increases incidence of renal stones, but does not change high prevalence of gall stones in patients with a short bowel. *Gut*. 1992; **33**: 1493–7.
7. AGA Technical Review on Celiac Sprue. *Gastroenterology* 2001; **120**: 1526–40.
8. National Institutes of Health Consensus Development Conference Statement on Celiac Disease, June 28–30, 2004. *Gastroenterology* 2005; **128**: S1–S9.

9. Attar A, Flourié B, Rambaud J, Franchisseur C, Ruszniewski P, Bouhnik Y. Antibiotic efficacy in small intestinal bacterial overgrowth-related chronic diarrhea: A crossover, randomized trial. *Gastroenterology* 1999; **117**: 794–7.

10. Loftus EV. Clinical epidemiology of inflammatory bowel disease: incidence, prevalence, and environmental influences. *Gastroenterology* 2004; **126**: 1504–17.

11. John Cambier. Immunosenescence: a problem of lymphopoiesis, homeostasis, microenvironment, and signalling. *Immunol Rev.* 2005; **205**: 5–6.

12. Prelog M. Aging of the immune system: A risk factor for autoimmunity? *Autoimmun Rev.* 2006; **5**: 136–9.

13. Mitsuoka T. Intestinal flora and aging. *Nutritional Reviews*. 1992; **50**: 438–46.

14. Earle E, Rowe R. Ulcerative disease of the large intestine in patients more than 50 years old. *Diseases of the Colon and Rectum* 1972; **15**: 33–40.

15. Gurudu S, Fiocchi C, Katz JA. Inflammatory Bowel Disease. *Best Practice & Research Clinical Gastroenterology* 2002; **16**: 77–90.

16. Travis SPL, Stange EF, Le'mann M, Oresland T, Chowers Y, Forbes A, D'Haens G, Kitis G, Cortot A, Prantera C, Marteau P, Colombel J-F, Gionchetti P, Bouhnik Y, Tiret E, Kroesen J, Starlinger M, Mortensen NJ, for the European Crohn's and Colitis Organisation (ECCO). European evidence based consensus on the diagnosis and management of Crohn's disease: current management. *Gut* 2006; **55**(Suppl I): i16–i35.

17. Otley A, Steinhart AH. Budesonide for induction of remission in Crohn's disease. *Cochrane Database Syst Rev.* 2005; (4):CD000296.

18. Akobeng AK, Gardener E. Oral 5-amino salicylic acid for maintenance of medically-induced remission in Crohn's Disease. *Cochrane Database Syst Rev.* 2005;(1): CD003715.

19. Candy S, Wright J, Gerber M, Adams G, Gerig M, Goodman R. A controlled double blind study of azathioprine in the management of Crohn's disease. *Gut* 1995; **37**: 674–8.

20. Sandborn WJ, Targan SR. Biologic therapy of inflammatory bowel disease. *Gastroenterology* 2002; **122**: 1592–1608.

21. Hanauer SB, Feagan BG, Lichtenstein GR, Mayer LF, Schreiber S, Colombel JF, Rachmilewitz D, Wolf DC, Olson A, Bao W, Rutgeerts P. Maintenance infliximab for Crohn's disease: the ACCENT I randomised trial. *Lancet* 2002; **359**: 1541–9.

22. Rutgeerts P, Sandborn WJ, Feagan BG, Reinisch W, Olson A, Johanns J, Travers S, Rachmilewitz D, Hanauer SB, Lichtenstein GR, de Villiers WJ, Present D, Sands BE, Colombel JF. Infliximab for induction and maintenance therapy for ulcerative colitis. *N Engl J Med.* 2005; **353**: 2462–76.

23. Lichtenstein GR. Use of laboratory testing to guide 6-MP/Azathioprine therapy. *Gastroenterology* 2004; **127**: 1558–64

24. Fraser AG, Orchard TR, Robinson EM, Jewell DP. Long-term risk of malignancy after treatment of inflammatory bowel disease with azathioprine. *Aliment Pharmacol Ther.* 2002; **16**: 1225–32.

25. Young-Fadock TM, Roberts PL, Spencer MP, Wolf BG. Colonic diverticular disease. *Current Problems in Surgery* 2000; **37**: 457–514.

26. Jensen DM, Machicado GA, Jutabha R, Kovacs TOG. Urgent Colonoscopy for the Diagnosis and Treatment of Severe Diverticular Hemorrhage *N Engl J Med* 2000; **342**: 78–82.

27. Rockey DC. Lower Gastrointestinal Bleeding. *Gastroenterology* 2006; **130**: 165–171.

28. Aldoori WH, Giovannucci EL, Rimm EB, Wing AL, Trichopoulos DV, Willett WC. A prospective study of diet and the risk of symptomatic diverticular disease in men. *Am J Clin Nutr* 1994; **60**: 757–64.

29. Stollman N, Raskin JB. Diverticular disease of the colon. *Lancet* 2004; **363**: 631–9.

30. Place RJ, Simmang CL. Diverticular disease. *Best Practice & Research Clinical Gastroenterology* 2002; **16**: 135–48.

31. Green BT, Tendler DA. Ischemic colitis: A clinical review. *Southern Medical Journal* 2005; **98**: 217–22.

32. AGA Technical Review on Intestinal Ischemia. *Gastroenterology* 2000; **118**: 954–68.

33. Thompson WG, Longstreth GF, Drossman DA, Heaton KW, Irvine EJ, Muller-Lissner SA. Functional bowel disorders and functional abdominal pain. *Gut* 1999; **45** Suppl 2: II43–7.

34. A Attar, M Lémann, A Ferguson, M Halphen, M-C Boutron, B Flourié, E Alix, M Salmeron, F Guillemot, S Chaussade, A-M Ménard, J Moreau, G Naudin, and M Barthet

Comparison of a low dose polyethylene glycol electrolyte solution with lactulose for treatment of chronic constipation. *Gut* 1999; **44**: 226–30.

35. de Wit N, Rubin G, Jones R. Irritable bowel syndrome. *Clin Evid*. 2005 Jun; (13): 556–63.

36. Gangarosa RE, Glass RI, Lew JF, Boring JR. Hospitalizations involving gastroenteritis in the United States, 1985: the special burden of the disease among the elderly. *American Journal of Epidemiology* 1992; **135**: 281–90.

37. Thomas PD, Forbes A, Green J, Howdle P, Long R, Playford R, Sheridan M, Stevens R, Valori R, Walters J, Addison GM, Hill P, Brydon G. Guidelines for the investigation of chronic diarrhoea, 2nd edition. *Gut* 2003; **52**(Suppl V): v1–v15.

38. Donowitz M, Kokke FT, Saidi R. Evaluation of patients with chronic diarrhea. *N Engl J Med* 1995; **332**: 725–9.

39. AGA Technical Review on the Evaluation and Management of Chronic Diarrhea. *Gastroenterology* 1999; **116**: 1464–86.

40. American Gastroenterological Association Technical Review on the Diagnosis and Treatment of Hemorrhoids. *Gastroenterology* 2004; **126**: 1463–73.

41. Alonso-Coello P, Mills E, Heels-Ansdell D, Lopez-Yarto M, Zhou Q, Johanson JF, Guyatt G. Fiber for the treatment of hemorrhoids complications: a systematic review and meta-analysis. *Am J Gastroenterol*. 2006; **101**: 181–8.

29 Abdominal malignancies

Sarah Zaidi and Guy Chung-Faye

Department of Gastroenterology, King's College Hospital, London, UK

INTRODUCTION

Cancer is predominantly a disease of the elderly with two thirds of new cases diagnosed in people aged 65 and over and more than three quarters of cancer deaths occurring in people aged over 65, with the mortality rate increasing with age (Figure 29.1) (1). In adults under the age of 75 years, deaths from cancer outnumber deaths from diseases of the circulatory system, including ischaemic heart disease and stroke. With an ageing population, the cancer workload is steadily rising, especially as we are increasingly able to offer multi-modality therapy. The four main abdominal cancers (colorectal, oesophagus, gastric and pancreatic) account for 24 % of all cancer deaths in the United Kingdom. Although surgery remains the mainstay of treatment, many cancers in the elderly are diagnosed at a late, inoperable stage or the patient may not be fit for surgery because of co-morbidities. Therefore, chemotherapy and/or radiotherapy is increasingly utilized with curative intent or in the palliative setting. Chemotherapy regimens for abdominal cancers are rapidly evolving and the latest drug combinations offer improved survival with better symptom control and quality of life.

Although cancers occur predominantly in the elderly, the elderly are under-represented in chemotherapy clinical trials. However, evidence suggests that chemotherapy is as safe and efficacious in fit, elderly patients as in younger patients (2, 3). Despite this, a large proportion of older persons diagnosed with cancer do not undergo what is often viewed as invasive treatment with a view to offering cure. A higher likelihood of poor general health, co-morbid illness, patient refusal and difficult social circumstances are cited as the main reasons behind this (2) and there is an increasing demand on the management of these patients in palliative care. Therefore, a comprehensive understanding of the issues regarding drug therapy for palliative symptom control in cases of advanced abdominal malignancies is important for physicians in primary and secondary care. This is covered in Chapter 46 (Palliative Care in the Elderly).

Finally, although chemo-radiotherapy regimes are highly specialized and guided by the oncologists, general physicians regularly manage patients undergoing chemo-radiotherapy, who are suffering from its complications or side effects. This is particularly relevant in the elderly because of an increased susceptibility due to reduced drug clearance and/or interaction with other medications.

EPIDEMIOLOGY

Colorectal cancer

An estimated 1 million cases of colorectal cancer were diagnosed worldwide in 2002,

Prescribing for Elderly Patients Edited by Stephen Jackson, Paul Jansen and Arduino Mangoni
© 2009 John Wiley & Sons, Ltd

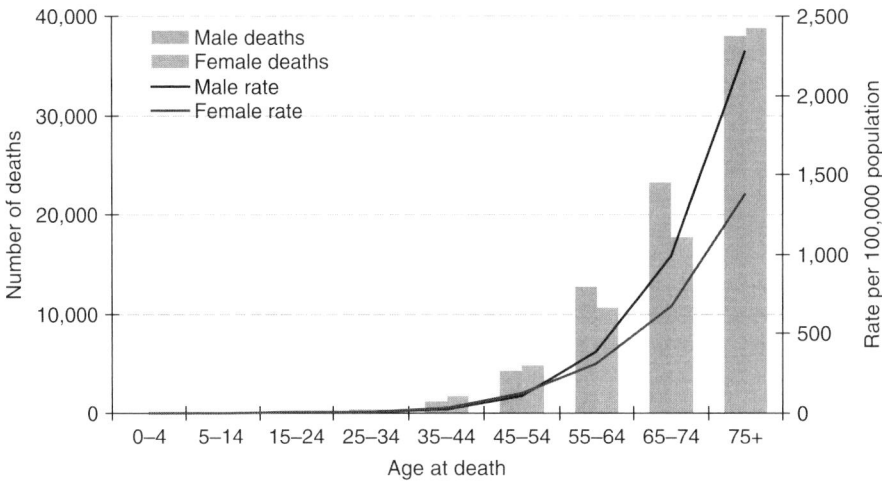

Figure 29.1. Mortality/mortality rate by age and sex, all malignant neoplasms, UK 2003. Reproduced with permission from Cancer Research UK website (http://info.cancerresearchuk.org/cancerstats/mortality/age/?a=5441)

accounting for more than 9 % of all new cancer cases (4). Incidence rates vary considerably, with the highest rates in developed countries and the lowest in Africa and Asia. In 2001, the UK had 34 539 new cases of colorectal cancer (63 % colon and 37 % rectal) (5–8). The incidence of colorectal cancer is strongly related to age, with nearly 85 % of cases arising in people who are 60 years or older.

Colorectal cancer is the second most common cause of cancer deaths in most developed countries. In the UK, there were 16 107 deaths from colorectal cancer (2003, see weblink (2)). There have been significant improvements in five-year survival from colon cancer in the UK over the last decade and is now of the order of 50 %, although it still lags behind the USA and most of Western Europe. One of the reasons for this, is late presentation, as early-stage disease (Dukes' stage A/B or TNM stage I/II) have a good/excellent (65–95 %) five-year survival with surgery alone but only 40 % of all colorectal cancers are diagnosed at early stages.

Oesophageal cancer

Oesophageal tumours (squamous cell and adenocarcinoma) are the fifth most common cancers worldwide (4). In the UK, ~7400 oesophageal cancers are newly diagnosed with ~7200 deaths, annually. It has a male preponderance and 80 % of cases are in people aged over 60 years (5–8). Squamous cell carcinoma of the upper/mid-oesophagus is the most common oesophageal tumour worldwide. However, in developed countries, this has been superseded by oesophageal adenocarcinoma, originating in the oesophago-gastric junction (OGJ). There has been a five-fold increase in OGJ adenocarcinomas since the early 1970s in the USA. A postulated explanation for this phenomenon is the increasing obesity epidemic leading to increased gastro-oesophageal reflux and Barrett's oesophagus, a pre-malignant condition.

Overall, the 5-year survival remains disappointingly poor and ranges from 10–20 %. Potential cure is possible by surgical resection in limited disease; however, less than 40 % of patients have potentially resectable disease at presentation. Furthermore, oesophageal resection carries a relatively high morbidity and mortality and a significant proportion of elderly patients are not suitable for resection due to poor performance status or co-morbidity.

Gastric tumours

Until the 1980s, gastric adenocarcinoma was one of the leading causes of cancer mortality worldwide. Currently, it is the seventh and eighth commonest cause of cancer deaths in the UK and worldwide, respectively (4–8). There is a marked geographic variation in incidence with markedly high rates in South East Asia (Japan and South Korea) due to dietary factors. Gastric cancer occurs predominantly in the elderly with the median age at diagnosis of 70 and 74 years for men and women, respectively. At diagnosis, 75 % of gastric tumours have spread at least to involve regional lymph nodes and the overall prognosis remains poor with a five-year survival of 13 % in England and Wales (5–7).

Pancreatic carcinoma

In the UK, there are ∼7000 newly-diagnosed and 7000 deaths from pancreatic cancer each year (5–8). Around 85 % of cases are diagnosed in the over 60s age group. The prognosis is poor with one and five-year survival rates of 12 % and 3 %, respectively. This is because the vast majority of tumours present at a late, inoperable stage with only 4 % of all patients suitable for surgical resection, which has a high peri-operative morbidity and mortality.

Less common tumours of the GI tract

Small cell carcinoma. The most common extra-pulmonary site for small cell tumours is the oesophagus and these represent less than 5 % of all oesophageal tumours. They are also rarely seen in the stomach but are extremely rare in the lower GI tract. As with other small cell tumours, early metastasis means the vast majority are diagnosed at an advanced stage. However, they are highly sensitive to chemotherapy, which can dramatically improve median survival and relieve symptoms.

Gastro-intestinal Stromal Tumour (GIST). GISTs are uncommon tumours of the GI tract and are thought to originate from the interstitial cells of Cajal (part of the autonomic nervous system). Although these cancers can arise anywhere in the GI tract, they most commonly occur in the stomach (60–70 %) and less commonly in the small intestine (20–30 %).

The remainder occur in the oesophagus and lower GI tract. Most cases of GISTs occur between the ages of 40 to 80 years (9).

Carcinoid tumour. Carcinoid tumours are neuro-endocrine tumours usually arising from enterochromaffin-secreting cells originating from neural crest derived cell populations. They are relatively common throughout the GI tract, especially within the upper GI tract and mid-gut (appendix). They often go undetected for long periods, unless they present with obstruction or bleeding. Metastases to the liver results in the carcinoid syndrome due to the systemic release of neuro-endocrine factors. Surgical resection, even at the metastatic stage, can have a favourable outcome. Somatostatin analogues, such as octreotide, offer good pharmacological management of the symptoms of carcinoid syndrome.

Lymphoma. The most common primary lymphomas are found in the stomach. Gastric lymphomas represent approximately 3–6 % of all gastric neoplasms. Over 95 % of these are Non-Hodgkins lymphomas (NHL), usually of B-cell origin. Primary lymphomas of the oesophagus are rare but are seen in the HIV-affected population. More commonly, lymphomas can involve the oesophagus as a result of extrinsic compression from mediastinal nodes. Mucosa-associated lymphoid tissue (MALT) (e.g. tonsils, Peyer's patches) can be associated with malignancies and are called MALT lymphomas or MALTomas. Most MALTomas are of low grade and occur in the stomach, and roughly 70 % of gastric MALTomas are associated with *Helicobacter pylori* infection and can sometimes be treated by *H. pylori* eradication alone, as well as conventional chemotherapy (10).

Pancreatic Endocrine Tumours. These include gastrinomas, insulinomas, VIPomas, somatostatinomas and glucagonomas. Also known as islet cell tumours, they present with an array of symptoms related to the active endocrine substances produced and are often associated with the MEN syndromes (types I, IIa and IIb) With the exception of glucagonomas, they usually occur in younger patients.

Table 29.1. Additional risk factors

Stomach	Previous gastric resection
	H. *pylori* →atrophic gastritis→intestinal metaplasia→dysplasia→cancer
	Pernicious anaemia
	Peutz-Jeghers syndrome
	Smoking, Alcohol
Oesophagus	
Adenocarcinoma	Longstanding GORD → Barrett's oesophagus
Squamous cell	Alcohol/smoking, aflatoxins, ↓Vit. A/C, achalasia, coeliac disease, Tylosis
Colorectal	Inflammatory bowel disease
	Colonic polyps
	Western diet (low fibre, high saturated fat and red meat)
Pancreas	Gastrectomy,
	Chronic pancreatitis,
	Alcohol, Smoking,
	Long standing diabetes

AETIOLOGY

Like almost all malignancies, the aetiology behind GI tumours appears to be multi-factorial. Genetic, environmental, dietary and lifestyle factors are all implicated. Common genetic abnormalities in colorectal cancers have been relatively well characterised and include APC, *K-ras*, p53 and DCC mutations. Additional risk factors implicated in abdominal tumours are shown in Table 29.1.

SYMPTOMS AND SIGNS

Common signs and symptoms are summarised in Table 29.2.

New onset dyspepsia is common in the elderly. However, in the absence of alarm symptoms, it is rarely a presentation of an underlying gastric malignancy. It should be initially treated symptomatically or with a 'test and treat' approach (H. *pylori* testing and eradication) and the patient reviewed. An endoscopy is indicated if the patient remains symptomatic or develops 'alarm' symptoms (urgent). Dysphagia is a serious 'alarm' symptom and warrants an urgent gastroscopy.

A change in bowel habit is another common symptom in the elderly and in the majority of cases does not signify the presence of cancer. Chronic constipation (rarely a presenting symptom of colorectal cancer) and diverticular disease, are common in this age group. Increased stool frequency or looser stools, particularly if associated with rectal bleeding, are more suggestive of an underlying malignancy. However, further assessment is usually necessary if the symptoms are persistent (>6 weeks) despite treatment and also the presence of any

Table 29.2. Common presentations of abdominal cancers

Oesophageal	Gastric	Colorectal	Pancreatic
Dysphagia/ odynophagia	Progressive/persistent dyspepsia, unresponsive to treatment	Altered bowel habit >6 weeks (loose, ↑ frequency)	Jaundice
Persistent vomiting	Persistent vomiting	Rectal bleeding (particularly without anal symptoms)	Weight loss
Iron deficiency anaemia	Iron deficiency anaemia	Iron deficiency anaemia	Abdominal pain
Weight loss	Weight loss Early satiety/fullness	Right sided abdominal mass/mass on PR examination Tenesmus/obstruction	Steatorrhoea

additional alarm symptom should prompt urgent investigations.

Anaemia is another common finding in the elderly and the causes are myriad. Anaemia of chronic disease, vitamin B12 and folate deficiency are more prevalent. The haematinics needs be measured and iron deficiency anaemia in men and post-menopausal women should prompt further investigations. Iron deficiency anaemia is present in ~60 % of all colorectal tumours and ~80 % of right-sided cancers (11). Serum ferritin is the most powerful predictor of iron deficiency but can sometimes be misleading and some studies have suggested that transferrin saturation may be a more accurate measure of iron status in the elderly (11).

Weight loss is another common symptom in the elderly. After excluding dietary and other non-GI causes (chest, thyroid, diabetes), unintentional weight loss needs further investigations as it can indicate an upper GI and less commonly a pancreatic or colorectal cancer (although it is rarely the sole feature unless disease is advanced).

Special diagnostic considerations for the elderly

Oesophageal, gastric and colonic neoplasms are usually diagnosed through endoscopy. Biphasic (arterial and venous phase) computed tomography (CT) provide accurate assessment of pancreatic tumours. Endoscopic retrograde cholangio-pancreaticography (ERCP) is an alternative for head of pancreas tumours, particularly if jaundice is present, as it can also be therapeutic, albeit with a lower sensitivity than with CT.

CT colonography is increasingly becoming available. As a diagnostic tool, it has a sensitivity of >95 % for colon cancers (12). It can be useful where colonoscopy is not possible because of strictures due to severe diverticular disease or malignancy. However bowel preparation is still required for CT colonography and a subsequent colonoscopy may be necessary for histological confirmation.

Fitness to undergo endoscopy can be problematic in the elderly and sometimes require hospital admission prior to endoscopy. Important considerations are related to:

- risks associated with use of sedation (especially with significant respiratory disease);
- fasting before endoscopy (diabetics);
- need for bowel preparation for colonoscopy (tolerability of preparation, mobility);
- higher prevalence of diverticular disease making colonoscopy technically difficult;
- provision of transport and adequate social support before and after the procedure;
- ability to give consent.

THERAPY

After diagnosis, the proposed treatment regimen depends on the tumour staging and individual case factors. Individual patient factors would include:

- performance status (fitness for surgery and/or chemo-radiation);
- presence of significant co-morbid illness;
- social circumstances;
- patient choice.

Performance status is an assessment of overall functional level and is widely utilized in determining patient suitability for proposed treatments. Various scoring systems have been proposed but the most widely used scoring system is the Eastern Cooperative Oncology Group (ECOG) (13) or Zubrod score used by the World Health Organisation and in clinical trials (Table 29.3). Performance status is graded from 0 to 5. Other scoring systems include the *Karnofsky score*. This score is measured from 100 % (perfect health) to 0 % (death) and allows for a slightly more detailed assessment of functional level in intervals of 10 (14).

The treatment of the various tumour types are summarized in Table 29.4.

Surgery in the elderly

Surgery in the elderly carries increased risks because of additional co-morbidities. Furthermore, oesophageal resection carries a significantly higher morbidity and mortality compared to colorectal resection because of the site of the tumour and logistical operative

Table 29.3. ECOG Performance status

Grade	ECOG
	ECOG performance status
0	Fully active, able to carry out all pre-disease performance without restriction
1	Restricted in physically strenuous activity but ambulatory and able to carry out work of a light or sedentary nature, e.g., light house work, office work
2	Ambulatory and capable of all selfcare but unable to carry out any work activities. Up and about more than 50% of waking hours
3	Capable of only limited self care, confined to bed or chair more than 50% of waking hours
4	Completely disabled. Cannot carry out any self-care. Totally confined to bed or chair
5	Dead

Table 29.4. Treatment

	Early (I)	Mid stage (II-III)	Late stage (IV)
Oesophagus (squamous cell/ adenocarcinoma)	Resection	Resection or Pre-operative (neo-adjuvant) chemotherapy + resection	Palliative chemo-radiation Metal stent Symptom control
Gastric	Resection	Pre-operative (neo-adjuvant) chemotherapy + resection	Palliative chemotherapy Symptom control
Colorectal	Resection	Resection + post-operative (adjuvant) chemotherapy (stage III)	Palliative chemotherapy Symptom control
Pancreas	Resection	Resection	Palliative chemotherapy Biliary metal stent
GIST	Resection	Resection	Imatinib

problems involving either a trans-hiatal or trans-thoracic approach. As a result of this, a significant proportion of elderly patients are not suitable for resection due to poor performance status or co-morbidity, however, some studies have suggested that carefully selected fit, elderly patients can have similar post-operative mortality rates when compared to younger patients (2). The results of a retrospective review of 505 consecutive patients who were operated on by a single surgical team over 17 years found no difference in the perioperative mortality, median survival, or palliative benefit of oesophagectomy on dysphagia when the group of patients older than 70 years were compared to their younger peers (15). Therefore, age alone should not determine therapy for patients with potentially resectable disease.

The use of neo-adjuvant (pre-operative) chemotherapy has shown improved over-all survival rates for oesophageal cancer (see Table 29.5) (16). However even with successful surgery, survival rates are still considerably poorer compared to those for colorectal carcinoma. Moreover, the majority of patients are not suitable for resection owing to advanced stage at diagnosis or poor performance status (18).

The mainstay of treatment for gastric cancers is adequate surgical resection. However, it has recently been shown that neoadjuvant chemotherapy improves survival compared to surgery alone (17). Although, gastric resection and gastrectomy are slightly better tolerated than radical oesophageal surgery, they still carry a relatively high mortality and morbidity (18). As for oesophageal tumours, a higher proportion of elderly patients diagnosed with gastric cancer do not undergo curative resection.

Table 29.5. Combination therapy regimes [5-fluorouracil (5-FU), folinic acid (FA), Radiotherapy (DXT)]

Tumour Site	Pre-operative/post-operative	Palliative/2nd Line
Oesophagus	5-FU/cisplatin (pre-op)	DXT/5-FU/cisplatin combination
Gastric	Epirubicin/5-FU/cisplatin	Epirubicin/5-FU/cisplatin combination (palliative)
Colorectal	5-FU + folinic acid (post-op)	Continuous 5-FU/FA
		Capecitabine (oral)
		Irinotecan +/−5-FU/FA
		Oxaliplatin + 5-FU/FA
Pancreatic		Gemcitabine
GIST		Imatinib

CHEMOTHERAPY

Important considerations in the elderly

Cancer chemotherapy carries some of the highest toxicity profiles of all pharmacological agents. Moreover, because of the relatively high doses required for tumour cytotoxicity, there is significant toxicity to other rapidly dividing cells, such as the GI tract and bone marrow. The elderly are at particular risk to these effects owing to the effects of ageing on the pharmacokinetics and pharmacodynamics of these agents.

- *Altered Volume of distribution of drug (Vd).* Ageing leads to an increase in fat content and a reduction in intracellular water, causing the Vd of lipid-soluble drugs to increase, while the Vd of water-soluble drugs decreases. This has an effect on peak concentrations of drugs and can prolong half-life if the Vd is increased. In addition a reduction in plasma albumin and higher incidence of anaemia can alter the Vd of those drugs that are either protein or RBC-bound (19).
- *Altered Renal Excretion.* Many chemotherapy drugs rely on renal elimination.

Glomerular filtration rate declines by 1 ml/minute for every year over the age of 40 leading to a significant decline with age (20). Also renal impairment due to cardiovascular disease or diabetes is more prevalent and the risk of toxicity, even with mildly reduced creatinine clearance, can be high, eg platinum compounds.

- *Poor stem cell reserve.* Stem cell reserve is reduced with age and may be responsible for increased bone marrow toxicity with chemotherapy (21–23). Chemotherapy- induced neutropaenia is more common in the elderly and is also associated with increased morbidity and mortality than in younger patients (23–25).

The toxicity and interactions of cytotoxic agents for abdominal cancers are summarised in table 29.6.

Thymidylate synthase inhibitors

5 Fluorouracil (5-FU) is the most widely used chemotherapy agent (adjuvant, neoadjuvant and palliative) for the common GI cancers (colorectal, gastric and oesophageal). It is usually co-administered with folinic acid (leucoverin),

Table 29.6. Toxicity and interactions of cytotoxic drugs for abdominal cancers

Drug	Class/Mode of action	Toxicity	Drug interactions
5-Fluorouracil	Thymydilate Synthase inhibitor	Mucositis Bone marrow toxicity Hand foot syndrome Diarrhoea Cerebellar syndrome	Allopurinol Metronidazole (enhanced toxicity) Warfarin (increased anti-coagulant effect)
Capecitabine	Thymidylate synthase inhibitor (oral precursor metabolised to 5-FU)	As for 5-FU	As for 5-FU

Table 29.6. (*continued*)

Drug	Class/Mode of action	Toxicity	Drug interactions
Gemcitabine	Nucleoside analogue inhibits DNA synthesis	Diarrhoea Bronchospasm Renal impairment (interstitial nephritis HUS proteinuria, haematuria Peripheral oedema)	Warfarin (increased anticoagulant effect)
Oxaliplatin	Platinum compound—prevents DNA replication by cross linking DNA	Peripheral neuropathy GI upset Ototoxicity Renal impairment	Aminoglycosides Vancomycin (renal toxic and ototoxic effects enhanced)
Cisplatin	Platinum compound—prevents DNA replication by cross linking DNA	Peripheral Neuropathy Ototoxicity Nephrotoxicity Nausea (severe) hypomagnesaemia	As for oxaliplatin
Irinotecan	Topo-isomerase 1 inhibitor	Cholinergic symptoms (diarrhoea) Hyperbilirubinaemia Marrow toxicity	

which has been shown to double tumour response rates (26–28). It blocks DNA synthesis by inhibiting the production of thymidine (through inhibition of thymidylate synthase). It also inhibits RNA synthesis and is cell cycle specific (S-phase), hence its efficacy (and side effects) in rapidly dividing cells. It is catabolised predominantly by the liver (80%) so it is contraindicated in hepatic impairment (bilirubin >85 mmol/L).

Evidence suggests that elderly patients with good performance status can tolerate 5-FU almost as well as younger patients. However there are some reports of higher incidences of mucositis and more profound leucopaenia in the elderly (3, 19).

Capecitabine is an oral fluoropyrimidine carbamate precursor of 5-FU. It is licensed as first-line monotherapy for metastatic colorectal cancer (28) but is more effective in combination chemotherapy. It is converted via enzymatic steps to give intratumoural release of 5-FU as the final enzyme involved in its conversion (thymidine phopshorylase) is found in higher concentrations in tumour tissue. It is administered orally and is as effective as conventional intravenous 5-FU therapy. (27, 29). It is predominantly renally

excreted so a dose reduction is advised in renal impairment (19).

Platinum compounds

Cisplatin is one of the alkylating agents. It binds covalently to DNA and inhibits DNA, RNA and protein synthesis. It is used, in combination with 5-FU, for gastric and oesophageal adenocarcinomas. It has over 90% renal elimination and a 5% risk of renal impairment (30). It is also highly emetogenic necessitating both pre and post treatment anti-emetics. The most effective agents are serotonin (5-HT$_3$) antagonists and premedication with steroids (dexamethasone). Elderly patients are at higher risk of peripheral neuropathy although concomitant use of amifostine can protect against toxic side-effects (19).

Oxaliplatin is licensed for use in metastatic colorectal cancer in combination with 5-FU and folinic acid (31). It is less nephrotoxic and better tolerated in the elderly (32).

Other agents

Irinotecan inhibits topo-isomerase 1, an essential enzyme for DNA replication. Irinotecan is used alone as 1st line adjuvant therapy for colorectal cancer or in combination with 5-FU (32). It is primarily metabolized in the liver and excreted in bile. A dose reduction is necessary in mild hepatic impairment and it is contraindicated when bilirubin is greater than 35 mmol/L (30). Irinotecan can cause profound diarrhoea. Early onset diarrhoea typically occurs within 24 hours and is part of a cholinergic syndrome. Late onset diarrhoea occurs between 5–11 days and is due to abnormal ion transport in injured intestinal mucosa leading to increased secretion of water and electrolytes (30).

Gemcitabine is a pyrimidine analogue and is incorporated into DNA, leading to inhibition of DNA synthesis and induction of apoptosis. It is used for inoperable pancreatic cancers (33). It is renally excreted and the dose is reduced in renal impairment. Acute pulmonary and renal toxicity have been reported (19, 30).

Imatinib binds to activated *c-KIT* receptors (tyrosine kinase growth factor receptor expressed in most GISTs), thereby blocking the tyrosine kinase mediated cell signal- transduction pathway to prevent uncontrolled cell proliferation. Imatinib was first licensed for treating chronic myeloid leukaemia but was also found to be effective in GISTs. In GISTs, 54 % of patients achieved a partial response with imatinib (34).

KEY POINTS

- GI malignancies are common in the elderly.
- An increased prevalence of co-morbidities in the elderly may preclude therapy.
- Surgical resection, the mainstay of treatment in early disease, offers the best chance of curative treatment.
- However, most cancers in the elderly present at late stages, necessitating adjuvant or palliative chemo-radiotherapy.
- There are now increasing multi-modality treatments to offer fit elderly patients.
- Chemotherapeutic agents for abdominal cancers carry significant toxicity, particularly in the elderly.
- Reduced renal excretion, hepatic dysfunction and decreased stem cell reserve are important factors to consider for elderly patients receiving chemotherapy as these increase the risk of toxicity.
- Carefully selected, fit elderly patients tolerate surgery and/or chemotherapy as well as younger patients and age alone should not preclude treatment.

LINKS

1. http://info.cancerresearchuk.org/cancerstats/mortality/age/?a=5441.
2. http://info.cancerresearchuk.org/cancerstats/mortality/cancerdeaths/?a=5441.
3. Office for National Statistics, Cancer Statistics registrations: Registrations of cancer diagnosed in 2001, England. Series MB1 no.32. 2004, National Statistics: London. http://www.statistics.gov.uk/statbase/Product.asp?vink=8843 & More=N.
4. ISD Online. 2004, Information and Statistics Division, NHS Scotland. http://www.isdscotland.org/isd/servlet/FileBuffer?namedFile=Cancer_in_Scotland_summary_m.pdf&pContentDispositionType=inline.
5. Welsh Cancer Intelligence and Surveillance Unit, Cancer Incidence in Wales 1992-2001. 2002. http://www.statistics.gov.uk/statbase/Product.asp?vink=8843&More=N.
6. Northern Ireland Statistics & Research Agency, 2004. http://www.nisra.gov.uk/.
7. http://www.nice.org.uk.
8. http://www.bccancer.bc.ca/.

REFERENCES

1. http://info.cancerresearchuk.org/cancerstats/mortality/age/?a=5441.
2. Ginsberg RJ. Cancer treatment in the elderly. *J Am Coll Surg*. 1998; **187**: 427–8.
3. Popescu RA, Norman A, Ross PJ, Parikh B, Cunningham D. Adjuvant or Palliative chemotherapy for colorectal cancer in patients 70 years or older. *Journal of Clinical Oncology* 1999; **17**: 2412.

4. GLOBOCAN 2000. Cancer Incidence, Mortality and Prevalence Worldwide (2000 estimates); 2001. http://www-dep.iarc.fr/.

5. Office for National Statistics, Cancer Statistics registrations: Registrations of cancer diagnosed in 2001, England. National Statistics: London: Series MB1 No. 32; 2004. http://www.statistics.gov.uk/statbase/Product.asp?vink=8843&More=N.

6. ISD Online. 2004, Information and Statistics Division, NHS Scotland. http://www.isdscotland.org/isd/servlet/FileBuffer?namedFile=Cancer_in_Scotland_summary_m.pdf&pContentDispositionType=inline.

7. Welsh Cancer Intelligence and Surveillance Unit, *Cancer Incidence in Wales 1992–2001*; 2002.

8. Northern Ireland Statistics & Research Agency; 2004. http://www.nisra.gov.uk/.

9. http://www.cancer.org/docroot/CRI/content/CRI_2_4_1x_What_Are_Gastrointestinal_Stromal_Tumors.asp?sitearea=.

10. Miki H, Kobayashi S, Harada H, Yamanoi Y, Uraoka T, Sotozono M et al. Early stage gastric MALT lymphoma with high-grade component cured by Helicobacter pylori eradication. *J Gastroenterol* 2001; **36**: 121–4.

11. Beale AL, Penney MD, Allison MC. The prevalence of iron deficiency among patients presenting with colorectal cancer. *Colorectal Disease* 2005; **7**: 398.

12. Halligan S, Altman DG, Taylor SA, Mallett S, Deeks JJ, Bartram CI et al. Computed tomographic colonography (virtual colonoscopy) for detection of colorectal polyps and cancer: meta-analysis. *Eur Radiol* 2004; **14** (suppl).

13. Oken MM, Creech RH, Tormey DC, Horton J, Davis TE, McFadden ET et al. Toxicity And Response Criteria Of The Eastern Cooperative Oncology Group. *Am J Clin Oncol*. 1982; **5**: 649–55.

14. Karnofsky DA, Burchenal JH. The Clinical Evaluation of Chemotherapeutic Agents in Cancer. In: MacLeod CM (Ed), *Evaluation of Chemotherapeutic Agents*. Columbia Univ Press, 1949: 196.

15. Ellis FH Jr, Williamson WA, Heatley GJ. Cancer of the Oesophagus and cardia: does age influence treatment selection and surgical outcomes? *J Am Coll Surg*. 1998; **187**(4): 345–51.

16. Medical Research Council Oesophageal Cancer Working Party. Surgical resection with or without preoperative chemotherapy in oesophageal cancer: A randomized controlled trial. *Lancet* 2001; **359**: 1727–33.

17. Cunningham D, Allum W, Stenning S, Thompson J, Van de Velde C, Nicolson M, Scarffe H, Lofts F, Falk S, Iveson T, Smith D, Langley R, Verma M, Weeden S, Chua Y, for the MAGIC Trial Participants. (2006) Perioperative Chemotherapy versus Surgery Alone for Resectable Gastroesophageal Cancer. *New Engl J Med*. **355**(1): 11–20.

18. Enzinger PC. Gastrointestinal cancer in older patients. *Seminars in Oncology* 2004; 206.

19. Wasil T, Lichtman SM. Clinical pharmacology issues relevant to dosing and toxicity of chemotherapy drugs in the elderly. *The Oncologist* 2005; **10**: 602–12.

20. Brenner BM, Meyer TW, Hostetter TH. Dietary protein intake and the progressive nature of kidney disease: the role of hemodynamically mediated glomerular injury in the pathogenesis of progressive glomerular sclerosis in aging, renal ablation, and intrinsic renal disease. *N Engl J Med* 1982; **306**: 652–9.

21. Boggs DR, Patrene KD. Hematopoiesis and aging III: Anemia and a blunted erythropoietic response to hemorrhage in aged mice. *Am J Hematol*. 1985; **19**: 327–38.

22. Rothstein G, Christensen RD, Nielsen BR. Kinetic evaluation of the pool sizes and proliferative response of neutrophils in bacterially challenged aging mice *Blood* 1987; **70**: 1836–41.

23. Baraldi-Junkins CA, Beck AC, Rothstein G. Hematopoiesis and cytokines. Relevance to cancer and aging. *Hematol Oncol Clin North Am*. 2000; **14**: 45–61.

24. Crawford J, Dale DC, Lyman GH. Chemotherapy-induced neutropenia: risks, consequences, and new directions for its management. *Cancer* 2004; **100**: 228–37.

25. Schild SE, Stella PJ, Geyer SM Bonner JA, McGinnis WL, Mailliard JA et al. The outcome of combined-modality therapy for stage III non-small-cell lung cancer in the elderly. *Clin Oncol*. 2003; **21**: 3201–6.

26. The Meta-analysis group in cancer: modulation of fluorouracil by leucovorin in patients with advanced colorectal cancer: an updated meta-analysis. *Journal of Clinical Oncology* 2004; **22**: 18: 3766–75.

27. Van Cutsem E, Hoff PM, Harper P, Bukowski RM, Cunningham D, Dufour P et al. Oral capecitabine vs intravenous 5FU and leucoverin; integrated efficacy data and novel analyses

from 2 large randomized phase III clinical trials. *Br J Cancer* 2004; **90**: 1190–7.

28. http://www.nice.org.uk.

29. Feliu J, Escudero P, Llosa F, Bolaños M, Vicent JM, Yubero A et al. Capecitabine As First-Line Treatment for Patients Older Than 70 Years With Metastatic Colorectal Cancer: An Oncopaz Cooperative Group Study. *Journal of Clinical Oncology* 2005; **23**: 3104–11.

30. http://www.bccancer.bc.ca/.

31. Carreca I, Comella P, Maiorino L. Oral capecitabine plus oxaliplatin in elderly patients with advanced colorectal carcinoma. Southern Italy Cooperative Oncology Group phase II study. *Proc Am Soc Clin Oncolol*. 2003; **22**: 2939a.

32. National Institute for Clinical Excellence Overview. The use of irinotecan, oxaliplatin and Ralitrexed in the treatment of advanced colorectal cancer. Review of Technology Appraisal No. 33.

33. Burris HA 3rd, Moore MJ, J Andersen J, Green MR, Rothenberg ML, Modiano MR et al. Improvements in survival and clinical benefit with gemcitabine as first line therapy for patients with advanced pancreas cancer: a randomized trial. *J Clin Oncol*. 1997; **15**: 2403–13.

34. Demetri GD, von Mehren M, Blanke CD, Van den Abbeele AD, Eisenberg B, Roberts PJ et al. Efficacy and safety of imatinib mesylate in advanced gastrointestinal stromal tumors. *N Engl J Med*. 2002; **347**(7): 472–80.

30 Liver diseases in the elderly

Réme Mountfield and Alan J. Wigg

Department of Gastroenterology and Hepatology, Flinders Medical Centre, Adelaide, Australia

INTRODUCTION

Liver disease in older people is becoming increasingly common. This is attributed to improved management of both life-threatening extrahepatic disease and that of chronic liver disease. In this chapter the important physiological changes of the liver associated with ageing are discussed along with the most common and important liver diseases in this age group. A number of other important hepatobiliary disease (genetic hemochromatosis, cholestatic liver disease, hepatocellular carcinoma and bile duct stones) are not discussed in this chapter.

PHYSIOLOGICAL CHANGES ASSOCIATED WITH AGEING

Hepatic volume and blood flow decrease with ageing, with no significant change in parenchymal arrangement. This has clinically significant effects on drugs with a high hepatic extraction ratio such as morphine, sertraline, venlafaxine, promethazine, levadopa, verapamil, midazolam and nitroglycerine. The increased bioavailability of these orally administered drugs implies a necessity for dose reduction in older patients.

Phase 1 metabolism (cytochrome P450 oxidation) is significantly altered by ageing due to a number of physiological changes. These include reduction in hepatic concentration of smooth endoplasmic reticulum, decreased overall microsomal content of CYP450, reduced activity of several microsomal enzymes like mono-oxygenases and glucose-6-phosphatase and decreased number of mitochondria in each hepatocyte. These changes have important implications for drug selection and dosage in the elderly, who are the predominant consumers of drugs dependent on oxidative metabolism for their clearance such as propranolol, amitriptyline, verapamil, theophylline and morphine. Although definitive quantitative data are not available to direct dose modification for most drugs, the reduction in hepatic clearance of such drugs is in the order of 10 to 50 % (1).

Phase 2 metabolism (conjugation by addition of polar groups to increase water solubility) is relatively spared by ageing and disease processes, thus benzodiazepines subject to glucuronidation (oxazepam, lorazepam and temazepam) or nitroreduction (nitrazepam) have minimal age related change in clearance, thus do not require dose reduction in the elderly for pharmacokinetic reasons.

Decreased regenerative capacity of the liver is also noted associated with ageing, conferring a tendency toward prolonged and often incomplete recovery after viral or toxic injury in older people (2).

Biochemical changes in the elderly often reflect systemic dysfunction rather than intrinsic

Prescribing for Elderly Patients Edited by Stephen Jackson, Paul Jansen and Arduino Mangoni
© 2009 John Wiley & Sons, Ltd

hepatic pathology. Isolated elevation in serum alkaline phosphatase should prompt investigation for bone and renal disease, intestinal malabsorption, malignancy and sepsis. Decreased albumin is another frequent biochemical abnormality which may be mistakenly attributed to liver dysfunction. In the context of sepsis albumin may decline due to its behaviour as a negative acute phase reactant. Albumin may also decline in the healthy elderly due to age related reduction in RNA translation and protein synthesis. Transaminase changes in the elderly should be regarded as an indicator of a disease process rather than attributed to ageing itself.

Despite these age related changes rendering the liver vulnerable to insult and altering drug pharmacokinetics, ageing alone is not responsible for clinically significant hepatic dysfunction.

DRUG INDUCED LIVER DISEASE

Introduction

This is a common and under recognised phenomenon in older patients, often resulting in inappropriate invasive investigation such as liver biopsy. In addition to the metabolic age related changes described above, altered plasma protein binding, smaller volumes of distribution and a greater prevalence of renal impairment further predispose older patients to hepatoxicity from drugs. Polypharmacy is also more common in aged populations, rendering kinetics less predictable and lowering the toxicity threshold for many medications.

Common culprit agents

A large number of drugs may cause hepatotoxicity but some common culprits include; non steroidal anti-inflammatory drugs, methotrexate, amiodarone, flucloxacillin, amoxycillin/clavulanic acid, isoniazid.

Mechanisms

While hepatocellular toxicity is most common, many drugs have a predilection for damage to bile ducts/canaliculi and vascular endothelium. All sites and types of medication induced damage can progress to chronicity and irreversibility, sometimes despite withdrawal of the offending agent. Two major categories of toxicity are recognized; intrinsic and idiosyncratic hepatotoxicity. Intrinsic hepatotoxicity is dose-dependent, predictable liver derangement secondary to direct chemical reactions within the hepatocyte. Idiosyncratic toxicity is unpredictable, unrelated to dose and duration of therapy, and recurs on rechallenge, often with deleterious consequences. Intrinsic/idiosyncratic hepatotoxicity may present in a systemic manner with fever, rash, joint pains and lymphadenopathy, analogous to infectious mononucleosis.

Symptoms and Signs

Older patients often under report symptoms related to adverse effects of medication, hence the need for vigilance on the part of the prescriber and careful consideration of the perceived risk to benefit ratio before commencing any new drug in this age group. Most commonly hepatotoxicity is discovered by review of liver function tests as part of a screening tool in the assessment of systemic illness.

Diagnosis

A careful medication history with attention to temporal course, cessation and rechallenge and knowledge of common culprit agents is the most effective method of diagnosis. This should be followed by assessment of serial liver biochemistry after medication cessation. Rechallenge should generally be avoided. Hepatic imaging may be appropriate to exclude other pathologies. Liver biopsy should be reserved for patients in whom the diagnosis of hepatotoxicity is in doubt and to exclude significant histological liver injury in situations where the suspected hepatotoxin is unable to be withdrawn. It should be noted that identifying the offending drug may be difficult in the elderly due to polypharmacy with multiple potential hepatotoxic drugs and delayed onset of hepatotoxicity.

Therapy

Identification and withdrawal of the offending agent is the ideal therapy. Selection of alternative, less toxic medication may be possible. However, the clinician must also assess the risks and benefits of medication cessation for each situation and decisions may not be straightforward. An example is amiodarone hepatotoxicity, where continuation of the drug in the presence of asymptomatic, mild biochemical abnormalities may better serve the patients long term health outcome.

Key Points

- Medications primarily dependent upon phase 1 hepatic metabolism for their clearance should be avoided or dose reduced in older patients.
- The manifestations of hepatotoxicity in older patients may be less specific than in the young.
- Hepatotoxicity may have intrinsic or idiosyncratic mechanisms.
- Liver biochemistry should be monitored regularly with the introduction of hepatotoxic drugs.
- Rechallenge with previous hepatotoxins should be avoided.

CIRRHOSIS

Introduction

Cirrhosis and portal hypertension is a major cause of morbidity and mortality worldwide. The prognosis for elderly patients with cirrhosis is often more influenced by their co morbid conditions rather than their liver disease. One study comparing patients older and younger than 80 years found that only 37 % of deaths amongst elderly cirrhotics were liver related (3). However, cirrhotic patients had much higher mortality than non cirrhotic elderly patients (19 % versus 69 % survival at nine years) (3).

Aetiology

The most common causes of cirrhosis in Western societies are alcohol, chronic hepatitis C, non-alcoholic steatohepatitis and haemochromatosis. Worldwide chronic hepatitis B is the most common cause of cirrhosis. Other important causes include cholestatic liver disease (primary biliary cirrhosis, primary sclerosing cholangitis), autoimmune hepatitis, Wilson's disease and alpha-1-antitrypsin deficiency.

Symptoms and signs

Well compensated cirrhotic patients may be asymptomatic and undiagnosed. Lethargy, stigmata of chronic liver disease (spider telangiectasia, palmar erythema, gynecomastia) malnutrition, osteoporosis may be early clinical features. With progressive decompensation, jaundice and symptoms and signs of portal hypertension including ascites, hepatic encephalopathy, variceal bleeding and splenomegaly become apparent.

Diagnosis

Histological diagnosis with liver biopsy remains the gold standard for diagnosis and may provide aetiological clues. In the presence of characteristic radiological findings (small, nodular liver with signs of portal hypertension) liver biopsy may not be required. Contraindications to percutaneous liver biopsy frequently exist in decompensated liver disease (coagulopathy, thrombocytopaenia, ascites) and in situations where biopsy is still necessary transjugular liver biopsy should be considered.

Therapy and drugs in cirrhosis

Other than therapy of the specific disease the principles of active management in cirrhotic patients include screening for varices, HCC, malnutrition and osteoporosis. Antibiotic prophylaxis for patients with prior spontaneous bacterial peritonitis and referral for liver transplantation assessment in decompensated patients are other important considerations in cirrhotic patients.

Endoscopic screening for oesophageal varices in cirrhotic patients is important as propranolol has been shown to reduce recurrent variceal bleeding and mortality in medium and large sized varices (4). The recommended dose is 40 mg bd, increasing to 80 mg bd orally according to pulse rate, aiming for a 25% reduction compared with baseline. The risk benefit ratio in older patients, however, is altered by propranolol's propensity to exacerbate postural hypotension already present in many older patients due to concurrent antihypertensive medication and autonomic dysfunction, leading to falls in a population predisposed to osteoporotic fractures. It is also contraindicated in other common conditions such as chronic obstructive pulmonary disease with reversibility, heart block, severe peripheral vascular disease and uncontrolled congestive cardiac failure. Daily dosing with longer acting non-selective β-blockers, such as nadolol, may improve compliance.

Screening for HCC in elderly cirrhotic patients is often not appropriate particularly if detection would not result in any form of therapeutic intervention. Referral for transplantation assessment is inappropriate if patients have significant other co-morbidities and are older than 65 years, as outcomes are poor in this subgroup.

Spironolactone and frusemide, commonly used in ascites management, often cause electrolyte disturbances and renal dysfunction in older patients, and these drugs require careful monitoring.

Key points

- Elderly cirrhotic patients have a higher mortality than elderly non-cirrhotic patients.
- Liver biopsy remains the gold standard for diagnosis but characteristic radiological findings of cirrhosis and portal hypertension are often sufficient for diagnosis.
- Cirrhotic patients should be investigated for oesophageal varices, malnutrition and osteoporosis.
- Primary prophylaxis, using non-selective β-blockers, of medium to large oesophageal varices reduces the risk of variceal bleeding but may not be tolerated in elderly patients.
- Selected cirrhotic patients may be appropriate for HCC surveillance.

ALCOHOLIC LIVER DISEASE

Introduction

Alcohol abuse is common in the elderly. One German study found the prevalence of alcohol problems in NH residents was 7.4% (5). Elderly patients who present to hospital with alcoholic liver disease are more likely to have cirrhosis on presentation (80% over 60 years versus 25% under 60 years) and have higher one year mortality relative to their younger counterparts (75% over 75 years versus 5% under 60 years) (6).

Symptoms and signs

Elderly patients with alcoholic liver disease may present atypically with symptoms such as poor sleep, anxiety, depression, falls and cognitive impairment. Those with acutely decompensated liver disease or alcoholic hepatitis may have characteristic biochemical abnormalities including leukocytosis, elevated transaminases (usually under 300 U/L with an AST/ALT ratio >2), elevated bilirubin and GGT. Initial presentation with decompensated chronic liver disease is also common in the elderly.

Diagnosis

As alcohol abuse is often unrecognized in the elderly a high index of suspicion is required. Simple alcohol screening questionnaire's such as CAGE and AUDIT are useful to detect problem drinkers in the primary care setting and the need for a more detailed alcohol assessment. In those patients with chronic liver disease a search for co-factors for liver injury, such as hepatitis C or haemochromatosis, is prudent.

Therapy

Abstinence from alcohol is the mainstay of therapy. This may be harder to achieve in elderly patients with longstanding patterns of alcohol use. There is evidence from randomized controlled trials that that brief interventions (assessment of alcohol intake, feedback on level of harm and clear advice to stop drinking) can change drinking behaviour in up to 30 % of cases (7). Those with more serious, dependent patterns of alcohol use, need referral to alcohol specialists for long-term support. Three drugs (acamprosate, naltrexone and disulfiram) may be useful adjunctive therapies in combination with alcohol counselling. These drugs should only be used in those who are alcohol free, motivated and compliant and have a history of prior relapses. Acamprosate (effects on GABA-ergic and glutamate neurotransmitter systems) and naltrexone (endogenous opiod antagonist) have been shown to reduce alcohol craving and intake and to prolong abstinence following detoxification (8). Disulfiram (blocks aldehyde dehydrogenase leading to accumulation of acetaldehyde and unpleasant flushing reaction) has also been used to maintain alcohol abstinence. Due to multiple drug interactions and contra-indications in cardiovascular disease disulfiram is less suitable in elderly patients.

In patients with severe alcoholic hepatitis, pharmacotherapy also appears to have a role. Meta-analyses and multiple randomised controlled trials of corticosteroid use have given conflicting results but they are likely to be beneficial in carefully selected patients with severe alcoholic hepatitis (Maddrey's discriminant function >32) without infection, gastro-intestinal bleeding, diabetes or pancreatitis. A four week course of prednisolone (40 mg daily) followed by tapering is the recommended regime. More recently pentoxyfylline, a non-selective phosphodiesterase inhibitor, has also demonstrated benefits in severe alcoholic hepatitis. Significantly reduced four-week mortality and frequency of hepatorenal syndrome have been reported (9). The dose used in this trial was 400 mg tds for 4 weeks. The mechanism of action of this drug is unclear but probably relates to modification of cytokine effects.

Most alcoholic patients will have nutritional deficiencies and therefore nutritional investigation and support is of paramount importance. Vitamin supplementation (thiamine, magnesium, multivitamins) and high protein dietary supplements are frequently required for several months following cessation of drinking.

Key points

- Alcohol abuse is common in the elderly and alcoholic liver disease may have an atypical presentation in this age group.
- Alcohol abuse is often unrecognized in the elderly and questionnaires such as CAGE and AUDIT are useful tools to detect problem drinking in the primary care setting.
- Patients with severe, dependent alcohol abuse require referral to specialist alcohol programs for longterm care and counselling.
- A number of drug therapies (acamprosate, naltrexone, disulfiram) can assist in maintaining abstinence following detoxification in selected patients.
- Corticosteroids and pentoxyfylline can reduce mortality in selective patients with severe alcoholic hepatitis.

NON-ALCOHOLIC STEATOHEPATITIS (NASH)

Introduction

With a growing obesity epidemic in Western countries non-alcoholic fatty liver disease and steatohepatitis has become the most common cause of abnormal liver function tests in patients presenting to liver clinics.

Aetiology

Although a minority of NASH can be caused by drugs, disorders of lipid metabolism, TPN, most cases are associated with obesity and underlying insulin resistance. NASH is increasingly viewed as a hepatic manifestation of the metabolic syndrome (abdominal obesity, diabetes, hypertension and dyslipidaemia).

Symptoms and signs

The usual presentation of NASH is an asymptomatic elevation of liver function tests. However, symptoms of mild right upper quadrant discomfort, malaise and fatigue may also be present. NASH usually presents between the ages of 40 and 60, thus it is a common diagnosis in older patients. A female preponderance has been noted in most studies.

Diagnosis

A thorough alcohol history is necessary and less than 40 g a week supports diagnosis of NASH. Classical liver function test abnormalities include elevations of AST and ALT, with the AST:ALT ratio <1. Signs of the metabolic syndrome are often present. Ultrasound may demonstrate an echogenic liver, although this is a non-specific finding and also present in cirrhosis. The gold standard for the diagnosis of NASH is liver biopsy which demonstrates macrovesicular fatty change and inflammation. Although clinical and laboratory evaluation have a poor predictive value for the diagnosis of NASH, liver biopsy is usually restricted to groups with warning signs of cirrhosis (hard liver edge, low albumin, low platelet count, AST > ALT, ultrasound suspicious of cirrhosis). Older age has consistently been shown to be an independent risk factor for fibrosis in NASH and therefore patients over 45 who are obese or diabetic should also be considered for liver biopsy (10).

Prognosis

NASH is a benign liver disease in most patients with a much better long-term prognosis than alcoholic hepatitis. However, prospective histological studies have suggested progression to cirrhosis in about 15 % of patients and NASH is an important cause of "cryptogenic" cirrhosis in elderly diabetic women (11). Population based studies have also demonstrated a higher overall mortality rate in NASH patients compared with the normal populations and a higher rate of liver related deaths (12).

Therapy

A number of pharmacological agents (Vitamin E, metformin, pioglitazone, rosiglitazone, probuchol, betaine, ursodeoxycholic acid, losartan, pentoxyfylline) have been investigated in NASH patients. Although improvements in liver function tests and histology has been demonstrated by some of these agents in small trials, their routine use in clinical practice is currently

premature. The mainstay of therapy in most patients is slow weight loss. A weight loss programme with formal dietician involvement and increased physical activity is recommended due to the difficulty of achieving lifestyle modification in the majority of patients. In the morbidly obese patient (BMI > 35 kg/m^2) with NASH and significant fibrosis, more aggressive weight loss interventions such as obesity surgery have been shown to improve liver histology (13).

Key points

- NASH is a common cause of liver function test abnormalities in Western societies.
- It is usually associated with abdominal obesity, insulin resistance and the metabolic syndrome.
- The AST:ALT ration <1 is characteristic.
- NASH can progress to cirrhosis in a minority of patients and old age is an independent risk factor for fibrosis.
- Gradual weight loss is the mainstay of therapy.

HEPATITIS C

Introduction

The prevalence of chronic hepatitis C is increasing in older people, as the cohort of patients exposed to blood products prior to screening programmes and administered drugs with non-disposable, inadequately sterilized needles grows older. In western societies cirrhosis due to HCV and alcohol are the most frequent causes of cirrhosis in older people, and the prevalence of HCV is expected to rise over the next 20 years. HCV acquired over age 65 confers increased chance of progression to cirrhosis (43 % >60 yrs, 7 % under 40 yrs), faster progression and increased mortality rate, especially in males with significant alcohol intake (14). The reason for more rapid progression of fibrosis in older patients in unknown but may relate to decreasing immune function.

Aetiology

In western societies the major mode of transmission is via infected blood or body fluids, the major risk factors in all ages being injection drug use. Migration from endemic hepatitis C areas provides another significant pool of HCV patients in western societies.

Symptoms and signs

Acute infection is usually asymptomatic with progression to chronicity in 80–85 % of cases. Extrahepatic manifestations such as depression, arthritis and glomerulonephritis can occur. Although HCV may present with decompensated liver disease, more frequently it is diagnosed following testing in asymptomatic individuals with abnormal liver function tests and risk factors for HCV.

Diagnosis

Elevation of transaminases (ALT > AST) in patients with risk factors for HCV should be initially investigated with antibody testing. Positive antibody tests should be confirmed with molecular PCR testing for HCV RNA. Genotype testing and liver biopsy are useful investigations which help guide decision making with respect to antiviral treatment.

Treatment

The current antiviral therapy for HCV consists of combination pegylated interferon injected weekly combined with daily oral ribavirin. Doses and duration of therapy vary with genotype and degree of fibrosis but favourable genotypes (2 and 3) will usually receive 24 weeks treatment whereas the initial aim will be 48 weeks of therapy for unfavourable genotypes (1 and 4). Testing for a rapid virological response following 4 weeks of therapy is now the standard of care. A rapid virological response at 4 weeks has been been shown to be the most powerful predictor of a sustained virological response. Testing for early viral response is usually performed at 12 weeks in unfavourable genotypes, and the absence of a 2 log drop in viral load at this point suggests that viral response is unlikely and that treatment should be discontinued. Presence of HCV RNA at 24 weeks in unfavourable genotypes is also an indication to cease anti-viral therapy. Current

trial data suggest a 76 % and 46 % sustained viral response rate for genotypes 2/3 and genotype 1 patients respectively. Sustained viral response is associated with reversal of fibrosis improved liver related morbidity and mortality.

Pegylated interferon and ribavirin therapy has a considerable toxicity profile and the higher rate of co morbid disease in older patients mandates a careful risk/benefit assessment before commencement of interferon in elderly patients.

The main toxicity of ribavirin is haemolytic anaemia, which is poorly tolerated in the elderly due to decreased cardiopulmonary reserve, and is relatively contraindicated in those with cardiac disease. Careful monitoring of haemoglobin with dose reduction following significant falls in haemoglobin is required. As ribavirin is predominantly renally cleared, it is poorly tolerated in patients with a GFR <50 mL/min. In this setting substantial dose reduction and careful monitoring is required. Pegylated interferon has the advantage of weekly administration with possible compliance benefits but toxicity does not appear to be reduced compared with standard interferon. The main toxicities of pegylated interferon include malaise and myelosuppression. Exacerbation of depression can increase suicide risk and requires early recognition.

There is limited evidence to guide treatment with pegylated interferon and ribavirin for HCV in elderly people and the decision to treat must be individualized. Although community based studies suggest that HCV is a slowly progressive and benign disease in the majority of patients therapy may be of greater benefit in elderly patients given faster progression of disease in this group. Treatment is usually contraindicated in the presence of decompensated liver disease, active alcohol, significant co-morbidities and age >70 and is of uncertain benefit in patients with histologically mild disease and persistently normal liver function tests.

There is considerable current interest surrounding the use of protease inhibitors and other small molecules in combination with interferon and ribavirin therapy. Such triple combination therapy has shown considerable promise in early studies, with further improvements in sustained viral responses described. More definitive clinical studies are awaited before such regimens enter clinical practice.

Key points

- Patients who acquire HCV infection at an older age have more rapid progression of fibrosis.
- The major risk factor for HCV infection is injection drug use in western societies.
- Diagnosis is achieved with positive antibody test and confirmatory molecular PCR testing for HCV RNA.
- Current therapy for HCV includes combination pegylated interferon and ribavirin.
- Toxicity of combination antiviral therapy and co-morbidities of elderly patients often prohibits therapy in this group.

HEPATITIS B

Chronic hepatitis B is a major worldwide global health problem with an estimated 350 million carriers worldwide and 1 million deaths annually. In Caucasian populations the most common mode of infection is to adults via injection drug use and sexual intercourse. Spontaneous clearance of the virus occurs in over 90 % of cases. By contrast infection in endemic areas usually occurs peri-natally or in early childhood and progression to chronic hepatitis is more common.

Three major categories of infection exist in patients who are hepatitis B surface antigen (HBsAg) positive. Chronic inactive carrier, E antigen positive chronic hepatitis and E antigen negative chronic hepatitis. Chronic inactive carriers are characterized serologically by HBsAg positivity with low ($<10^5$ copies/ml) or undetectable hepatitis B DNA (HBV DNA) and normal liver function tests. These patients usually seroconvert with time from E antigen (HBeAg) to E antibody (anti-HBe). Such patients may reactivate infection and require infrequent monitoring of liver function tests. HBeAg positive patients are characterised by absence of anti-HBe and detectable HBV

DNA($>10^5$ copies/ml). This subgroup has more predictable responses to antiviral therapy in the setting of elevated transaminases. The third major group is chronic HBeAg antigen negative hepatitis (often called pre-core mutants). This group is characterized serologically by absence of HBeAg, presence or absence of anti-HBe, and detectable HBV DNA. This group often have fluctuating levels of HBV DNA and may be confused with chronic inactive carriers if HBV DNA becomes undetectable and liver function tests normalize. The response of this group to antiviral therapy is less predictable and long-term therapy is frequently required.

Management of chronic hepatitis B is complex and evolving due to the recent introduction of pegylated interferons and newer nucleoside analogues (adefovir, tenofovir, entecavir). Usually observation only is required in the absence of significant (>2 times upper limit of normal) transaminase elevation or histological liver injury, as therapy is rarely effective in this setting. Newly diagnosed, well compensated, E antigen positive hepatitis with elevated transaminases should also be observed for three to six months as activity may represent spontaneous HBeAg seroconversion.

Current treatment options are between pegylated interferons (poor tolerability but definite end point of therapy and higher chance of durable HBsAg seroconversion) and nucleotide/nucleoside analogues (good tolerability but often longterm therapy required leading to resistance). Although lamivudine has been associated with very high resistance rates with long-term therapy, resistance appears to be a lesser problem with newer agents (adefovir, tenofovir, entecavir). For elderly patients the better tolerability of nucleoside/nucleotide analogues and the reduced need for very long term therapy due to more advanced age with subsequent resistance issues, often makes them a more attractive therapeutic option in this setting. The usual commencing dose for lamivudine is 100 mg daily and for adefovir is 10 mg daily. An important practice point is the need for dose reduction in renal impairment for GFR < 50 ml/min.

LIVER TRANSPLANTATION

Increasing demand for liver transplantation in elderly patients is now occurring and the numbers of patients being transplanted over 60 years of age is increasing. Although intensive care and hospital stays have usually been longer, most studies have not demonstrated worse patient or graft survival rates at 12 months following transplantation. However, longer term five-year survival data have usually demonstrated significantly poorer outcomes in older patients with the most common cause of death being malignancy in this age group.

Data from the Australian and New Zealand Transplant registry illustrates these points with one-year and five-year survival of 85 % and 61 % respectively in patients over 65 years. While the one-year survival is equivalent to younger age groups the five-year survival is almost 20 % worse than for patients younger than 60. However, a 61 % five-year survival still remains above the 50 % five-year survival mark, which has been widely accepted as the threshold below which liver transplantation should be considered futile.

It seems reasonable therefore not to consider age as an absolute contra-indication for transplantation. However, patients above 65 years should be highly selected for transplantation and only those without significant co-morbidities should be considered.

One interesting observation has been the lower rates of rejection associated with elderly patients, possibly due to the associated decline in immune function associated with ageing.

REFERENCES

1. Regev A, Schiff ER. Liver disease in the elderly. *Gastroenterology Clinics of North America* 2001; **30**(2): 547–63.
2. Sanz N, Diez-Fernandez C, Alvarez AM, Fernandez-Simon L, Cascales M. Age-related changes on parameters of experimentally-induced liver injury and regeneration. *Toxicology & Applied Pharmacology* 1999; **154**(1): 40–9.
3. Hoshida Y, Ikeda K, Kobayashi M, Suzuki Y, Tsubota A, Saitoh S, et al. Chronic liver disease in the extremely elderly of 80 years or more: clinical characteristics, prognosis and patient survival analysis. *Journal of Hepatology* 1999; **31**(5): 860–6.
4. Hayes PC, Davis JM, Lewis JA, Bouchier IA. Meta-analysis of value of propranolol in prevention of variceal haemorrhage. [see comment] [erratum appears in Lancet 1990 Aug 4;336 (8710):324]. *Lancet* 1990; **336**(8708): 153–6.
5. Weyerer S, Schaufele M, Zimber A. Alcohol problems among residents in old age homes in the city of Mannheim, Germany. *Australian & New Zealand Journal of Psychiatry* 1999; **33**(6): 825–30.
6. Potter JR, James OF. Clinical features and prognosis of alcoholic liver disease in respect of advancing age. *Gerontology* 1987; **33**: 380–7.
7. Wallace P, Cutler S, Haines A. Randomised controlled trial of general practitioner intervention in patients with excessive alcohol consumption. *BMJ* 1988; **297**(6649): 663–8.
8. Graham R, Wodak AD, Whelan G. New pharmacotherapies for alcohol dependence. [see comment]. *Medical Journal of Australia* 2002; **177**(2): 103–7.
9. Akriviadis E, Botla R, Briggs W, Han S, Reynolds T, Shakil O. Pentoxifylline improves short-term survival in severe acute alcoholic hepatitis: a double-blind, placebo-controlled trial. [see comment]. *Gastroenterology* 1637; **119**(6): 1637–48.
10. Angulo P, Keach JC, Batts KP, Lindor KD. Independent predictors of liver fibrosis in patients with nonalcoholic steatohepatitis. *Hepatology* 1356; **30**(6): 1356–62.
11. Lee RG. Nonalcoholic steatohepatitis: a study of 49 patients. *Human Pathology* 1989; **20**(6): 594–8.
12. Adams LA, Lymp JF, St Sauver J, Sanderson SO, Lindor KD, Feldstein A, et al. The natural history of nonalcoholic fatty liver disease: a population-based cohort study. [see comment]. *Gastroenterology* 2005; **129**(1): 113–21.
13. Dixon JB, Bhathal PS, Hughes NR, O'Brien PE. Nonalcoholic fatty liver disease: Improvement in liver histological analysis with weight loss. *Hepatology* 1647; **39**(6): 1647–54.
14. Roudot-Thoraval F, Bastie A, Pawlotsky JM, Dhumeaux D. Epidemiological factors affecting the severity of hepatitis C virus-related liver disease: a French survey of 6,664 patients. The Study Group for the Prevalence and the Epidemiology of Hepatitis C Virus. *Hepatology* 1997; **26**(2): 485–90.

31 Disorders of the lower urinary tract

Adrian Wagg

University College Hospital, London, UK

Urinary incontinence and the associated lower urinary tract symptoms (LUTS) constitute one of the giants of geriatric medicine, but the management of the underlying disorders contributing to these is often neglected. The prevalence of urinary incontinence and LUTS increases with increasing age. This reflects a combination of physiological change, an increased incidence of lower urinary tract disease and the influence of associated morbidity in older people. It is both a marker of dependency, of poorer health related outcomes and also leads to an increased likelihood of institutionalization.

An understanding of the approaches to drug treatment of urinary incontinence and lower urinary tract disease can be aided by an understanding of the anatomy and physiology of the micturition system. The smooth muscle fibres of the detrusor muscle of the bladder appear to be randomly arranged over the dome of the bladder but funnel at the bladder neck to be continued into the urethra as longitudinal fibres forming a tube. In the male these fibers are inserted into the verumontanum, but in the female they terminate in the distal urethra. Contraction of the detrusor results in a rise in bladder pressure associated with shortening of the urethra; contraction of the muscle of the trigone, the triangular baseplate with its apex at the bladder neck, and base running between both ureters results in funneling of the bladder neck. There are some fibres which are inserted into the external surface of the trigone, distally. These pull the distal margins of the trigone apart, thus opening the bladder neck.

In normal circumstances the detrusor is highly compliant. This means that it is normal for a bladder to be filled to 500 mL, and more, without an increase in intravesical pressure, other than the pressure head resulting from the volume of the fluid in the bladder, which would be approximately 8 cm H_2O at 500 mL. If the wall tension in the detrusor increases in association with filling but then fails to relax (stress relaxation), then the bladder is said to "lack compliance". "Low compliance" may result from fibrosis, detrusor hypertrophy or an increased resting tone secondary to reduced neural inhibition (1).

Control of the bladder and urethra depends upon a complex supraspinal neuronal network which allows voluntary postponement of voiding and the ability to empty the bladder at a socially convenient time, even if there is little need to void. In adults, the normal mechanism for activating contraction of the detrusor is the release of acetylcholine from parasympathetic nerves, stimulated by a spinobulbospinal micturition reflex. Tension receptors in the detrusor activate afferents traveling in the pelvic nerves. These afferents pass through the lumbosacral dorsal roots to ascending tracts where they synapse in the midbrain periaqueductal gray (PAG). Their signalling intensity increases as the bladder fills and fibres from the PAG descend to the pontine micturition centre (PMC),

Prescribing for Elderly Patients   Edited by Stephen Jackson, Paul Jansen and Arduino Mangoni

causing excitation. This causes activation of the descending motor efferents which cause co-ordinated detrusor contraction and urethral relaxation. However, afferent signals from the bladder do not automatically trigger the micturition reflex, but are relayed via the forebrain where a voluntary decision to empty the bladder can be made.

Since higher cerebral centres tend to inhibit the pontine micturition center, lesions above this are associated with detrusor overactivtiy of neurogenic origin. Frontal lobe lesions are associated with frequency, urgency and urgency incontinence with a loss of warning of impending micturition. Strokes are often associated with detrusor overactivity, excepting those which primarily affect the occipital lobes. Any spinal cord injury which disrupts the normal connection between the sacral spinal cord and the supraspinal pathways controlling micturition will cause bladder dysfunction. Lesions of the spinal cord below the pons, but rostral to the sacral nuclei, result in bladder areflexia initially, lasting days to weeks before detrusor overactivity develops. However, if a spinal lesion involves complete destruction of the sacral nuclei, bladder areflexia will be permanent.

The external urethral sphincter is the principal mechanism for maintaining urethral continence in both sexes although the smooth muscle and epithelium of the urethra is also important, particularly in women. The striated muscles of the pelvic floor and the external sphincter are supplied by somatic efferents originating in the anterior horns of the sacral cord segments S2–S4. The motor neurons are grouped in a specific region called Onuf's nucleus. The axons originating from Onuf's nucleus pass to the periphery through the pudendal nerve and the pelvic nerves. External sphincter activity is supported by the adrenergic smooth muscle of the urethra.

The sympathetic innervation for the lower urinary tract comes from postganglionic nerves traveling in the hypogastric plexus, the pelvic nerves, and the pudendal nerves. This sympathetic innervation inhibits the detrusor, providing an active component to relaxation and also stimulates the urethral smooth muscle and the sphincters. The inhibitory noradrenergic receptors on detrusor cells are β_3 subtype. Motor activation of the detrusor in healthy humans is achieved by the stimulation of muscarinic receptors by acetylcholine. Ligand studies of the M2 and M3 muscarinic receptors in the bladder have shown that the greater proportion (85 %) are M2 receptors with only 15 % being M3. All of the contractile activity appears to be attributed to the M3 receptor in healthy humans. It has been found that some muscarinic antagonists prove selective for the bladder, but this tissue specificity does not appear to be associated with either M2 selectivity or lack of M3 selectivity (2).

Acetylcholine and noradrenaline are not the only significant neurotransmitters in the lower urinary tract. Nonadrenergic noncholinergic (NANC) neurotransmitters are neuropeptides which modulate the actions of the classical transmitters and may act as transmitters themselves. Neuropeptide-Y and vasoactive intestinal polypeptide are important neuromodulators which are released at neuromuscular junctions so as to influence the release and uptake of acetylcholine and noradrenaline. Adenosine triphosphate (ATP) is thought to be an important neurotransmitter, co-released with acetlycholine and it is known to cause depolarization of the detrusor. While in the normal human bladder ATP is not important, there is evidence that in diseased states the activating mechanisms of the detrusor change and that NANC transmitters exert a much greater influence on the bladder, the ATP being broken down less effectively in overactive detrusor.

As far as bladder outflow tract obstruction is concerned, the main drug targets have been the alpha adreno-receptor, which are abundant in the prostatic stroma and in the bladder. The alpha 1_A appears to be the primary regulator of smooth muscle tone in the prostate and bladder neck, the alpha 1_D subtype is associated with detrusor contraction. The population of these receptors in the detrusor also increases with detrusor overactivity but there appears to be no value in pharmacological manipulation. The other main target has been the inhibition of testosterone 5 alpha–reductase, leading to a regression in prostate size.

PATHOPHYSIOLOGY

Urgency incontinence is the commonest cause of urinary incontinence in elderly people, this being due chiefly to detrusor overactivity. This is particularly the case in elderly people living in institutions. Among outpatients presenting with lower urinary tract symptoms, 75–85 % of women aged 75 and over and 85–95 % percent of similarly aged men have detrusor overactivity. Some observed changes associated with greater age in men and women with lower urinary tract symptoms undergoing cystometry are listed in Table 31.1.

Men with lower urinary tract symptoms do not demonstrate all of the age-related changes associated with women. This probably relates to the higher urethral resistance caused by the prostate gland, causing detrusor muscle hypertrophy. In elderly people of both sexes detrusor overactivity is associated with lower bladder capacities than in those with normal bladders. Contrary to expectations, lower bladder capacities, more aggressive detrusor overactivity, and older age do not appear to be associated with a poorer therapeutic prognosis.

Both sexes void less successfully in late life and voiding is associated with higher residual urine volumes and a higher proportion of patients with incomplete bladder emptying. The explanations for this are probably complex. Obstruction will play a part in men but it is by no means the only explanation. There is evidence for a reduced speed of detrusor shortening in late life as well as problems in sustaining adequate voiding contractions. The transmission of force from the detrusor in later life is damped by an accumulation of collagen and connective tissue, giving the impression of "impaired contactility" a common misnomer.

INCONTINENCE SUBTYPES

The majority of incontinence can be classified as either: Urgency urinary incontinence, usually due to an *"overactive bladder"*; this is a disorder characterized by urinary urgency, with or without urgency incontinence, usually with frequency and nocturia. This is the commonest cause of incontinence in later life and usually maps onto the observation of involuntary detrusor contractions during filling cystometry, termed *detrusor overactivity*. This disorder may co-exist with *stress urinary incontinence*, that is, incontinence on effort or exertion, indicative of urethral sphincter incompetence. *Mixed urinary incontinence* indicates the coexistence of symptoms of stress and of urgency incontinence. *Overflow urinary incontinence* is characterized by the almost constant loss of small amounts of urine and is related to gross retention of urine and leakage as intravesical pressure overcomes urethrel pressure. *Functional incontinence* denotes that which is related to disorders outside the lower urinary tract, usually due to cognitive or physical disability, leading to an inability to toilet appropriately. The main other significant condition for which pharmacotherapy has a significant role is bladder outflow tract obstruction presumed secondary to benign prostatic enlargement in the male.

Table 31.1. Physiological changes in the lower urinary tract associated with increasing age

Decreased
Urinary flow rate,
Speed of contraction of detrusor
Collagen:detrusor ratio ($\female$ only)
Maximum bladder capacity
Functional bladder capacity
Sensation of filling

Increased
Post void residual volume of urine
Urinary frequency
Outflow tract obstruction ($\male$ only)

TREATMENT CESSATION

No treatise on the management of these problems would be complete without considering the withdrawal or alteration of drug treatment which might worsen symptoms or lead to the condition. Table 31.2 lists the medications which may either precipitate or contribute to incontinence.

Table 31.2. Medications which may predispose an older person to become incontinent

Medications	Effects on continence
Alpha adrenergic agonists	Increase smooth muscle tone in urethra and prostatic capsule and may precipitate obstruction, urinary retention, and related symptoms
Alpha adrenergic antagonists	Decrease smooth muscle tone in the urethra and may precipitate stress urinary incontinence in women
Angiotensin converting enzyme (ACE) inhibitors	Cause cough that can exacerbate incontinence
Agents with anti-muscarinic properties	May cause constipation that can contribute to incontinence. May cause cognitive impairment and reduce effective toileting ability
Calcium channel blockers	May cause constipation that can contribute to incontinence. May cause dependent oedema which can contribute to nocturnal polyuria
Cholinesterase inhibitors (cognitive enhancers)	Associated with detrusor overactivity and may precipitate urgency incontinence
Diuretics	Cause diuresis and precipitate incontinence
Lithium	Polyuria due to diabetes insipidus like state
Opioid analgesics	May cause urinary retention, constipation, confusion, and immobility—all of which can contribute to incontinence
Sedatives Hypnotics Antipsychotics	May cause confusion and impaired mobility and precipitate incontinence
Histamine₁ receptor antagonists	Some agents have anticholinergic effects
Selective serotonin re-uptake inhibitors	Increase cholinergic transmission and may lead to urgency urinary incontinence
Gabapentin Glitazones Non-steroidal anti-inflammatory agents	Can cause oedema, which can lead to polyuria while supine and exacerbate nocturia and nighttime incontinence

ASSESSMENT WITH A BEARING ON DRUG ADDITION OR WITHDRAWAL

Urinalysis and the diagnosis of urinary tract infection

This should be done for all patients with urinary incontinence at first presentation, or if there is a change in symptoms suggesting infection of the urine. The presence of frank blood indicates the need for action to be taken. The best dipstick tests to use are those with leucocytes and nitrite test pads; if both tests are negative the chance of there being an infection is low when compared to laboratory evidence of a UTI based upon microscopic pyuria and bacteriuria. Large amounts of glucose or ketones in the urine can make the nitrite test falsely negative. If there are lower urinary tract symptoms or the patient

has a delirium then a mid-stream specimen of urine should be obtained if at all possible. For the very frail, there are pads which are similar to those used in paediatric practice which enable the collection if urine. For those doubly incontinent, an in and out catheter may be the only way of reliably obtaining a specimen.

Asymptomatic bacteriuria is common in older women (reports suggest up to 25 %) and treating this will have no effect on incontinence. Antibiotic treatment will merely add to the likelihood of developing resistance to the antibiotic and expose the individual to antibiotic related side effects. If the patient is already known to be chronically incontinent then eradicating the bacteria will not help.

If dipstick-positive blood is found it should be followed up by sending a sample for microscopy. If there is true microscopic haematuria then a referral for investigation should be made as this can result from having urinary tract stones or a tumour. Clearly glycosuria, indicating either a low renal threshold for glucose or poorly controlled diabetes mellitus requires further investigation and will cause polyuria.

RECTAL EXAMINATION

Although there is no published evidence that performing a rectal examination alters outcomes for the treatment of incontinence in women, expert opinion suggests that a loaded rectum may, because of its size, lead to voiding difficulty or the presence of a significant post-void residual volume. Additionally, an assessment of prostate size and consistency in men will help to guide medical treatment. Occasionally, faecal impaction will lead to acute retention, resolution of which will lead to normal voiding.

VAGINAL EXAMINATION

This is an important part of a continence assessment. However, this should only be undertaken by a professional with the necessary competence and probably as part of a specialist rather than generalist assessment. A visual examination though might reveal conditions such as urogenital atrophy or prolapse that can cause urinary symptoms.

THE PHARMACOLOGICAL TREATMENT OF URINARY INCONTINENCE

An absolute cure for incontinence cannot be achieved for many older, frailer people but the best that any clinician might aim for is resolution of symptoms leading to a return to normal bladder habits and a normal lifestyle. Data from randomized, controlled studies for

older people are available but often exclude the frail elderly, thus exptrapolations have to be made. In some instances, these may be perfectly valid but sometimes caution needs to be taken.

The hypotheses underlying drug treatment for OAB have undergone a revolution over the last eight years; it was widely held that the action of antimuscarinic agents was to suppress overactive contractions of the bladder acting via M3 receptors. It has become established that there is considerable sensory dysfunction associated with OAB and that M_2 receptors, found in the suburothelium, have a significant effect on the appreciation of urinary urgency. Newer drugs are now targeted to control urinary urgency, a central feature of the symptom complex which has a major impact on quality of life. The role of antimuscarinics in patients with cognitive impairment is discussed later.

Oxybutynin is the most established antimuscarinic drug in use today. Trials comparing oxybutynin with placebo have consistently shown a reduction in symptoms with the active drug. Studies in older people, using lower doses than the licensed dose (5 mg three times daily), show some efficacy with a concomitant reduction in the adverse effects, which at normal dosing resulted in up to 60% of subjects being unable to take it (3). Oxybutynin is also effective when used in combination with prompted voiding schedules in the nursing-home environment. However, the drug had no effect on the requirement for nursing intervention in the management of incontinence. Extended-release oxybutynin is also effective in elderly patients, with 31% remaining free of urge incontinence in one 12-week study. However, 58.6% of subjects reported dry mouth, with 23.0% rating it moderate or severe, but despite this, only 1.6% of subjects withdrew (4).

Oxybutynin is also available in a transdermal preparation which is effective and avoids most antimuscarinic side-effects associated with the oral preparation. Side-effects associated with transdermal delivery include local application-site irritation or erythema, generally managed by appropriate rotation of application site.

Solifenacin is a long-acting once-daily non-selective antimuscarinic agent which is effective in the treatment of OAB. A pooled analysis of results from older subjects taking solifenacin showed the drug to be effective in reducing urinary frequency, the number of urgency episodes, and sensation of urgency, with a restoration of continence in up to 49 % of people (5). In the pooled analysis, 13.5 % of people on 5 mg reported dry mouth, which was mild to moderate. At the higher dose, a third of people complained of dry mouth and in 1.9 % this was reported as severe. In a randomized controlled trial vs tolterodine extended-release, solifenacin was shown to be equivalent in terms of reduction in micturition frequency. There appeared to be no lessening of effect in those subjects aged >65 years (6).

Tolterodine is a non-selective antimuscarinic agent which appears to have some functional selectivity and greater affinity for bladder muscarinic receptors over those in the salivary glands. This appears to explain the lower incidence of dry mouth and the reduction in withdrawals from treatment seen with the use of the drug. The extended-release form of the drug gives greater tolerability and better efficacy than the immediate-release compound, which should be reserved for those older people with significant hepatic impairment. An effect of therapy can be seen within a week but the maximum effect is seen after five to eight weeks of treatment. Tolterodine does not appear to significantly worsen the postvoid residual urine volume and is been effective in treating men with both OAB and bladder outflow tract obstruction. An evening dose of the drug is effective in reducing nocturnal voids and has been shown to be more tolerable (7).

Propiverine hydrochloride has combined antimuscarinic and calcium channel-blocking actions. Comparative trials against flavoxate and placebo, and oxybutynin and placebo, showed that propiverine has a similar efficacy to oxybutynin. Propiverine has a similar efficacy in treatment of symptoms to oxybutynin 5 mg twice daily, but with a statistically significantly milder, and less common incidence of dry mouth. Although there are no specific data in older people, the elderly were not specifically excluded from studies. However, up to 20 % of patients have adverse effects, which are mainly anticholinergic.

Trospium chloride is a quaternary ammonium salt derived from atropine. The drug was assessed in studies vs placebo and standard release oxybutynin, and was better in effect to placebo and equivalent in efficacy to oxybutynin, when treating DO, at doses of 5 mg three times daily. Adverse effects occur less commonly with trospium than with oxybutynin. The drug has no significant drug–drug interactions and does not normally cross the blood–brain barrier and thus it is unlikely to have an adverse effect on cognition. Trospium might therefore be a useful drug where there is coexisting polypharmacy or concern about significant cognitive dysfunction.

Darifenacin is an antimuscarinic agent which has 50-fold selectivity for M3 over M2 receptors, but only nine-fold for M3 over M1. The drug has been specifically tested in older people in randomized controlled trials, and is effective in terms of objective and subjective variables and quality of life. Pooled data from the population aged >65 years show a similar effect size to the younger groups (8). In cognitively intact older people darifenacin does not adversely affect cognition, probably due to its lack of M1 receptor activity, and its CNS tolerability appears to be similar to placebo. The major side-effects are constipation, affecting 24 % of subjects at a dose of 15 mg, and dry mouth.

Fesoterodine, a pro-drug which is converted into the active metabolite of tolterodine (5-hydroxymethyl tolterodine) has recently been launched in Europe and is due for launch in the US in 2009. It is statistically significantly better than placebo in all of the objective disease variables and has a favourable effect on quality of life. For some outcome measures the 8 mg dose appears to be more effective than the 4 mg dose (9). The side effect side-effect profile appears much the same as other available antimuscarinics with the exception of a lower incidence of reported constipation.

COGNITION AND ANTIMUSCARINCS

It is recognized that total serum anticholinergic activity is related to sub-clinical cognitive dysfunction in otherwise well community dwelling older people. The newer antimuscarinic medications have been subjected to studies of their effect on the elderly. However, the subjects in these studies have been cognitively intact and perhaps at less risk of developing cognitive dysfunction. Only relatively recently have data concerning the effect of these drugs on people on cholinesterase inhibitors been published (10); these data reveal that only in those with the highest level of functional ability can any deterioration in function be detected. Clearly whilst data on the cognitively frail are awaited it is wise to initiate treatment at low dose and review patients frequently.

BLADDER OUTFLOW TRACT OBSTRUCTION

Alpha blockers

All of the commonly used alpha blockers vary in their subtype selectivity and are associated with different side effect profiles. The main concern with using these drugs in older people is the incidence of cardiovascular side effects. They have the potential to cause orthostatic hypotension, dizziness, pre-syncope or syncope. Terazosin and doxazosin were originally designed as anti-hypertensives and are not subtype selective. Both are significantly associated with a higher incidence of vasodilatory side effects than either tamsulosin or alfuzosin and both require careful titration if used. Although alfuzosin is non-subtype selective, it appears to be uro-selective, and is associated with fewer of this type of side effect. Tamsulosin is selective for $\alpha 1_A$ and $\alpha 1_D$ receptor and is associated with a reduced level of these side effects. A recent meta-analysis found that all of the available compounds were associated with an increase in vasodilatory side effects, although the increase associated with tamsulosin were not statistically significant. Tamsulosin and terazosin were

associated with an increase in abnormal ejaculation (11). All of the alpha blockers are equally effective in relieving the symptoms associated with Benign Prostatic Enlargement (BPE) thus for older men the choice should be made upon the likelihood of adverse events, the associated co-morbidities and the ease of administration. Alpha-blockade has no effect on the natural history of prostatic enlargement.

5α-reductase inhibitors

These drugs act by the inhibition of testosterone 5α-reductase which converts testosterone to dihydrotestosterone, the hormone which appears to be implicated in prostate growth. The enzyme is present in two isotypes, type 1 and 2, of which type 2 is found predominantly in the genitalia and prostate. Of the two commercially available drugs, finasteride inhibits the action of the type 2 isoenzyme and dutasteride, both.

In one study of 613 subjects aged between 45–80 years, finasteride was associated with a significant decrease in AUA score and increase in urinary flow rate vs. placebo. Additionally, mean prostate size decreased by 21 % versus 8.1 % in the placebo group (12).

Dutasteride has been associated with improvements in symptom scores, increased in flow rates and reduction in the requirement for surgery of a similar magnitude to finasteride (13). The side effects of these compounds are mainly related to sexual functioning; impotence, decreased libido, abnormal ejaculation and gynaecomastia. These side effects appear to occur in the first year of therapy, after which the incidence is no greater than in a placebo group.

Combination therapy

The combination of alpha-adrenoreceptor blockade and 5-α reductase inhibition in the MTOPS study resulted in a 66 % reduction in a compound end point (decrease in AUA score, incontinence, renal impairment or recurrent UTI) compared to placebo over 4.5 years. The reduction with doxazosin was 39 % and finasteride 34 % (14). The combination of tamsulosin and dutasteride has also been studied in a six month trial, originally designed to assess whether the alpha blocker could be stopped without deterioration in urinary symptoms. This study recruited subjects with moderate to severe symptoms thought to be due to prostatic enlargement. The results showed that, following cessation of the alpha blocker; there was no deterioration in urinary symptoms (15).

Botulinum toxin

Inradetrusor injection of botulinum toxin A following failure of antimuscarinic therapy for detrusor overactivity of either idiopathic or neurogenic origin is gaining in popularity amongst urologists. The action of botulinum toxin prevents fusion of neurotransmitter vesicles with the neuronal cell membrane. Release of acetylcholine into the synaptic cleft becomes impossible, causing a functional denervation. This effectively prevents spontaneous contraction of the detrusor but, for the majority, does not cause paralysis. However, the main side effect is ineffective voiding and urinary retention, which although temporary, may last months. Subjects need to be counselled regarding this side effect and should ideally be taught to perform self catheterisation before the procedure. Because of the increased incidence of impaired voiding in older people; this adverse effect may be commoner and some dosage adjustment may be required.

OTHER PHARMACOLOGICAL MEASURES

Although there is no evidence for oestrogen therapy being of use in the treatment of incontinence in women, there are data to support the use of topical oestrogens for treating OAB in postmenopausal women. One systematic review of studies involving 430 subjects found benefits in all of the relevant symptoms associated with the condition (16). It may, however, have a role in the management of recurrent urinary infection. Oestrogen withdrawal is associated with a fall in the levels of intravaginal glycogen on which lactobacilli depend. These

bacteria cease to colonize the vagina, which is then occupied by colonic organisms that thrive in the higher pH associated with this change. The atrophy of the urothelium encourages colonization by Gram-negative faecal organisms and the bacteria adhere more easily. There is some evidence that oestrogen replacement therapy may reverse this process and give protection to elderly women with recurrent urinary tract infection.

Topical oestrogen therapy appears to be associated with a negligible risk of endometrial hyperplasia and certainly, our onconlogists are happy for its use even in those women with a previous breast cancer. A minimum of three months use is required as a trial of efficacy.

Desmopressin (synthetic antidiuretic hormone with no effect on blood pressure) can be useful in those individuals with nocturnal frequency or nocturnal polyuria. Its use might be hampered by drug–drug interactions, predisposing to hyponatraemia or excessive drinking habits. More recent data have been offered in support of careful, supervised use of desmopressin in older individuals (17). In one meta-analysis of available trial data, dilutional hyponatraemia occurred in 7 % of patients, all within the initial phase of dose titration (18). Given that this decrease in serum sodium may occur within 72 h, it is worthwhile checking the levels before and 72 h after initiation. Levels should be then checked again if there is any change to the disease state or treatment taken by the patient.

STRESS URINARY INCONTINENCE

Until recently there were no drug treatments with evidence of efficacy in the treatment of stress urinary incontinence. However, duloxetine, a combined serotonin and noradrenaline reuptake inhibitor was licensed in Europe in 2004. It is thought to act by increasing the tone of the urethral sphincter. There are data from randomized, controlled trials supporting its efficacy in women (it is not licensed for use in men) but there are no specific data in the elderly. The main side effect of the drug in clinical practice is nausea in 24% of women (19). The drug has not been considered by the FDA. In England and Wales, NICE does not recommend the drug for the treatment of stress urinary incontinence in women, on grounds of cost effectiveness.

SUMMARY

There has been much progress in the pharmacotherapeutics of lower urinary tract disorders over the last ten year. There are ongoing efforts to improve the efficacy of currently available drugs and to utilize different mechanisms of action, for example, β_3 adrenoreceptor agonists, neurokinin 1 and 3-receptor antagonists. The efficacy of botulinum toxin in idiopathic detrusor overactivity still needs to be proven; randomized, controlled studies are in progress.

REFERENCES

1. Brading, A.F. and W.H. Turner, The unstable bladder: towards a common mechanism. *Br J Urol* 1994; **73**(1): 3–8.
2. Eglen, R., Reddy, H, Watson, N, Challis, JRA., Muscarinic acetylcholine receptor subtypes in smooth muscle. *Trends. Pharmacol Sci* 1994; **15**: 114–19.
3. Bemelmans, B.L., L.A. Kiemeney, and F.M. Debruyne, Low-dose oxybutynin for the treatment of urge incontinence: good efficacy and few side effects. *Eur Urol* 2000; **37**(6): 709–13.
4. Gleason, D.M., et al., Evaluation of a new once-daily formulation of oxbutynin for the treatment of urinary urge incontinence. Ditropan XL Study Group. *Urology* 1999; **54**(3): 420–3.
5. Wagg, A., J.J. Wyndaele, and P. Sieber, Efficacy and tolerability of solifenacin in elderly subjects with overactive bladder syndrome: a pooled analysis. *Am J Geriatr Pharmacother* 2006; **4**(1): 14–24.
6. Chapple, C.R., et al., A comparison of the efficacy and tolerability of solifenacin succinate and extended release tolterodine at treating overactive bladder syndrome: results of the STAR trial. *Eur Urol* 2005; **48**(3): 464–70.
7. Rackley, R., et al., Nighttime dosing with tolterodine reduces overactive bladder-related nocturnal micturitions in patients with overactive bladder and nocturia. *Urology* 2006; **67**(4): 731–6.
8. Foote, J., et al., Treatment of overactive bladder in the older patient: pooled analysis of three phase III studies of darifenacin, an M3 selective receptor antagonist. *Eur Urol*; 2005; **48**(3): 471–7.
9. Khullar, V., et al., Fesoterodine dose response in subjects with overactive bladder syndrome. *Urology* 2008; **71**(5): 839–43.
10. Lackner, T.E., et al., Randomized, placebo-controlled trial of the cognitive effect, safety, and tolerability of oral extended-release oxybutynin in cognitively impaired nursing home residents with urge urinary incontinence. *J Am Geriatr Soc* 2008; **56**(5): 862–70.
11. Nickel, J.C., S. Sander, and T.D. Moon, A meta-analysis of the vascular-related safety profile and efficacy of alpha-adrenergic blockers for symptoms related to benign prostatic hyperplasia. *Int J Clin Pract* 2008; **62**(10): 1547–59.
12. Nickel, J.C., et al., Efficacy and safety of finasteride therapy for benign prostatic hyperplasia: results of a 2-year randomized controlled trial (the PROSPECT study). PROscar Safety Plus Efficacy Canadian Two year Study. *CMAJ* 1996; **155**(9): 1251–9.
13. Roehrborn, C.G., et al., Efficacy and safety of a dual inhibitor of 5-alpha-reductase types 1 and 2 (dutasteride) in men with benign prostatic hyperplasia. *Urology* 2002; **60**(3): 434–41.
14. McConnell, J.D., et al., The long-term effect of doxazosin, finasteride, and combination therapy on the clinical progression of benign prostatic hyperplasia. *N Engl J Med* 2003; **349**(25): 2387–98.
15. Barkin, J., et al., Alpha-blocker therapy can be withdrawn in the majority of men following initial combination therapy with the dual 5alpha-reductase inhibitor dutasteride. *Eur Urol* 2003; **44**(4): 461–6.
16. Cardozo, L., et al., A systematic review of the effects of estrogens for symptoms suggestive of overactive bladder. *Acta Obstet Gynecol Scand* 2004; **83**(10): 892–7.

17. Kuo, H., Efficacy of desmopressin in treatment of refractory nocturia in patients older than 65 years. *Urology* 2002; **59**: 485–9.

18. Weatherall, M., The risk of hyponatremia in older adults using desmopressin for nocturia: a systematic review and metaanalysis. *Neurourol Urodyn* 2004; **23**: 302–5.

19. Dmochowski, R.R., et al., Duloxetine versus placebo for the treatment of North American women with stress urinary incontinence. *J Urol* 2003; **170**(4 Pt 1): 1259–63.

32 Management of benign prostatic hyperplasia in elderly men

Ming Liu [1] and Gordon H. Muir [2]

[1] Department of Urology, Beijing Hospital, Beijing, China
[2] Department of Urology, King's College Hospital, London, UK

ASSESSMENT

Benign prostatic hyperplasia (BPH) is one of the most common diseases of the ageing male affecting more than 50 % of men aged over 60 years (1). Clinically, it is characterized by lower urinary tract symptoms (LUTS), including urinary frequency, urgency, a weak and intermittent stream, needing to strain, a sense of incomplete emptying, and nocturia. These symptoms may affect quality of life, interfering with normal daily activities and sleep patterns. BPH can also lead to some complications, including acute or chronic retention, infection, bleeding, or renal impairment. Careful recording of symptoms, with emphasis on how they interfere with the patient's quality of life, as well as the use of selected tests, constitutes the mainstay of making a correct diagnosis. The International Prostate Symptom Score (www.gp-training.net/protocol/docs/ipss.doc) may be helpful in establishing symptom severity (see Figure 32.1).

In men with moderate to severe symptoms, or where there is concern over bladder emptying, the use of urine flow rates and bladder ultrasound may help guide therapy.

This chapter will look at assessment and treatment options: because most studies have addressed a relatively elderly trial population most treatments need no modification for elderly men.

We will address a few areas of diagnostic uncertainty, then deal with treatment options.

PROSTATE SPECIFIC ANTIGEN (PSA)

PSA testing may detect early prostate cancer in 2 % to 3 % of men aged 50 to 65 years but it will fail to detect some early tumours. An evaluation of serum PSA in the adult male population is no longer limited to the diagnosis of prostate cancer. New information has become available that there is a clear correlation between prostate size and higher serum PSA levels (2). PSA testing is appropriate in older men with symptomatic BPH since the presence of prostate cancer would alter management in most case. However there is no evidence for screening in men with a life expectancy of less than 10 years (3).

URINARY RETENTION

Acute urinary retention refers to the sudden inability to pass urine and is always painful. Men in their 70s have a one in ten chance of developing acute urinary retention in the subsequent five years. If they have urinary symptoms, the risk is greater. Three other factors increase the risk

Prescribing for Elderly Patients Edited by Stephen Jackson, Paul Jansen and Arduino Mangoni
© 2009 John Wiley & Sons, Ltd

Name: Date:

	Not at all	Less than 1 time in 5	Less than half the	About half the time	More than half the	Almost always	**Your score**
Incomplete emptying Over the past month, how often have you had a sensation of not emptying your bladder completely after you finish urinating?	0	1	2	3	4	5	
Frequency Over the past month, how often have you had to urinate again less than two hours after you finished urinating?	0	1	2	3	4	5	
Intermittency Over the past month, how often have you found you stopped and started again several times when you urinated?	0	1	2	3	4	5	
Urgency Over the last month, how difficult have you found it to postpone urination?	0	1	2	3	4	5	
Weak stream Over the past month, how often have you had a weak urinary stream?	0	1	2	3	4	5	
Straining Over the past month, how often have you had to push or strain to begin urination?	0	1	2	3	4	5	

	None	1 time	2 times	3 times	4 times	5 times or more	**Your score**
Nocturia Over the past month, many times did you most typically get up to urinate from the time you went to bed until the time you got up in the morning?	0	1	2	3	4	5	

Total IPSS score	

Quality of life due to urinary symptoms	Delighted	Pleased	Mostly satisfied	Mixed - about equally satisfied and dissatisfied	Mostly dissatisfied	Unhappy	Terrible
If you were to spend the rest of your life with your urinary condition the way it is now, how would you feel about that?	0	1	2	3	4	5	6

Total score: 0–7 Mildly symptomatic; 8–19 moderately symptomatic; 20–35 severely symptomatic.

Figure 32.1. International prostate symptom score (IPSS) — from (http://www.gp-training.net/protocol/docs/ipss.doc)

of acute urinary retention: a large prostate, low peak urine flow rate, and abnormally high level of serum prostate specific antigen (4). One randomized study has shown that finasteride reduces the risk of acute urinary retention from 7 % to 3 % (5). Usually acute urinary retention is treated by urethral catheterization, although sometimes the suprapubic approach is needed. Some urologists regard acute urinary retention and previous lower urinary tract symptoms as an absolute indication for prostatectomy and others tend to allow most men a trial of voiding, often with alpha-blocking drugs (6).

Chronic urinary retention occurs over a long period, leading to recurrent urinary tract infections, hydronephrosis and renal impairment. Men presenting with acute or chronic urinary retention tend to be older and less fit for operation than men presenting for elective prostatic surgery. They have significantly longer post-operative hospital stay, and a higher post-operative morbidity and mortality (7).

NOCTURNAL FREQUENCY

Nocturia is a common symptom in the elderly, which profoundly influences the quality of life in all patients, and can increase the risk of falls in the elderly. Sommer and colleagues found that the percentage number reporting three or more voiding episodes at night increased among both males and females from adolescence (0 %) to the age of 60–70 years (11 %) (8). It is partly because of a reduced bladder capacity, and partly because of nocturnal polyuria. The total 24-hr urine output in adult men is about 1600 ± 300 ml and does not change substantially with increasing age. In contrast, the distribution of the urine output during the 24-hr period changes considerably, which manifest mainly by the increased amount of urine output at night without a corresponding increase in voiding in the daytime. The reason of this change is the disturbance in the vasopressin system, with a lack of nocturnal increase in plasma vasopressin. Some other diseases, such as diabetes insipidus, diabetes mellitus and congestive heart failure, are also causes of nocturnal polyuria (9).

TREATMENT

The aims of treatment are to alleviate LUTS, to improve quality of life, to prevent complications and to minimize the adverse effects of treatment.

Only symptomatic BPH needs to be treated (unless men have asymptomatic chronic retention.) Men with mild or moderate symptoms not experiencing complications are ideal candidates for the lifestyle changes or medical treatment. For those with persistent symptoms or complications, more invasive forms of treatment need to be considered.

Lifestyle changing

Untreated BPH does not always progress. Indeed, the placebo response in clinical BPH is comparatively high. One review by Isaacs showed that 16 % of those with untreated BPH had no changes in symptoms and 38 % were better, with a follow-up of 2.6–5 years (10). Especially in those with mild or moderate symptoms, the disease progresses slowly. So patients with mild symptoms should consider a regime composed of some lifestyle changes. These include reducing fluid intake in the evening, reducing caffeine and alcohol intake, and reviewing prescribed drugs with the potential to inhibit bladder function (tricyclics, anticholinergics). There is no consensus on the need for regular follow-up of patients with LUTS managed conservatively, but annual assessment and review of renal function would seem sensible to detect the small number of men who may develop retention.

Medical treatment

Phytotherapy

Phytotherapeutic agents are composed of various plant extracts: it may be difficult to identify which component has the major biological activity. About 30 different compounds are available in different countries, based on seven major plant extracts: Curcubita pepo (pumpkin) seed, Hypoxis rooperi (South African star grass), Pygeum africanum (African Plum tree), Serenoa repens (Saw palmetto berry), Urtica dioica (stinging nettle root) and Opuntia (cactus flower extracts) (11). Although a few short term randomized trials have shown clinical efficacy for some of these, without major side effects, the longer term durability remains unproven (12, 13). It is unknown whether there is a need for dose adjustment in the elderly.

Alpha-adrenergic blockade

LUTS are secondary to both the static effect (increased enlargement) and the dynamic effect (increased tone) of BPH. Alpha-blocker therapy points to the dynamic effect caused by α-adrenergic-mediated contraction of the smooth muscle, predominantly in the capsule of the prostate and bladder neck (14). The α-blocker has advanced from the first antagonising $\alpha 1$ and $\alpha 2$ adrenoreceptors to the short acting $\alpha 1$ antagonist only (15), which may reduce cardiovascular side effects. It seems that there is no significant difference in symptom control among different type of $\alpha 1$-blockers.

Randomized controlled trials have found a greater improvement in symptoms with α-blockers than with placebo. They have rapid onset (within days or weeks), increase maximal flow rate in 40% and produce on average 4–6 point improvement in IPSS symptom index (16). Furthermore, the efficacy of α 1-blockers seems not to correspond to disease severity. There is no limitation to efficacy depending on prostate size, and efficacy does not relate to baseline PSA levels (17). Other studies have shown that α-blockers have favourable effect on acute urinary retention (AUR) 18, both in preventing it, and also increasing the success rates of trial without catheter and successful voiding in men presenting in AUR (19). The main side effects include headache, dizziness, drowsiness, postural hypotension and rarely syncope.

Further characterization of the α-1 receptor indicates that three receptors subtypes exist in humans (A, B and C). Their different distribution between urinary tract and cardiovascular tissues has provided a strategy for the development of improved therapeutic agents. Since excessive activity of $\alpha 1a$ receptor and $\alpha 1c$ receptor appears to be a common feature in symptomatic BPH and

α-1a receptor is rich in prostatic tissue, drugs that demonstrate high $\alpha 1a$ receptor selectivity have attracted attention (20).

All α-blockers have the potential to induce hypotension, particularly postural hypotension, and this side effect may be more pronounced in the elderly and in particular those on concomitant anti-hypertensive medication. This is a particular concern in those men who have significant nocturnal frequency as there is a very real risk of night-time falls. While initial clinical trials suggested lower rates of postural hypotension with the selective α-blockers such as tamsulosin, this has not been confirmed in later studies.

In men with hypertension there may be a place for considering the use of doxazosin, which may allow for treatment of both conditions with a single pill.

For those patients also utilising oral treatment for erectile dysfunction it should be noted that potential exacerbation of hypotension can exist for patients using alpha blockers and phosphodiesterase type 5 (PDE-5) inhibitors. Interestingly this has not been shown to be a problem with sildenafil, although caution is advised in patients using tadalafil and vardenafil with some of the α blockers (this may amount in some countries to a formal contraindication for treatment.)

Some patients notice a dry orgasm with α blockers: although this is rarely a significant problem in the elderly it can, if needed, be avoided by prescribing alfuzosin.

Five α-reductase inhibitors

Within many cells, the enzyme 5α-reductase converts testosterone to dihydrotestosterone (DHT), a more potent androgen. Within the prostate, 90% of testosterone is converted to DHT. 5α-reductase has two isoforms. Type I isoenzyme is expressed in liver, skin, sebaceous glands and most hair follicles. Type II is highly expressed in prostate (where type I is also thought to be present) (21). Finasteride is mainly a type II 5-α reductase inhibitor, which is only weakly active against type I. It reduces serum DHT levels by 65–70% and by 85–90% in the prostate. Finasteride causes atrophy of the prostatic glandular epithelial cells, which results in a 20–30 % reduction in volume. The onset of action is slow (three to six months), but durable (22). Randomized controlled trials have shown that finasteride improves quality of life, decrease prostatic volume, and decrease the risk of urinary retention or prostatic surgery (23). It seems to work best in patients with extremely enlarged prostates. The main side effects include ejaculatory dysfunction (2–8 %), loss of libido (1–10 %), and impotence (3.4–16 %) (24).

Even after treatment with finasteride, the prostate still receives an androgenic stimulus from the 30 % of serum DHT and 10 % of intraprostatic DHT converted by type I isoenzyme, and intraprostatic testosterone rises to physiologically significant levels. The newly released compound dutasteride is a dual 5α-reductase inhibitor which shows a 60-fold greater inhibition of type I isoenzyme than does finasteride, as well as being potent against the type II isoenzyme (25). Dutasteride seems to have a broadly equivalent effect on the symptoms, prostatic volume and flow rates as finasteride, although its speed of effect may be more rapid (26). However, until dutasteride and finasteride have been compared in a randomized controlled trial the effect of the dual inhibition is not clear.

The most bothersome side effects of 5α-reductase inhibitors tend to be sexual, with loss of libido, erectile dysfunction and dry orgasm being troublesome to some men. No dose modification is required in the elderly.

Combined treatment with α-blocker and 5-α reductase inhibitor

The results of a multicentre trial (MTOPS trial) have assessed the combination of finasteride and doxazosin (27). Combination therapy was superior to either drug alone in reducing AUA symptom scores, in increasing median maximal flow rates, and in reducing the likelihood of AUR and surgery. The follow-up period of the MTOPS trial was four and a half years. In another study examining combination therapy, it was shown that patients with LUTS and moderately enlarged prostates initially receiving combination therapy were likely to experience no significant symptom

deterioration after discontinuing the α-blocker following nine to 12 months of combination therapy (28).

The relatively modest benefits of continuing dual therapy need to be set against possible costs, compliance and side effects in the elderly population.

Surgical treatment

Surgical treatments have a much higher rate of disobstructing patients than any of the medical therapies, and deliver improvements in symptom scores and flow rates of greater than 100 %. Possibilities are:

Endoprostatic stents

Endoprostatic stents designed either for permanent or for temporary placement. The duration of use in temporary stents varies from several weeks to six months. Characteristic of permanent stents is that they allow epithelial ingrowth, and thus reduce the chances of infection and encrustation. Several studies show that permanent stents can remain patent for four to seven years (29).

Open prostatectomy

Open prostatectomy is performed in less than 1 % of patients now (usually in glands over 100g).

Transurethral resection of prostate (TURP)

This is often used as the "standard" against which to compare other therapies. The absolute indications for surgical intervention in patients with LUTS should be urinary retention, recurrent gross haematuria caused by benign prostatic enlargement (BPE), renal failure or bladder stones from bladder outlet obstruction (BOO), large bladder diverticula, or recurrent urinary tract infections ascribable to BOO (30). "Relative" indications should take account of the patients' symptoms, result of examination, comorbidity and expectations.

Long term complications include urethral stricture (1–29 %), bladder neck contracture, impotence (5–10%), and retrograde ejaculation (60–90%) (31).

Laser prostatectomy

Currently two laser technologies are challengers to the position of TURP as the standard treatment: Holmium laser enucleation of the prostate (HoLEP) and high-powered potassium-titanyl-phosphate (KTP) laser vaporization of the prostate.

HoLEP has been shown to be as effective as TURP in terms of symptom relief, improvement in peak urinary flow rates, potency and continence at a follow up of 48 months (32). The length of hospital stay and time to catheter removal are less with HoLEP. Despite the potential advantages of HoLEP over TURP, it has been slow to gain popularity as a front-line surgical treatment for BPH, possibly because of the long learning curve associated with this procedure and the difficulty many centres have had in obtaining good results.

The KTP laser uses laser energy to vaporize the prostatic adenoma. The main advantage of KTP laser is the virtually bloodless procedure (33). Our group and others have confirmed the safety of the procedure in frail, elderly and anticoagulated patients (34). Even elderly patients with retention of urine can usually go home on the say of surgery, often without a catheter (35).

Other minimal invasive therapies

Other minimal invasive therapies, such as transurethral microwave therapy (TUMT), transurethral needle ablation of the prostate (TUNA), high intensity focused ultrasound (HIFU) all show benefits equivalent to or superior to medical therapy. As yet however none seems to be equivalent to TURP.

Long time catheterization

When medical therapies fail to give acceptable result for patients in a poor general condition and not suitable for invasive treatments, long time catheterisation remains an option. We would stress however that there are few patients with good cognitive function who are not candidates for consideration of modern surgical techniques. Long term catheterisation carries a significant morbidity from urinary sepsis, apart from its inconvenience and discomfort. In general, a long term suprapubic catheter is more comfortable and less prone to infection than a transurethral one for those patients who fail surgery or are not candidates.

REFERENCES

1. Barry MJ. Epidemiology and natural history of benign prostatic hyperplasia. *Urol Clin North Am* 1990; **17**: 495–507.
2. Wright EJ, Fang J, Metter EJ, et al. Prostate specific antigen predicts the long-term risk of prostate enlargement: results from the Baltimore Longitudinal Study of Aging. *J Urol* 2002; **167**: 2484–88.
3. Scolarikos A, Thorpe AC, Deal DE. Lower urinary tract symptoms and benign prostatic hyperplasia. *Minerva Urol Nefrol* 2004; **56**: 109–122.
4. Licher M, Fowler J, Castellanos R, et al. PSA is the strongest predictor of BPH related outcomes: results of a 4-year placebo controlled trial. *J Urol* 1998; **159**(Suppl): 107.
5. McConnell JD, Bruskewitz R, Walsh P, et al. The effect of finasteride on the risk of acute urinary retention and need for surgicalo treatment among men with benign prostatic hyperplasia. *N Engl J Med* 1998; **338**: 557–63.
6. Mark E, Ken A. Acute urinary retention in men: an age old problem. *BMJ* 1999; **318**: 921–25.
7. Thorpe AC, Cleary R, Coles J, et al. Deaths and complications following prostatectomy in 1400 men in the northern region of England. *Br J Urol* 1994; **74**: 559–65.
8. Sommer P, Nielsen KK, Bauer T, et al. Voiding patterns in men evaluated by a questionnaire survey. *Br J Urol* 1990; **65**: 155–160.
9. R Asplund. Nocturia, nocturnal polyuria, and sleep quality in the elderly. *Journal of Psychosomatic Research* 2004; **56**: 517–25.
10. Isaacs JT. Importance of the natural history of benign prostatic hyperplasia in the evaluation of pharmacologic intervention. *Prostate Supplement* 1990; **3**: 1–7.
11. Christopher RC. Pharmacological therapy of benign prostatic hyperplasia/lower urinary tract symptoms: an overview for the practising clinician. *BJU* 2004; **94**: 738–44.

12. Lowe FC, Fagelman E. Phytotherapy in the treatment of benign prostatic hyperplasia. *Curr Opin Urol* 2002; **12**: 15–18.

13. Debruyne F, Koch G, Boyle P, et al. Comparison of a phytotherapeutic agent (Permixon) with an α-blocker (Tamsulosin) in the treatment of benign prostatic hyperplasia: a 1-year randomized international study. *Eur Urol* 2002; **41**: 497–506; discussion 506–07.

14. Lepor H. The pathophysiology of lower urinary tract symptoms in the aging male population. *Br J Urol* 1998; **81**: 29–33.

15. Kirby RS, Coppinger SW, Corcoran MO, et al. Prazosin in the treatment of prostatic obstruction: a placebo controlled study. *Br J Urol* 1987; **60**: 136–42.

16. Narayan P, Evans CP, Moon T. Long term safety and efficacy of tamsulosin for the treatment of lower urinary tract symptoms associated with benign prostatic hyperplasia. *J Urol* 2003; **170**(2 Pt 1): 498–502.

17. Kirby R, Roehrborn C, Altwein JE, et al. Impact of prostate size on response to medical therapy for benign prostatic hyperplasia (BPH): results of the PREDICT trial. *J Urol* 1999; **161** (Suppl.): 266.

18. Speakman M. Tamsulosin reduces the risk of acute urinary retention. *J Urol* 2002; **167**: 375.

19. McNeill SA, Daruwala PD, Mitchell ID, et al. Sustained release alfusosin and trial without catheter after acute urinary retention: a prospective, placebo controlled trial. *BJU Int* 1999; **84**: 622–27.

20. Claus GR, Debra AS. α 1 adrenergic receptors and their inhibitors in lower urinary tract symptoms and benign prostatic hyperplasia. *J Urol* 2004; **171**: 1029–35.

21. Russell DW, Wilson JD. Steroid 5 alpha-reductase: two genes/two enzymes. *Annu Rev Biochem* 1994; **63**: 25–61.

22. Lam JS, Romas NA, Lowe FC: Long-term treatment with finasteride in men with symptomatic benign prostatic hyperplasia: 10-year follow-up. *Urology* 2003; **61**: 354–58.

23. Roehrborn CG, Bruskewitz R, Nikel GC, et al. Urinary retention in patients with BPH treated with finasteride or placebo over 4 years. Characterization of patients ultimate outcomes. The PLESS study group. *Eur Urol* 2000; **37**: 528–36.

24. Wessells H, Roy J, Bannow J, et al. PLESS Study Group. Incidence and severity of sexual adverse experiences in finasteride and placebo-treated men with benign prostatic hyperplasia. *Urology* 2003; **61**: 579–84.

25. Bartsch G, Rittmaster RS, Klocker H. Dihydrotestosterone and the concept of 5alpha-reductase inhibition in human benign prostatic hyperplasia. *World J Urol* 2002; **19**: 413–25.

26. Roehrborn CG, Andriole G, Nickel C, et al. Effect of dutasteride, a novel dual 5-alpha-reductase inhibitor, on BPH related signs and symptoms. *J Urol* 2002; **167**(Suppl 4).

27. McConnel JD. The long-term effects of medical therapy on the progression of BPH: results from the MTOPS trial. *J Urol* 2002; **167**: 264.

28. Baldwin KC, Ginsberg CG, Harkaway RC, et al. Discontinuation of α-blockade after initial treatment with finasteride and doxazosin in men with lower urinary tract symptoms and clinical evidence of benign prostatic hyperplasia. *Urology* 2001; **58**: 203–09.

29. Rakesh K, Evangelos N, Liatsikos, et al. Endoprostatic stents for management of benign prostatic hyperplasia. *Current Opinion in Urology* 2000; **10**: 19–22.

30. Chatelain C, Denis L, Foo KT, et al. *Proceedings of the 5th international consultation on BPH*. Plymouth: Plymbridge Distributors Ltd, 1998.

31. Roos NP, Wennber JE, Malenka DJ, et al. Mortality and reoperation after open and transurethral resection of the prostate. *New Engl J Med* 1989; **320**: 1120–24.

32. Westenberg A, Gilling P, Kennett K, et al. Holmium laser resection of the prostate: results of a randomized trial with 4-year minimum long-term followup. *J Urol* 2004; **172**: 616–19.

33. Andrew HT, Peter JG. Lasers in the treatment of benign prostatic hyperplasia: an update. *Curr Opin Urol* 2005; **15**: 55–58.

34. Oliver R, Alexander B, Michael S, et al. High power (80W) potassium-titanyl-phosphate laser vaporization of the prostate in 66 high risk patients. *J Urol* 2005; **173**: 158–160.

35. Gómez Sancha F, Bachmann A, Choi BB, Tabatabaei S, Muir GH. Photoselective vaporization of the prostate (GreenLight PV): lessons learnt after 3500 procedures. *Prostate Cancer Prostatic Dis* 2007; **10**(4): 316–22.

33 Management of erectile dysfunction in the elderly

Kevin Dennison

King's College Hospital, London, UK

INTRODUCTION

Erectile dysfunction, (ED), or impotence, is the term now used for the consistent inability to get or maintain an erection of sufficient rigidity for satisfactory sexual intercourse to the mutual satisfaction of both partners (1). It is a serious condition and one that can affect both partners in a relationship, regardless of age. It is of course important to realize what is meant when men report erection difficulties: almost all men will have transient failures associated with life events, but if the problem is persistent reassurance alone will not do as treatment.

It is often not realized that many men presenting with ED have potentially serious underlying medical conditions, leading to the prospect of early intervention for such conditions as diabetes, cardiovascular disease and depressive illnesses. The attention of the patient to his erection is also a powerful aid to reinforcing advice on general lifestyle changes.

This chapter looks at the available diagnostic and treatment options and their place in management of this distressing condition, in the elderly. It will not seek to address any arguments over use of resources in managing non life threatening issues in older patients: it is our view that if a man seeks professional help over an embarrassing issue he deserves to be taken seriously.

PREVALENCE AND AETIOLOGY OF ED

Erectile dysfunction is common in all age groups, with the incidence increasing, as men get older. While this was first demonstrated by Kinsey in 1948, probably the most significant study of recent years is that of the Massachusetts Male Ageing Study (2), which ultimately showed that the incidence of complete erectile dysfunction rose from 5.1 % at the age of 40, to 15 % at the age of 70. Despite this decline, the elderly remain sexually active, with more than 75 % of men in their 60s having intercourse more than once a month (3). In fact 29 % of men over the age of 80 are still sexually active (4).

Alongside the potential for co-morbidities causing erectile difficulties in the elderly, there are also the physical manifestations that naturally occur in the elderly man such as the general length of time it takes to achieve an erection due to generalized vascular changes, the fact that the elderly tend to take longer to get aroused in the first instance and that they may also require more physical as opposed to psychogenic stimulation. As opposed to women, age as been shown to be a determinant in associated sexual problems in men (5).

In contrast to the commonly held belief that ED is more common in older men due to decreasing androgen levels, impotent elderly men

Prescribing for Elderly Patients   Edited by Stephen Jackson, Paul Jansen and Arduino Mangoni
© 2009 John Wiley & Sons, Ltd

do not seem to have significantly lower serum androgens than potent age matched controls. Thus it would seem that an underlying increase in the frequency of co-morbidity is likely to be to blame.

Men with impotence have a significantly increased risk of suffering from cardiac and other arterial disease, diabetes and depression, and ED may be a predictor of other avoidable cardiovascular events.

PHYSICAL OR PSYCHOGENIC?

Most men with erectile dysfunction will present a mixed picture of physical and psychogenic origin. While differentiation may be made (see below) on the grounds of the history, it is inappropriate to make a value judgement about whether or not a man deserves treatment based on this. We do not refuse to treat patients with chronic pain syndromes for which no physical cause is obvious!

Every study which has looked at the psychological impact of ED has found a negative correlation between the presence of impotence and general well being and quality of life. Anxiety and depression, along with self-esteem, are adversely affected. Treatment is capable of reversing these problems.

DIAGNOSIS AND ASSESSMENT OF ED IN PRIMARY CARE

The main place of physical examination and investigation in the management of primary care is, arguably, in diagnosing underlying disease. A brief and structured approach is outlined below.

History

In terms of the history that should be taken, a few brief and direct questions need to be asked. Be aware that different patients have different ideas of what sexual dysfunction means, so the direct approach is mandatory both to get an accurate picture and to avoid wasting time on the interview. It may be difficult at first for the physician to be very direct with patients in these matters, and one must be realized that in some cases these are matters doctors do not feel comfortable discussing even with their own partners. Patients who are questioned directly and without embarrassment will however feel less embarrassed and more secure themselves.

Examination

The examination can be limited to an assessment of the patient's blood pressure and external genitals. Further examination will be dictated by the doctor's own interest in screening the patient for co-morbidity.

In our practice we check:

- the breasts (to exclude gynaecomastia);
- carotid, aortic and femoral pulses (major peripheral vascular disease);
- knee, ankle and bulbo-urethral reflexes (undiagnosed neuropathy);
- The prostate (prostate disease is no more common in impotent men than controls, but we would feel foolish sending an undiagnosed prostate cancer back to our GP colleagues!)

This examination can be carried out in only a few minutes.

Laboratory tests

The only mandatory test is of a *urine or blood sample* for **glucose.**

It is most unusual to find a man with significantly low **testosterone** in the presence of a normal libido and secondary sexual characteristics. If these exist, it is important to check the level of sex hormone binding globulin (SHBG), since the ratio between this carrier molecule and testosterone is what determines the biologically available testosterone. Further investigation of men with low testosterone is most appropriately carried out in a specialist centre.

If signs of general ill health are present then checks on renal and hepatic function are appropriate, along with a full blood count and possibly thyroid function check.

An argument can be made for checking both the serum lipids and the PSA depending on local and national screening guidelines.

Patients who should always be referred or discussed with a specialist are:

- young men who have never been able to have an erection;
- patients with a sudden onset of impotence liked to trauma;
- men with genital or prostatic abnormalities;
- those with abnormalities found on any of the screening tests above;
- patients who fail to respond to first line medical therapy.

Thus the majority of elderly men initially presenting with ED do not need specialist involvement

TREATMENT OPTIONS

It is essential that the patient be involved in the choice of management, along with his partner where possible.

This is particularly pertinent in the elderly population, as whereas a younger couple would not hesitate to seek help and appropriate treatment for erectile dysfunction, occasionally an elderly male patient will seek advice independently, which, if the problem has existed for a significant period of time, can sometimes be off putting for his partner. The high response rate with the available options makes treatment very rewarding: these patients are grateful for success!

Treatments can broadly be divided into psychological, pharmaceutical and physical therapies. All of the drugs available act by increasing the blood flow in the cavernous bodies and allowing tumescence then rigidity.

Counselling

Most men have some degree of psychological involvement in their erectile dysfunction. Equally, many men with a psychological problem will also have a co-existent physical one. The history is most important in making this distinction.

Counselling must involve a significant investment of time and commitment by the patient, with well-motivated patients in good centres

achieving benefits in up to 80 % of cases. Default rates can however be high, and the desirability of involving the partner may be seen as either a good or a bad thing depending on the individual.

Few controlled studies on counselling outcomes exist, and the availability of services in different parts of the country varies.

Where counselling is effective it is a non-invasive therapy, which can address the underlying problems both with an individual patient and in a relationship.

The place of a combination of counselling and medical therapy, (mirroring treatment in depressive illness), has not really been addressed but may be of considerable interest in the future.

Oral treatment: PDE-5 inhibitors

The advent of sildenafil, a selective inhibitor of phosphodiesterase type 5, dramatically changed the face of therapy in erectile dysfunction in 1998. It has been demonstrated in well-conducted placebo control studies to be significantly superior to placebo, giving good results in 46–88 % of users depending on the patient group. Interestingly, patients deemed to have "primary psychogenic impotence" are among the best responders to the drug. Despite the enormous amount of media hype, which surrounded the drug and its safety profile, follow up of millions of men who have taken the drug shows no obvious cardiac or other risk associated with its use.

Since the advent of sildenafil two other PDE-5 inhibitors have come onto the market; tadalafil and vardenafil. There have predictably been numerous pieces of work conducted in comparing the three drugs, and patient satisfaction rates: many of these studies have been confounded by potential conflicts of interest, making an overview difficult. It should be noted that tadalafil has a significantly longer half-life than the other two drugs, and may be active for up to 36 hours, making it a very popular treatment option in younger men.

It must be stressed that by virtue of potentiation of the effects of nitric oxide, PDE-5 inhibitors are absolutely contraindicated in men taking any nitrate drugs. Profound systemic hypotension can result, and patients should be aware that amyl nitrate ("poppers") used recreationally would have the same risk: elderly men of any sexual orientation are not immune to using recreational drugs! Ironically despite the initial concern regarding taking a PDE-5 inhibitor and its effect upon a patient's cardiac status, it is more pertinent to assess the individual patient's exercise tolerance. They should ideally be able to walk up two flights of stairs having been gently mobilising beforehand or walk a mile without getting breathless. Caution should also be taken when prescribing a PDE-5 inhibitor concurrently with an ACE inhibitor. While this combination is certainly not contra-indicated, it should be ascertained that the patient is not unduly hypotensive from taking the ACE inhibitor prior to being prescribed the PDE-5 inhibitor.

Sildenafil is available in three doses (25 mg, 50 mg and 100 mg) with a dose response evident both from trials and from patients' preferences. Men take the drug one to two hours prior to planned intercourse. In the elderly the dose should commence at 25 mg, with a view of increasing this dose to 50 mg and then to 100 mg if required.

Tadalafil commences at 10 mg in the elderly, and can be doubled to 20 mg. The advantage of tadalafil is that unlike the other two PDE-5 inhibitors it I is less sensitive to patients having eaten prior to taking it.

Vardenafil should commence at 5 mg in the elderly, increasing to 10 mg and then 20 mg as appropriate.

All drugs are best taken approximately 30 minutes to an hour prior to an erection being achieved. There has been work looking at optimal time from taking the drug to achieving an erection but especially in the elderly, when foreplay may not be as important as for a younger couple, the added time span may help.

Sildenafil and vardenafil must be taken on an empty stomach, and where possible, if sexual intercourse is planned, then any food taken prior to taking the drug should be low in fat.

It must be stressed to patients that sexual stimulation is essential for erection with all the PDE-5 inhibitors, and patients should realize that it may take up to eight to ten attempts

at taking any of the PDE-5 inhibitors before they achieve a reliable response to a given dose. In order to reduce any performance anxiety, it may be pertinent for a patient to 'practise' taking the drug alone, in order to build up confidence, using erotic materials to help with self stimulation if needed.

Other oral agents

Oral apomorphine has is also available, although since the introduction of the other PDE-5 inhibitors, it has generally slipped into the background of treatment options. Apomorphine acts by central stimulation of the parasympathetic erectile stimulus. This drug is administered sublingually, which gives a much faster onset of action than sildenafil. In trials it is well tolerated at doses that give a positive response in around 40–50 % of patients. It may be very effective in younger men with anxiety and in patients with spinal injuries. At present it seems likely that it may be used for patients in whom a PDE-5 inhibitor is contraindicated, and who don't wish to inject intra-cavernosally.

Apomorphine has not yet been evaluated in patients following radical prostatectomy or radiotherapy, but it will not in general be expected to have an effect in men who have a complete subsacral nerve lesion since the parasympathetic stimulus will not be deliverable. It may however be of help in some men with a partial nerve injury.

One minor drawback with apomorphine is that it requires sexual stimulation, but due to the man having to allow the drug to dissolve sub-lingually, kissing is in effect excluded from the couple's foreplay technique. This may be less acceptable to older men.

Until recently, the drug yohimbine was commonly prescribed for men without a significant physical component to their impotence. It has a side effect profile significantly higher than that of the newer agents and there is only weak evidence for its efficacy, so as an unlicensed drug its use cannot be recommended.

Injection therapy

Direct intracavernosal injection of vasoactive agents has been practised for some years now.

While many agents have been used with success, the only freely available licensed product at present is prostaglandin E1. Over 75 % of men will be able to attain an erection with intracavernosal therapy; while an automatic erection is obtained, concomitant sexual stimulation will enhance the effects.

Obviously there are drawbacks to the use of such treatment, not least being the reaction of most men on being invited to put a needle into their own penis! The injection itself in fact rarely hurts, although around 5 % of men experience burning pain or discomfort afterwards. It is also a problem in men who have visual or co-ordination difficulties and this remains true despite the efforts of the pharmaceutical companies in adapting the delivery systems to become more patient friendly.

Perhaps the main reason that up to 40 % of users will no longer be injecting after a year is the feeling of a physical barrier that any external device can create between a couple. That aside, this is a relatively discreet drug to administer, and while the couple engage in foreplay, the man will develop a good, strong erection that gives the whole process a semblance of normality.

It is likely that higher dose formulations, possibly in combination with other vasoactive agents, will be developed for those men in the future who fail to respond to oral agents.

At present the dose of intra-cavernosal alprostadilcomes in 10 mcg, 20 mcg, 30 mcg and 40 mcg doses. It is always good practise to start at the lowest dose and increase sequentially, until the correct dose is obtained. This also gives the clinician the knowledge that if a certain dose does indeed achieve the intended effect, if in the future this fails, the patient's technique can be observed.

Transurethral prostaglandin E1

This system (MUSE) consists of a prostaglandin pellet absorbed after urethral insertion and transmitted to the corpora cavernosa by venous communications. While the applicator is small, discrete and easy to use it is handicapped by a significant minority of men who report burning and discomfort after use; despite this sensation indicating that the drug is being absorbed

effectively, the effect does prevent some patients from having intercourse. Penile pain is the most common side effect with 9.1 % of men to 18.3 % reporting this (6). Although high doses of prostaglandin are used, the effectiveness seems less easy to predict than using the intracavernosal route, although up to 70 % of men can achieve an erection strong enough for intercourse (7). The route of administration is also of considerable interest for a number of possible drugs.

MUSE comes in 250 mcgs, 500 mcgs and 1000 mcg doses, and should be titrated from the lowest dose up as appropriate. After the drug is administered it needs to be massaged in a downward motion, heading towards the base of the penis. It can take up to 15 minutes for the drug to become absorbed, and another factor that help this process is a slight increase in cardio-vascular activity, such as walking up and down a flight of stairs.

In younger patients. MUSE is very much seen as a 'bridge' between the PDE-5 inhibitors, and intra-cavernosal injections, the latter of which are predictably not as attractive a treatment option in the first instance. In the elderly, care should be taken to assess whether the individual patient is likely to tolerate such a treatment which requires a degree of manual dexterity, hasn't got the highest success rate of treatments and may make patients despondent and more likely to give up on treatment altogether.

Physical therapies

Some men will not respond to any of the above therapies, and may need to consider surgical or non-surgical techniques. While counselling may be beneficial for men with relationship problems, its place is limited in elderly men with erectile dysfunction. While psychosexual counselling may help men with accepting the "medical" aspect of their problem, or suggesting alternative techniques of making love which do not centre around physical penetration.

Vacuum pumps

These devices use a cylinder with a pump by which negative pressure induces an erection, following which a constriction ring at the base of the penis maintains rigidity. Vacuum pumps work for nearly all men. The resulting erection may sometimes feel heavy or cold, but many men using pumps are very satisfied, particularly men in a stable relationship.

Surgical options

Vascular penile surgery has an extremely limited place in younger patients, and is almost never justified in elderly men: where carried out it should be in specialist centres as part of ongoing clinical studies.

With new implant technology, implantation of a penile prosthesis gives a reliable and effective long-term solution. This does require surgery, but has only a small chance of infection, and are associated with very high patient satisfaction rates.

KEY POINTS

- Erectile dysfunction is an under-diagnosed and under-resourced condition, which causes distress to men and their partners.
- Evaluation and diagnosis are simple, inexpensive and may pick up a number of serious co-morbid conditions at an early stage.
- Treatment is relatively simple for most men and rewarding for patient and physician alike. Most treatments need little dose modification in the elderly.

- Elderly men and their partners often find a physical relationship rewarding and essential to their happiness: treatment to allow this should not be based on any value judgements.

REFERENCES

1. Eardley I and Sethia K. *Erectile Dysfunction – Current Investigation and Management.* (2nd edn) 1998. London: Mosby-Wolfe.
2. Feldman HA et al. Massachusetts Male Ageing Study. *Journal of Urology* 1994; **151**: 54–61.
3. Hashmi FH et al. Sexually Disinhibited Behaviour in the Cognitively Impaired Elderly. *Clinical Geriatrics* 2000; **8**(11): 61–68.
4. Bloom P. Sex in the Elderly. Global Action on Aging, March 2000. (from http://www.globalaging.org/health/us/sexelderly.htm)
5. Lauman EO et al. Sexual Problems Among Women and Men Ages 40 – 80: Prevalence in the Global Study of Sexual Attitudes and Behaviours. *International Journal of Impotence Research*, 2005; **17**: 39–57.
6. Hellstrom WJ et al. A Double-Blind, Placebo-Controlled Evaluation of the Erectile Response to Transurethral Alprostadil. *Urology* 1996; **48**: 851–856.
7. Padma-Nathan H et al. Treatment of Men with Erectile Dysfunction with Transurethral Alprostadil, Medicated Urethral System for Erection (MUSE), Study Group. *New England Journal of Medicine* 1997; **336**: 1–7.

34 Benign gynaecological disorders

Maria Vella, James Balmforth and Linda Cardozo

Department of Urogynaecology, King's College Hospital, London, UK

UROGENITAL ATROPHY

Urogenital atrophy occurs secondary to oestrogen withdrawal. It can occur perimenopausally but may start for the first time up to 10 years after the last menstrual period. Oestrogen is known to affect the lower urinary tract. In fact the bladder, urethra and the vagina have all been shown to have both oestrogen and progesterone receptors (1).

Oestrogen deficiency is therefore associated with urinary symptoms such as frequency, urgency, nocturia, incontinence and recurrent infection. These may co-exist with symptoms of vaginal atrophy (dysparunia, itching, burning and vaginal dryness).

Low dose local oestrogen replacement therapy has a role in the treatment of urogenital symptoms. Being topical local low dose oestrogen avoids the risk of endometrial proliferation and the necessity of providing endometrial protection with progestogens (1).

A review of oestrogen therapy used for managing urogenital atrophy (2) was performed by the Hormones and Urogenital Therapy Committee Meta-analysis of ten placebo-controlled trials proved the importance of oestrogens in treating women with urogenital atrophy. Route of administration, type of oestrogen used and dosage were all studied. The vaginal route was found to produce best symptomatic relief. Oestrdiol was the oestrogen preparation found to be the most effective. Low dose vaginal oestradiol was found to be most efficacious.

A continuous low dose oestradiol-releasing silicone vaginal ring (known as Estring) releases 5–10 μg oestradiol/24 hrs, has shown a significant beneficial effect on symptoms of vaginal itchiness, dryness, dyspareunia and urinary urgency (3).

PROLAPSE

Pelvic organ prolapse is a common and distressing condition. It occurs when there is a weakness in the supporting structures of the pelvic floor allowing the pelvic viscera to descend. Whilst usually not life threatening, prolapse is often associated with a deterioration in quality of life and may contribute to bladder, bowel and sexual dysfunction. Extended life expectancy and an expanding elderly population mean that prolapse is an increasingly prevalent condition.

Pelvic organ prolapse is more common following childbirth although it is frequently asymptomatic. Studies have estimated that 50 % of parous women have some degree of urogenital prolapse, and of these, 10–20 % are symptomatic (4). Only 2 % of nulliparous women are reported to have prolapse, and this is usually uterine rather than vaginal (5).

Prescribing for Elderly Patients   Edited by Stephen Jackson, Paul Jansen and Arduino Mangoni
© 2009 John Wiley & Sons, Ltd

Classification of Prolapse

Urogenital prolapse has traditionally been classified by the degree of anatomical deformity, depending on the site of the defect and the presumed pelvic viscera that are involved. The large number of different grading systems that have been used is reflective of the difficulty in designing an objective, reproducible system of grading prolapse. Intra and inter-observer variability is often poor. This makes it difficult to compare successive examinations over time in the same woman or between different women.

TRADITIONAL ANATOMICAL SITE PROLAPSE CLASSIFICATION

- **Urethrocele**
  Prolapse of the lower anterior vaginal wall involving the urethra only.
- **Cystocele**
  Prolapse of the upper anterior vaginal wall involving the bladder. Generally there is also associated prolapse of the urethra and hence the term cystourethrocele is often used.
- **Uterovaginal prolapse**
  This term is used to describe prolapse of the uterus, cervix and upper vagina.
- **Enterocele**
  Prolapse of the upper posterior wall of the vagina usually containing loops of small bowel.
- **Rectocele**
  Prolapse of the lower posterior wall of the vagina involving the rectum bulging forwards into the vagina.

The other problem with this terminology, is that it implies an unrealistic certainty as to the structures on the other side of the vaginal bulge. This is often a false assumption, particularly in women who have had previous prolapse surgery. The terms '**anterior vaginal wall prolapse**', '**posterior vaginal wall prolapse**' and '**apical prolapse**' are therefore often preferred because of the uncertainty as to the anatomical structures on the other side of the vaginal bulge.

Symptoms

Most women complain of a feeling of discomfort or heaviness within the pelvis in addition to a 'lump coming down'. Symptoms tend to become worse with prolonged standing and towards the end of the day. They may also complain of dyspareunia, difficulty in inserting tampons and chronic lower backache. In cases of advanced, long-term prolapse there may be epithelial ulceration and lichenification which results in a symptomatic vaginal discharge or bleeding. Pelvic organ prolapse may be associated with lower urinary tract symptoms of urgency and frequency of micturition in addition to a sensation of incomplete emptying which may be relieved by digitally reducing the prolapse.

Signs

An abdominal examination should be performed to exclude the presence of an abdominal or pelvic tumour that may be responsible for the prolapse. Pelvic examination to assess the degree of prolapse is usually performed with the patient in either the left lateral position using a Simms' speculum or in a semi recumbent position in an examination chair. In addition, digital examination of the woman in a standing position allows an accurate assessment of the degree of urogenital prolapse, and in particular of vaginal vault support.

Management

In women who also complain of concomitant lower urinary tract symptoms urodynamic studies or a post-micturition bladder ultrasound should be performed in order to exclude a chronic residual due to associated voiding difficulties. In such cases a mid-stream specimen of urine should be sent for culture and sensitivity. Since occult urodynamic stress incontinence may be unmasked by straightening the urethra following surgical repair of the anterior vaginal wall, this should be simulated by the insertion of a ring pessary or tampon to reduce the cystocele. Studies have described an occult stress incontinence rate after various methods of reducing the prolapse (6, 7) during preoperative testing, of 23–50 %. If stress incontinence is demonstrated then the possibility of performing a simultaneous continence procedure, such as colposuspension or insertion of tension free vaginal tape (TVT) should be discussed.

In cases of severe prolapse, in which there may be a degree of ureteric obstruction, it is important to evaluate the upper urinary tract either with a renal tract ultrasound or intravenous urogram.

Treatment

Prevention

In general any factor that leads to chronic increases in abdominal pressure should be avoided. Consequently care should be taken to avoid constipation which has been implicated as a major contributing factor to urogenital prolapse in Western society (8). In addition the risk of prolapse in patients with chronic chest pathology such as obstructive airways disease and asthma should be reduced by effective management of these conditions. Hormone replacement therapy may theoretically also decrease the incidence of prolapse although to date there are no studies which have tested this effect. Smaller family size and improvements in antenatal and intra-partum care have been implicated in the primary prevention of urogenital prolapse. The role of caesarean section may also be important. One large study of over 21 000 Italian women demonstrated a significant association between vaginal delivery and subsequent uterine prolapse (4). Antenatal and post-natal pelvic floor muscle training has not yet been shown to conclusively reduce the incidence of prolapse, although there are logical reasons to think that it may be protective.

Physiotherapy

Pelvic floor muscle training has a role in cases of mild prolapse, especially in younger women who have not yet completed their family and may find an intravaginal device unacceptable. Education about pelvic floor exercises may be supplemented with the use of a perineometer and biofeedback allowing quantification of pelvic floor contractions. In addition vaginal cones and electrical stimulation may be used.

Intravaginal Devices

Intravaginal devices are available in a wide variety of sizes and designs. Ring pessaries made of silicone or polythene, are currently the most frequently used. They are available in a number of different sizes (52 mm–120 mm) and are designed to lie horizontally in the pelvis with one side in the posterior fornix and the other just behind the pubis, hence providing support the uterus and upper vagina. Fitting is usually done by trial and error. A properly fitted pessary should allow a finger to fit between the pessary and the vaginal wall, thus aiding and ensuring easy removal. Wood advises starting with the largest pessary that can be comfortably admitted into the introitus but not protrude out of the orifice (9). A vaginal lubricant is usually applied to the pessary surface to minimize the discomfort of fitting. Pretreatment with vaginal oestrogen for two to three weeks prior to the insertion appointment is the best way to enhance vaginal lubrication, to decrease atrophy and thereby minimize discomfort at the time of fitting.

Pessaries should be changed every six months and long-term use may be complicated by vaginal ulceration and hence a low dose topical oestrogen may be helpful in postmenopausal women.

Pessaries offer an effective conservative line of therapy for women who do not wish to undergo or are unfit for surgery. They are also suitable for women who suffer with pelvic organ prolapse during pregnancy and the puerperium and may offer symptomatic relief in women awaiting surgery.

Surgery

Surgery offers the best chance of a long-term cure, but as with all forms of surgical treatment it is not entirely risk free. In particular the risk of post-operative dyspareunia, both in the short-term, and occasionally as a long-term complication, need to be discussed. As in other forms of pelvic surgery patients should receive prophylactic antibiotics, to reduce the risk of post-operative infection, as well as thromboembolic prophylaxis in the form of low dose heparin and anti-thromboembolic (TED) stockings. All women should also have a urethral catheter inserted at the time of the procedure unless there is a particular history of voiding dysfunction, in which case a supra-pubic catheter may be more appropriate. This allows the residual urine volume to be checked following a void without the need for re-catheterisation.

Women having pelvic floor surgery are positioned in lithotomy with hips abducted and flexed. To minimize blood loss local infiltration of the vaginal epithelium is performed using 0.5 % xylocaine and 1/200 000 adrenaline although care should be taken in patients with co-existent cardiac disease. At the end of the procedure a vaginal pack may be inserted and removed on the first post-operative day.

URINARY INCONTINENCE

Urinary incontinence, the 'complaint of any involuntary leakage of urine' (10) is a common and distressing condition known to adversely affect quality of life (11). Whilst the prevalence of urinary incontinence has been found to vary widely depending on the definition used a recent large scale epidemiological study found that 25 % of women complain of urinary leakage and 7 % had significant incontinence that was bothersome (11).

The major causes of chronic incontinence are listed below:

- Urodynamic stress incontinence
- Detrusor overactivity
- Mixed incontinence
- Overflow incontinence
- Fistula
- Congenital Abnormality
- Urethral Diverticulum
- Functional Incontinence

Urodynamic stress incontinence (USI), detrusor overactivity (DO), and overflow incontinence are by far the commonest causes of incontinence in the developed world. In the Norwegian EPINCONT community-based survey, 25 % of all respondents had some urinary leakage, the prevalence being age related. Of the women studied, 50 % complained of stress incontinence, 11 % had urge incontinence and 36 % had mixed incontinence (12).

Urodynamic stress incontinence is the leakage of urine per urethram during periods of raised intra-abdominal pressure in the absence of a detrusor contraction. Normal urethral function maintains a positive urethral closure pressure even in the presence of raised intra-abdominal pressure, although detrusor overactivity may overcome it. An incompetent urethra allows leakage of urine in the absence of a detrusor contraction. Damage to the pubo-urethral ligaments and levator ani muscles may allow bladder neck hypermobility and descent of the bladder neck and proximal urethra, so that they are no longer within the intra-abdominal pressure zone. Intrinsic damage to the rhabdosphincter, or scarred drainpipe urethra that cannot occlude properly, may occur after vaginal surgery, previous incontinence surgery, urethral dilatation, chronic urethritis, or radiotherapy (13). The hermetic closure properties of the proximal urethra are lost, and USI may result.

DETRUSOR OVERACTIVITY

Detrusor overactivity (DO) is a urodynamic observation characterised by involuntary detrusor contractions during the filling phase that may be spontaneous or provoked. Sufferers usually complain of urgency, perhaps with urge incontinence, frequency of micturition, and nocturia. The pathophysiology of DO is poorly understood, and an underlying cause is rarely found, leading to the term idiopathic DO. USI and DO can co-exist as mixed incontinence, and DO can arise after incontinence surgery. The process of toilet training in young children requires learning of cortical inhibition of detrusor contractions, and some authorities believe that idiopathic DO may be due to "un-learning" or poor initial learning of this control. Any neurological lesion or condition that interrupts cortical inhibition of detrusor contractions can result in neurogenic DO, e.g. multiple sclerosis and spinal cord lesions. Urethral outflow obstruction can lead to incomplete bladder emptying, and subsequent symptoms of urgency and frequency.

Functional incontinence includes cases of urinary incontinence where no organic cause can be found and may be due to problems with mobility. Restricted mobility may alter the balance between coping and not coping with lower urinary tract symptoms, simply by limiting the ability of an individual to reach the toilet in time. A simple urinal or bedside commode or other lifestyle adaptations may resolve the problem.

Several other factors may be responsible for incontinence due to interference with voiding behaviour. These include cognitive factors such as dementia and learning difficulties as well as physical factors such as immobility and disability. Constipation can cause urinary incontinence, especially in elderly patients and children. Removing impacted stool may restore continence. Additionally, constipation and straining at stool as a young adult is a risk factor for the development of pelvic organ prolapse and stress incontinence in later life (14).

Transient (acute) incontinence is uncommon in young women, but relatively common in the elderly. It should be considered in the differential diagnosis, as it may only require treatment of the underlying cause. Untreated, it is likely to become persistent, but it is not considered chronic, simply because it is long-standing. These causes have been summarized by the acronym "DIAPPERS", as shown below:

- Delirium
- Infection
- Atrophic Change
- Pharmacological
- Psychological
- Excess urine output
- Restricted mobility
- Stool Impaction

Investigation

The diagnosis of urinary incontinence starts with a thorough history and examination. Considering other medical conditions and their treatment may help, by changing medication to an alternative that has fewer side effects on the lower urinary tract, by improving the control of conditions affecting lower urinary tract function for example diabetes mellitus. Simple tests may be invaluable in identifying associated causal factors not immediately apparent. Urinalysis allows detection of urinary tract infection (UTI) and diabetes mellitus; culture of the urine will identify bacterial and fastidious organism UTI; a frequency volume chart may reveal excessive fluid intake, or those drinking large quantities of alcohol or caffeine. Simple lifestyle interventions can often reduce symptoms significantly.

'**Urodynamics**" is a term used to describe a combination of tests that measure the ability of the bladder to store and expel urine. These consist of uroflowmetry and pressure flow studies, cystometry and tests of urethral function. It is most important to differentiate between symptoms and diagnoses, commonly by conventional laboratory urodynamics using retrograde bladder filling, (or ambulatory urodynamics using physiological filling, whilst reproducing everyday activities). Symptoms of lower urinary tract dysfunction are often misleading. Studies have repeatedly shown the greater value of urodynamics over symptoms alone in diagnostic accuracy (15, 16).

Management

A conservative approach is often justified, especially if symptoms are only mild, or easily manageable. When a woman's family is incomplete, or when symptoms manifest during pregnancy, surgery should be avoided. If surgery is considered unwise because of medical illness, when surgery is refused, or if the waiting time for surgery is long, the symptoms may be ameliorated by appropriate conservative interventions.

Lifestyle interventions

The frequency-volume chart (FV chart), or urinary diary, is an important tool in the investigation of patients with lower urinary tract symptoms and voiding dysfunction (17). This facilitates history taking regarding frequency, nocturia and volume voided, and has been shown to be valuable and reliable for the assessment of micturition patterns. There is poor correlation between subjective estimates of diurnal and nocturnal urinary frequency and objective charted measurements (18). Moderation of fluid intake to 1–1.5 litres per day reduces urine production and can ease symptoms. Alcohol, caffeine, and medications such as diuretics are major causes of acute incontinence, especially in the elderly (19). Drug regimens avoiding diuretics, control of chronic cough and constipation, cessation of smoking, exclusion or treatment of urinary tract infection, and weight reduction are desirable.

Physiotherapy

Urodynamic stress incontinence The mainstay of conservative treatment for USI is still physiotherapy, with recourse to surgery when indicated. Physiotherapy includes pelvic floor muscle training, with or without adjuvant electrical stimulation, vaginal cones, and the use of biofeedback. Physical therapies represent the least invasive, but effective option for treating stress urinary incontinence. For this reason they are commonly used as first line treatment. The advantage of this approach is that many women's symptoms are cured or improved to the point where they do not require surgery, with its potential complications. Morkved et al showed that objective cure rate at 6 months can be up to 50 % (20), although most randomized controlled studies have shown that pelvic floor exercises has result in a 60–70 % improvement or cure rate for stress incontinence (21). A recent Cochrane review of 43 randomized trials in women with a symptomatic or a urodynamic diagnosis of stress, urge and mixed incontinence who underwent pelvic floor exercises, showed that pelvic floor exercises are better then no treatment or placebo in women with mixed or urge incontinence and that "intensive" therapy is better then "standard" (21).

In addition, the success of future operative procedures is not adversely affected. Pelvic floor exercises (PFE) provide, in addition to an increase in strength and tone of the pelvic floor, enhancement of cortical awareness of muscle groups, and hypertrophy of existing muscle fibres. Patients need instruction, motivation, and an understanding of the pelvic floor musculature.

"The knack" is a consciously timed pelvic floor contraction coinciding with the need to cough. It has been shown that a pelvic floor muscle contraction in preparation for, and throughout, a cough can augment proximal urethral support during stress, thereby reducing the amount of dorso-caudal displacement of the bladder neck and proximal urethra (22). Within one week of learning the technique, 98.2 % of selected women with mild-to moderate SUI can acquire the skill of using a properly timed pelvic floor muscle contraction to reduce urine leakage during a medium cough.

Pelvic floor muscle training was shown to be more effective than electrical stimulation or vaginal cones in a single blind, randomized controlled trial (23). Postnatal women given advice at regular intervals had a lower prevalence of urinary and faecal incontinence at 1 year and an increase in pelvic floor strength (24). However, at five to seven years follow-up, there was no difference in urinary incontinence, number of pads used, severity of incontinence and frequency of performing pelvic floor exercises, compared to those women who were not given intensive protracted PFEs (25).

Detrusor overactivity Behavioural therapy for detrusor overactivity was first reported by Jeffcoate and Francis who, in the 1960s advocated the practice of voiding "by the clock" for urge incontinence (26). Treatment frequently consists of bladder re-training by "bladder drill", to re-learn the cortical inhibition of detrusor contractions. This may be time consuming and frustrating–correct diagnosis is necessary to ensure maximum patient compliance with treatment. Behavioural modification improves central control of bladder function, avoiding at the same time the complications of surgery and the side-effects of drug treatment.

However, this type of treatment requires high levels of motivation and encouragement, and suffers from high relapse rates.

Studies of "bladder drill" lack consistency in their nomenclature and methodology. However, in a review of the randomised clinical trials of conservative treatments, Berghams et al. (27) showed strong evidence that bladder drill is more effective than no treatment, and weak evidence that bladder drill is better then drug therapy. There is insufficient evidence, though, of the efficacy of bladder drill with drug therapy, bladder drill with pelvic floor exercises and biofeedback, or biofeedback and behavioural therapy, due to inadequate clinical trials.

DRUG THERAPIES

Urodynamic stress incontinence

A drug has been recently marketed, specifically for the treatment of stress urinary incontinence. Duloxetine is a potent dual serotonin and no-radrenaline reuptake inhibitor (SNRI) that enhances urethral striated sphincter activity via a centrally mediated pathway (28).

Clinical trials have shown a significant decrease in incontinence episode frequency and an improvement in quality of life in women taking duloxetine 40 mg bd when compared to placebo (29, 30).

The safety and efficacy of duloxetine has been evaluated in four 12-week placebo- controlled clinical trials, including almost 2000 women (31). The commonest side-effects were nausea, dry mouth, fatigue, insomnia and constipation.

Detrusor overactivity

Most patients with DO will require drug therapy, which is the mainstay of treatment. Many drugs have been tried over the years in the treatment of DO–none is completely satisfactory, and many have been abandoned due to lack of efficacy, or dangerous, or unpleasant, side-effects. Even then the placebo response can be so large that clinical effect is difficult to distinguish.

The main transmitter in the parasympathetic nervous system is acetylcholine. Voluntary and involuntary bladder contractions are mediated via muscarinic receptors in the bladder smooth muscle. Anti-muscarinic agents act by competitive inhibition at the post-ganglionic receptor sites and therefore suppress both types of contraction, irrespective of the activation of the efferent part of the reflex.

Oxybutynin has been available for the last 25 years. It has well-documented efficacy in the treatment of detrusor overactivity but has a poor side-effect profile. However new and novel delivery systems like the oxybutynin patch have attempted to overcome this (32). Oxybutynin and tolterodine are currently the first line medication for patients with DO.

Tolterodine is a potent and competitive antagonist of muscarinic receptors. However, it has no selectivity for the subtypes of muscarinic receptor, but seems to show selectivity for the bladder over the salivary glands (33). The therapeutic effect of tolterodine is bolstered by the similar activity of its metabolite (34, 35). Tolterodine and oxybutynin immediate release preparations have similar benefit in reducing incontinence episodes and urinary frequency, but the side-effect profile appears to favour tolterodine.

Tolterodine ER 4 mg is currently the most widely used formulation. Studies have shown that it is more effective than immediate release and has a lower rate of dry mouth (36).

A transdermal preparation of oxybutynin has been shown to be well tolerated and efficacious when compared with placebo (32). This study also found that the incidence of dry mouth was not significantly different from placebo- patch site pruritus was the commonest side-effect. Intra-vesical administration allows effective absorption from the bladder, with serum concentrations at least as high as with oral administration.

Anticholinergic therapy is typically limited by patient complaints of dry mouth. Anticholinergics may also be responsible for producing a degree of cognitive impairment, particularly in the elderly. This has been partly addressed by the development of sustained release (ER) preparations of both oxybutynin and tolterodine, and development of newer selective anti-muscarinic drugs, such as solifenacin or darifenacin. The development of bladder selective M3 specific antagonists offers the possibility of increasing efficacy whilst minimizing adverse effects.

Solifenacin has been shown to cause a reduction in frequency, urgency and urge incontinence and to significantly improve quality of life (37). In the STAR trial, where it was directly compared to tolterodine, there was a significantly greater decrease in incontinence episodes and urgency. Solifenacin can be used in doses of 5 and 10 mg. Side effects are dose dependent, suggesting that solifenacin 5 mg once daily may offer the best compromise between efficacy and tolerability (38).

Trospium chloride is a quaternary ammonium compound which is nonselective for muscarinic receptor subtypes and shows low bioavailability (39). In a recent placebo-controlled, randomised double-blind, multicentre trial trospium chloride produced significant improvements in maximum cystometric capacity and bladder volume at first unstable contraction (40). Trospium chloride has also been compared to oxybutynin in a randomised, double-blind, multicentre trial. There were no statistically significant differences between the two treatment groups. Those taking Trospium had a lower incidence of dry mouth and were also less likely to withdraw from treatment when compared to the group receiving oxybutynin (41).

Propiverine has been shown to combine anticholinergic and calcium channel blocking actions (42). Open studies in patients with detrusor overactivity have demonstrated (43) increased bladder capacity in comparison to placebo. Dry mouth was experienced by 37 % in the treatment group as opposed to 8 % in the placebo group with dropout rates being 7 % and 4.5 % respectively (44).

Imipramine and other tricyclic antidepressants have been shown to have systemic anticholinergic effects (45) and block re-uptake of serotonin. Their role in detrusor overactivity

remains of uncertain benefit although they are often useful in patients complaining of nocturia and bladder pain.

Desmopressin (DDVAP), a synthetic vasopressin with potent antidiuretic effect, has been shown to be effective in reducing nocturia in patients with both neuropathic and non-neuropathic bladders (46). Recent studies have also demonstrated benefit in daytime urinary frequency and urinary incontinence (47).

Intra-vesical instillations of capsaicin, a neurotoxin extracted from red chilli peppers (48), have significant effect over placebo in the treatment of neurogenic DO. Its analogue resiniferatoxin (49) has been shown to have fewer side effects, with an increase in bladder capacity. However, the place of these neurotoxins in clinical practice is still uncertain.

Surgery

Urodynamic stress incontinence The traditional aims of incontinence surgery were to elevate the bladder neck and proximal urethra, to support them and prevent funnelling, and to align the bladder neck to the postero-superior aspect of the symphysis-pubis, and sometimes to increase outflow resistance.

Over the last 20 years, attention has been directed at developing less invasive procedures, which replicate the high cure rates of conventional slings and the Burch colposuspension but with reduced morbidity, hospital stay, and time taken to return to normal activities. Three types of surgical intervention characterise the current trend towards less invasive surgical treatments for female stress urinary incontinence:

- Laparoscopic colposuspension.
- Mid-urethral tape procedures, e.g. Tension free vaginal tape (TVT), Intravaginal slingoplasty (IVS) tuneller, suprapubic arc sling procedures (SPARC), transobturator tapes (TOT).
- Injectable peri-urethral bulking agents.

In a meta-analysis of eight trials, five of which compared open and laparoscopic colposuspension, there was a lower objective success rate for laparoscopic colposuspension (RR 0.89, CI 0.82–0.98) with a higher risk of complications and a longer operating time (50).

Of the minimally invasive, mid-urethral supports, tension free vaginal tape (TVT) has been the most extensively investigated. In a multi-centre, randomized trial to compare TVT with colposuspension as a primary treatment for stress incontinence, 344 women with USI were randomized to TVT or colposuspension. At two years no significant difference was found between the groups for cure rates. However, surgery with TVT was associated with more operative complications than colposuspension, mainly bladder perforation. However, colposuspension was associated with more postoperative complications and longer recovery (51). Eleven year data are now available and suggest that TVT and colposuspension have a similar cure rate.

Transobturator tapes have been developed to avoid the retro-pubic space and reduce the risk of bladder, urethral, and intrabdominal trauma. In an outcome study of the "inside-out" TVT-O(Gynaecare) transobturator tape, assessment with visual analogue scale showed improvement in 49 of 52 women. No lower urinary tract injuries were reported.

The SPARC procedure utilizes a similar mid-urethral placement of a monofilament polpropylene mesh but with an abdominal approach to passage of the needles. In a series of 104 women receiving a SPARC, the objective cure rate was 90.4% with subjective cure of 72% (52). No objective difference was seen between the cure rates of urodynamic stress incontinence and mixed incontinence. There was, however, a significant increase in risk of bladder injury if previous continence surgery had been undertaken (36.3% vs 7.5%, p<0.001). 12 women (11.5%) developed de novo urgency. In a non-randomized, case-controlled series of 37 SPARC and 69 TVT placements (53), no significant differences were seen for subjective cure/improvement, satisfaction, or symptoms of incontinence.

Coaptation of the urethral epithelium is an important part of the continence mechanism. If it fails, reduced pressures are needed to overcome the continence mechanism, and peri-urethral bulking agents aim to create artificial cushions at the bladder neck. The only comparison of peri-urethral bulking agents against placebo was by Lee et al. (54) comparing autologous fat with saline. They showed no significant difference in outcome, although it must be noted that the study was terminated early due to the death of a patient from fat embolus, and was therefore underpowered. The effectiveness of peri-urethral bulking agents is, as yet unproven; they may be most useful where co-morbidity is a problem, due to their low complication rates.

The most commonly used injectable material consists of micronised silicone rubber particles suspended in a non-silicone carrier gel (56). Marketed in Europe as Macroplastique (Uroplasty), the large particle size of this material makes migration and displacement less likely. In addition, the inert nature of the material makes a local inflammatory reaction less problematic. The silicone particles are designed to act as a bulking agent with local inflammatory response removing the carrier gel. This results in encapsulation of the silicon in fibrin and treplacement of the gel with collagen fibres.

Detrusor overactivity Surgical solutions for DO include Botulinum toxin A ("Botox"), sacral neuromodulation, detrusor myectomy, augmentation cystoplasty, or urinary diversion.

Botox has been successfully used to overcome outflow obstruction in patients with voiding difficulty (57) and to treat detrusor-sphincter dyssynergia after spinal cord injury (57). It is currently the subject of research to assess its efficacy in the suppression of detrusor overactivity, although the long term effects of repeated cystoscopic injections are not known.

Stimulation of the S3 nerve root by an implanted electrical pulse generator can provide effective relief from frequency-urgency symptoms. In a prospective randomised trial of sacral neuromodulation versus delay, incontinence episode frequency (IEF), severity, and pad use were all reduced in the active arm (p<0.0001). 47% were dry, and 29% reported a reduction in IEF of more than 50% at six months (58). Neuromodulation is, however, very expensive. Patients need expert assessment, and management–although it is not suitable for routine use, sacral neuromodulation appears to be useful for a selected minority. The stimulator is a small electrical pulse generator, approximately the same size as a cardiac pacemaker, and is commonly implanted in the upper outer quadrant of the buttock. Complications most commonly reported are generator site pain (15.9%) and implant site pain (19.1%). Lead migration may occur in up to 7%. The surgical revision of technical failures and complications was 32.5% (58). This may be expected to reduce in the future as the technological development of generators and implant leads progresses.

Augmentation cystoplasty is used to increase the size of the urinary reservoir and render the bladder less contractile. It is indicated in patients who lack adequate bladder capacity or detrusor compliance; who manifest debilitating frequency-urgency symptoms, with urge incontinence, UTIs or renal insufficiency; who have failed to derive benefit from medical therapy; whose lifestyle is severely limited; or with high pressure urine storage endangering the upper renal tracts.

The operation most frequently used is the "clam" cystoplasty. A cure rate up to 90% has been reported (59) which compares very favourably with alternatives, such as Ingelman-Sundberg bladder denervation (54% complete response at 44 months) and detrusor myectomy (63% showed improvement of compliance and/or resolution of detrusor contractions). Post-operative complications include a significant risk of post-operative voiding difficulty, presumably secondary to a failure to generate adequate voiding pressures. This may be overcome by teaching the patient clean intermittent self-catheterisation. Mucus production by the ileal segment may cause distress, especially when passed per urethram. This may be ameliorated by the ingestion of cranberry juice, which decreases mucus viscosity. Additionally there is an increased risk of urolithiasis. Of those who develop stones, there is a 30% risk of further stone formation within two years. Electrolyte and acid-base balance may become disturbed resulting in a metabolic acidosis. Malignant change occasionally occurs within the ileal segment. Urinary nitrites, produced by recurrent bacterial infection, may also contribute to the increased risk of malignancy. The carcinogenic effects of this and nitrosamines have been implicated in tumours of urinary conduits and those with uretero-sigmoidostomy.

In some patients, the bladder becomes severely contracted due to severe long-term detrusor-overactivity. In these cases, drug therapy and behaviour modification are of little or of no benefit, and augmentation cystoplasty is inappropriate and technically difficult. Relief for intractable detrusor overactivity, especially of neurogenic origin may eventually require a urinary diversion procedure with an ileal conduit. The management of a stoma may be easier than constantly changing and washing wet underwear and incontinence pads.

LICHEN SCLEROSIS

Lichen sclerosis is characterised by epithelial thinning, inflammation, and histological changes in the dermis. It is the commonest cause of vulval itching in postmenopausal women. Its aetiology is unknown although it is thought to be associated with autoimmune disorders (60).

Women generally present with intractable vaginal itching although it may be asymptomatic. The skin generally appears thinned and has white lesions on it. The vulva appears to have a crinkled surface and there may be loss of the labia minora.

A clinical diagnosis can generally be made although ideally a vulval biopsy is taken whenever possible as there is a small risk (about 4%) of developing vulval carcinoma.

Management is generally targeted towards symptomatic relief. If the patient is asymptomatic no treatment is required. Mild itching may be helped by an aqueous cream or a 1% hydrocortisone preparation three times a day. In more severe cases short courses of more potent steroids may be used.

LICHEN PLANUS

Lichen planus can be an acute or a chronic condition affecting the skin or mucous membranes or both. Its appearance changes according to its location. On the vulva the lesions are usually purple-white papules with a shiny surface and a regular outline.

This is a self limiting and often asymptomatic condition. The diagnosis is generally made on histology. Treatment tends to involve topical steroids.

REFERENCES

1. Iosif S, Batra S, Elk A, Astedt B. Oestrogen receptors in the human female lower urinary tract. *Am. J. Obstet. Gynaecol.* 1981; **141**: 817–20.

2. Cardozo LD, Bachmann G, McClish D, Fonda D, Birgeron L. Meta-analysis of oestrogen therapy in the management of urogenital atrophy in postmenopausal women. Second report of the hormones and urogenital therapy committee. *Obstet Gynaecol.* 1998; **1992**: 722–7.

3. Bachmann G. Oestradiol releasing vaginal ring delivery system for urogenital atrophy. Experience over the last decade. *J. Reprod Med* 1998; **43**: 991–8.

4. Progetto Menopausa Italia Study Group Risk factors for genital prolapse in non-hysterectomized women around menopause, results from a large cross-sectional study in menopausal clinics in Italy. *Eur J Obstet Gynecol Reprod Biol* 2000; **93**: 125–40.

5. Samuelsson EC, Victor FTA, Tibblin G. Signs of genital prolapse in a Swedish population of women 20 to 59 years of age and possible related factors. *Am J Obstet Gynecol* 1999; **180**: 299–305.

6. Chaikin DC, Groutz A, Blaivas JG. Predicting the need for antiincontinence surgery in continent women undergoing repair of severe urogenital prolapse. *J Urol* 2000; **163**: 531–4.

7. Gallentine ML, Cespedes RD. Occult stress urinary incontinence and the effect of vaginal vault prolapse on abdominal leak point pressures. *Urol* 2001; **57**: 40–4.

8. Spence-Jones C, Kamm MA, Henry MM, Hudson CN. Bowel dysfunction: a pathogenic factor in uterovaginal prolapse and urinary stress incontinence. *Br J Obstet Gynaecol* 1994; **101**: 147–52.

9. Wood N. The use of vaginal pessaries for uterine prolapse. *Nurse Pract* 1992; **17**: 31–8.

10. Abrams P, Cardozo L, Fall M, Griffiths D, Rosier P, Ulmsten U et al. The standardisation of terminology of lower urinary tract function. Report from the standardization committee of the International Continence Society. *Neurourol Urodynam* 2002; **21**: 167–78.

11. Kelleher CJ, Cardozo LD, Khullar V, Salvatore S. A new questionnaire to assess the quality of life of urinary incontinent women. *Br J Obstet Gynaecol* 1997; **104**: 1374–9.

12. Hannestad YS, Rortveit G, Sandovik H, Hunskaar S, A community-based epidemiological survey of female urinary incontinence: the Norwegian EPINCONT study. Epidemiology of incontinence in the county of Nord-Trondelag. *J. Clin Epidemiol* 2000; **53**: 1150–7.

13. Kelleher C. Epidemiology and classification of Incontinence. In Cardozo LD (Ed.) *Urogynaecology*. Churchill Livingstone, 1997: 3–23.

14. Spence-Jones C, Kamm M A, Henry M M, Hudson C N. Bowel dysfunction: a pathogenic factor in utero-vaginal prolapse and urinary stress incontinence. *Br J Obstet Gynaecol* 1994; **101**(2): 147–52.

15. Jarvis GJ, Hall S, Stamp S, Millar DR. An assessment of urodynamic investigation in incontinent women. *Br J Obstet Gynaecol* 1980; **87**: 873–96.

16. James M, Jackson S, Shepherd A, Abrams P. Pure stress leakage symptomatology: is it safe to discount detrusor instability? *Br J Obstet Gynaecol* 1999; **106**: 1255–8.

17. Larsson G, Victor A. Micturition patterns in a healthy female population, studied with a frequency-volume chart. *Scandinavian Journal of Urology and Nephrology Supplementum* 1988; **114**: 53–7.

18. McCormack M, Infante-Rivard C, Schick E. Agreement between clinical methods of measurment of urinary frequency and functional bladder capacity. *Br J Urol* 1992; **9**(1): 17–21.

19. Linjakumpu T, Hartikainen S, Klaukka T, Koponen H, Kivela SL, Isoaho R. Psychotropics among the home dwelling elderly–increasing trends. *International Journal of Geriatric Psychiatry* 2002; **17**(9): 874–83.

20. Morkved S, Bo K, Fjortoft T. effect of adding biofeedback to pelvic floor muscle training to treat urodynamic stress incontinence. *Obstet Gynecol* 2002 Oct; **100**(4): 730–9.

21. Hay-Smith EJ, Bo Berghman's LC, Hendricks HJ, de Bie Ra, van Waalwijk van Doorn ES.

Pelvic Floor muscle training for urinary incontinence in women. *Cochrane Systematic Review* 2001; (1): CD001407.

22. Miller JM, Ashton-Miller JA, DeLancey JO. A pelvic muscle precontraction can reduce cough related urine loss in selected women with mild SUI. *J Am Geriatr Soc* 1998; **46**(7): 870–4.

23. Bo K, Talseth T, Holme I. Single blind, randomised controlled trial of pelvic floor exercises, electrical stimulation, vaginal cones, and no treatment in management of genuine stress incontinence in women. *BMJ* 1999; **318**(7182): 487–93.

24. Morkved S, Bo K. Effect of postpartum pelvic floor muscle training in prevention and treatment of urinary incontinence: a one-year follow-up. *BJOG* 2000; **107**(8): 1022–8.

25. Wilson P, Herbison P, Glazener C et al. Obstetric practice and urinaryu Incontinence 5–7 years after delivery. *Neurourol Urodynam* 2002; **21**: 284–300.

26. Jeffcoate TN, Francis WJ. Urgency incontinence in the female. *Am J Obstet Gynecol* 1966 Mar 1; **94**(5): 604–18.

27. Berghams LC, Hendriks HJ, De Bie RA, van Waalwijk van Doorn ES, Bo K, van Kerrebroeck PE. Conservative treatment of urge urinary incontinence in women: a suystematic review of randomised clinical trials. *BJU Int* 2000; **85**(3): 254–63.

28. Thor KB, Katofiasc MA. Effects of duloxetine, a combined serotonin and norepinephrine reuptake inhibitor, on central neural control of lower urinary tract function in the cloralose-anaesthetised female cat. *J Pharmacol Exp Ther* 1995; **274**: 1014–24.

29. Norton PA, Zinner NR, Yalcin I, Bump RC; Duloxetine versus placebo in the treatment of stress urinary incontinence. *Am J Obstet Gynaecol* 2002; **187**(1): 40–8.

30. Millard R, Moore K, Yalcin I, Bump R. Duloxetine vs.placebo in the treatment of stress urinary incontinence: a global phase 3 study. *Neurol Urodynam* 2003; **22**: 482–3.

31. *Duloxetine Summary of product characteristics*. Eli Lilly and company, p. 5

32. Dmochowski RR, Davila GW, Zinner NR et al. Efficacy and safety of Transdermal oxybutynin in patients with urge and mixed urinary incontinence. *J. Urol* 2002; **168**(2): 580–6.

33. Abrams P, Freeman R, Anderstom C et al. Tolteridone, a new anti-muscarinic agent: as effective but better tolerated than oxybutynin in patients with an overactive bladder. *Br J Urol* 1998; **81**: 801.

34. Stahl MMS, Ekstrom B, Sparf B et al. Urodynamic and other effects of Tolteridone: a novel antimuscarinic drug for the treatment of detrusor overactivity. *Neurourol Urodyn* 1995; **14**: 647.

35. Brynne N, Stahl MMS, Hallen B. Pharmacokinetics and Pharmacodynamics of tolteridone in man: a new drug in the treatment of urinary bladder overactivity. *Int J Clin Pharmacol Ther* 1997; **35**: 287.

36. Van Kerrebroek P, Kreder K, Jonas U, Zimmer N, Wein A; Tolteridone Study Group, Tolteridone once daily: superior efficacy and tolerability in the treatment of the overactive bladder. *Urology* 2001; **57**(3): 414.

37. Cardozo L, I Kuzmin, M I Lisek and European YM905 Study Group. Solifenacin in symptomatic Oveactive Bladder. YM905 Results of a Phase 3, Randomised, Placebo-controlled Trial.

38. Chapple CR, Rechberger T, Al-Shukri et al. Randomised double-blind placebo and tolteridone-controlled trial of the once-daily antimuscarinic agent solefanicin in patient with symptomatic overactive bladder. *BJU Int* 2004; **93**(3): 303–10.

39. Schladitz Keil G, Spanh H, Mutschler e. Determination of bioavailibilty of the quaternary ammonium compound trospium chloride in man for the urinary excretion data. *Arzneimittel Forsch/Drug Res*. 1986; **36**: 984–7.

40. Cardozo LD, Chapple CR, Toozs-Hobson P et al. Efficacy of trospium Chloride in patients with detrusor instability: a placebo- controlled, randomized, double-blind multi-centre clnical trial. *BJU Int* 2000; **85**(6): 659–64.

41. Madersbaher H, Stoher M, Richter R, Burgdorfer H., Hachen HJ, Murtz G. Trospium chloride versus oxybutynin: a randomized, double-blind multicentre trial in the treatment of detrusor hyperreflexia. *Br J Urol* 1995; **75**(4): 452–6.

42. Haruno A, Yamasaki Y, Miyoshi K et al. Effects of Propiverine hydrochloride and its metabolites on isolated guinea pig urinary bladder. *Folia Pharmacol Japon* 1989; **94**: 145–50.

43. Mazur d, whnert J., Dorshner W, Schubert G, Herfurth G, alken RG. Clinical and urodynamic effects of propiverine in patients suffering from urgency and urge incontinence. *Scan J. Urol Nephrol* 1995; **29**: 289–94.

44. Stoher M, Madersbacher H., Richter R, Wehnert J, Dreikorn K. Efficacy and safety of propiverine in SCI-patients suffering

from detrusor hyper-reflexia: a double-blind, placebo-controlled clinical trial. *Spinal Cord* 1999; **37**(3): 196–200.

45. Baldessarini KJ. Drugs in the treatment of psychiatric disorders. In: Gilman et al. (Eds) *The Pharmacological Basis of Therapeutics*, 7th edn, McMillan Publishing Co., 1985, pp. 387–445.

46. Hilton P, Hertogs K, Stanton SL. The use of Demopressin (DDVAP) for nocturia in women multiple sclerosis. *J. Neurol Neurosurg Psychiatry* 1983; **46**: 854–5.

47. Robinson D, Cardozo L, Akeson M et al. Women take control; desmopressin–a drug for daytime urinary incontinence. *Neurourol Urodyn* 2002; **21**: 385–6.

48. de Seze M, Wiart L, Joseph PA et al. Caspaicin and neurogenic detrusor hyperreflexia: a double blind placebo-controlled study in 20 patients with spinal cord lesions. *Neurourol Urodyn* 1998; **17**(5): 513–23.

49. Lazzeri M, Beneforti P, Turini D. Urodynamic effects of intra-vesical resiniferatoxin in humans: preliminary results in stable and unstable detrusor. *J Urol* 1997; **158**(6): 2093–7.

50. Moehre B, Carey M, Wilson D. Laparoscopic colposuspension: a systemtic review. *BJOG* 2003; **110**(3): 230–5.

51. Ward K, Hilton P; United Kingdom and Ireland Tension-free Vaginal Tape and colposuspension as primary treatment for stress incontinence. *BMJ* 2002; **325**(7355): 67.

52. Deval B, Levardon M, Samain E et al. A French multicentre clinical trial of SPARC for stress urinary incontinence. *Eur Urol* 2003; **44**(2): 254–8.

53. Dietz HP, Foote AJ, Mak HL, Wilson PD. TVT and SPARC Suburethral Slings: a case-control series. *International Urogynaecology Journal* 2004; **15**(2): 129–31.

54. Lee PE, Kung RC, Drutz HP. Periurethral autologous fat injection as treatment for female stress incontinence: a randomized, double-blind controlled trial. *J Urol* 2001; **165**(1): 153–8.

55. Chapple C, Sultan AH, Cervigni M. Efficacy and safety of the Zuidex system for the treatment of stress urinary incontinence: 6-month results of an open, multicentre study. Proceedings of the 34th Annual Scientific Meeting of the International Society, Paris, France. August 2004. Abstract No. 314.

56. *Macroplastique Implants Technical Overview*. Maastricht, The Netherlands: Uroplasty BV; 1995.

57. Phelan MW, Franks M, Somogyi GT, Yokoyama T, Fraser MO, Lavelle JP, Yoshimura N, Chanellor MB. Botulinum toxin urethral sphincter injection to restore bladder emptying in men and women with voiing dysfunction. *J.Urol* 200 **165**(4): 1107–10.

58. Schmidt RA, Jonas U, Oleson KA, Janknegt RA, Hassouna MM, Siegel SW, van Kerrebroek PE. Sacral nerve stimulation for treatment of refractory urinary re incontinence. Sacral Nerve Stimulation Study Group. *J Urol* 1999; **162**(2): 352–7.

59. Mark SD, McRae CU, Arnold EP, Gwland SP. Clam cystoplasty for the overactive bladder: a review of 23 cases. *Aust NZ J Surg* 1994; **64**(2): 88–90.

60. Meyrick Thomas RH, Ridley CM, McGibbon DH, Black MM. Lichen sclerosis and autoimmunity: a study of 350 women. *British Journal of Dermatology* **118**: 41–6.

35 Breast cancer in elderly patients

Bogda Koczwara

Department of Medical Oncology, Flinders Medical Centre, Adelaide, Australia

INTRODUCTION

Breast cancer is the most common cancer affecting older women. Its treatment involves a broad range of therapeutic approaches which take into account not only the biology of cancer but also physiological changes of aging that may impact on pharmacokinetics and pharmacodynamics of cancer drugs in an elderly patient. As such, breast cancer management can serve as a model of cancer therapeutics in an elderly patient in general.

Approximately 45 % of new breast cancers are detected after the age of 65 and the risk increases steadily with age (1). As western (and recently eastern) population ages, breast cancer incidence is increasing. In contrast rates of death have been declining slightly, presumably reflecting effectiveness of breast cancer screening and treatment.

Management of breast cancer in an elderly patient requires careful consideration of the biology of this disease, risks and benefits of treatment and appreciation of the impact of age-related physiological changes and comorbidities on the treatment tolerability and overall life expectancy. Unfortunately, for many breast cancer treatments little data is available on their specific efficacy of breast cancer treatments in elderly women. As a result, controversy exists on almost every aspect of breast cancer management in the elderly population. Even less data exists for treatment of breast cancer in males and the general approach follows that of women.

Breast cancer in elderly patients may actually be more indolent than in the younger patients. Despite its favorable characteristics (Table 35.1) survival studies are conflicting. This may be because of comorbidities that prevent elderly patients from tolerating cancer treatment. However, there is also data that elderly women receive less treatment, even after adjusting for women's treatment preferences, health status, and comorbidity(2). In recent years, clinical trials focused specifically on treatment of elderly women with breast cancer are being designed, which may provide more evidence to support treatment approaches for these patients.

PRESENTATION AND DIAGNOSIS—SPECIAL CONSIDERATIONS IN ELDERLY PATIENTS

Presentation of breast cancer in elderly patients can vary from asymptomatic early stage breast tumour detected as part of the screening process to symptoms related to advanced metastatic disease.

Although the positive predictive value of screening tests becomes more accurate with increasing prevalence of cancer, value of screening of older individuals may be limited because of their shorter life expectancy. As yet, no study conclusively demonstrated that screening mammography decreases the breast cancer-related mortality for women aged 70 and older. It is however possible that elderly

Prescribing for Elderly Patients Edited by Stephen Jackson, Paul Jansen and Arduino Mangoni

Table 35.1. Breast cancer biology in elderly women (as compared to younger women)

- lower grade
- higher hormone receptors concentration
- less local recurrence
- less visceral metastases
- more bone metastases

women with higher risk of breast cancer and long life expectancy may still benefit from a mammography.

Many women continue screening with mammography throughout their later life and changes on mammography (microcalcification, architectural distortion and density changes) can lead to a diagnosis of an early stage cancer. For others with early stage breast cancer, the process of diagnosis is initiated following a discovery of a breast lump or redness, as is the case with inflammatory breast cancer. Redness and swelling of the breast is often difficult to diagnose as breast cancer as a lump is frequently absent and inflammatory breast cancer is sometimes mistaken for mastitis. Sadly, some elderly women present with gross advanced breast masses which are often no longer amenable to surgical treatment.

Patients with metastatic disease may either present with symptoms relating to the primary site (breast lump) or to the metastatic involvement in other organs—most frequently bone (pain and fractures), liver (pain, nausea, jaundice), lung (cough and shortness of breath) or any other organs. In some cases patients presenting with metastatic breast cancer do not have distinct breast pathology and all women who present with axillary node involvement with cancer but no distinct breast abnormality should be treated as breast cancer.

Evaluation of an elderly patient with suspected breast cancer consists of three distinct elements—confirmation of pathologic diagnosis, staging of cancer and assessment of patient's fitness to be treated.

Confirmation of tissue diagnosis usually involves a biopsy—either fine needle or core of a breast mass and or redness which has previously been assessed by mammography and frequently breast ultrasound, or in case of obvious metastatic involvement of other organ—a

biopsy of a metastatic lesion may be more appropriate—for example a liver biopsy.

Staging of cancer involves assessment of liver function; chest X-ray and a bone scan for patients who present with early stage disease. Patients suspected of metastatic disease should have imaging of relevant organs ideally using a CT scan or in case of spinal disease a MRI or bone scan.

Assessment of patient's fitness to be treated involves assessment of end organ function, co-morbidities as well as assessment of patient functional capacity including both cognitive and physical capacity. This comprehensive geriatric assessment includes assessment of comorbidities, socioeconomic conditions, functional dependence, and emotional and cognitive conditions, along with an estimate of life expectancy and the recognition of frailty, increasingly effective simple screening tools are being developed which allow a rapid assessment to be undertaken to identify those patients requiring a more detailed assessment. Essential elements of assessment of an elderly patient with breast cancer are summarised in table 35.2.

MANAGEMENT OF BREAST CANCER

Approach to management of breast cancer in elderly patients is based on same principles as approach to all patients with cancer (table 35.3). It requies firstly a careful consideration of prognosis and goals of treatment (cure versus palliation) in order to estimate expected benefit of treatment and secondly, an assessment of any comorbidities that may impact on life

Table 35.2. Assessment of an elderly patient with breast cancer

- tumour factors - size, lymph nodes, grade, receptor status, stage
- end organ function and comorbidity - including bone marrow reserve, renal function, drug interactions, nutrition
- functional status
- depression
- cognition
- social supports

Table 35.3. Approach to management of a woman with breast cancer

- assess prognosis and goals of treatment (cure versus palliation)
- evaluate and manage comorbidities that may affect quality of life and tolerance of treatment
- involve patient in decision making

expectancy and add to treatment toxicity. Consideration of these issues needs to involve the patient to the extent that is acceptable to, and desired by the patient and that allows for informed decision making.

MANAGEMENT OF EARLY BREAST CANCER

Management of breast cancer in an elderly patient is broadly based on the same principles as in younger women. Early stage disease is treated with surgery followed by adjuvant radiotherapy and systemic therapy in women at high risk of recurrence. However the magnitude of benefit of adjuvant therapies in elderly women may not be as high as in younger women.

Surgery

While elderly women can tolerate elective surgery well, avoidance of axillary lymph node dissection in the older woman has been advocated to prevent additional morbidity, especially in frail women. It is possible that, with increased prevalence of the sentinel lymph node sampling, axillary dissection may be eliminated for a number of patients.

Radiotherapy

Radiation therapy to the breast is equally well tolerated in older and younger patients but the magnitude of benefit from radiotherapy may be affected by the existence of comorbidities, which may impact on their risk of dying from other causes. The recent metaanalysis concluded that survival benefit from RT would likely to be unfavorable for older women since the risk of dying of other causes other than breast cancer

outweighs the benefits of radiotherapy(3). As the local recurrence rate of breast cancer after partial mastectomy declines with patient age the final decision of whether postoperative irradiation can be avoided is based on patient's risk of recurrence, life expectancy, and patient's preference.

Adjuvant systemic therapy: hormonal versus chemotherapy

The objective of adjuvant systemic therapy is to reduce risk of cancer recurrence and improve cure rate by eradicating any remaining micrometastases that exist after surgery. While both chemotherapy and hormonal therapy has been shown to be effective in reducing the risk of recurrence and risk of death, there is a paucity of chemotherapy data pertaining to women older than 70 years. Benefits of adjuvant chemotherapy appear smaller than those of tamoxifen and decline with age (4). The controversy remains about the value of chemotherapy in an adjuvant setting for women with high risk, receptor negative tumours, who would not benefit from tamoxifen. The Early Breast Cancer Trialists Collaborative Group metaanalysis concluded that postoperative tamoxifen in women with receptor positive tumours reduced odds of recurrence and death by 47% and 26% respectively for women irrespective of age or nodal status (5). Recent studies demonstrated increased benefit of aromatase inhibitors in adjuvant setting using aromatase inhibitors (6).

For patients who display overexpression of a HER2 receptor, there is emerging data that herceptin (trastuzumab) may be beneficial in improving freedom from disease and survival (7). The detailed approach to management of patients with early breast cancer is summarized in Figure 35.1.

TREATMENT OF ADVANCED BREAST CANCER

Although advanced breast cancer cannot be cured, with appropriate treatment strategies, it is possible to obtain durable palliation. Women with bone only metastases and

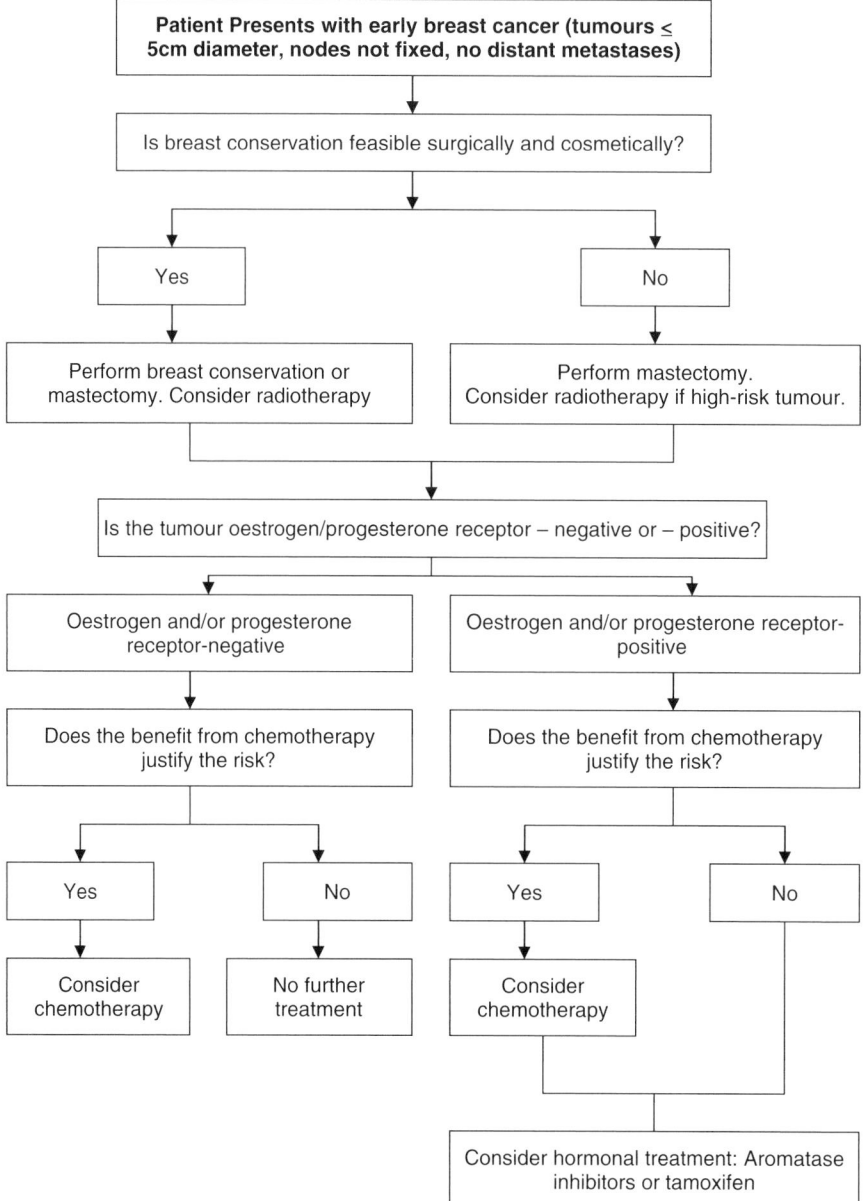

Figure 35.1. Management of early breast cancer in an elderly patient

hormone positive tumours frequently respond to hormonal treatments of tamoxifen or newer aromatase inhibitors (letrozole, anastrazole and examestane).

Women with metastatic disease involving the viscera, especially those with receptor negative tumours may require treatment with chemotherapy. Assuming that dose adjustments for organ dysfunction, especially age associated decline in glomerular filtration rate (GFR) are made, the tolerability and efficacy of chemotherapy is likely to be similar to younger women. Newer drugs with better toxicity profiles including vinorelbine (oral and intravenous), capecitabine (oral), liposomal doxorubicin, monoclonal antibodies directed against HER2/neu protein (8) and newer schedules (with weekly taxanes or anthracyclines) may offer better tolerability and ultimately quality of life for these patients.

In addition to cytotoxic management strategies, supportive measures using bis-phosphonates (pamidronate, zoledronate and clodronate) have been shown to reduce bony morbidity and improve quality of life (9). Detailed approach to management of patients with advanced breast cancer is summarized in Figure 35.2.

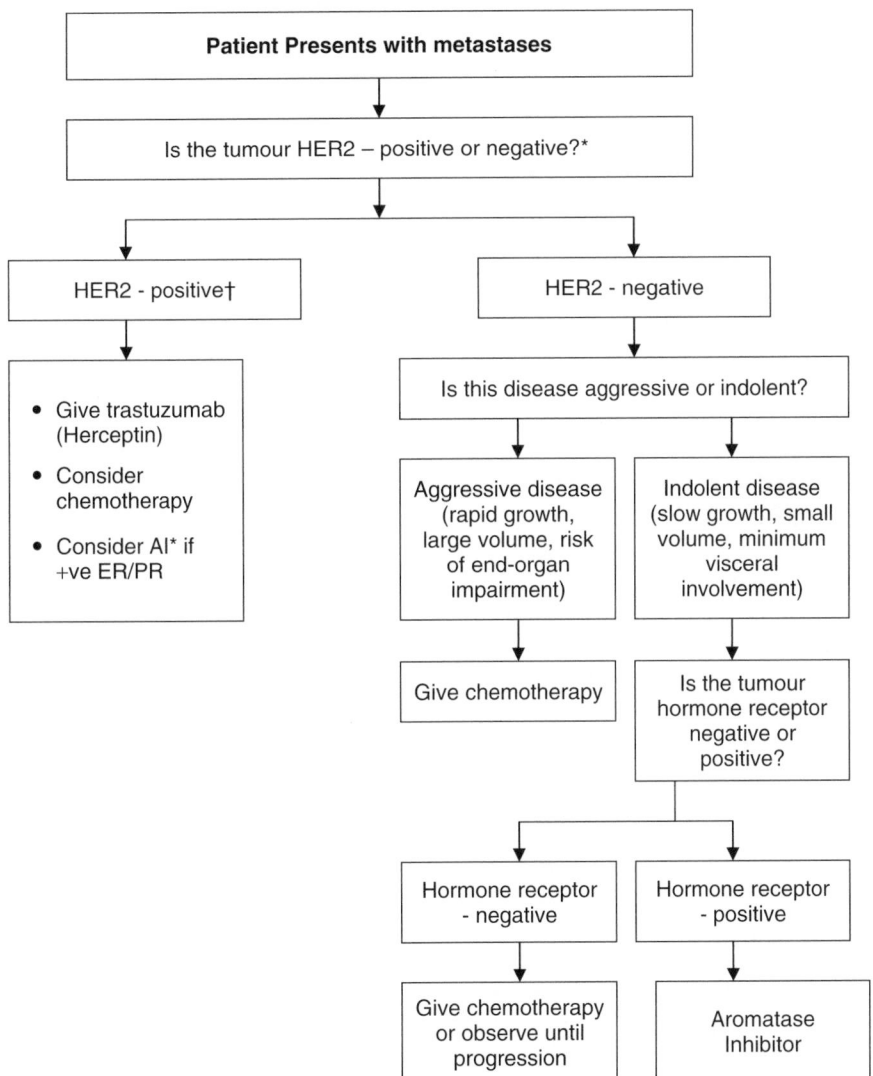

†HER2 – human epidermal growth factor receptor 2 - the majority of patients with HER2 – positive disease have hormone receptor – negative disease.

Figure 35.2. Management of metastatic breast cancer in an elderly patient

SUPPORTIVE CARE DURING BREAST CANCER TREATMENT

The use of cytotoxic chemotherapy frequently necessitates treatment with antiemetics including 5HT antagonists, metoclopramide and dexamethasone. These drugs can be associated with increased side effects in elderly patients including constipation and rarely confusion and delirium. Steroids can also precipitate glucose intolerance and unmask latent diabetes.

Recent guidelines have stressed the need for early and adequate treatment of anemia in older patients to maintain a hemoglobin level of approximately 12 g/dl as anaemia is associated with impaired outcome (10). Chemotherapy-induced neutropenia also seems to be more common and associated with a higher rate of complications, and a higher mortality in elderly individuals necessitating consideration of growth factor supports when myelotoxic chemotherapy is used.

BREAST CANCER THERAPEUTICS IN AN ELDERLY PATIENT

Specific consideration regarding the use of specific drugs used in elderly patients are summarized in Table 35.4. The key principles of breast cancer therapeutics in this population of patients relate to selecting the least toxic agent given using the most convenient schedule for the patient and making appropriate adjustments for end organ function in particular hepatic and renal clearance.

As renal function declines with age, many patients need to be evaluated for their ability to handle renally excreted drugs. The reduction in GFR may not be reflected by an increase in serum creatinine because of the simultaneous loss of muscle mass. To calculate creatinine clearance the Wright equation may provide more accurate estimates in an elderly patient. Dosing modifications is recommended to avoid

toxicity in older patients with moderate renal impairment particularly in patients treated with methotrexate (used as part of the CMF regime) and capecitabine. Similar considerations may be needed for zoledronic acid and other bisphosphanates.

Patients with severe renal impairment should not be treated with capecitabine.

Patients with liver impairment may require dose reductions of taxanes and anthracyclines or weekly administration, which is generally well tolerated in elderly patients.

CONCLUSION

Breast cancer is an important health problem in an elderly patient. Its management of breast cancer is based on similar principles as that of younger women, but in addition requires consideration of overall life expectancy, comorbid condition and functional status. Comprehensive decision-making process involving the patient is essential to identify an appropriate management strategy for individual patients.

KEY POINTS

- Breast cancer risk increases with age but the likelihood of dying of breast cancer declines with age as risks of competing comorbidities rises.
- Older women receive less treatment for breast cancer.
- Principles of treatment of breast cancer in an elderly patient are the same as in the young but require adjustments for comorbidities and functional status that influence life expectancy and treatment toxicity.
- Adjuvant hormonal therapy and for some patients chemotherapy reduce risk of recurrence and death.
- Newer chemotherapy regimes can be better tolerated in elderly patients.

Table 35.4. Selected drugs used in elderly patients* designates medications particularly well tolerated in the elderly population

Cytotoxics	Dose	Half life	Metabolism	Interactions	Important adverse events	Other tips
Capecitabine*	1250/m2 BD × 14 days every 21 days	0.85 hrs	Metabolism in liver and then in tumour	warfarin phenytoin	Hand and foot syndrome Diarrhoea Coronary spasm	Dose reduction for renal impairment Dose reduction may be useful in very elderly pts
Cyclophosphamide	500–600 mg/m2 IV every 3–4 weeks usually in combination regimes (CMF, AC, FEC) or 100 mg/m2 × 14 days as part of the oral CMF regime	2–9 hrs	Activated by hepatic microsomal enzymes to alkylating metabolism Excretion—mainly renal	warfarin ciprofloxacin	Alopecia Nausea and vomiting Myelosuppression Pneumonitis Hemorrhagic cystitis	May need dose reduction for moderate renal impairment
Docetaxel	75–100 mg/m2 every 3 weeks	11 hrs	Needs dose reduction if elevated transaminases and bilirubin	cyclosporine ketoconazole erythromycin	Fluid retention Nail changes Bone marrow suppression alopecia	
Doxorubicin	50–90 mg/m2 every 3–4 weeks or 15–30 mg/m2 weekly	16–24 hrs	Liver CYP450 Needs dose reduction for liver And in severe renal impairment	propranolol ca channel blockers cyclosporine digoxin	Bone marrow suppression Mucositis Alopecia Nausea and vomiting Cardiac impairment	Vesicant
Epirubicin	50–120 mg/m2 every 3 weeks or 25 mg/m2 weekly	30–40 hrs	As above In severe renal impairment	—	Bone marrow suppression Mucositis Alopecia Nausea and vomiting Cardiac impairment	Vesicant Weekly treatment well tolerated in elderly

(continued overleaf)

Table 35.4. (*continued*)

Cytotoxics	Dose	Half life	Metabolism	Interactions	Important adverse events	Other tips
5FU	350–600 mg/m2 weekly	10–20 min	Dose reduction for moderate hepatic impairment and in severe renal impairment	allopurinol cimetidine metronidazole warfarin	Mucositis Diarrhoea Rare neurologic Dysfunction	
Gemcitabine*	1000 mg/m2 weekly × 3 followed by week	0.7–12 hrs	Rapid metabolism in liver kidney 99 % excreted in urine dose reduction in cr cl < 30 ml	warfarin	Pulmonary toxicity	In breast cancer treatment used with paclitaxel
Liposomal Doxorubicin*	40–50 mg/m2 every 4 weeks	74 hrs	Dose reduction for liver impairment and high bili	barbiturates digoxin quinolones	Diarrhea, hep-ato/nephrotocixity Bone marrow suppression	Vesicant
Methotrexate	Variable depending on schedule	8–15 hrs	Mainly excreted by kidneys Dose reduction if cr cl low Bound to albumin	salicylates tetracyclines phenyton NSAIDs—delayed clearance	Bone marrow suppression Mucositis Diarrhea Renal impairment Liver dysfunction pneumonitis	Reversed by administration of leucovorin
Paclitaxel	175 mg/m2 every 3 weeks or 90 mg weekly	6–12 hrs	Hepatic	famotidine ketoconazole	Neuropathy Hypersensitivity reaction alopecia	Premedication with steroids required
Vinorelbine*	25–30 mg/m2 weekly	More than 40 hrs	Hepatic metabolism	CYP450 metabolised drugs	Myelosuppression Vesication Neuropathy Constipation	Vesicant

Tumour antibodies	*Dose*	Pharmacokinetics	Metabolism	Interactions	Important adverse events	Other tips
Trastuzumab	Weekly and every 3 weeks Load with 4 mg/kg 2 mg/kg weekly maintenance	6–21 days	Protein bound	anthracyclines paclitaxel warfarin	Cardiotoxicity Fever chills Pulmonary toxicity	

Hormonal preparations	*Dose*	Pharmacokinetics	Metabolism	Interactions	Important Adverse Events	Other tips
Anastrazole	1 mg daily PO	50 hrs	Hepatic	cimetidine warfarin	Osteoporosis Musculoskeletal pains	
Examestane	25 mg daily PO	24 hrs	Hepatic	CYP450	Osteoporosis Musculoskeletal pains	
Letrozole	2.5 mg daily PO	48 hrs	Hepatic	CYP450	Osteoporosis Musculoskeletal pains	
Tamoxifen	20 mg daily PO	5–7 days	Hepatic	warfarin digoxin phenytoin	Venous thromboembolism	Less bone loss than aromatase inhibitors

Bisphosphanates	*Dose*	Pharmacokinetics	Metabolism	Interactions	Important adverse events	Other tips
Pamidronate	90 mg IV every 3–4 weeks	27 hours	Renal excretion	loop diuretics	Osteonecrosis of jaw Renal impairment Hypocalcaemia fever	
Zoledronate	4 mg IV every 3–4 weeks	146 hrs	Renal excretion	loop diuretics	Osteonecrosis of jaw Renal impairment Hypocalcaemia fever	

REFERENCES

1. Yancik R, Ries LG, Yates JW. Breast cancer in aging women. A population-based study of contrast in stage, surgery and survival. *Cancer* 1989; **63**: 976–81.

2. Mandelblatt JS, Hadley J, Kerner JF, et al. Patterns of breast carcinoma treatment in older women: Patient preference and clinical and physician influences. *Cancer* 2000; **89**: 561–73.

3. Early Breast Cancer Trialists' Collaborative Group. Favourable and unfavourable effects on long-term survival of radiotherapy for early breast cancer: an overview of the randomised trials. *Lancet* 2000; **355**: 1757–70.

4. Early Breast Cancer Trialists' Collaborative Group. Tamoxifen for early breast cancer: an overview of the randomised trials. *Lancet* 1998; **351**: 1451–67.

5. Early Breast Cancer Trialists' Cooperative Group. Polychemotherapy for early breast cancer: an overview of the randomised trials. *Lancet* 1998; **352**: 930–41.

6. Howell A, Cuzick J, Baum M et al. Results of the ATAC (Arimidex, Tamoxifen, Alone or in Combination) trial after completion of 5 years' adjuvant treatment for breast cancer. *Lancet* 2005; **365**: 60–2.

7. Romond EH, Perez EA, Bryant J, Suman VJ, Geyer CE Jr, Davidson NE, Tan-Chiu E, Martino S, Paik S, Kaufman PA, Swain SM, Pisansky TM, Fehrenbacher L, Kutteh LA, Vogel VG, Visscher DW, Yothers G, Jenkins RB, Brown AM, Dakhil SR, Mamounas EP, Lingle WL, Klein PM, Ingle JN, Wolmark N. Trastuzumab plus adjuvant chemotherapy for operable HER2-positive breast cancer. *N Engl J Med*. 2005 Oct 20; **353**(16): 1673–84.

8. Slamon DJ, Leyland-Jones B, Shak S et al. Use of chemotherapy plus a monoclonal antibody against HER2 for metastatic breast cancer that overexpresses HER2. *New England Journal of Medicine* 2001; **344**: 783–92.

9. Hortobabyi GN, Theriault RL, Porter L, et al. Efficacy of pamidronate in reducing skeletal complications in patients with breast cancer and lytic bone metastases. *New England Journal of Medicine* 1996; **335**: 1785–91.

10. Balducci L, Yates J. General guidelines for the management of older patients with cancer. *Oncology* (Williston Park) 2000; **14**: 221–7.

36 Pharmacological management of endocrine conditions in the elderly patient

Nikolai Petrovsky

Department of Endocrinology, Flinders Medical Centre, Adelaide, Australia

INTRODUCTION

Endocrine problems common in elderly patients include hypogonadism, osteoporosis, multinodular goiter and endocrine tumours. However, by far the most common endocrine disease in this group is diabetes mellitus. Up to 50 % of individuals over the age of 75 demonstrate impaired glucose tolerance or frank type 2 diabetes. Complications of diabetes include hyperosmolar coma, renal failure, vision loss, peripheral nerve damage, vascular disease and increased risk of infection, all common problems in elderly patients. Special challenges with dealing with diabetes and other endocrine disorders in elderly patients arise as a consequence of altered drug metabolism, coexistent diseases and general problems of frailty and immobility. The first half of this chapter will focus on diabetes in the elderly with the second half dealing with other endocrine conditions affecting elderly patients.

DIABETES AETIOLOGY

Type 2 diabetes is by far the most prevalent form of diabetes in elderly patients with an approximate ratio of at least 10:1 compared to type 1 diabetes. Whilst most elderly patients with type 1 diabetes will have developed it when young, type 1 diabetes can present at any age, leading to the naming of a new entity called LADA (latent autoimmune diabetes of adults). It is estimated that up to 10 % of adults initially diagnosed with type 2 diabetes in fact have LADA. Type 2 diabetes results from the combination of peripheral insulin resistance with impaired beta cell insulin secretion. Whilst most individuals with type 2 diabetes may have a genetic predisposition to insulin resistance, the major factor driving development of type 2 diabetes in elderly subjects is increased central visceral obesity. Insulin resistance increases in direct proportion to increased intra-abdominal fat. As people age they tend to exercise less while maintaining a similar caloric intake as when they were young and more active. This imbalance between food consumption and energy expenditure translates into increased body fat stores as people age and thereby increased insulin resistance. Conditions that impair exercise capacity in elderly patients including arthritis, cardiac failure, airways disease, muscle weakness, or reduced vision or balance increase the risk of accumulating excess body fat and type 2 diabetes (Table 36.1).

Prescribing for Elderly Patients   Edited by Stephen Jackson, Paul Jansen and Arduino Mangoni
© 2009 John Wiley & Sons, Ltd

Table 36.1. Potential causes of diabetes mellitus
in the elderly

Primary type 2 diabetes
    Obesity
    Inactivity
Secondary type 2 diabetes
    Chronic pancreatitis
    Acromegaly
    Cushing's syndrome or glucocorticoid
      medication
    Haemochromatosis
    Mitochondrial myopathy
Other
    Latent autoimmune diabetes of adults (LADA)

The cause of impaired beta cell insulin secretion in elderly individuals developing type 2 diabetes is less well understood. Metabolic factors including high blood glucose and free fatty acids have been shown to induce beta cell apoptosis (death) and may be the cause of beta cell loss in type 2 diabetes. Other causes of diabetes should also be considered in elderly subjects. Chronic pancreatitis can be overlooked as a cause of diabetes mellitus and should be considered in the setting of known alcohol or drug abuse, or diabetes occurring in the setting of malnourishment or malabsorption. Other secondary forms of diabetes that need to be considered include thyroid disease and endocrine tumours causing insulin resistance. In particular, growth hormone excess due to acromegaly or glucocorticoid excess due to Cushing's syndrome may underly hyperglycaemia. Rarer causes of diabetes in the elderly include haemochromatosis, pancreatic tumours or beta cell failure due to mitochondrial or other rare genetic disorders (Table 36.1).

DIABETES SYMPTOMS AND SIGNS

It is estimated that up to 50 % of adults with type 2 diabetes in the community remain undiagnosed at any one time. Given that type 2 diabetes prevalence increases with age, this means that the majority of undiagnosed cases of diabetes will be in elderly patients. Type 2 diabetes often develops insidiously, with the classic symptoms of hyperglycaemia namely thirst and polyuria only occurring very late in the disease process. Thus, routine screening even in the absence of symptoms is the best method for early detection. Also, a high index of clinical suspicion of diabetes should be maintained when elderly patients present with tiredness, confusion, or recurrent infections such as urinary tract infections, candidiasis or skin infections.

DIABETES DIAGNOSIS

Because of its insidious nature, all elderly patients presenting with obesity, hypertension, hyperlipidaemia, cardiovascular, cerebrovascular or peripheral vascular disease should be screened for diabetes given the close association of metabolic syndrome, diabetes and vascular disease. At the other end of the spectrum elderly patients with unrecognized type 2 diabetes who become dehydrated may present in a hyperosmolar coma. This is a state of extremely high blood sugar levels due to haemoconcentration and reduced intravascular volume, and is associated with an extremely high mortality rate. Non-ketotic hyperosmolar coma commonly occurs in the setting of an elderly person with unrecognized diabetes, who becomes increasingly hyperglycaemic, e.g. in response to infection, develops secondary polyuria due to the osmotic effect of increased urinary glucose, and who because of confusion or frailty is unable to drink or access sufficient fluids to prevent dehydration. Increasing dehydration causes the blood and urine glucose levels to rise which in turn increases the level of dehydration in a vicious cycle. Not surprisingly this is a particular problem of frail elderly people, particularly those living alone, and hence the importance of screening at risk elderly subjects for type 2 diabetes on a regular basis.

Differences exist in diagnostic criteria for diabetes mellitus, under guidelines of international bodies including the World Health Organisation and American Diabetes

Association (ADA). Whilst bodies such as ADA recommend reliance on fasting glucose levels for diagnosis of diabetes, namely a fasting plasma glucose greater or equal to 7.0 mmol/L, other guidelines continue to emphasize the importance of the oral glucose tolerance test (OGTT), with a two hour post 75 gram-OGTT plasma glucose greater or equal to 11.1 mmol/L, being diagnostic of diabetes.

TYPE 2 DIABETES MANAGEMENT

Just as in young patients, the mainstay of type 2 diabetes management when presenting in elderly patients should be exercise, diet and weight reduction. Surprisingly, the Diabetes Prevention Study found the greatest reductions in progression to type 2 diabetes in subjects over the age of 65, when compared to younger subjects, in response to an exercise and diet regime. The results of this study dispel the myth that diet and exercise are impractical or ineffective when applied to elderly patients with type 2 diabetes. Whilst many elderly patients with type 2 diabetes will benefit from diet, exercise and weight loss management, a significant proportion will continue to have significant hyperglycaemia despite these benefits and will consequently require pharmacological treatment.

Ageing is commonly associated with decreased hepatic or renal clearance of drugs and care should be taken when introducing hypoglycaemic agents in elderly patients. Death caused by drug-induced hypoglycaemia is an ongoing but avoidable problem in elderly diabetic patients. The dangers of over-treatment of diabetes in the elderly may be considerably greater than the consequences of under-treatment. Compounding the normal age-related decline in renal and hepatic function that reduces clearance of drugs in the elderly is the specific damage to the kidneys and liver as a result of diabetes itself.

The recommended first line agent in type 2 diabetes, both young and elderly, is metformin. This is because metformin works as an insulin sensitiser improving hepatic insulin sensitivity. In addition, metformin has other advantages over other hypoglycaemic medications in that its use is not associated with significant hypoglycaemia and it is an anorexiant that induces weight loss rather than weight gain. This in turn improves insulin sensitivity and overall diabetes control. Serious side effects of metformin are rare with the most common side effect being mild gastrointestinal upset manifesting as bloating, indigestion, diarrhoea or constipation which often abates over time even when the drug is continued. The risk of gastrointestinal side effects of metformin can be minimized by first introducing metformin at a relatively low dose, for example 500 mg per day, and then slowly increasing the dose on a fortnightly basis as tolerated with the aim of achieving an effective dose of 1.5–3 g per day. Metformin is renally excreted and therefore lower doses should be used in elderly subjects with significantly reduced renal function. Whilst many pharmacology textbooks state that metformin may cause lactic acidosis, in fact this was a problem restricted to an earlier drug phenformin, and a recent published Cochrane review found no evidence of an association between metformin and lactic acidosis in subjects with normal renal function. In addition, in the United Kingdom Prospective Diabetes Study, a group of obese subjects commenced on metformin as a first line agent had a significant and very major reduction in cardiovascular events, a feature not seen with patients initiated on sulphonylureas or insulin. This suggests that over and above its ability to reduce blood glucose levels metformin also has a cardioprotective effect. For the above reasons and because it doesn't cause life threatening hypoglycaemia, metformin remains one of the safest diabetes drugs for use in elderly patients. It should be noted that whilst the weight reducing effects of metformin make it an ideal drug for use in obese individuals with type 2 diabetes, it is also effective in non-overweight individuals with type 2 diabetes, and therefore its use as a first line agent should not be restricted to only those who are obese. As metformin is renally excreted dose reductions should be made in individuals with reduced renal function and metformin is contraindicated in those with a glomerular filtration rate <30 ml/min.

In a significant proportion of patients, metformin alone may be insufficient to control hyperglycaemia in which case a second line hypoglycaemic agent needs to be added. Traditionally, sulphonylureas were used as second line agents although over recent years the thiazolidenediones are also being used as second line agents. Whilst sulphonyureas might be effective at lowering blood sugar levels, their use is associated with significant risks and side effects, most particularly weight gain usually of the order of 3–5 kg, and an increased risk of serious and prolonged hypoglycaemia, occasionally leading to coma or death. Both weight gain and hypoglycaemia are major problems for elderly patients taking sulphonyureas, and the risk of sulphonyurea-induced hypoglycaemia is increased in the presence of hepatic or renal impairment given that sulphonyureas are excreted via both routes.

Thiazolidenediones, principally pioglitazone, are also used as a second line agents in type 2 diabetes. The advantages of thiazolidenediones are that they like metformin are insulin sensitizers, working at the level of fat, muscle and to a lesser extent liver to increase insulin sensitivity. Hence when given alone or in combination with metformin they do not cause hypoglycaemia, unlike sulponylureas. The most common side effect of thiazolidenediones is weight gain of 1–3 kg due to fluid retention, and this may be associated with marked ankle oedema in up to 10 % of individuals taking them. Since this drug induced fluid retention can precipitate acute pulmonary oedema in individuals with underlying heart disease, thiazolidenediones should be avoided in elderly subjects with known heart disease.

Other oral hypoglycaemic agents include meglitinides, a class of drugs that work by inducing insulin secretion and acarbose, a unique drug that works by inhibiting gut carbohydrate absorption and commonly causes excess flatulence and gastrointestinal symptoms.

Another downside to both meglitinides and acarbose is that they are both short-acting and therefore need to be taken at least three times a day with each meal, and this may lead to reduced compliance.

Another recent advance in type 2 diabetes is the development of a new class of drugs working on the incretin pathway, the first example of which is exenatide. Many drugs that work through the incretin pathway are in late stage development and these are either incretin analogues like exenatide or work through inhibiting the major endogenous enzyme dipeptidyl peptidase IV that breaks down endogenous incretins. In either case the effects of elevating incretin levels is to stimulate postprandial insulin and suppress glucagon secretion, and slow down gastric emptying. Other important positive effects of incretin drugs acting are that like metformin they induce beneficial weight reduction. Furthermore, incretins have been shown at least in animal models to stimulate growth of new beta cells. However at this stage experience of incretin use in the elderly population remains limited.

The final therapeutic option in type 2 diabetes if all else fails is insulin. Insulin is the most potent currently available hypoglycaemic agent and approximately 30 % of individuals with type 2 diabetes will receive insulin at some point in their disease. These days it is routine to continue oral insulin sensitisers, namely metformin in subjects with type 2 diabetes commencing insulin unless there is a clear contraindication. Co-administration of insulin sensitisers is associated with improved glycaemic control compared to insulin alone, reduces the total amount of insulin required to be injected, and in the case of metformin, reduces the marked weight gain seen with insulin initiation which is typically of the order of 5–8 kg. Apart from the problems of weight gain the other serious downside to insulin therapy in the elderly diabetic patient is the increased risk of serious hypoglycaemia. This risk is particularly high in elderly subjects with either hepatic or renal insufficiency as the half life of insulin is increased in renal impairment and the ability of the liver to compensate for hypoglycaemia by gluconeogenesis and glycolysis is reduced in the presence of liver disease. If insulin is to be used in the elderly diabetic then consideration should be given to introduction of a single daily dose of Glargine insulin, which is a peakless synthetic analogue insulin with 24 hour duration and which is associated with less hypoglycaemia and less weight gain than isophane insulins or pre-mixed insulins.

The objectives of diabetes treatment in very elderly patients should be increasingly skewed towards symptom control and avoidance of serious drug-related side effects. Overzealous treatment of glucose levels particularly in those over the age of 70 years or those frail and incapacitated, has the potential of doing more harm than good. A recent study showed no significant increase in mortality rates when people diagnosed with type 2 diabetes at 70 years of age or older were compared to non-diabetic peers. Thus excess mortality in elderly subjects with diabetes is almost totally concentrated in those who developed diabetes at a much younger age, indicating that type 2 diabetes must be present for many years before detrimental effects manifest. Thus there is little justification for overly aggressive hypoglycaemic therapy in elderly new-onset diabetes patients, and any hypoglycaemic therapy should be tempered against the patient's age of diabetes onset and expected life expectancy in the absence of diabetes. Reduction of mortality in elderly subjects with new onset type 2 diabetes is better achieved from aggressive blood pressure and lipid lowering than from an undue focus on glycaemic control as there is currently little data that better glycaemic control alone has major effects on reducing mortality rates in elderly diabetes subjects as compared to treatment with statins, aspirin, angiotensin converting inhibitors, and other antihypertensive agents.

Prior to commencement of oral hypoglycaemics a full assessment needs to be undertaken, including cardiovascular examination and biochemical assessment of renal and hepatic function, to identify those most at risk of drug associated side effects. Hypoglycaemic medication should be started judiciously and at low dose, and then progressively increased with the aim of firstly controlling hyperglycaemic symptoms, i.e thirst and polyuria, and only secondarily if life expectancy justifies it, tighter glycaemic control with the objective of preventing or slowing long-term diabetes complications, e.g. retinopathy, nephropathy and neuropathy.

If hypoglycaemic therapy is felt justified then metformin is the preferential first line agent with sulphonylureas or thiazolidenediones being used as second or third line and insulin when all else fails. For particular patients acarbose or meglitinides may also be useful in some cases. If insulin is required then a single daily dose of glargine in addition to continuing insulin sensitizers is preferred. Given that diabetes control can be improved by reductions in insulin resistance, drugs or interventions that reduce weight and body fat such as sibutramine, orlistat or gastric banding can also be used to help control obesity and type 2 diabetes in the elderly.

Figure 36.1 illustrates current recommendations for treatment of diabetes in the elderly.

PHARMACOKINETIC AND PHARMACODYNAMIC DATA OF DIABETES MEDICATIONS IN ELDERLY PATIENTS

Elderly subjects commonly have multiple medical problems rather than just diabetes alone and this need to be taken into consideration when commencing therapy. In particular, elderly diabetic patients may also have vascular disease, kidney and liver impairment, degenerative arthritis, and dementing processes all of which may impact upon and interact with diabetes drug therapy. This has implications for drug plasma protein binding, metabolism, and clearance and also greatly increases the risk of potential drug-drug interactions. The presence of multiple disease states in the one elderly individual increases overall frailty and thereby increases the risk of drug associated morbidity and mortality. For example, a fall

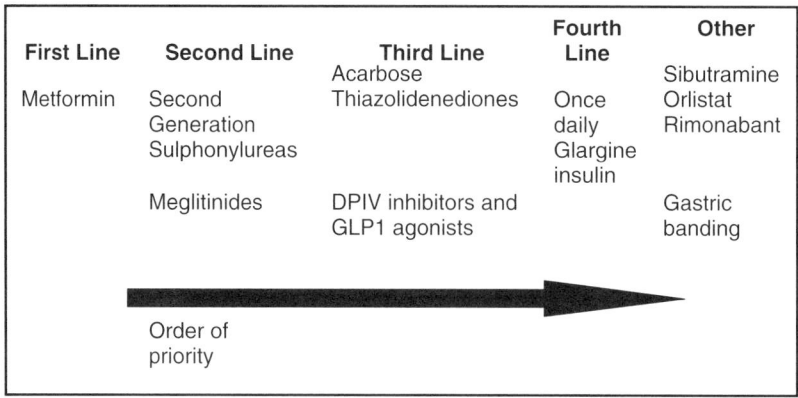

First Line	Second Line	Third Line	Fourth Line	Other
		Acarbose		Sibutramine
Metformin	Second Generation Sulphonylureas	Thiazolidenediones	Once daily Glargine insulin	Orlistat Rimonabant
	Meglitinides	DPIV inhibitors and GLP1 agonists		Gastric banding

Order of priority

Figure 36.1. Relative preference of diabetes drugs in elderly patients

in an elderly diabetic subject caused by hypoglycaemia from sulphonylurea therapy may result in an osteoporotic hip or vertebral fracture which in turn may result in death of the patient.

CLINICALLY IMPORTANT DRUG INTERACTIONS WITHIN DIABETES DRUGS

The aim of diabetes management in elderly patients should be directed towards control of hyperglycaemic symptoms and prevention of premature mortality by reduction of vascular risk factors. If hyperglycaemic symptom control is not achieved with monotherapy then an additional hypoglycaemic medication will need to be added, as no one oral hypoglycaemic medication is any more potent than the other, with maximal doses of metformin, sulphonylureas or thiazolidenediones all reducing blood sugar levels by the same approximate amount. Where possible, given the possible that they will be on multiple other medications and are at increased risk of confusion regarding their medications, there is clear benefit from testing whether symptom control can be achieved by optimizing the dose of one hypoglycaemic medication in elderly patients rather

than introduction of dual hypoglycaemic therapy too early.

GENERAL ADVERSE EFFECTS OF DIABETES MEDICATIONS IN ELDERLY PATIENTS

Diabetes drugs are very commonly prescribed especially in the elderly group where diabetes prevalence is extremely high. Adverse drug events relating to diabetes medications are common and cause hospital admission, major morbidity and excess mortality in elderly diabetes patients. The common side effects of diabetes agents are generally well known, with hypoglycaemia being the most frequent and common to all diabetes medications with the possible exception of metformin and thiazolidenediones. Diabetes medications are thus major culprits for adverse drug events, particularly the long acting sulphonylureas and insulin because of their ability to induce life threatening hypoglycaemia. Another common adverse effect of diabetes drugs is weight gain, with sulphonylureas or thiazolidenediones causing 3–4 kg of weight gain and insulin upwards of 5–8 kg of weight gain. Other common side effects of diabetes medications include gastrointestinal upset and allergic skin reactions.

SPECIFIC ADVERSE EFFECTS AND CLINICALLY-IMPORTANT DRUG INTERACTIONS OF DIABETES DRUGS

Adverse drug events may occur due to inter-action between diabetes drugs and other agents or diseases, for example cerebral haemorrhage caused by commencement of sulphonylureas in a patient on warfarin due to the sulphonylureas ability to interfere with the metabolism of war-farin.

The adverse effects of sulphonylureas apart from weight gain, include gastrointestinal upset, a disulfiram-like syndrome, skin reactions, haema-tological abnormalities and the syndrome of in-appropriate secretion of antidiuretic hormone. Common drug interactions are seen with sulpho-nylureas given their metabolism by the liver cy-tochrome P450 system. Meglitinide metabolites and thiazolidinediones are also highly depen-dent on the liver cytochrome P450 system for their metabolism and are therefore also prone to drug-drug metabolic interactions. Amongst rele-vant agents with which P450 related drug-drug in-teractions may occur include statins, gemfibrozil and angiotensin converting enzyme inhibitors, all of which may potentiate the hypoglycaemic effect of sulphonyureas, meglitinides or the thi-azolidenediones by reducing their metabolism. Other potentially important interactions may oc-cur between these oral hypoglycaemic drugs and digoxin and warfarin.

It is relevant to note that there are no clini-cally relevant drug-drug interactions with met-formin, because metformin is not metabolized by the liver and does not inhibit the metabolism of other drugs, making it ideal for use in el-derly type 2 diabetes patients who are already on large numbers of medications and are at high risk of adverse effects due to drug-drug inter-actions. Metformin, particularly if the dose is escalated too rapidly, has the potential to cause major discomfort from gastrointestinal distur-bance and diarrhoea, although in many cases this abates with dose reduction and longer-term usage. Although lactic acidosis is highlighted as a major risk in all pharmacology textbooks when discussing metformin, despite millions of years of patient use experience, there are very few reports of metformin induced lactic acidosis, a conclusion highlighted by a recent Cochrane review and several editorials on this topic.

Fluid retention is a common adverse effect of thiazolidenedione therapy with potential to precipitate pulmonary oedema in patients with pre-existing cardiac disease. Recently, thiazo-lidinediones have been associated with increased bone fracture risk. Also, rosiglitazone has been associated with increased risk of ischemic heart disease. Acarbose, a competitive inhibitor of in-testinal alpha-glucosidases, is rarely if at all asso-ciated with major life-threatening adverse effects but does commonly cause gastrointestinal distur-bances particularly excess flatulence.

The most serious adverse effect of insulin is hypoglycaemia, with potential to result in death particularly in elderly frail patients living alone. Lesser adverse effects are injection site reac-tions and/or bruising or pain on injection and rarely allergic skin reactions which are typically to one of the incipients in which the insulin is formulated. Angiotensin converting enzyme inhibitors, angiotensin 2 receptors inhibitors, other antihypertensive agents and statins are so frequently used in management of individuals with type 2 diabetes that they could also be re-garded as true diabetes drugs. Specific adverse effects of drugs blocking the renin-angiotensin system includes angiooedema, cough, hyper-kalaemia and renal dysfunction and of statins include myopathy and hepatitis.

PITUITARY ADENOMAS

Although the vast majority (>90%) of pitu-itary adenomas occur in people under the age of 65, of the adenomas that do occur in el-derly patients there is an overrepresentation of non-secreting adenomas. Because they are non secreting these adenomas will only be identified when they become large macroadenomas with space compressing effects, or are picked up coincidentally during cranial imaging for other reasons. In addition, even where a macroadenoma does occur in elderly patients, it may be missed because its symptoms overlap with other comorbidities that the patient may have. Thus, for example subtle visual field defects due to optic chiasm compression could be missed in elderly patients who have known age-related eye disease. This is highly relevant because visual impairment is the most common form of clinical presentation of pituitary tumours in elderly patients with the next more common presentation being symptoms of endocrine hormone excess or deficiency. Headache is noted by up to a quarter of patients particularly those with acromegaly but is a non-specific symptom. Other rare presentations include pituitary apoplexy or cranial nerve palsy.

The symptoms of hormone hypersecretion are dominated by growth hormone hypersecretion (acromegaly) since prolactin hypersecretion commonly causes no symptoms in postmenopausal women or elderly men. Hypopituitarism is clinically underestimated in elderly patients because they are less likely than in younger patients to have classical symptoms and in any case symptoms of pituitary hypofunction may overlap with symptoms of ageing. Given the marked decline in IGF-1 levels with age, age-corrected IGF-1 levels should be used in elderly patients with suspected acromegaly. Similarly, androgen deficiency in elderly men may be difficult to interpret in order to distinguish true hypogonadotropic hypogonadism due to an adenoma suppressing LH production from normal age-related decline in testosterone levels in elderly men.

Therapy of adenomas in elderly patients needs to be appropriate to their age, physical condition, comorbidities and life expectancy. Most adenomas are slowly growing and treatment therefore should be directed towards control of the disease while taking care to maintain or improve the patient's quality of life. Therapeutic options are the same as in younger patients including surgery,

medical therapy with dopamine-agonists or somatostatin analogues or radiotherapy. Any hormone replacement for hypopituitarism should be tailored to the patient's age and physical condition. Thus, for example, caution should be used when replacing thyroid hormone in elderly patients with TSH deficiency particularly where they might have ischaemic heart disease as a co-morbidity, as overaggressive replacement may aggravate their ischaemia via increased metabolic oxygen demand. Treatment for central hypothyroidism should always be preceded by assessment of adrenal function and where required adequate glucocorticoid hormone replacement to avoid risk of precipitating an adrenal crisis.

Transphenoidal surgery is the treatment of choice for elderly patients presenting with major visual disturbances or severe acromegalic symptoms if their overall condition is suitable for surgery. Interestingly, recovery of hypopituitarism postoperatively appears to be less frequent in elderly patients. Dopamine agonists are first choice for prolactinomas, as they both normalize prolactin and shrink prolactinomas in the majority of cases. Caution needs to be taken however when using dopamine agonists since the side effects of dizziness and postural hypotension may cause particular problems in this group. In general, microprolactinomas rarely increase in size over time and elderly women with isolated hyperprolactinaemia due to an adenoma that does not exhibit space occupying effects probably do not require treatment with a dopamine agonist. Radiotherapy of the pituitary is a less commonly utilized modality of treatment in elderly patients, given that it can take up to five years to become effective, which may be beyond the life expectancy of the patient anyway.

THYROID DISEASE

Thyroid function problems increase with age and therefore is extremely common in elderly patients, where it may go undiagnosed due to non-specificity of symptoms and signs. In a study in Levanto, thyroid function alterations were discovered in approximately an eight of elderly patients admitted to an hospital and in those with a thyroid function alteration almost half had hypothyroidism and under a quarter, hyperthyroidism. Hypothyroidism can be difficult to diagnose in the elderly as symptoms such as tiredness, fatigue, and weight gain can easily be overlooked as symptoms of ageing. As noted above, therapy of hypothyroidism should be undertaken with caution in the elderly due to the risk of aggravating comorbitities such as ischaemic heart disease. Furthermore, the appropriate replacement dose of thyroid hormone tends to be less in the elderly due to a reduction in thyroid hormone metabolism. Hyperthyroidism is also common in elderly patient, and may present atypically, e.g. with cardiac symptoms. Definitive treatment of hyperthyroidism due to autoimmune thyroid disease or toxic multinodular goitre is usually with radioactive iodine, after a course of antithyroid drugs to render the patient euthyroid, surgery being largely reserved to those elderly patients who have co-existing compressive symptoms from their toxic multinodular goitre.

Apart from thyroid hormone disturbances, thyroid masses are extremely common in elderly patients most commonly due to thyroid nodules. Most thyroid nodules in the elderly are not malignant but careful attempts must be made to distinguish those that are. Ultrasound and where necessary fine needle aspiration for cytology are the most commonly used tools to make the distinction of which nodules require surgery, with thyroid nucleotide scanning having little or no role. Although the majority thyroid tumours in elderly patients are well-differentiated papillary cancers just as in the young, there is a higher relative incidence of undifferentiated cancers and thyroid lymphomas in elderly patients. Multinodular goiter is extremely common in elderly patients and if asymptomatic rarely requires intervention. Where compressive symptoms occur, if mild these may be alleviated by radioiodine that can cause gland shrinkage by the order of up to 20 %, but if compression is severe surgery is the only answer. Patients found to have papillary cancer at surgery, would normally have total thyroid resection followed by radioactive iodine ablation after being rendered hypothyroid to maximise the uptake of radioiodine. Thyroid cancer in elderly patients has a worse prognosis than for younger patients. In the elderly, because of the increased risk of severe symptoms from hypothyroidism, with the availability of recombinant TSH, this provides an alternative to avoid the need for induction of hypothyroidism in elderly patients.

HYPERPARATHYROIDISM

Primary hyperparathyroidism is a common coincidental finding in elderly patients due to the increased prevalence of regular biochemical screening including serum calcium levels in these age groups. Secondary hyperparathyroidism commonly occurs in a setting of vitamin D deficiency and this should be screened for and treated in all patients with elevated levels of parathyroid hormone. Although hyperparathyroidism is curable by surgery, elderly patients with asymptomatic hypercalcaemia due to hyperparathyroidism commonly do well with conservative follow up, with no good evidence being available of any benefit to these patients from early surgery. Thus, surgery is normally reserved for those elderly patients who are fit enough for the procedure, and who either have kidney stones, significant osteoporosis greater than expected for their age or total serum calcium over 3.0 mmol/L.

HORMONE REPLACEMENT

Elderly men exhibit age related declines in production of testosterone, albeit not as abrupt as the loss of oestrogen in women passing the menopause. The loss of androgens contributes to the symptoms of ageing including loss of muscle and bone mass. Similarly there is a progressive decline in both women and men in growth hormone and IGF1 levels with age, which has been linked to some of the skin and muscle changes of ageing. Fierce debate still rages as to whether these changes of ageing can be slowed or arrested by appropriate androgen or growth hormone replacement and, if so, whether the potential side effects of such therapy, such as the increased risk of prostate cancer with testosterone therapy, outweigh the benefits. In absence of resolution of this debate one way or the other, it must be left to the clinician and the individual elderly patient to decide whether such hormone replacement therapy is warranted or not.

ENDOCRINE DISEASE IN THE ELDERLY—KEY POINTS

- Diet and exercise are often overlooked in the management of type 2 diabetes.
- Optimal management of type 2 diabetes must include minimisation of vascular risk factors including adequate control of hypertension and hyperlipidaemia.
- Goals of treatment of hyperglycaemia should primarily be directed towards symptom control and only secondarily towards long-term complication avoidance in those whose life expectancy justifies it.
- Benefits of reduction of asymptomatic hyperglycaemia in elderly patients need to be weighed against risks of major adverse reactions and drug-drug reactions.
- There is strong evidence in favour of metformin as the preferred treatment for initial monotherapy of type 2 diabetes in elderly patients.
- Insulin may ultimately be required to control hyperglycaemia in up to 30 % of individuals with type 2 diabetes, but side effects of insulin including major weight gain and life-threatening hypoglycaemia remain powerful negatives against use of insulin particularly in the elderly frail population.
- Visual field defects are the most common presenting sign of pituitary adenomas in elderly patients, with the other common presentation

being as an incidentaloma discovered during brain imaging for another reason.
- Elderly patients require lower doses of thyroid hormone replacement due to reduced metabolism and may get exacerbation of co-morbid ischaemic heart disease if replacement is too rapid.
- Adrenal function should always be assessed and where necessary replaced before commencement of thyroid hormone replacement to avoid risk of precipitating an adrenal crisis.
- Hyperparathyroidism in elderly patients is commonly associated with vitamin D deficiency which should be screened for and treated.
- The restoration of falling androgen and growth hormone levels in elderly patients to retard the effects of ageing remains highly controversial and is best managed on a case by case basis.

FURTHER READING

Salas M, Caro JJ. Are hypoglycaemia and other adverse effects similar among sulphonylureas? *Adverse Drug React Toxicol Rev*. 2002; **21**(4): 205–17.

Scheen AJ. Drug interactions of clinical importance with antihyperglycaemic agents: an update. *Drug Saf*. 2005; **28**(7): 601–31.

GC Jones J P Macklin, W D Alexander Editorials: Contraindications to the use of metformin–Evidence suggests that it is time to amend the list. *BMJ* 2003; **326**: 4–5.

Barnett, K. McMurdo, M. et al. Mortality in people diagnosed with type 2 diabetes at an older age: a systematic review. *Age and Ageing* 2006; **35**: 463–8.

Sakharova OV, Inzucchi, SE Treatment of diabetes in the elderly. Addressing its complexities in this high-risk group *Postgrad Med*. 2005; **118**(5): 19–26, 29.

Holstein A, Stumvoll M. Contraindications can damage your health–is metformin a case in point? *Diabetologia*. 2005; **48**(12): 2454–9. Epub 2005 Nov 11.

Oiknine R, Mooradian AD. Drug therapy of diabetes in the elderly 2003; **57**(5–6): 231–9.

Knowler WC, Barrett-Connor E, Fowler SE, Hamman RF, Lachin JM, Walker EA, Nathan DM; Diabetes Prevention Program Research Group. Reduction in the incidence of type 2 diabetes with lifestyle intervention or metformin. *N Engl J Med*. 2002 7; **346**(6): 393–403.

Minniti G, Esposito V, Piccirilli M, Fratticci A, Santoro A, Jaffrain-Rea M-L Diagnosis and management of pituitary tumours in the elderly: a review based on personal experience and evidence of literature. *European Journal of Endocrinology*, **153**(6): 723–35.

37 Rheumatoid arthritis, osteoarthritis, polymyalgia rheumatica, gout and pseudogout

E. Michael Shanahan[1] and Stephen Hedger[2]

[1]*Department of Rheumatology, Flinders Medical Centre and Repatriation General Hospital, Adelaide, Australia*
[2]*Department of General Medicine, Flinders Medical Centre, Adelaide, Australia*

RHEUMATOID ARTHRITIS

Introduction

Rheumatoid arthritis (RA) is the commonest form of inflammatory arthritis, with an overall population prevalence of between 0.5 and 2 %. The prevalence increases with increasing age, with mean age of onset in the fourth and fifth decades possibly reaching a peak at around 85 years (1). The prevalence in the population who are over 60 years is reported to be approximately 2 % (2).

Despite current treatment strategies, RA remains an important cause of morbidity, functional disability and premature death.

Aetiology

The aetiology of RA remains unknown. A combination of genetic and environmental factors (possibly including infection) appears to play a major role in its aetiology. There is a strong association with major histocompatibility complex class II allele human leukocyte antigen (HLA)-DR4, and also HLA-DR-1 and DR 14.

The pathophysiology of RA at the joint involves the development of synovitis and subsequent joint destruction. Tissue necrosis factor alpha (TNF-α) and interleukin-1 are important cytokines enhancing synovial proliferation and they also stimulate the secretion of matrix metalloproteinases, other inflammatory cytokines and adhesion molecules. Proinflammatory cytokines in the disease process are produced by activated T-cells, macrophages and fibroblasts.

Symptoms and signs

Rheumatoid arthritis is a systemic illness with multiple clinical manifestations. Classically it presents as a small joint, symmetrical polyarthritis which may be rapidly destructive, with 60 % of patients developing erosions on x-ray within two years of diagnosis (3).

Elderly onset rheumatoid arthritis (EORA) is sometimes recognized as a subset of RA. Features that may distinguish EORA from younger onset disease include a possible higher prevalence in males, a higher likelihood of acute onset, more systemic features including weight loss, a higher prevalence of shoulder joint involvement (sometimes resembling polymyalgia rheumatica [PMR]) and a rapid functional

Prescribing for Elderly Patients   Edited by Stephen Jackson, Paul Jansen and Arduino Mangoni
© 2009 John Wiley & Sons, Ltd

decline (4). However, diagnostic imprecision may account for some of the previously reported heterogeneity of the disease in elderly populations (1). The syndrome of remitting seronegative symmetrical synovitis with pitting oedema (RS3PE) is a relatively benign steroid responsive polyarthritis which occurs specifically in elderly patients and may represent a subgroup of RA.

RA that has developed many years previously is commonly seen in older patients. In these cases the clinical picture reflects the duration of the disease and the adequacy of the control over that period. The clinical picture may include varying degrees of active synovitis, joint destruction and deformity, joint replacement surgery and the effects of long term therapy (including long term steroid use). In addition, multi-organ disease effects on the lung, skin, vascular and nervous system and kidney in particular may result in considerable morbidity.

Diagnosis

The diagnosis of RA can be difficult in the elderly population. Systemic symptoms and large joint involvement may dominate over the more typical findings of a symmetrical, small joint synovitis. Some serological markers such as rheumatoid factor (RF) and erythrocyte sedimentation rate (ESR) are less specific in elderly patients (5). Anticyclic citrullinated antibody (anti-CCP) may be more specific (6). C-reactive protein (CRP) is of value in monitoring disease activity. Other laboratory indicators such as hypergammaglobulinemia, anaemia, occasional hypocomplementaemia, thrombocytopaenia and eosinophilia are more commonly seen in more severe RA and are also seen in conditions more common in elderly patients. Radiographs are of limited utility in the early diagnosis of RA and typical features of peri-articular osteopaenia, soft tissue swelling and (later) loss of joint space and joint erosions can be difficult to distinguish in the presence of other joint changes in the elderly patient.

RA in elderly patients should be distinguished from other common causes of polyarthritis in this age group including PMR,

crystal arthropathies, osteoarthritis and paraneoplastic syndromes.

Therapy

Pharmacotherapy remains the cornerstone of RA management in elderly patients. However it should be remembered that a multi-disciplinary approach including appropriate physical therapy, the provision of aids, timely surgical intervention and environmental modification can all play significant roles in reducing morbidity and maintaining independence.

The therapeutic aims of disease management in elderly patients are to maintain function, relieve pain and minimize disease progression. Management of RA in elderly patients requires flexibility and is complicated by the presence of co-morbidities, altered age-related physiology and pharmacokinetics and also issues of polypharmacy including drug compliance and drug interactions.

Disease modifying anti-rheumatic drugs (DMARDS) are the most important group of drugs used in the management of RA. Drugs in this group are used as single agents or increasingly in combination to suppress the disease process. Table 37.1 outlines the major DMARDS in use currently, and summarises some special considerations for their use in elderly patients. Other drugs commonly used include non-steroidal anti-inflammatory drugs (NSAIDS), oral and parenteral corticosteroids, and simple analgesics. These groups of drugs are discussed more fully elsewhere in this chapter.

The most widely used DMARD in the US, Australia and Europe is methotrexate (MTX). MTX is an antifolate agent and inhibits dihydrofolate reductase, thereby impairing the conversion of dihydrofolate to tetrahydrofolate. It has good efficacy, acceptable tolerability and significant cost advantages over some of the more recently developed "biological" agents. MTX has a bioavailability of 70–75 % and a half life of 8–24 hours, though MTX glutamates have a half life of up to one week. 50 %–80 % of MTX is cleared at the kidney, and 10–30 % through the bile. Important gastrointestinal adverse effects include nausea and

Table 37.1. The principle DMARDS, used in the management of RA, appropriate monitoring when stable and special considerations for their use in elderly patients

Drug	Start dose	Maintenance dose	Interactions	Pharmacokinetics/ metabolism	Monitoring requirements*	Special considerations in elderly patients
Methotrexate	7.5 mg/week	7.5–25 mg/week	Cotrimoxazole increases bone marrow suppression, probenecid decreases excretion.	Plasma level peak 1–2 hours, clearance within 24 hours, principally renal excretion	LFTS, CBC every 1–2 months	May require lower maintenance dose especially in the presence of renal impairment. Regular monitoring of renal function advised.
Sulfasalazine	500 mg/day	1–3 gms/day	Decreases digoxin levels by 25%, azathioprine (leucopenia)	T 1/2 4–14 hours 20% biliary secreted 80% Split into sulfapyridine and 5-aminosalacylic acid. Sulfapyridine n-acetylated and renally excreted	CBC, LFTs every 2 months	Increased risk of gastrointestinal side-effects. Consider enteric coated preparations.
Leflunomide	Loading possible 100 mg daily for 3 days	10–20 mg/day	Inhibits CYP2C9—may reduce metabolism of warfarin and phenytoin	t1/2 15–18 days enterohepatic recirculation and renal excretion	LFTS, CBC, creat every 1–2 months	No dosage adjustment needed for age. Possible increased risk of pancytopenia.
Hydroxychloroquine	200–400 mg/day	200–400 mg/day	Monoamine oxidase inhibitors, may increase digoxin concentrations		Pre-treatment and annual eye examination	Retinal toxicity increases with age and cumulative dose.

(continued overleaf)

Table 37.1. (*continued*)

Drug	Start dose	Maintenance dose	Interactions	Pharmacokinetics/metabolism	Monitoring requirements*	Special considerations in elderly patients
Azathioprine	1 mg/kg/day	Up to 2.5 mg/kg/day, Usual 50–150 mg/day	Allopurinol. Reduce dose of azathioprine by 50–75 %, Thiazides and frusemide.	T1/2 0.2–0.5 hours Most metabolised to 6 mercaptopurine and eliminated as oxidized thiouric acid	CBC, LFTS every 2 months. Check TMT enzyme def. before therapy	No dose adjustment required with age.
Cyclosporine	3 mg/kg/day	4 mg/kg/day	Nephrotoxic agents, K+, K+ sparing diuretics, ACE-I, ACE-II antagonists	T1/2 6–20 hours. Biotransformed to 15 metabolites. Mainly biliary excretion	ELU, uric acid, LFTS monthly for 6 months, then 2 monthly, monitor blood pressure closely	Contraindicated in renal failure. Potentially difficult to use in elderly patients particularly because of drug interactions.
Gold	10 mg week 1, 25 mg week 2	50 mg weekly to 2 gms, then 50 mg 2nd weekly	Penicillamine, phenylbutazone, ACE-I	40 % excreted in first week, steady-state achieved 6–8 weeks 70 % renal excretion	Urinalysis, CBC platelets every 2 months	Rarely used due to toxicity

*commencement or changes of therapy may require closer monitoring.
LFTs- liver function tests, CBC—complete blood count, ELU—serum electrolytes, TMT—thiopurine methyltransferase

vomiting (which can sometimes be managed through a change to parenteral administration), abdominal pain, stomatitis, mouth ulcers and elevation of liver enzymes. Transient elevation in liver function tests occur in up to 50 % of users of MTX but a persistent elevation of greater than two to three times baseline is an indication for ceasing the drug. Alcohol intake, diabetes and obesity are considered risk factors for hepatotoxicity (7). Other important side effects include leucopenia, anaemia and thrombocytopaenia, pneumonitis (<1 %), photosensitivity, alopecia and headache. Infections, especially in severe RA, are a recognized problem with MXT use and occur in about 25 % of patients on the drug (8).

Teratogenesis and decreased sperm counts are of less relevance in the elderly population. Clinically important drug interactions in elderly patients may include the concomitant use of NSAIDs, especially in the presence of reduced renal function. Co-trimoxazole and MTX can interact to produce life-threatening haematological abnormalities. The co-administration of folic acid is usual practice and may reduce the incidence of mouth ulcers and other side effects.

Sulfasalazine (SSZ) is sometimes preferred to MTX in milder disease as it is felt to have a slightly less toxic profile. Principle side effects are gastroenterological, although fatal agranulocytosis has been reported. Hydroxychloroquine is sometimes used in mild disease but more commonly used in combination with MTX or SSZ. Leflunomide is a relatively new drug that acts by inhibiting dihydroorotate dehydrogenase in the intramitochondrial pyrimidine biosynthesis pathway. It can be used alone or in combination with MTX. Diarrhoea is a significant side effect of leflunomide and may necessitate dose reduction or cessation. Loading with leflunomide was initially recommended but is becoming less popular. Cyclosporine is used in refractory cases of RA but its renal and hypertensive side effects can make it difficult to use, especially in elderly patients. Also, it is a substrate of both cytochrome P450 and P-glycoprotein in the gut and liver

which may interfere with the metabolism of other drugs. Azathioprine is rarely used alone but may be used in low doses in combination with other DMARDS. Dose reduction of azathioprine is required with concomitant use of allopurinol. Parenteral gold therapy was the earliest of the DMARDs in use, but is now infrequently commenced. It requires monitoring of urinalysis and complete blood count including platelet count. Alkylating agents (cyclophosphamide and chlorambucil) are generally reserved for the most intractable cases because of the great risk of significant adverse events.

Biological therapeutic agents that target various specific components of the inflammatory process are relatively recent additions to the management of RA. There are currently three TNF-α blockers (infliximab, etanercept and adalimumab) available and one IL-1 receptor antagonist (anakinra) although a number of other agents and therapeutic targets are in development. They are sometimes used in combination with MTX but should not be used in combination with each other. Because of the clearly increased risk of tuberculosis on the TNF-α blocking therapies, patients should be screened prior to commencement for prior TB exposure. The British Thoracic Society has recently developed a guideline for this purpose (9). Reported side effects of the TNF-α blockers include increased risk of infection, drug induced SLE, demyelinating disease, cytopaenias, injection site reactions, cardiac failure and possibly lymphoma. Side effects of anakinra include injection site reactions, headache, infections and neutropaenia. Overall these agents are well tolerated and represent a significant advance in the management of RA. Early data suggests they are reasonably well tolerated in elderly patients (10). Various guidelines have been published to assist in the rational prescribing of these drugs (11).

Oral (especially low dose) and parenteral corticosteroids have a role in the management of RA in elderly patients. The use of oral NSAIDs is becoming less popular for long term use. Finally, the consumption of omega-3 fpolyunsaturated fatty acids found in fish can reduce the inflammatory metabolites of arachidonic acid and may reduce requirement for NSAIDs in patients with RA (12).

KEY POINTS IN RHEUMATOID ARTHRITIS

- RA may present differently in elderly patients and be more difficult to diagnose.
- Medical management in elderly patients is complicated by issues relating to the presence of co-morbidities, altered pharmacokinetics and polypharmacy
- Methotrexate remains the mainstay of DMARD therapy in elderly patients and is mostly well tolerated.
- New biological agents hold promise for future treatment in elderly patients, though their safety in this group is not currently well established.

OSTEOARTHRITIS

Introduction

Osteoarthritis (OA) is probably the leading cause of disability among adults in developed countries (13). Age is the most significant risk factor for the development of OA, with greater than 75 % of people over the age of 65 years having radiographic evidence of OA (14). Other risk factors include obesity, previous joint trauma and joint overload. OA accounts for more disability among older people than any other disease.

Aetiology

OA is currently defined by the American College of Rheumatology as "a heterogeneous group of conditions that leads to joint symptoms and signs which are associated with defective integrity of articular cartilage, in addition to related changes in the underlying bone at the joint margins". The aetiology of OA is unknown however it is now recognized that an active disease process characterized by derangement

in the process of healthy cartilage maintenance with a sustained increase in degradative activity relative to synthetic activity leads to OA. There are inflammatory, metabolic, genetic and mechanical factors involved in the process. In the slowly progressing inflammatory reaction cytokines such as IL-1 and TNF-α are significant contributors to the process (15).

Symptoms and signs

Joint pain is the hallmark symptom of OA. This is generally insidious in onset, worsened by activity and improved with rest. Short term joint stiffness and "gelling" of joints after inactivity is sometimes seen. Bony swelling can develop and interfere with normal joint range of movement. Herberden's nodes (distal interphalangeal joints [DIP]) and Bouchard's nodes (proximal interphalangeal joints [PIP]) are common findings. Most joints can be affected but knees, hips, feet, carpometacarpal joints of the thumbs, lumbar and cervical spines are most frequently involved. Crepitus, tenderness, joint swelling and deformity and limited range of joint movement are all clinical signs of OA.

Diagnosis

The diagnosis of OA is based on typical clinical findings with supportive imaging. Other laboratory investigations are of most use in excluding other diagnoses. Typical x-ray findings include loss of joint space, subchondral sclerosis, bony cysts and osteophytosis. The differential diagnosis can include seronegative RA (especially when the inflammatory findings are prominent) and psoriatic arthritis can mimic OA at the DIPs. OA of the hip and knee can be mimicked by a wide range of conditions including spondyloarthropathies, avascular necrosis, pigmented villonodular synovitis or chronic infection.

Therapy

The aim of treatment is to relieve pain and maintain function. Issues of mobility and the consequent maintenance of independence are frequently the most important goals for elderly patients.

Non pharmacotherapies

Non pharmacotherapies are very important in the management of OA. These therapies include the provision of walking aids, weight reduction, patient education, physical therapies such as exercise therapies, topical heat and cold applications, transcutaneous nerve stimulation (TENS) arch supports and environmental modification. The judicious use of joint replacement surgery is of major benefit in hip and knee osteoarthritis in particular.

Pharmacotherapies

Table 37.2 outlines the major classes of pharmacotherapeutic agents used in the management of OA and special considerations for their use in elderly patients.

Paracetamol (Acetaminophen)

Paracetamol is an effective, cheap and relatively safe therapy for mild to moderate pain from OA. It is generally regarded as first line therapy especially in elderly patients and the dose should not exceed 4 grams per day. Paracetamol is principally an analgesic and anti-pyretic and has no anti-inflammatory affect. Its mechanism of action is uncertain but may involve a central nervous system reduction in cyclooxygensase (COX) (16). Dose reductions may be required in regular users of alcohol. Potential side effects include heptotoxicity and nephrotoxicity. Slow release preparations of paracetamol are available and may have some advantages in terms of dose schedules.

Non-steroidal Anti-inflammatory Drugs (NSAIDs)

For pain not adequately controlled with paracetamol the use of a NSAID can be considered. NSAIDs are effective in treating pain from OA including rest pain, night pain and pain associated with inflammation. NSAIDS work through the inhibition of cyclooxygenase and subsequently prostaglandin synthesis. Various NSAIDs have varying degrees of COX-2 inhibition selectivity and the side effect profile of the individual NSAID depends to some degree on the COX-2 selectivity. The choice of NSAID prescribed depends on dosage schedule, response, cost, side effect profile and physician and patient preference. The principle of "start low, go slow" in prescribing of NSAIDS in the elderly is important, and short term, intermittent use for flares is recommended in preference to protracted use. Efficacy and side effect profiles may vary across agents in any particular individual, so it is appropriate to trial more than one NSAID before concluding the class to be ineffective. The side effect profile of NSAIDs is significant and includes GI effects such as peptic ulceration and haemorrhage, cardiovascular effects of hypertension, and cardiac failure and renal toxicity. Recently concerns about an increase in acute cardiovascular and thrombotic adverse effects have led to the withdrawl of rofecoxib, a so called COX-2 selective agent. Celecoxib, another COX-2 selective agent now comes with a warning concerning the potential for such events. If the long term use of non-selective NSAIDs is necessary, then the concomitant use of a proton pump inhibitor is recommended (17). NSAIDs are contraindicated in those with a significant history of peptic ulceration, hypertension, heart failure or renal impairment, limiting their use in elderly patients. Potential drug interactions include warfarin, cyclosporine, lithium and digoxin. Patients on long term NSAIDs should have a baseline complete blood count and biochemistry, and these tests should be repeated at one month and at least annually thereafter.

Opioids

A number of opioid preparations are available for the treatment of moderate to severe pain from OA refractory to other therapies. These include morphine, methadone, codeine, hydromorphone, oycodone and the atypical opioid tramadol. Tramadol is a synthetic agent structurally unrelated to other opioids which appears to have actions on the serotonergic, noradrenergic and GABAergic systems, as well as the opioid mu receptor. It can be used in combination with paracetamol and NSAIDs. Use with monoamine oxidase inhibitors and selective serotonin reuptake inhibitors are contraindicated because of the risk of serotonin

Table 37.2. The main groups of pharmacotherapies used in the management of OA and special considerations in elderly patients

Treatment	Starting dose	Maintenance dose	Interactions	Pharmacokinetics/ metabolism	Monitoring requirements	Special considerations in elderly patients
Paracetamol (acetaminophen)	1 gm 4/24	Max dose 4 gms/day	Anticoagulant dosage may require reduction with prolonged use	T1/2 1–4 hours. Hepatically metabolised and renally excreted.	nil	Preferred first line management— low gastrointestinal and renal toxicity
NSAIDs	Individualise Depending on preparation	individualise	Multiple—warfarin, lithium, digoxin, diuretics, other NSAIDS, antihypertensives etc	Depends on preparation	Baseline Complete blood count and biochemistry, then at 1 month and annual thereafter	Potential cardiovascular, renal and GI toxicity limit their utility in the elderly
Opioids	5 mg morphine (or equivalent) 4 hourly	Lowest effective dose	CNS depressants, muscle relaxants, MAO-I, cimetidine, diuretics, St Johns Wort	Variable. Extensive 1st pass metabolism. T1/2 variable (4 hours), hepatic metabolism and renal excretion.	nil	Constipation, sedation, confusion and nausea are particular problems. Lower doses in the frail elderly patient.
Intra-articular Corticosteriods	Intra-articular dose depends on joint size and preparation used	For example 2.5–5 mg triamcinolone in small joints, 10–40 mg in large joints	Few interactions when given intra-articularly. May transiently raise blood sugars		nil	Intra-articular injection in affected joints may have fewer side effects than some systemic therapies.
Glucosamine and chondroitin	1.5 gm. glucosamine sulphate daily	1.5 gm glucosamine daily			nil	Adverse effects rare, contraindicated in shellfish allergy.
Viscosupplementation	16 mg intra-articular weekly hylan G-F 20 for 3 weeks	Max of two courses in 6 months.			nil	Useful for knee OA, contraindicated in infection or inflamed joints
Topical analgesics or capsaicin cream	Apply 2–4 times daily for 14 days, then review	2–4 times daily			nil	Appropriate adjunctive or monotherapy

syndrome. Seizures, nausea, vomiting and dizziness have all been reported with tramadol. All opioid analgesics have a range of side effects that can be particularly troublesome in elderly patients. Constipation is common and should be managed with appropriate prophylaxis. Drowsiness, respiratory depression, confusion or myoclonus may limit the use of this class of drug in elderly patients. Again the treatment should commence at low dose (equivalent of 5 mg (intramuscularly) of morphine 4 hourly) and titrated slowly. Doses may need to be lower in the frail elderly patient. Side effects may necessitate a change in opioid. Fentanyl transdermal patches can be useful and the topical route of administration is often popular with patients. Combinations with paracetamol or NSAIDs can be considered. Patients may require different regimens for baseline pain and breakthrough pain. The therapeutic index of most opioids is reduced in the presence of renal or hepatic impairment and in these situations dose reduction and/or increased dosage intervals may be required. Significant drug interactions can occur with benzodiazepines, some antibiotics, H_2 antagonists, and some anticonvulsants, tricyclic antidepressants and serotonin reuptake inhibitors.

Other therapies

Glucosamine and chondroitin sulphate are generally classed as dietary supplements and may have a role in the management of OA, especially of the knee. However evidence for the use of these agents is inconsistent (18). Viscosupplementation is a therapy which consists of injecting hyaluronan into affected joints (especially the knee). Repeated injections may delay the progression of OA (19) though the mechanism is uncertain. Topical agents acting as counter-irritants can be effective and safe in the management of OA pain. Finally, monoarticular pain and swelling can be managed with intra-articular steroids. Usually these should be restricted to no greater than 4 injections in any one joint per year.

KEY POINTS IN OSTEOARTHRITIS

- Osteoarthritis is the leading cause of disability in elderly patients.
- Paracetamol remains first line therapy for mild-moderate OA.
- NSAIDs should be used with caution in elderly patients and stomach protection is strongly advised.
- Opioid analgesia can be used in elderly patients with moderate to severe OA though dose modification may be required.
- Non-pharmacotherapies including arthroplasty are important in the management of osteoarthritis.

POLYMYALGIA RHEUMATICA

Introduction

Polymyalgia rheumatica (PMR) is a common inflammatory disease in adults over the age of 50, with an annual incidence estimated at 50/100 000 in this population (20). It is twice as common in women as men and is related to giant cell arteritis (GCA), although the precise relationship between the two conditions is unknown. PMR occurs in about 50 % of patient with GCA, while approximately 5–15 % of patients with PMR as the primary diagnosis have GCA. This section will confine itself to the topic of PMR.

Aetiology

The aetiology of PMR is unknown. The cause of symptoms is inflammation but the site of inflammation is disputed.

Symptoms and signs

Characteristic symptoms of PMR are aching and stiffness affecting the shoulder and hip girdles. Pain can involve the neck, shoulders, upper arms, lower back and thighs. Small joints of the hands and feet are occasionally involved. The onset may be abrupt and symptoms are usually symmetrical. Patients may complain of difficulty getting out of bed or standing from the seated position. Fatigue, malaise and depression may accompany the other features of disease. Clinical signs are few, with tenderness and restriction of shoulder and hip range of movement. Muscle strength is usually normal although interpretation may be difficult because of pain. Occasionally pitting oedema develops in the upper and lower limbs and may result in carpal tunnel syndrome. Atypical presentations include younger patients or patients with asymmetrical symptoms.

Diagnosis

Diagnosis is based on the clinical presentation and supportive laboratory findings. Elevated inflammatory markers (ESR and CRP) are the only abnormal laboratory findings although rarely patients with PMR can present with a normal ESR and CRP. The exclusion of other conditions such as rheumatoid arthritis, infection, endocrinopathies, polymyositis, drug-induced myopathies or para-malignant syndromes is important. Degenerative disease such as cervical spondylosis and/or rotator cuff disease can occasionally mimic PMR. As PMR is exquisitely sensitive to corticosteroids, a rapid and complete resolution of symptoms after the commencement of therapy often confirms the diagnosis.

Treatment

Patients with PMR respond dramatically to relatively low doses of corticosteroids. The dose chosen depends on the patient's weight and severity of symptoms. Usually a dose of 7.5–20 mg of oral prednisolone can be trialled and patients should respond quickly (often after the first dose). The dose can be increased if a rapid and satisfactory response is not achieved.

Dose reduction should be commenced quickly, that is approximately two to four weeks after symptoms are controlled. The rate of dose reduction needs to be individualized but as a guide by approximately 10 % every two to four weeks to achieve the minimum dose required to suppress symptoms. Once the dose is reduced to 10 mg per day, a slower reduction of 1 mg every one to 2 months is usual. Relapse occurs in 25–50 % of patients, sometimes related to a too rapid reduction of steroid. Relapses are managed by an increase in the oral prednisolone dose. Prednisolone can be withdrawn from most patients eventually, but a small subset requires ongoing treatment with very low dose oral prednisolone.

The side effects of long term ongoing oral steroid therapy are significant and every effort should be made to reduce the dose as soon as possible. In addition, every effort should be made to minimize side effects with appropriate prophylaxis. Osteoporosis is a particular issue in elderly women. Patients should be evaluated for osteoporosis by DEXA as soon as possible after commencement of the drug. Supplemental calcium 1200 mg/day and Vitamin D 400 to 800 IU/day are recommended for those with normal bone density. Anti-resorptive therapy such as a bisphosphonate should be considered when there is evidence of osteoporosis. Bone density requires annual assessment while on oral corticosteroids. Blood glucose should be monitored during therapy with oral corticosteroids and treatment of hyperglycaemia may be required. Those with known diabetes may require an increase in therapies. Occasionally patients on oral hypoglycaemics need to be managed on insulin during the course of their therapy. Patients should also be monitored for hyperlipidaemia, hypertension, myopathy and occasionally cataracts. Patients should be advised about the potential for adrenal suppression during and after any prolonged course of steroids.

KEY POINTS IN PMR

- PMR is common over the age of 60 years.
- Treatment with long term oral corticosteroids is effective.
- Long term treatment with oral corticosteroids is associated with multiple side effects and requires careful monitoring and prophylaxis.
- Prognosis is generally excellent.

GOUT AND CALCIUM PYROPHOSPHATE DISEASE (CPPD)

Introduction

Crystal associated arthritis is common in the elderly. The two most recognized forms are gouty arthritis caused by the deposition of monosodium urate (MSU) and calcium pyrophosphate disease (CPPD) or pseudogout. The prevalence of both these conditions increases with age. Gout is more frequently seen in males, while pseudogout is more common in women. The prevalence of gout in people over 65 is approximately 5 % in men and 2 % in women (14). CPPD is a disease of the elderly, with the prevalence of chondrocalcinosis (the radiographic marker of calcium pyrophosphate deposition) approximately 40 % in patients over 80 (21).

Aetiology

Gout is a syndrome caused by the deposition of MSU in tissues and around joints and a subsequent inflammatory response. The crystal deposition is a result of hyperuricemia, which is often present for decades prior to the development of clinical gout. The presence of crystals then leads to an activation and release of pro-inflammatory cytokines and chemotactic factors which recruit phagocytic cells that engulf and ingest the crystals.

Hyperuricemia can result from either decreased renal excretion (80–90 % of primary gout) or increased production (10–20 %) of uric acid. There is a genetic component to gout, with approximately 40 % of patients reporting a family history, probably relating to multiple genes involving production and excretion of uric acid (22). A number of other factors commonly seen in the elderly predispose to hyperuricemia. Hypertension, obesity, renal impairment and metabolic syndrome are all associated with higher uric acid levels. In addition the use of some drugs such as thiazide and loop diuretics and aspirin increases the risk of hyperuricemia.

CPPD is caused by the deposition of calcium pyrophosphate crystal in articular and periarticular tissues and a subsequent inflammatory reaction to those crystals. The cause of crystal deposition is uncertain but is associated with locally elevated levels of calcium or pyrophosphate and/or an abnormal substrate of matrix collagen and proteoglycan promoting crystal deposition.

Signs and symptoms

The typical attack of acute gout is reasonably easy to identify. The initial attack of gout is monoarticular in 85–90 % of cases and usually affects lower extremity joints. First Metatarsophalangeal joint involvement (podagra) occurs in 50 % of first attacks. Typically upon awakening the patient suffers from the sudden onset of exquisite pain, joint swelling and redness with maximum symptoms over several hours, and the attack (untreated) lasts days to one to two weeks. Any joint can be affected, and extra-articular involvement at sites such as the Achilles tendon or the olecranon bursa occasionally occurs. Without treatment, following an "intercritical" period of weeks to months, a second attack will occur in 78 % of patients within two years, and 93 % within 10 years. Attacks usually occur with increasing frequency and often become polyarticular. Attacks may be associated with fever, delirium, leukocytosis and elevated inflammatory markers and over many years tophaceous deposits appear over the elbows, fingers, ears and other sites. Risk factors for the development of tophaceous gout includes alcohol abuse, thiazide diuretic use, poor compliance, longer and under-treated disease, frequent attacks and a higher uric acid level (23). Tophi may ulcerate or become infected. Chronic polyarticular gout may develop and chronic hyperuricemia may impact negatively on the kidney.

The presentation of gout in the elderly may differ from younger patients. These differences include a higher prevalence of polyarticular gout and a larger proportion of women being affected. In addition, gout in the elderly tends to involve the small joints of the fingers more commonly and tophi occur more frequently. Finally the use of diuretic therapy and the presence of renal disease are higher in the elderly.

Radiographic changes in gout vary. Characteristic well-defined lytic and erosive lesions in or around joints with characteristic overhanging edges can occur. Early in the disease there may be little or no change, and late in the disease the destructive arthropathy can be difficult to distinguish from other forms of inflammatory arthritis or from osteoarthritis.

The differential diagnosis of gout includes infection, other crystal arthropathies, RA, and osteoarthritis. When systemic features are prominent, acute bacterial infections should be considered.

Clinical features of CPPD may mimic gout or other inflammatory and non-inflammatory forms of arthritis. CPPD may also co-exist with these conditions. CPPD can present as acute attacks of mono or polyarthritis or as a chronic arthropathy often associated with osteoarthritis. Chondrocalcinosis may be an incidental finding on x-ray. The most commonly involved joints include the knee, wrist, shoulder and hip. Attacks sometimes occur after surgery, medical illness or trauma. Chronic CPPD can be a symmetrical arthritis though symptoms are generally restricted to a few joints. Plain radiography demonstrating chondrocalcinosis can help with the diagnosis, although it is not diagnostic of the condition.

Diagnosis

The diagnosis of gout is made on the detection of negatively bi-refringent urate crystals under polarized light microscopy aspirated from a joint during an attack. Crystals detected from joints previously affected, or from possible tophi can be helpful. An elevated uric acid level is not diagnostic of gout, as many individuals with hyperuricemia do not develop the disease, and up to 50% of people may have normal uric acid levels during an acute attack of gout. Likewise, the examination of synovial fluid for crystals is essential for the diagnosis of CPPD. CPPD crystals are pleomorphic and may be intracellular or extra-cellular, and are weakly positively birefringent. CPPD can be difficult to distinguish from RA, although the absence of erosive disease can be helpful. In patients with CPPD, endocrine and metabolic diseases such

as hyperparathyroidism and haemochromatosis should be considered.

Treatment

Gout can be among the most satisfying forms of inflammatory arthritis to manage. The aim of treatment should be to terminate acute attacks and if possible prevent further attacks. In older patients the presence of co-morbid conditions may dictate modification of standard therapies. Table 37.3 outlines the major pharmacotherapeutic agents used in the management of gout and special considerations for their use in elderly patients.

Lifestyle modification can significantly reduce hyperuricemia in many patients with gout (24). Moderation of heavy alcohol intake may be of benefit in some cases. Patients should be encouraged to lose weight where appropriate and offered treatment for hyperlipidemia. Advice concerning the restriction of purine ingestion is likely to be of benefit in only a minority of cases. The cessation of thiazide and loop diuretics should be considered where possible. Occasionally the cessation of low dose aspirin should be considered.

The management of acute attacks involves the short term use of NSAIDs, corticosteroids (oral, intra-articular or parenteral), colchicine and occasionally corticotropin (ACTH). The need for caution with the use of NSAIDS in elderly patients has already been discussed. Oral corticosteroids (prednisolone 20–50 mg daily, tapering quickly over a week) or intra-articular corticosteroid use is effective and may be a safer alternative, although should be used cautiously in the presence of diabetes. Colchicine should be used cautiously in elderly patients, especially those with hepatic or renal impairment. It has a narrow therapeutic index and gastrointestinal side effects (sometimes severe) in higher doses occur in the majority of patients. Bone marrow suppression and sudden death has been reported with colchicine use and intravenous therapy with this drug should be avoided.

Following an acute attack of gout, patients remain at increased risk for another attack for several weeks. For this reason prophylaxis with

Table 37.3. Therapies available for gout and special considerations in elderly patients

Treatment	Starting dose	Maintenance dose	Interactions	Pharmacokinetics/metabolism	Monitoring	Special considerations in elderly patients
NSAIDS	Individualise Depending on preparation	Individualize	Multiple—warfarin, lithium, digoxin, diuretics, other NSAIDS, antihypertensives etc	Depends on preparation	Baseline Complete blood count and biochemistry, then at 1 month and annual thereafter	Useful in acute attacks. Potential cardiovascular, renal and GI toxicity limit their utility in elderly patients
Corticosteroids	20–50 mg prednisolone daily	Taper rapidly to 0	Multiple—anatacids, antidiabetic agents, digoxin, diuretics, drugs inducing hepatic enzymes etc	T1/2 3–4 hours, conjugated in the liver, excreted in the urine.	Blood sugar monitoring may be required	Intra-articular, parenteral or oral. Acute attacks. May be safer than NSAIDs in the elderly. Diabetes may limit use.
Colchicine	Acute 1 mg—then 500 µg every 2–3 hours until pain relief or side effects. Max 6 mg	500 µg i–ii daily. 1/2 dose if creatinine clearance <50 ml/min	Cyclosporine, erythromycin, CNS depressants, NSAIDS, alcohol, immunosuppressants, anticoagulants	T1/2 4–5 hours. Acetylated in the liver, predominantly excreted in the faeces, 10–20 % urine excreted	Complete blood counts periodically in chronic dosing	Side effects (diarrhoea, toxicity) limit use in acute setting. Low dose therapy for prophylaxis can be used cautiously. Special caution in hepatic or renal impairment.
Allopurinol	100 mg daily increasing by 100 mg daily each month according to response	100–300 mg daily	Azathioprine/ mercaptopurine Reduce dose of azathioprine or mercaptopurine by 50–75 %.	Metabolised to oxypurinol (active metabolite) T1/2 1–2 hours. 20 % faecal excretion. Mainly renally excreted.	Periodic uric acid levels, complete blood count and electrolytes	May need dose reduction based on renal function.
Uricosuric agents eg probenecid	Probenecid 250 mg twice daily	500 mg twice daily	Aspirin contraindicated with probenecid. May need to reduce methotrexate doses. May potentiate oral sulfonylureas and thiazide diuretics	Probenecid T 1/2 6–12 hours Both glomerular filtration and active secretion by proximal tubule.	Uric acid levels	Rarely used. Angiotensin converting enzyme inhibitors (losartan) and/or lipid lowering agents (fenofibrate) may have a moderate uricosuric effect.

low dose colchicine, NSAIDS or corticosteroids is sometimes used.

The lowing of serum urate levels is central to the effective management of gout. This should be considered in all patients with more than a single attack of proven gout and especially in those with tophaceous disease or radiographic changes of joint damage. Tophi can be resorbed over time with a sustained lowering of hyperuricemia into the normal range and recurrent attacks effectively prevented (25). Allopurinol is effective in the majority of patients in lowering serum uric acid levels. It is a xanthine-oxidase inhibitor and dosage should be adjusted in elderly patients based on reduced renal function. Commencement of allopurinol, or dose increases may occasionally precipitate an attack of gout and this may lead to poor compliance. Dose adjustments should therefore be undertaken under prophylaxis cover. Standard doses of allopurinol 300 mg/day should be reduced to 200 mg/day for glomerular filtration rates (GFR) below 60 ml/min, and to 100 mg/day below 30 ml/min. A dose of 100 mg alternate days can be used for GFR less than 10 ml/min (22). Up to 5 % of patients are unable to tolerate allopurinol, usually because of rash. Allopurinol intolerance in the form of hypersensitivity can sometimes be managed with a desensitization regimen. Interactions with some other drugs (eg azathioprine) may require dose reduction of those drugs.

There are a number of new agents in development for the management of gout including new xanthine oxidase inhibitors, and improved understanding of the pathogenesis of the disease is likely to lead to new management approaches in the future (26).

There is no role for uric acid lowering strategies in the management of CPPD. NSAIDS, corticosteroids (oral, intra-articular or parenteral) and colchicine may all be used for the management of this condition.

KEY POINTS IN GOUT AND CPPD

- Gout is among the most manageable of all rheumatic diseases.

- Lifestyle modification can have a significant role in the treatment of gout.
- Most therapies for acute gout or the long term management of hyperuricemia involve dose adjustment in elderly patients.

LINKS

There are a multitude of links available to investigate these topics further. Some of these include:

- The American College of Rheumatology: http://www.rheumatology.org
  This website allows access to a number of guidelines including the management of RA and OA.
- The British Society for Rheumatology: http://www.rheumatology.org.uk.
  The website has a number of guidelines available on multiple topics and has useful links to a number of patient support groups.
- RheumatologyLinx; http://www.mdlinx .com/rheumatologylinx/index.cfm.

REFERENCES

1. Tutuncu Z, Kavanaugh A. Rheumatic Disease in the Elderly: Rheumatoid Arthritis. *Clin Geriatr Med* 2005; **21**: 513–25.
2. Rasch EK, Hirsh R, Paulose-Ram, et al. Prevalence of rheumatoid arthritis in persons 60 years of age and older in the United States. Effects of different methods of case classification. *Athritis Rheum* 2003; **48**: 917–26.
3. Van der Heijde DM, van Leeuwen MA, van Riel PL et al, Radiographic progression on radiographs of hands and feet during the first 3 years of rheumatoid arthritis measured according to Sharp's method (van der Heijde modification). *J Rheumatol* 1995; **22**(9): 1792–6.
4. van Schaardenburg D. Rheumatoid Arthritis in the Elderly. *Drugs and Aging* 1995; **7**(1): 30–7.
5. van Schaardenburg D, Breedweld FC. Elderly-onset rheumatoid arthritis. *Semin Arthrtis Rheum* 1994; **23**(6): 367–78.
6. Palosuo T, Tilvis R, Standberg T et al. Filaggrin related antibodies among the aged. *Ann Rheum Dis* 2003; **62**: 261–3.

7. Rau R Methotrexate. In Firestein GS, Panayi GS, Wallheim FA eds. *Rheumatoid Arthritis; new frontiers in pathogenesis and treatment*. Oxford: Oxford University Press, 2000.

8. Weinblatt ME, Trentham DE, Fraser PA. Long-term prospective trial of low-dose methotrexate in rheumatoid arthritis. *Arthritis Rheum* 1988; **31920**: 167–75.

9. British Thoracic Society. BTS recommendations for assessing risk, and for managing *M. tuberculosis* infection and disease in patients due to start anti-TNF-α treatment. London: British Thoracic Society, 2004 (http://www.brit-thoracic.org.uk). To be published in *Thorax* and *Rheumatology*.

10. Fleischman RM, Baumgartner SW, Tindall EA et al. Response to Etancercept (enbrel) in elderly patients with rheumatoid arthritis: a retrospective analysis of clinical trials. *J Rheumatol* 2003; **30**(4): 691–6.

11. J. Ledingham and C. Deighton on behalf of the British Society for Rheumatology Standards, Guidelines and Audit Working Group (SGAWG) Update on the British Society for Rheumatology guidelines for prescribing TNFα blockers in adults with rheumatoid arthritis (update of previous guidelines of April 2001) *Rheum* 2005; **44**(2): 157–63.

12. Cleland LG, James MJ, Proudman SM. The role of fish oils in the management if rheumatoid arthritis. *Drugs* 2003; **63**(9): 845–53.

13. Prevalence of disabilities and associated health conditions among adults-United States 1999, *MMWR Morb Mortal Wky Rep. 23* 2001; **50**: 120–5.

14. Lawrence RC, Helmick CG, Arnettt FC et al. Estimates of the prevalence of arthritis and selected musculoskeletal disorders in the United States. *Arthritis Rheum* 1998; **41**: 778–99.

15. Goldring MB. The role of chondrocyte in osteoarthritis *Arthritis Rheum* 2000; **43**: 1916–26.

16. Botting R, Ayoub SS. COX-3 and the mechanism of action of paracetamol/acetaminophen. *Prostaglandins Leukot Essent Fatty Acids* 2005 Feb; **72**(2): 85–7.

17. American College of Rheumatology. Recommendations for the Management of Osteoarthritis of the Hip and Knee. *Arthritis Rheum* 2000; **43**(9): 1905–15.

18. Towheed TE, Maxwell L, Anastassiades TP, Shea B, Houpt J, Robinson V, Hochburg MC, Wells G. Glucosamine therapy for treating osteoarthritis (Cochrane Review). *Cochrane Database System Rev*. 2005 April **18**; (2): CD002946.

19. Listrat V, Ayral X, Francesca P et al. Arthroscopic evaluation of potential structural modifying activity of hyluronan (Hyalgan) in osteoarthritis of the knee. *Osteoarthritis Cartilage* 1997; **5**: 153–60.

20. Chuang TY, Hunder GG, Ilstrup DM, Kurland LT: Polymyalgia rheumatica: a 10-year epidemiologic and clinical study. *Ann Intern Med* 1982; **97**: 672–80.

21. Neame RL, Carr AJ, Muir et al. UK community prevalence of knee chondrocalcinosis: evidence that correlation with osteoarthritis is through a shared association with osteophyte. *Ann Rheum Dis* 2003; **62**(6): 513–8.

22. Wise CM. Crystal-associated Arthritis in the Elderly. *Clin Geritr Med* 2005; **21**: 491–511.

23. Nakayama DA, Bathelemy C, Carrera G, et al. Tophaceous gout: A clinical and radiographic assessment. *Arthritis Rheum* 1984; **27**(4): 468–71.

24. Wortmann RL. Gout and hyperuricemia. *Curr Opin Rheumatol* 2002; **14**: 281–6.

25. Shoji A, Yamanaka H, Kamatani N. A retrospective study of the relationship between serum urate level and recurrent attacks of gouty arthritis; evidence for reduction of recurrent gouty arthritis with antihyperuricemic therapy. *Arthritis Rheum* 2004; **51**(3): 321–5.

26. Bieber JD, Terkeltaub RA. Gout. On the brink of novel therapeutic options for an ancient disease. *Arthritis and Rheum* 2004; **50**(8): 2400–14.

38 Falls, Osteoporosis, Paget's disease and Osteomalacia

Harald J.J. Verhaar and Paul Jansen

Department of Geriatric Medicine, University Medical Centre Utrecht, The Netherlands

FALLS AND OSTEOPOROSIS

Introduction

One in three elderly people living at home and half of the people living in nursing homes fall at least once a year. Although most falls do not result in serious injury, in some cases admission to hospital or nursing home is needed. One percent of those who fall sustain a hip fracture, 5 % another fracture, and 5 % soft tissue damage. Falls are the main cause of accidental death among people older than 65 years. A loss of self-confidence after a serious fall can lead people to become less active, because of a fear of falling. This in turn leads to a deterioration of functioning in daily life and to social isolation.

Risk factors for and causes of falls

Two or more falls in the previous year is an important predictor of new falls. Extrinsic factors, such as environmental factors (e.g., poor lighting), are involved in 40 % of falls. Intrinsic factors for falls are summarized in Table 38.1. (1) Both acute disorders (such as pneumonia) and chronic disorders can adversely affect balance, leading to falls. Aging is accompanied by several pathophysiological changes, which increase the risk of falling, such as visual problems, slowed reaction time, diminished

muscle strength, and diminished joint flexibility. The muscle strength of healthy older individuals is between 20 % and 40 % of that of younger individuals and much lower in chronically ill individuals living in nursing homes.

The central processing and integration of afferent sensory information and its translation into efferent muscle and joint action must occur rapidly and smoothly to respond adequately to changing input during motion. However, central processing functions less well with advancing age, which increases the risk of falls. It may have an even greater role in patients who are confused or suffer from dementia. Impairments of spatial insight and orientation also play a role.

Dizziness is often mentioned as a symptom in the context of falls. This may be "rotational" dizziness, or true vertigo, with a vestibular origin, such as benign positional vertigo, acute labyrinthitis, or Menière's disease, or "light-headedness" as a result of cardiovascular problems, hyperventilation, orthostatic hypotension, medication, anxiety, or depression. A "drop attack" is a sudden fall without loss of consciousness or dizziness and is often triggered by a sudden movement of the head. Such attacks are caused by vertebrovestibular insufficiency, but other pathophysiological mechanisms may be involved. Syncope, an acute loss of consciousness followed by

Prescribing for Elderly Patients   Edited by Stephen Jackson, Paul Jansen and Arduino Mangoni

Table 38.1. Causes of falls in the elderly

Cause	% Home-living elderly (7 studies, 2,312 fall incidents)	% Nursing homes (4 studies, 1076 fall incidents)
I. Extrinsic factors (accident/environ- mental factors)	41	16
II. Intrinsic factors	53	80
a. Muscle weakness, balance and/or walking disturbance	13	26
b. (Acute) confusion	2	10
c. Poor eye sight	0.8	4
d. Orthostatic hypotension	1	2
e. Dizziness or light-headedness	8	25
f. Drop attack	13	0.3
g. Syncope	0.4	0.2
h. Acute illness (e.g. pneumonia)/CVA/ parkinsonism/osteoarthritis	14	12
III. Unknown	6	4

spontaneous recovery, can be caused by diminished perfusion of the brain. In elderly people the most common causes of syncope are vasovagal reactions, cardiac arrhythmias, and orthostatic hypotension. A fall occurring after a person looks up or sideways may be caused by carotid sinus compression, with a drop in blood pressure and/or sinus bradycardia as result. Neurological disorders that can lead to falls include parkinsonism, cerebrovascular diseases, normal pressure hydrocephalus, and dementia.

Risk factors for hip fracture

A history of low-impact trauma, corticosteroid use, early menopause, low weight (body mass index $<19 \text{kg/m}^2$), and a mother with previous hip fracture increase the risk of a hip fracture, in addition to the above-mentioned risk factors (Table 38.2). Bone mineral density (BMD), an important risk factor for fractures, is only marginally lower in patients with a hip fracture than in age-matched controls. Thus factors other than osteoporosis have a role in the pathogenesis of hip fractures. The EPI-DOS (Epidémiologie de l'ostéoporose) study in France investigated the predictive value of certain risk factors for falls and a low BMD on the incidence of hip fractures in 7575 independently living women older than 75 years (2). The predictive value for hip fractures of a

Table 38.2. Risk factors for a hip fracture

- A positive family history, e.g. having a mother with a hip fracture
- 'Low-trauma' fracture in past history
- Low 'body mass index' (BMI $<19 \text{kg/m}^2$)
- Poor vision
- Reduced walking speed and/or balance disturbance
- Use of corticosteroids (>7.5 mg daily, >3 months)
- Underlying disorder associated with osteoporosis (malabsorption due to inflammatory bowel disease, chronic renal insufficiency, etc.)

high risk of falls and a low BMD was similar but was larger when the two factors were combined.

Diagnostic approach to high-risk patients

History

In the first instance, patients should be asked whether they have fallen before. An earlier fall without injury is often not mentioned but may be of importance for determining the predisposing factors. The time and place where the fall occurred, and whether it was associated with a specific activity, are important for determining the cause of the fall. Is there an association between the fall and getting up quickly (orthostatic hypotension), tripping or slipping (gait, balance, vision disturbance, or environmental obstacle), coughing or urination (reflex hypotension), a meal (postprandial hypotension), looking up or sideways (arterial or carotid sinus compression), or loss of consciousness (syncope or seizure)?

Symptoms preceding the fall can provide information about its cause, such as dizziness or light-headedness (orthostatic hypotension, vestibular problems, hypoglycemia, arrhythmia, or drug side effects), palpitations (arrhythmia), incontinence or tongue biting (seizure), asymmetric loss of strength (cerebrovascular accident), or chest pain (myocardial ischemia). Certain drugs have a sedative action and slow the reaction time (long-acting benzodiazepines), or lower blood pressure (diuretics, vasodilator agents, certain antidepressants), or cause parkinsonism (neuroleptics), thereby increasing the risk of a fall. Physicians should also be aware that a fall could be a geriatric presentation of several diseases, such as pneumonia.

Physical examination

Physical examination should focus on the possible existence of confusion, cognitive disturbances, orthostatic hypotension, nystagmus, presence of carotid bruit, arrhythmias, focal neurological signs, sensory disturbances, gait disorders, and musculoskeletal abnormalities. Special attention should be paid to orthopaedic problems, such as pain or deformity of the spinal column, joints, or feet. Gait or balance is best assessed by asking the patient to stand up from a chair, walk, turn around, and sit down again. Patients with kyphosis, bulging of the abdominal wall accompanied by a short ribcage-to-pelvis distance, which is suggestive of severe osteoporosis, have a high fall risk.

The nature of the gait disorder can provide clues. For example, patients with vascular parkinsonism walk slowly, with small shuffling but broad-based steps. Circumduction may be indicative of a cerebrovascular accident, a drop foot of a peroneal nerve lesion, and a waddling gait of proximal myopathy due to vitamin D deficiency. Often patients need to take more steps when turning to prevent loss of balance. Proprioception can be tested with the Romberg test, and physicians can gain an impression of the strength of the lower extremities by asking patients to walk on their toes and heels.

Laboratory investigations

Anaemia, infection, diabetes, vitamin B12 deficiency, and hypothyroidism should be excluded in patients with a high risk of falls. A normal erythrocyte sedimentation rate (ESR) and alkaline phosphatase concentration make malignancy less likely in patients with an osteoporotic fracture. TSH, calcium, and phosphate concentrations should be measured to exclude secondary causes of osteoporosis, such hyperparathyroidism. Vitamin D deficiency (25-hydroxyvitamin D_3 concentration <50 nmol/L) should be considered in older patients who do not go outdoors often.

Electrocardiogram

An electrocardiogram should be made if arrhythmia is suspected. A 24-hour or 48-hour ambulatory (Holter) electrocardiogram may be useful, but is not a standard part of the diagnostic work-up because transient arrhythmias are prevalent in older people and it is often difficult to establish a relationship between the two.

Imaging

Imaging (such as CT of the brain) is only relevant when there is a raised risk of falls in patients with focal neurological deficits. Radiography of the spine should be considered if osteoporosis is suspected.

Bone mineral density

BMD should be measured by dual energy X-ray absorptiometry (DEXA) to further define the risk of hip fracture in patients with one or more risk factors for a fall or osteoporosis. However, it is of little added value to measure BMD in older patients with an existing "osteoporotic" vertebral fracture because the risk of hip fracture is strongly increased in these patients.

Treatment and prevention

General measures to prevent falls

Before considering intervention, physicians should first investigate the cause of the fall and the presence of risk factors for falls (3, 4). Certain antihistamines and antiemetics should be prescribed with caution to patients who complain of dizziness because the potential sedative properties of these drugs can increase the risk of confusion in elderly individuals. People who suffer from orthostatic hypotension should be advised to raise the head-end of their bed, to wear support stockings, and to avoid heavy meals and physical exertion on warm days. Such patients should also be advised to get upright slowly and to sit on the edge of the bed for several minutes before standing. Additional salt in the diet or fludrocortisone may be prescribed to expand the circulating volume, but caution should be taken against overexpansion. Medications with a sedative action which slow reactions, or which lower blood pressure, or which cause parkinsonism should be stopped or replaced, where possible.

Physical therapy and occupational therapy

Exercise training, supervised by a physiotherapist, is recommended for muscle weakness and gait or balance disorders. Therapists can also teach people how to break a fall and to stand up, and give advice about walking aides (canes, walkers, etc) and "safe" footwear. Shoes with a thin, hard sole provide the greatest stability during walking. Older people at increased risk of falling should be advised to take regular physical exercise (e.g., walking for 30 minutes, five times a week) as a way to prevent falls and to improve muscle function, coordination (balance), and stamina. An occupational therapist can advise about improvements in the home environment (better lighting, handrails, raised toilet, etc).

Prevention of hip fractures

In addition to preventative measures to avert falls, physicians should consider treating older patients with osteoporosis with calcium, vitamin D and bisphosphonatesor strontium ranelate. A study in a nursing home in France showed that the incidence of hip fractures decreased when residents received supplements of calcium and vitamin D (5). A similar study in the Netherlands involving less vulnerable individuals did not find supplementation to be an effective intervention for preventing hip fractures (6). However, calcium supplements are indicated for older patients with osteoporosis and a low dietary calcium intake (500–1000 mg daily), and vitamin D supplementation (e.g., 400–800 U cholecalciferol, once or twice daily) should certainly be considered in immobile older patients with evident limited exposure to sunlight. The bisphosphonates alendronate (70 mg once weekly) and risedronate (35 mg once weekly) and the drug strontium ranelate (2 grams daily) have proved effective in lowering the incidence of hip fractures in approximately 50 % of postmenopausal women with severe osteoporosis (7–10). To achieve this, patients should to be prepared to take the drug for several years. Hip protectors should be considered in patients with a very high falls risk. When used correctly, hip protectors can reduce the incidence of hip fractures by 50 % (11).

PAGET'S DISEASE

Paget's disease, or osteitis deformans, is a local skeletal disorder characterized by substantial remodeling of one or more bones, leading to disorganization of the shape, structure, and function of affected bone. The disease is caused by an increased breakdown of bone by osteoclasts, which become not only more numerous but also larger, with multiple nuclei. The increased breakdown of bone leads to a secondary increase in bone formation, because of the coupling between the two processes. The rapid bone remodeling leads to structural disorganization of bone tissue, which is of poor quality with a higher risk of malformation and fractures. Paget's disease has a male:female ratio of 3:2 and its prevalence increases with age, such that 2–5 % of people older than 50 have the disease. After osteoporosis, it is the second most common bone disease among the elderly.

Pathogenesis

The prevalence of Paget's disease shows a geographical distribution. The disease mainly occurs in Europe, North America, some South American countries, Australia, and New Zealand. It is rare in Scandinavia and Asia. There is also evidence of a genetic predisposition. A study from the United States showed a 7-fold higher risk of disease among first-degree relatives of patients. A number of studies have reported a positive family history in 10–25 % of patients, and a recent detailed study from Spain reported that 40 % of 35 patients had at least one relative with Paget's disease. A possible association with chromosome 18 is being investigated.

While the cause of the disease is unknown, there are strong indications that the disease arises following an earlier viral infection with a "slow virus" of the paramyxovirus group, such as the measles virus, respiratory syncitial virus, or canine distemper virus.

Localization

Paget's disease can affect all the bones of the skeleton but it most frequently affects the pelvis (67 %), femur (35 %), spine (27 %), skull and jaw (29 %), and sacrum (26 %). The disease can affect more than one bone, and in about 65 % of patients Paget's disease affects at least two bones. The number of bone lesions does not change once the disease is established. This is an important point to emphasize to patients, who may be afraid that the disease will spread to other parts of the skeleton.

Clinical signs

Most patients are asymptomatic and in most cases the disease is detected incidentally, following the measurement of an increased alkaline phosphatase activity or the detection of radiographic abnormalities (12). A large study in England estimated the prevalence to be 4–5 %. More than 80 % of symptomatic patients report pain as the main symptom. The pain is usually dull but can be nagging or stabbing. In about 50 % of patients pain is caused by an active lesion; in the remaining patients it is due to osteoarthritis or malformations caused by the disease Fifteen percent of patients have bone deformities at the time of diagnosis, especially of the weight-bearing long bones such as the tibia and femur, but also of the skull and jaw. Deformities often cause abnormal loading of bone, which can lead to osteoarthritis of the large joints. A fracture is the first symptom in 9 % of patients. Such fractures are more common in the long bones and can be complete or pseudofractures. A serious but rare complication (less than 1 %) is the development of an osteosarcoma in the Paget's lesion. Neurological symptoms occur in 8–10 % of patients, such as hearing loss in a third of patients with Paget's disease of the skull. Other rare neurological complications are myelum compression and obstructive hydrocephalus. The increased vascularization of affected bone can lead to ischaemia of surrounding tissues ("steal syndrome"). Depending on the site involved, this may give rise to claudication in the legs, headache, or in rare cases dementia in patients with Paget's disease of the skull. The skin covering affected bone is often warm, red, and shiny as a result of the increased local circulation and bone formation. A raised skin temperature is often present when Paget's disease affects the long bones. Heart failure, which was often reported in patients with Paget's disease in the past, is rarely seen nowadays.

Imaging

On radiographs a decreased density of the affected bone is seen which sometimes appears as a wedge-shaped or "blade of grass"-shaped segment in the long bones. Translucent areas on the skull, osteoporosis circumscripta, may also be detected. This is a sign of early disease of the skull. Old lesions often have a mixed sclerotic and lytic appearance, the bone structure is irregular, and the bone volume is increased. Cyst-like lesions that disrupt the bone cortex and pseudofractures of the long bones are particularly important because of the high risk of fracture. Although these radiographic signs are usually pathognomic, it is sometimes difficult to distinguish these signs from those of bone metastases from prostate cancer or fibrous dysplasia. Skeletal scintigraphy is used to determine the extent of the disease. Although this technique is not specific, it is more sensitive than radiography.

Laboratory investigation

Paget's disease is characterized by increased bone remodeling, with an equilibrium between biochemical markers of bone resorption (excretion of hydroxyproline) and formation (serum alkaline phosphatase). However, levels of these markers are within the normal range in 10 % of patients with limited disease. Recently, more specific markers have been developed, such as N- and C-telopeptides, breakdown products of collagen type I and hence markers of bone resorption. New markers of bone formation include bone-specific alkaline phosphatase and osteocalcin and procollagen propeptide, which are produced by osteoblasts. These markers of remodeling are of value when evaluating subtle changes in bone metabolism but are not more informative than hydroxyproline or alkaline phosphatase in diagnosing and monitoring Paget's disease. Moreover, osteocalcin levels are within the normal range in about 50 % of patients with Paget's disease. Bone biopsy is usually not needed to establish the diagnosis but is useful if there is doubt. It should be borne in mind that, with the exception of the pelvis, bone biopsy could give rise to long-lasting and often disruptive pain in patients with Paget's disease. The incidence of secondary hyperparathyroidism and hypercalciuria is increased in Paget's disease.

Treatment

The aim of treatment is to inhibit the increased osteoclast activity. Several drugs are available, the best-known being calcitonin and the bisphosphonates. Less well known and used are the mithramycins (plicamycin, a highly toxic cytostatic antibiotic) and gallium nitrate.

Salmon calcitonin is the most effective drug. Calcitonin binds to specific receptors on mature osteoclasts, decreasing their activity. It produces both clinical and biochemical improvement, but the effect is incomplete and is rapidly lost after discontinuation of treatment. Moreover, patients can develop resistance to calcitonin. The adverse effects of parenteral calcitonin are nausea, vomiting, and hot flashes.

Bisphosphonates are currently the treatment of choice because a near-normalization of the raised bone resorption can be achieved and the effect is sustained after treatment discontinuation. The selectivity for active lesions, the specific inhibition of bone resorption, and the lack of circulating metabolites make bisphosphonates the ideal drug to treat patients with Paget's disease.

Bisphosphonates, such as alendronate, ibandronate, olpadronate, pamidronate, and risedronate, are the most effective, bringing about clinical, radiological, and histological improvement (13). Treatment with daily risedronate 30 mg tablets, for a period of two months, is usually sufficient to treat the disorder.

Bisphosphonates decrease pain in 80 % of patients if the pain is caused by disease activity and in 50 % of patients if the pain is due to deformity of the femur or tibia. Osteotomy is often needed for persistent pain. Only 25 % of patients with pain due to disease-associated osteoarthrits respond to bisphosphonates. Diminishing of myelum cord compression can be reached and the risk of fracture decreases. Although hearing problems do not improve, further deterioration is prevented. These results constitute an argument for early intervention to prevent complications.

Treatment effectiveness can be monitored by measuring serum alkaline phosphatase activity. Because treatment with bisphosphonates leads to a predictable change in bone remodeling, it is not necessary to continue treatment until alkaline phosphatase activity reaches a minimum. Complete inhibition of bone resorption leads to a slow decrease in alkaline phosphatase activity regardless of whether treatment is continued or not. It is important that physicians are aware of this, to prevent unnecessarily prolonged treatment.

Patients with lower levels of alkaline phosphatase activity after treatment have a longer remission. Remission can last for up to two to three years after a short treatment but remission lasting up to 10 years has been seen with the potent nitrogen-containing bisphosphonates. Recurrences occur slowly after complete biochemical remission. This means that it is necessary to monitor patients once or twice a year only, with measurement of alkaline phosphatase activity being sufficient. Treatment should be restarted if alkaline phosphatase activity increases beyond the normal range or if patients experience symptoms.

The first course of treatment with nitrogen-containing bisphosphonates can cause an acute-phase reaction, with a brief increase in temperature accompanied by flu-like symptoms and a decreased lymphocyte count. This reaction resolves spontaneously even though treatment is continued and never occurs with subsequent treatments. Because rapid parenteral administration of bisphosphonates can lead to the formation of nephrotoxic calcium complexes, the drug should be given slowly, by infusion.

OSTEOMALACIA

Osteomalacia is a disease of the mineralization of the matrix (osteoid) of both trabecular and cortical bone. It is accompanied by diffuse bone pain and proximal muscle weakness (14). The disease is generally caused by a deficiency of the active metabolite of vitamin D, usually as a consequence of malabsorption of vitamin D by the intestines, diminished synthesis in the skin, or dysregulated hydroxylation of vitamin D in the kidneys. The disease is thus usually treated with supplementary vitamin D. The disease was mentioned in the ancient Indian literature (Vagbhatta 500 AD), where it was described as persistent severe pain in the hip area accompanied by loss of muscle strength. However, most patients have only mild symptoms, which makes the diagnosis difficult.

Pathogenesis and histopathology

Adequate amounts of calcium and phosphate are essential for the appropriate mineralization of the organic matrix of trabecular and cortical bone. A shortage of the most biologically active metabolite of vitamin D, 1,25-dihydroxyvitamin D ($1,25(OH)_2D$), can lead to hypocalcaemia and hypophosphataemia as a result of diminished intestinal absorption. This can result in an increased volume of non-mineralized matrix and a decreased volume of calcified matrix. Hypocalcaemia stimulates the parathyroid gland to produce parathyroid hormone (PTH), which in turn stimulates osteoclasts to break down bone, increasing the blood levels of calcium and phosphate. The renal clearance of phosphate and the tubular resorption of calcium also increase under the influence of the raised levels of PTH, which also stimulate the renal conversion of 25-hydroxyvitamin D ($25(OH)D$) into $1,25(OH)_2D$. This in turn stimulates the intestinal absorption of calcium and phosphate.

The cause of myopathy (decrease in proximal muscle strength) in patients with osteomalacia is not fully known. It is possible that atrophy of "rapid" type 2 muscle fibers, which can be seen in biopsy specimens, has a role. The binding of calcium in the sarcoplasmic reticulum is also diminished in vitamin D deficiency, which leads to a decrease in contractile force. Vitamin D supplementation stimulates the binding of calcium in the sarcoplasmic reticulum and the expression of genes for contractile proteins such as actin. It also promotes the differentiation of myoblasts into myofibrils.

Causes

The main cause of osteomalacia is a shortage of the active metabolite of vitamin D as a result of its diminished synthesis or too little exposure to sunlight. Vitamin D shortage can also occur as a result of disturbed absorption of vitamin D due to celiac disease, partial gastric resection, intestinal resection or bypass, and disorders of the gall bladder.

The synthesis of the active metabolite $25(OH)D$ can become dysregulated in patients with liver disease, such as biliary cirrhosis. Anticonvulsants, such as phenytoin, phenobarbital, and carbamazepine increase the activity of certain liver enzymes, with the result that levels of biologically inactive vitamin metabolites increase, leading to insufficient formation of 25(OH)D.

The 1α-hydroxylation of 25(OH)D to 1,25(OH)$_2$D is diminished in certain renal diseases and malignancies. Mesenchymal tumors and prostate carcinoma can affect proximal tubule function—the tumor may secrete an as yet not identified toxic substance that disturbs the function of the proximal tubules. As a consequence, hypophosphataemia and low levels of 1,25(OH)$_2$D (due to dysregulated 1α-hydroxylation) develop, events that can be reversed by tumor resection.

In renal disease accompanied by glomerular filtration defects, phosphate levels rise, leading to a decrease in serum calcium levels and an increase in PTH levels, which triggers bone resorption. The diminished synthesis of 1,25(OH)$_2$D in the kidneys leads to a reduced intestinal absorption of calcium, which negatively affects bone mineralization.

Combinations of the above-mentioned factors can also lead to osteomalacia. Thus in immobile elderly individuals with a chronic disorder, a decreased exposure to sunlight in combination with diminished renal function can lead to altered bone mineralization.

Clinical signs

The clinical signs of osteomalacia are often mild, which can lead to a missed diagnosis. Diffuse skeletal pain, often centered on the hips, and proximal muscle weakness are the most common symptoms and can lead to diminished mobility and even long-lasting confinement to bed. It is often difficult to determine whether the diminished mobility is due to pain or muscle weakness. Other factors, such as secondary hyperparathyroidism, can also contribute to the myopathy. Rib fractures (patients are at increased risk of such fractures) can lead to deformity of the thorax, while collapse of the vertebral bodies leads to loss of height.

Diagnosis

In osteomalacia the trabeculae and the cortex of bone become thinner and some trabeculae are lost, which makes it difficult to distinguish the disease from osteoporosis. These changes diminish the intrinsic strength of bone and deformities, such as curvature of the lower extremities, may develop. Characteristic are the often multiple Milkman's pseudofractures, also termed Looser's zones, that occur symmetrically on the ribs, lateral edges of the shoulder blades, pelvic girdle, neck of the thigh bones, and fibula. These are radiolucent bands varying in width between several millimeters to centimeters that often run perpendicular to the bone surface. It is not know what causes these Looser's zones. The preferential sites for their occurrence are where arteries pass through bone, and it is possible that the mechanical pressure of the pulsations in these vessels causes these pseudofractures.

The disease underlying osteomalacia determines whether the serum levels of 25(OH)D and or 1,25(OH)$_2$D are normal, low, or high. Serum calcium levels are low or normal and phosphate and 25(OH)D levels are low in vitamin D deficiency. Indeed, the level of 25(OH)D can be used to determine the vitamin D status of a patient. The 1,25(OH)$_2$D level is usually normal in patients with osteomalacia as a result of secondary hyperparathyroidism. The raised levels of PTH stimulate the activity of osteoclasts, increasing bone resorption, which leads to an increased urinary excretion of hydroxyproline. This leads to a compensatory increase in the activity of osteoblasts, accompanied by an increase in serum alkaline phosphatase.

The need for bone biopsy has diminished because the incidence of osteomalacia has decreased and because the disorder can be diagnosed by other methods. If a biopsy specimen is needed, a trans-iliac specimen is best.

Treatment

If osteomalacia is caused by a dietary deficiency or limited exposure to sunlight vitamin D$_3$ should be given orally in daily doses of 1000–2000 IU for 6 to 12 weeks (15–17).

Thereafter maintenance dosing with 400–800 IU daily should be started. Muscle strength and mobility increase within weeks, and serum calcium and phosphate levels normalize. Alkaline phosphatase activity takes somewhat longer to decrease. Within weeks the pseudofractures start to heal, a process that is completed by about 6 months.

However, if the disorder is caused by intestinal malabsorption, and especially steatorrhea, higher doses are needed, varying between daily doses of 10,000 and 50,000 IU vitamin D_3 together with 4 g calcium. If the malabsorption is severe, it may be necessary to administer vitamin D parenterally, for instance 600,000 IU vitamin D_3 injected intramuscularly once a year or half the dose twice a year.

Patients with osteomalacia caused by anticonvulsant medication should be treated with up to 4,000 vitamin D_3 daily or even more during one month. A prophylactic dose of 800 IU vitamin D_3 daily should be given to patients treated with anticonvulsants who are at risk of osteomalacia.

Patients with osteomalacia as a result of diminished activity of 25-hydroxylase due to severe liver disease should be treated with $1,25(OH_2)D$. It is recommended that serum calcium levels should be closely monitored at the start of treatment with high doses of vitamin D.

KEY POINTS

- Two or more falls in the previous year is an important predictor of new falls.
- Bisphosphonates and the drug strontium ranelate have proved effective in lowering the incidence of hip fractures in approximately 50 % of postmenopausal women with severe osteoporosis.
- The selectivity for active lesions, the specific inhibition of bone resorption, and the lack of circulating metabolites make bisphosphonates the ideal drug to treat patients with Paget's disease.
- Osteomalacia is generally caused by a deficiency of the active metabolite of vitamin D, usually as a consequence of malabsorption

of vitamin D by the intestines, diminished synthesis in the skin, or dysregulated hydroxylation of vitamin D in the kidneys.
- If osteomalacia is caused by a dietary deficiency or limited exposure to sunlight, then vitamin D_3 should be given orally in daily doses of 1000–2000 IU for six to 12 weeks. Thereafter maintenance dosing with 400–800 IU daily should be started.

REFERENCES

1. Tromp A.M., Smit J.H., Deeg D.J.H., Bouter L.M., Lips P. Predictors for falls and fractures in the Longitudinal Aging Study Amsterdam. *J. Bone Miner. Res.* 1998; **13**: 1932–9.
2. Dargent-Molina P., Favier F., Grandjean H., Baudoin C., Schott A.M., Hausherr E., Meunier P.J., Bréart G., for EPIDOS Group. Fall-related factors and risk of hip fracture: the EPIDOS prospective study. *Lancet* 1996; **348**: 145–9.
3. Oliver D., Britton M., Seed P., Martin F.C., Hopper A.H. Development and evaluation of evidence based risk assessment tool (STRATIFY) to predict which elderly inpatients will fall: case-control and cohort studies. *BMJ* 1997; **315**: 1049–53.
4. Tinetti M.E., Baker D.I., McAvay G., et al. A multifactorial intervention to reduce the risk of falling among elderly people living in the community. *N. Engl. J. Med.* 1994; **331**: 821–7.
5. Chapuy M.C., Arlot M.E. Duboeuf F., et al. Vitamin D_3 and calcium to prevent hip fractures in elderly women. *N. Engl. J. Med.* 1992; **337**: 670–6.
6. Lips P., Graafmans W.C., Ooms M.E., Bezemer P.D., Bouter L.M. Vitamin D supplementation and fracture incidence in elderly persons. *Ann. Intern. Med.* 1996; **124**: 400–6.
7. Black D.M., Cummings S.R., Karpf D.B. et al. Randomised trial of effect of alendronate on risk of fracture in women with existing vertebral fractures. Fracture Intervention Trial Research Group. *Lancet* 1996; **348**: 1535–41.
8. McClung M.R., Geusens P., Miller P.D. et al. Effect of risedronate on the risk of hip fracture in elderly women. *N. Engl. J. Med.* 2001; **344**: 333–40.
9. Boonen S., McClung M.R., Eastell R. et al. Safety and efficacy of risedronate in reducing fracture risk in osteoporotic women aged 80 and older: implications for the use of antiresorptive

agents in the old and oldest old. *J. Am. Geriatr. Soc*. 2004; **52**: 1832–9.

10. Meunier P.J., Roux C., Seeman E. et al. The effects of strontium ranelate on the risk of vertebral fracture in women with postmenopausal osteoporosis. *N. Engl. J. Med*. 2004; **350**: 459–68.

11. Kannus P., Parkkari J., Niemi S. et al. Prevention of hip fracture in elderly people with use of a hip protector. *N. Engl. J. Med*. 2000; **343**: 1506–13.

12. Duursma SA, Raymakers JA, Verhaar HJJ. Osteoporosis, osteomalacia and Paget's disease of bone. *Reviews Clin Gerontol* 1997; **7**: 127–36.

13. Langston A.L., Ralston S.H. Management of Paget's disease of bone. *Rheumatology* (Oxford) 2004; **43**: 955–99.

14. Klein G.L. *Nutritional Rickets and osteomalacia. Primer on the metabolic bone diseases and disorders of mineral metabolism* (3rd edn). An official publication of the American Society for Bone and Mineral Research 1996: pp. 301–5.

15. Gloth III F.M., Smith C.E., Hollis B.W., Tobin J.D. Functional improvement with vitamin D replenishment in a cohort of frail, vitamin D-deficient older people. *J. Am. Geriatr. Soc*. 1995; **43**: 1269–71.

16. Janssen H.C.J.P., Samson M.M., Verhaar H.J.J. Vitamin D deficiency, muscle function, and falls in elderly people. *Amer. J.Clin. Nutrition* 2002; **75**, 611–15.

17. Holick M.F. High prevalence of vitamin D inadequacy and implications for health. *Mayo Clin. Proc*. 2006; **81**: 353–73.

39 Drugs and falls

Nathalie van der Velde and Tischa J.M. van der Cammen

Department of Internal Medicine, Erasmus University Medical Centre, Rotterdam, The Netherlands

INTRODUCTION

Falls are among the most common and serious problems facing older persons and are associated with considerable morbidity and mortality (1). Assessment of falls and fall risk is a complex matter. By now, over 20 risk factors have been identified and often there are multiple causes for falls in a given patient (see Chapter 38).

An important risk factor for falls is the use of certain drugs. Several drug groups have been identified which increase fall risk, with psychotropic drugs as the most well known (2, 3). In addition, an increased fall risk has been demonstrated for cardiovascular drugs and for polypharmacy (4). Polypharmacy in itself, however, is not a risk factor, unless it includes at least one fall-risk-increasing drug (5). Therefore, a check-up of the drug regimen should not just merely be an attempt to cut down the total number of prescribed drugs, but needs to optimize the drug regimen for the individual patient. This means that besides possible withdrawal (cessation or dose reduction) of certain drugs, adding new drugs may be necessary, in order to reach a maximum reduction of fall risk and other possible adverse events.

PATHOPHYSIOLOGY

The incidence of falls increases with age. Furthermore, it is generally assumed that the incidence rate of drug-induced falls also increases with age. Apart from an increased utilization of drugs in the elderly, this is attributed to the fact that physical reserves decrease with ageing. Changes in pharmacokinetics and pharmacodynamics make older persons more prone to adverse drug reactions, including fall incidents (6). Because of these changes, an adverse drug reaction can occur even without recent changes in the drug regimen (7). Drug-related falls are usually caused either via the pathway of reduced mobility or via negative effects on the cardiovascular system (Figure 39.1). In some instances both pathways are affected at the same time. Mobility can be hampered in several ways: through negative effects on muscle strength and balance, or on concentration and reaction time. Regarding the cardiovascular system, use of certain drugs may lead to hypotension or heart rhythm disorders, or give rise to vascular adverse events like orthostatic hypotension, carotid sinus hypersensitivity or vasovagal collapse. A recent trial looking at the effects of withdrawal of fall-risk-increasing drugs in older fallers showed that both improvement of mobility and amelioration of cardiovascular side effects, especially orthostatic hypotension, led to a decrease in the number of fall incidents (8–10). For the withdrawal of psychotropic drugs, the largest effect was on mobility. However, orthostatic hypotension also significantly lessened. For the withdrawal

Prescribing for Elderly Patients   Edited by Stephen Jackson, Paul Jansen and Arduino Mangoni
© 2009 John Wiley & Sons, Ltd

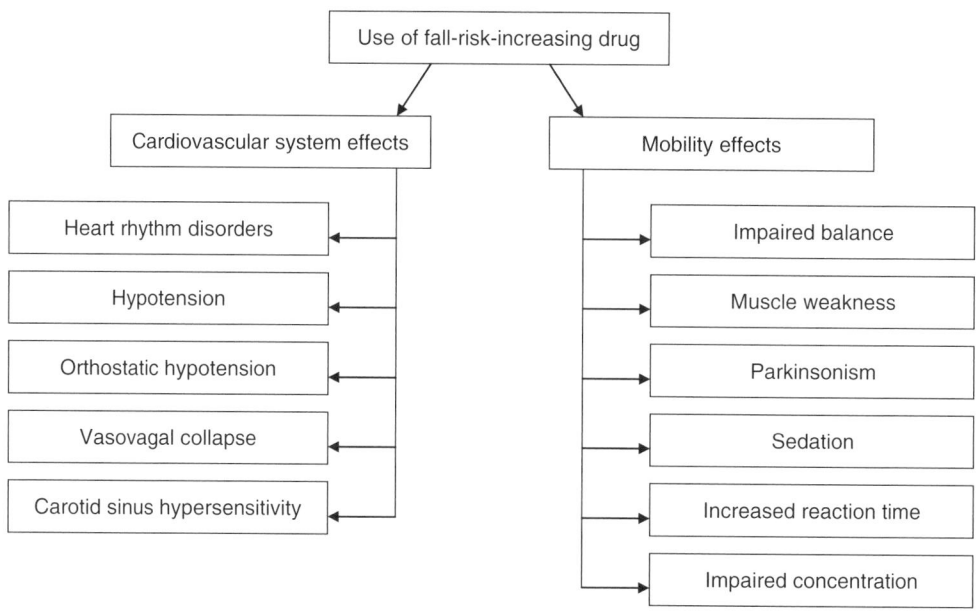

Figure 39.1. The main pathways of drug-related falls

of cardiovascular drugs, improvement of both orthostatic hypotension and carotid sinus hypersensivity was demonstrated, but mobility tests also appeared to show some improvement. Hence, both pathways seem to be involved in causing the increased fall risk for these drug categories.

FALL-RISK-INCREASING DRUGS

As mentioned above, there are several drug groups that can increase fall risk (Table 39.1). For psychotropic drugs, the increased fall risk is partly caused by the direct pharmacodynamic effects they have on the brain, giving rise to sedation, increased reaction time and impaired concentration. Furthermore, psychotropic drugs regularly cause cardiovascular adverse events like orthostatic hypotension. This is true for antipsychotics, sedatives, hypnotics, anxiolytics and antidepressants. In case of antidepressant use, it is important to realize that not only the older drug groups like the tricyclic antidepressants and monoamine oxidase inhibitors give a significant increase in orthostatic hypotension, but also the newer drugs, selective serotonin reuptake inhibitors (SSRIs) and serotonin

norepinephrine reuptake inhibitors, have these adverse effects. Furthermore, besides increasing fall risk, use of SSRIs also results in an extra increase in fracture risk, most likely caused by a negative effect on bone metabolism (11). When prescribing sedatives and hypnotics, the dose should be kept to the absolute minimum, since the beneficial effects are very limited and the negative effects are numerous. In prescribing, adhere to the lowest effective dose and keep the duration of the prescription limited, especially if prescribing hypnotics. If prescription can not be avoided, it is advisable to choose short-acting preparations, because with increasing age, the half-life of sedatives and hypnotics is prolonged and can be up to one or two weeks, both in short-acting and in long-acting benzodiazepines. With the use of antipsychotics, patients need regular follow-up, since mobility can become impaired if extrapiramidal symptoms and signs or other dyskinesias develop. This risk is highest for the classic antipsychotics, and in these cases the prescribed drug needs to be withdrawn. If a neuroleptic is still needed, clozapine or low doses of quetiapine can be considered.

As is to be expected, cardiovascular drugs mainly give rise to cardiovascular side effects.

Table 39.1. Drugs associated with an increased fall risk

Psychotropic drugs	
Sedatives	Benzodiazepines and others
Antipsychotics	D2 agonists and serotonin dopamine receptor antagonists
Antidepressants	Tricyclic antidepressants, selective serotonin reuptake inhibitors, serotonin norepinephrine reuptake inhibitors and monoamine oxidase inhibitors
Cardiovascular drugs	
Antihypertensives	Diuretics, beta-blockers, alpha-blockers, centrally acting antihypertensives, calcium channel blockers, angiotensin converting enzyme inhibitors and angiotensin receptor blockers
Anti-arrhythmics	Class IA anti-arrhythmics, digoxin and others
Vasodilators	Nitrates and others
Miscellaneous drugs	
Beta-blocker eye drops	
Analgesics	Especially opioids
Anticholinergic drugs	Anticholinergics, antispasmodics, mydriatics, tricyclic antidepressants, certain anti-arrhythmics, antihistamines, antipsychotics
Anti-vertigo drugs	
Anti-epileptics	
Antidiabetics	

This can either be a heart rhythm disorder, mainly tachy- or brady arrhythmias, or a vascular adverse event. As shown in a recent meta-analysis, fall risk is increased with the use of diuretics, type IA anti-arrhythmics or digoxine (4). However, all antihypertensives, vasodilators and anti-arrhythmics have been shown to give rise to negative cardiovascular effects like orthostatic hypotension, carotid sinus hypersensitivity and vasovagal collapse, thereby leading to an increased fall risk. When treating orthostatic hypotension, remember that hypertension itself can also cause or increase the severity of orthostatic hypotension (12). This stresses the importance of individualizing the drug-regimen, since, in this situation, some patients may need to start an antihypertensive or may need an increase in their dosage, whereas others may benefit from withdrawal of these drugs. Because it is thought angiotensin converting enzyme inhibitors and angiotensin receptor blockers have fewer adverse cardiovascular events, a switch to one of these drug groups can also be an effective option. But again, it has to be tested in the individual patient whether such a "switch" indeed results in the expected amelioration. For beta-blockers, there have been positive reports on their use in the treatment of vasovagal collapse and carotid sinus hypersensitivity. However, data regarding this issue are conflicting, since a negative association with carotid sinus hypersensitivity and vasovagal collapse has also been shown. These differing results underline the importance to individually test per patient, which drugs increase or decrease fall risk and other possible adverse events.

Not only oral or intravenous use of beta-blockers, but also use of beta-blocker eye drops carries a high risk of systemic adverse events. This is caused by the fact that eye drops enter the systemic blood flow directly via the naso-lacrimal duct, without undergoing the first pass effect of the liver. For this reason, even small ocular concentrations can lead to systemic relevant concentrations and thus possible adverse events (13). Other miscellaneous drugs with an increased fall risk are analgesics. Opioids have a negative effect on mobility via cerebral blunting effects and can also give rise to orthostatic hypotension. Non-steroidal anti-inflammatory drugs are also thought to increase fall risk, likely through adverse central nervous system effects (14). Anticholinergics significantly increase fall risk as well, through negative cerebral effects, leading to impaired mobility, and they can also induce orthostatic hypotension (15). For anti-vertigo drugs there is very limited evidence regarding their beneficial effects and this is pertained to Menière's disease. There are however many reports on adverse events, and this class of drugs may paradoxically lead to an increased fall risk, because they can induce dizziness. Therefore, these drugs seem better avoided in the majority of cases.

CLINICAL APPROACH

When assessing a patient who is referred because of a fall incident or fear of falling, a complete comprehensive geriatric assessment is warranted, including a full physical examination (blood pressure, orthostatic hypotension measurement, heart rhythm, hydration, etc.) and neurological examination (tremor, rigidity, postural reflexes, bradykinesia, etc.).

A rigorous review of the medication regimen is an essential part of the assessment (1, 8). If falling started after the prescription of a new drug or after a change of dosage of existing medication, then withdrawal of the new drug or re-assessment of the dosage of the existing medication are the first steps in the medication review.

Nonetheless, as mentioned above, due to changes in pharmacokinetics and pharmacodynamics with age, even drugs that have been used for several years can suddenly lead to adverse drug reactions, including fall incidents. Therefore, all fall-risk-increasing drugs should be considered for withdrawal. Furthermore, as mentioned above, the medical history and patient assessment are essential to determine the underlying reason for the fall incident (see Chapter 38), and to give direction towards the possible causative pathway. But since patients may not have or may not recognize preceding or accompanying symptoms of an imminent fall, mobility and cardiovascular tests can be of help in the diagnosis of the underlying mechanisms, and in the follow-up. Mobility can be easily tested with the Timed Up and Go

Test, which is also useful for follow-up (10). If needed, more extensive mobility testing can be performed by using the POMA (Performance Oriented Mobility Assessment) or other more extensive mobility tests. Orthostatic hypotension, carotid sinus hypersensitivity and vasovagal collapse are preferably tested using a tilt-table and a continuous blood pressure measurement system. This will ensure maximal reproducibility. Orthostatic hypotension tested with continuous blood pressure monitoring has also been shown to have a better association with fall incidents compared to measurements performed with a regular blood pressure measurement system (16).

TREATMENT: DRUG WITHDRAWAL

Withdrawal of medication needs to be performed under vigilant attention of the treating physician and starts with determining which drugs may be eligible for withdrawal. At the top of the list are the drugs that have been prescribed for the wrong indication or for which the indication is no longer present. Secondly, it needs to be established for which drugs the dosages possibly are too high and which drugs may remain effective if the dosage is lowered. Finally, safer alternatives should be considered for those drugs that are clinically necessary to be continued. Depending on the drug and on the indication, withdrawal may either be at once or in smaller steps, lowering the doses for example every few days. The patient needs to be well informed of the impending change in drug regimen, in order to reach maximum compliance and safety. Regarding the former, this is especially true for withdrawal of sedatives and hypnotics, since this requires a lot of effort from the patient. In our experience, success rate is fairly good if small steps are taken at a time and if there is regular supportive contact with the patient, for example once or twice a week by telephone. Regarding the safety of withdrawal, longer follow-up may be needed in order to ascertain for example a stable balance between intravascular hypovolemia and cardiac congestion or to verify that blood pressure remains within the desired ranges. Up to now, long term data regarding the safety of drug withdrawal in older fallers is scarce. However, if withdrawal is performed as is described above, safety can be assumed, especially if the short term health risks of the fall incidents are taken into account (17). Because of the high risk of adverse events—including fall incidents—with increasing age, we recommend that doctors when prescribing for older persons regularly, review the medication regimen of older fallers. In addition, if falls were to be recognized and accepted as adverse events, this would enhance the detection of drug-related fall incidents and would improve prescribing for older persons.

KEY POINTS

- Withdrawal of fall-risk-increasing drugs in older fallers effectively reduces the number of fall incidents.
- Not only psychotropic, but also cardiovascular drugs need to be targeted in order to maximally decrease fall risk.
- Polypharmacy in itself does not increase fall risk, unless it includes at least one fall-risk-increasing drug.
- An annual review of the medication regimen is advisable in older fallers.
- Recognizing falls as an adverse drug reaction would improve prescribing for older persons.

REFERENCES

1. American Geriatrics Society, British Geriatrics Society, and American Academy of Orthopaedic Surgeons Panel on Falls Prevention: Guideline for the prevention of falls in older persons. *J Am Geriatr Soc* 2001; **49**: 664–72.
2. Campbell AJ, Robertson AC, Gardner MM, Norton RN, Buchner DM: Psychotropic medication withdrawal and a home-based exercise program to prevent falls: a randomized, controlled trial. *J Am Geriatr Soc* 1999; **47**: 850–3.
3. Leipzig RM, Cumming RG, Tinetti ME. Drugs and falls in older people: a systemic review and meta-analysis I: Psychotropic drugs. *J Am Geriatr Soc* 1999; **47**: 30–9.
4. Leipzig RM, Cumming RG, Tinetti ME. Drugs and falls in older people: a systemic review and meta-analysis II: Cardiac and analgesic drugs. *J Am Geriatr Soc* 1999; **47**: 40–50.
5. Ziere G, Dieleman JP, Hofman A, Pols HAP, van der Cammen TJM, Stricker BHCh. Polypharmacy and falls in the middle age and elderly population. *Br J Clin Pharmacol* 2006; **61**(2): 218–23.
6. Turnheim K. Geriatric pharmacology: Pharmacokinetics and pharmacodynamics in the elderly, geriatric and nootropic drugs. *Wien Klin Wochenschr* 1995; **107**: 349–56.
7. Mannesse CK, van der Cammen TJM. Adverse drug reactions in three older patients, even without changes in medication. *Ned Tijdschr Geneesk* 2003; **147**: 585–7.
8. Van der Velde N, Stricker BHCh, Pols HAP, Van der Cammen TJM. Risk of falls after withdrawal of fall-risk-increasing drugs: a prospective cohort study. *Br J Clin Pharmacol* 2007; **63**(2): 232–7.
9. Van der Velde N, Stricker BHCh, Pols HAP, Van den Meiracker AH, Van der Cammen TJM. Withdrawal of fall-risk-increasing drugs in older persons: effect on tilt-table test outcomes. *J Am Geriatr Soc* 2007; **5**(5): 734–9.
10. Van der Velde N, Stricker BHCh, Pols HAP, Van der Cammen TJM. Withdrawal of fall-risk-increasing drugs in older persons: effect on mobility test outcomes. *Drugs Aging* 2007; **24**(8): 691–9.
11. Ziere G, Dieleman JP, van der Cammen TJ, Hofman A, Pols HA, Stricker BH. Selective serotonin reuptake inhibiting antidepressants are associated with an increased risk of nonvertebral fractures. *J Clin Psychopharmacol* 2008; **28**(4): 411–7.
12. Mukai S, Lipsitz LA. Orthostatic hypotension. *Clin Geriatr Med* 2002; **18**(2): 253–68.
13. Shell JW. Pharmacokinetics of topically applied ophthalmic drugs. *Surv Ophthalmol* 1982; **26**: 207–18.
14. Walker PC, Alrawi A, Mitchell JF, Regal RE, Khanderia U. Medication use as a risk factor for falls in hospitalized patients. *Am J Health Syst Pharm* 2005; **62**(23): 2495–9.
15. Aizenberg D, Sigler M, Wizman A, Barak Y. Anticholinergic burden and risk of falls among elderly psychiatric inpatients: a 4-year

case-control study. *Int Psychogeriatr* 2002; **14**: 307–10.

16. Van der Velde N, Van den Meiracker AH, Stricker BHCh, Van der Cammen TJM. Measuring orthostatic hypotension with the Finometer device: is a blood pressure drop of one heartbeat clinically relevant? *Blood Press Monit* 2007; **2**(3): 167–71.

17. Alsop K, MacMahon M. Withdrawing cardiovascular medications at a syncope clinic. *Postgrad Med J* 2001; **77**: 403–5.

40 Pressure ulcers

Rob J. van Marum

Department of Geriatrics, University Medical Centre Utrecht, The Netherlands

INTRODUCTION

A pressure ulcer is an area of localized damage to the skin and underlying tissue caused by pressure, shear, friction and or a combination of these. Pressure ulcers are classified according the extension of the damage (Table 40.1, Figure 40.1).

Pressure ulcers form an important problem in geriatric care. Incidence and prevalence figures in different health care settings show large variation. In the Netherlands prevalence figures were found varying from 20 % in home care and general hospital till around 34 % for nursing homes and institutions for the mentally retarded (1). For other countries comparable figures can be found.

Besides of being an obvious burden for the patient (e.g. pain, nasty smell, impairment of activities of daily living and (prolonged) hospitalisation), pressure ulcers are also a large problem for health care. Allman et al. found that incident pressure ulcers were associated with significantly higher hospital costs ($ 37 288 vs $ 13 924) and length of stay (30.4 vs 12.8 days). Patients who developed pressure ulcers also were more likely to develop nosocomial infections (45.9 % vs. 20.1 %) and other hospital complications (2). The cost of treating a pressure ulcer varies from £ 1064 (Grade 1) to £ 10 551 (Grade 4). Costs increase with ulcer grade because the time to heal is longer and the incidence of complications is higher in more severe cases. The total cost in the UK is £ 1.4–£ 2.1 billion annually (4 % of total NHS expenditure). Most of this cost is nurse time (3). In the Netherlands, the most conservative estimate is approximately 1 % of the total Dutch health care budget (4). Nowadays, pressure ulcer incidence is seen as an indicator of quality of care provided by health care facilities. This view has led to many lawsuits against health care providers related to pressure ulcers in which amounts up to $ 300 million have been awarded to pressure ulcer patients (5). Guidelines for pressure ulcer prevention and treatment from the American Agency for Healthcare Research and Quality (http://www.ahrq.gov/clinic/cpgonline.htm) and European Pressure Ulcer Advisory Panel (http://www.epuap.org) are easily accessible on the Internet and should form the basis of local protocols for pressure ulcer care.

THE ROLE OF PRESSURE IN PRESSURE ULCER DEVELOPMENT

Pressure ulcers are the result of tissue ischemia due to occlusion of blood flow. Pressure and shear forces attributed to the tissues are the key components in the development of pressure ulcers. Many other patient bound factors like malnutrition, anaemia, hypotension and fever may play a role by increasing the patients susceptibility for pressure ulcer development but their effect is limited compared to the effect of increased pressure. Intensity and duration are the two major components of pressure. A high intensity pressure applied to the tissues for a

Prescribing for Elderly Patients   Edited by Stephen Jackson, Paul Jansen and Arduino Mangoni
© 2009 John Wiley & Sons, Ltd

Table 40.1. Classification of pressure ulcers (European Pressure Ulcer Advisory Panel
(http://www.epuap.org/gltreatment.html)

Classification

Grade 1: non-blanchable erythema of intact skin. Discolouration of the skin, warmth, oedema, induration
  or hardness may also be used as indicators, particularly on individuals with darker skin.
Grade 2: partial thickness skin loss involving epidermis, dermis, or both. The ulcer is superficial and
  presents clinically as an abrasion or blister.
Grade 3: full thickness skin loss involving damage to or necrosis of subcutaneous tissue that may extend
  down to, but not through underlying fascia.
Grade 4: extensive destruction, tissue necrosis, or damage to muscle, bone, or supporting structures with or
  without full thickness skin loss.

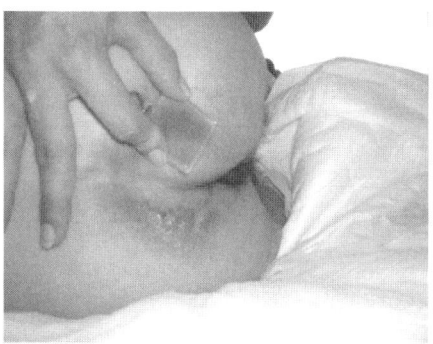

Grade 1 pressure ulcer

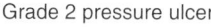

Grade 2 pressure ulcer

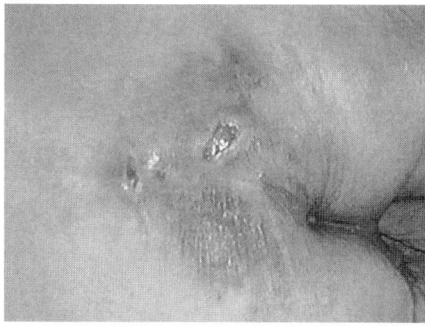

Grade 3 pressure ulcer

Grade 4 pressure ulcer

Figure 40.1. Classification of pressure ulcers

short period of time (e.g. patient on the oper-ation table for hip-replacement) can result in a high risk of pressure ulcer development. Also a low pressure intensity applied for a long pe-riod of time (e.g. patient bedridden on standard hospital mattress) can result in pressure ul-cer development. There is no critical occlusion pressure for all tissues. The often-mentioned threshold of 32 mmHg for tissue-interface pres-sure (the pressure between skin and upper

layer of a mattress) has no rationale basis. The pressure needed for total occlusion of capillar-ies will vary depending on the condition of the patient and body part exposed to pressure and can be as low as 11 mmHg.

A third component of pressure relevant for pressure ulcer development is the direction of pressure. Pressure applied perpendicular to tis-sues (lying or sitting on a stable surface) will concentrate just above bony prominences in the deep tissues (muscular and fat). This will lead to extensive damage to the deep tissues with no visible skin involvement. This effect is increased because the skin is mechanically stronger than the deeper tissues and can withstand longer periods of ischemia. Eventually, the skin will show discoloration and necrosis due to extension of the process. Shear forces, resulting from sliding downwards from a half sitting position in chair or bed, will result in distension of the perforating blood vessels responsible for skin blood supply. Since distension will occur at much lower pressure intensity than occlusion by perpendicular pressure application, shear forces will lead to pressure ulcers at a relatively low-pressure intensity. Besides these two types of pressure ulcers, originating in the deep tissues and extending to the skin leaving deep ulcers, another type of pressure ulcer is the one originating in and often limited to the skin. This type of pressure ulcer (excoriation and blister forming) can result from increased friction between skin and supporting layers (e.g. bed sheets). This superficial damage may eventually extend to deeper tissues, mainly as a result of secondary inflammation. Especially in patients with urinary or faecal incontinence or extensive sweating, the skin may become more vulnerable to friction leading to superficial pressure ulcers.

THE ROLE OF NUTRITION IN PRESSURE ULCER DEVELOPMENT

Malnutrition may also contribute to an increased risk of pressure ulcer development. Energy intake of less than 1500 kcal is found in almost 30 % of elderly women and 10 % of men in the general population. Prevalence figures for malnutrition in patients living in nursing homes vary from 19–59 % (6). Many factors can attribute to the impaired nutritional status of the elderly. One of the most important risk factors is an increased ADL-dependency (from impaired mobility, eyesight, cognition) leading to the inability to obtain, prepare and consume adequate nutrition. Also, impaired health is frequently associated with decreased appetite. Next

to this, gastro-intestinal problems caused by the use of medication can lead to decreased food intake. An association between impaired nutritional status and the risk of developing pressure ulcers is found in most cross-sectional and longitudinal studies. This relationship, however, is only found when global measures of malnutrition (e.g. clinical impression of health care workers) are used to assess nutritional status. The association with more defined parameters like weight-loss, laboratory values and anthropometrical measures and the risk of developing pressure ulcers is less well proven. Although conclusive studies regarding the causal relationship between malnutrition and pressure ulcer development are lacking, it is widely assumed that malnutrition is an important risk factor. However, compared to the influence of pressure on pressure ulcer risk, the effect of nutritional status is relatively small.

RISK ASSESSMENT

Early identification of patients with an increased risk of developing pressure ulcers is essential in prevention. For this purpose, many risk assessment scores have been developed in the past 40 years. The first widely used risk score was the Norton score, followed by many other risk scores such as the Braden and Waterlow scores. Most of these scores are based on the original Norton score, extended with items representing other supposed risk factors. Most scales show a poor balance between sensitivity and specificity. The Braden scale offers the best balance between sensitivity and specificity (57.1 %/67.5 %, respectively) and the best risk estimate (odds ratio = 4.08, CI 95 % = 2.56–6.48) (7). The Norton scale performed slightly less. Another problem with these scales is that much needless work is done and expensive material is wrongly allocated when prevention is exclusively based on these scales. If nurses act according to risk assessment scales, 80 % of the patients would unnecessarily receive preventive measures (8, 9).

However, using a risk assessment tool seems to be a better alternative than relying on the clinical judgement of the nurses (7, 9). Risk assessment should be used as an adjunct to clinical judgement and not as a tool apart from other clinical features. A full risk assessment should include: general medical condition, skin assessment, mobility, moistness and incontinence, nutrition and pain. Assessment should also be ongoing and frequency of re-assessment should be dependent on change in the patient's condition. In all patients considered at risk of developing pressure ulcers, daily inspection of the skin, especially over bony prominences (e.g. heels, ankles, knees, hips, sacrum) should be performed. Since ulceration may start in the deeper tissues before any visible skin defects can be found, this should not be limited to visual inspection but also include palpation of deeper tissue layers at risk sites.

PREVENTION

Pressure reducing devices Pressure reduction is the central element of prevention. Intensity of pressure application can be reduced by providing the patient with special supportive devices (e.g. mattresses and cushions). The question which mattress should be used in pressure ulcer prevention cannot easily be answered since compelling evidence from large randomized controlled trials are lacking. Specific foam mattresses seems to reduce the incidence of pressure ulcers in people at risk. The relative merits of alternating and constant low-pressure devices and of the different alternating pressure devices for pressure ulcer prevention are unclear (10). Furthermore, it is also not possible to indicate which chair cushion shows the best preventive characteristics. Lifting the heels by placing a pillow under the legs can prevent pressure application on heels in bedridden patients. Sheepskins do not reduce pressure. Donut-type devices should not be used since pressure redistribution often causes ulceration in tissues supported by these devices.

Repositioning Frequent repositioning of the patient in order to limit the amount of time spent on the same body surface is on the basic preventive measures. Turn at least every 2–4 hours on a pressure-reducing mattress or at least every two hours on a non pressure-reducing mattress. Special lifting devices can be used to assure that shear forces and friction of skin and bed sheets during repositioning are prevented. When positioning the patient on his side, a $35°$ position is preferred above the $90°$ position in which large pressure is applied to the hip. In the $35°$ position, most pressure is applied to the more muscular gluteal region which leads to a better pressure distribution. Devices such as pillows or foam wedges can be used to keep bony prominences (for example knees, heels or ankles) from direct contact with one another. For patients at risk sitting in (wheel)chairs, frequent shifting weight from one to the other buttock may help in preventing ischemia. Lifting of the chair bound patient for a few seconds is not sufficient for adequate restoration of blood flow.

Nutritional interventions Few methodological correct studies have been performed concerning the effects of nutritional interventions on pressure ulcer development or healing. Although the available studies suggest that nutritional interventions may be able to reduce the incidence of pressure ulcers, more evidence is needed to identify effective dietary interventions (6, 11, 12). In general an individual at risk for pressure ulcer development may require a minimum of 30–35 kcal/kg/day, with 1 to 1.5 g/kg/day protein required and 1 ml/kcal/day of fluid intake (13). Specific guidance on energy expenditure may be provided through equations such as the Harris-Benedict or Schofield formulae although it is recommended that advice is sought from a dietician. For the positive effects of supplementation of specific nutrients (e.g. arginine, zinc, ascorbic acid) on pressure ulcer healing, no evidence is found.

Other preventive measures. Attention must be paid to adequate skin care. Skin cleansing should occur at the time of soiling and at routine intervals. Avoid hot water, and use a mild cleansing agent that minimizes irritation and dryness of the skin. During the cleansing process, care should be utilized to minimize the force and friction applied to the skin. Patients with incontinence should use incontinence systems that must be replaced frequently. The use of a bladder catheter in pressure ulcer prevention is incorrect since it frequently generates new and serious health problems (e.g. infections, persistent incontinence). Use incontinence skin barriers as needed to protect and maintain skin integrity. Friction injuries may be reduced by the use of lubricants, protective films, dressings (such as hydrocolloids) and padding.

LOCAL TREATMENT

In case of pressure ulcer development, the first step must always be the re-evaluation and improvement of preventive measures taken. Without adequate reduction of pressure, local wound treatment will have little effect. Basically, local wound treatment consists of three principles: removing necrotic tissue, creating a moist wound bed and prevention of inflammation. Moist, necrotic tissue provides a medium for infection, initiates an inflammatory response and retards wound healing. Surgical removal of necrosis is preferred. Do not debride dry, black eschar on heels that are non tender, non fluctuant, non erythematous and non suppurative. After surgical necrotectomy, the remaining debris can be removed with the use of sodium hypochlorite in paraffin (Eusol: Edingburgh University Solution). This solution should be used three times a day for a short period (days) until the wound bed is largely free from debris and is showing red granulation tissue. The surrounding skin must always be protected with zinc oil. Dry eschar may also be removed with dressings like hydrocolloids and hydrogels that provide moist environment to encourage autolysis. The efficacy of enzymatic crèmes (collagenase) in wound cleansing has not adequately been proven. Cleanse wounds as necessary with tap water or saline. Use minimal mechanical force when cleansing or irrigating the ulcer. Showering is appropriate.

No good evidence exists for specific wound dressings (14). All dressings should primarily create a moist wound bed. In strongly exsudative wounds, a dressing with large absorptive characteristics (e.g. foams, alginates) can be chosen. These dressings are also suited for the filling of larger cavities. Hydrocolloids can be used in more superficial and medium exsudative wounds. In dry wounds, the addition of hydrogels can be necessary. In a healing wound, the dressing must be kept in place as long as possible (days). If there is leakage or strike through, it causes a break in the barrier that the dressing provides to external contamination, and so it should be changed. Wet-to-dry dressings (gauzes) adhere to devitalised tissue. One disadvantage of wet-to-dry dressings is that they remove both nonviable and viable tissues and are therefore potentially traumatic to granulation tissue and especially to new epithelial tissue. Wet gauzes can be used three to four times a day. However, this is more time consuming and can be painful for the patient. Since all wounds are colonised with multiple bacteria in general there is no rational for cultures. Only if there are clinical signs of infection cultures may be taken. In general, topical antibiotics are not recommended. Reasons for this include inadequate penetration for deep skin infections, development of antibiotic resistance, hypersensitivity reactions, systemic absorption when applied to large wounds, and local irritant effects leading to further delay in wound healing. Local inflammation can be treated with local antiseptics. All antiseptics are potentially cytotoxic and should only be used for a limited period of time until the wound is clean and surrounding inflammation reduced. The use of iodine containing preparations in large ulcers may lead to resorption of iodine with sensitisation and effects on thyroid function. Use systemic antibiotics in the presence of bacteremia, sepsis, advancing cellulitus, or osteomyelitis. The therapeutic efficacy of miscellaneous topical agents (e.g., sugar, vitamins, elements, hormones, other agents), growth factors, and skin equivalents has not yet been sufficiently established.

KEY POINTS

- The risk of developing pressure ulcers is primarily determined by the extend en duration of pressure applied to the tissues.
- The validity of special pressure ulcer risk scores is poor.

- An individual at risk for pressure ulcer development may require a minimum of 30–35 kcal/kg/day, with 1 to 1.5 g/kg/day protein required and 1 ml/kcal/day of fluid.
- Since ulceration may start in the deeper tissues before any visible skin defects can be found, skin assessment should not be limited to visual inspection but also include palpation of deeper tissue layers at risk sites.
- Pressure ulcer prevention must always include the attribution of special mattresses and cushions in combination with frequent repositioning.
- Local wound treatment consists of three principles: removing necrotic tissue, creating a moist wound bed and prevention of inflammation.

REFERENCES

1. Bours GJ, Halfens RJ, Abu-Saad HH, Grol RT. Prevalence, prevention, and treatment of pressure ulcers: descriptive study in 89 institutions in the Netherlands. *Res Nurs Health* 2002; **25**(2): 99–110.
2. Allman RM, Goode PS, Burst N, Bartolucci AA, Thomas DR. Pressure ulcers, hospital complications, and disease severity: impact on hospital costs and length of stay. *Adv Wound Care* 1999; **12**(1): 22–30.
3. Bennett G, Dealey C, Posnett J. The cost of pressure ulcers in the UK. *Age Ageing* 2004; **33**(3): 230–5.
4. Severens JL, Habraken JM, Duivenvoorden S, Frederiks CM. The cost of illness of pressure ulcers in The Netherlands. *Adv Skin Wound Care* 2002; **15**(2): 72–7.
5. Voss AC, Bender SA, Ferguson ML, Sauer AC, Bennett RG, Hahn PW. Long-term care liability for pressure ulcers. *J Am Geriatr Soc*. 2005; **53**(9): 1587–92.
6. Mathus-Vliegen EM. Old age, malnutrition, and pressure sores: an ill-fated alliance. *J Gerontol A Biol Sci Med Sci* 2004; **59**(4): 355–60.
7. Pancorbo-Hidalgo PL, Garcia-Fernandez FP, Lopez-Medina IM, Alvarez-Nieto C. Risk assessment scales for pressure ulcer prevention: a systematic review. *J Adv Nurs* 2006; **54**(1): 94–110.
8. Schoonhoven L, Haalboom JR, Bousema MT, Algra A, Grobbee DE, Grypdonck MH, Buskens E. Prospective cohort study of routine use of risk assessment scales for prediction of pressure ulcers. *BMJ*. 2002; **325**(7368): 797.
9. Defloor T, Grypdonck MF. Pressure ulcers: validation of two risk assessment scales. *J Clin Nurs* 2005; **14**(3): 373–82.
10. McInnes E, Bell-Syer SE, Dumville JC, Legood R, Cullum NA. Support surfaces for pressure ulcer prevention. *Cochrane Database Syst Rev*. 2008 Oct 8; (4):CD001735.
11. Langer G, Schloemer G, Knerr A, Kuss O, and Behrens J. Nutritional interventions for preventing and treating pressure ulcers (Cochrane Review). In: *The Cochrane Library*, Issue 4, 2003. Chichester: John Wiley & Sons, Ltd.
12. Stratton RJ, Ek A, Engfer M, Moore Z, Rigby P, Wolfe R, Elia M. Enteral nutritional support in prevention and treatment of pressure ulcers: a systematic review and meta-analysis. *Ageing Res Rev* 2005; **4**(3): 422–50.
13. Clark M, Schols JM, Benati G, Jackson P, Engfer M, Langer G, Kerry B, Colin D; European Pressure Ulcer Advisory Panel. Pressure ulcers and nutrition: a new European guideliner. *J Wound Care* 2004; **13**(7): 267–72.
14. Bradley M, Cullum N, Nelson EA, Petticrew M, Sheldon T, Torgerson D. Systematic reviews of wound care management: (2). Dressings and topical agents used in the healing of chronic wounds. *Health Technol Assess* 1999; **3**(17 Pt 2): 1–35.

41 Leg Ulceration

Gabrielle M. McMullin

South Sydney Vascular Centre, St. George Hospital, Sydney, Australia

INTRODUCTION

It is estimated that 1% of the population in industrial nations suffer from ulceration of the lower leg at some time. The overall prevalence is about 1.5 per 1000 but this increases to 3.6 per 1000 in those over 65 years of age and 20 per 1000 in those over 80 years (1).

The cost of leg ulcers is enormous due to lengthy admissions to hospital, frequent community nursing visits and increasingly expensive dressings. In addition antibiotics are frequently prescribed both orally and intravenously. Despite all this attention, leg ulcers frequently persist for months or years and frequently recur. Focus of treatment is almost invariably on dressings and control of infection, despite the lack of evidence to support either of these measures.

Effective treatment of leg ulcers depends on an accurate identification of the cause of the failure of the wound to heal.

AETIOLOGY

Arterial Insufficiency

Poor arterial supply to the lower leg is largely attributable to atherosclerosis. Smoking (including a past history of smoking), hyperlipidaemia and lack of exercise are the most important factors in the development of the disease. Diabetes is associated with early development of atherosclerosis but results in a different pattern of arterial involvement often with sparing of the larger arteries but occlusion of the more distal tibial arteries or arterioles. Diabetic arteries are also characterized by marked calcification. Arterial insufficiency is a factor in about 30% of leg ulcers.

Venous Hypertension

Venous hypertension may be caused by venous reflux in the deep or superficial veins; venous obstruction; poor calf muscle pump function (2) or by high venous pressure in the right side of the heart.

Varicose veins are present in 50% of people over the age of 50 and there is a high recurrence rate after both surgery and sclerotherapy.

Venous obstruction resulting from deep vein thrombosis is much less common since the introduction of heparin (3) and with early detection using duplex ultrasound scanning.

In the upright position, the action of foot and calf muscles in particular is essential for return of venous blood to the heart. In the recumbent position muscular action is not required. The decreasing ability to exercise effectively with age accounts for the high prevalence of venous ulceration in the elderly who spend long periods of time sitting with their legs dependant. In addition many are on medication such as steroids and antihypertensive agents that exacerbate lower limb oedema.

Venous hypertension may also result from back pressure at the level of the heart due to either right heart failure or pulmonary hypertension.

Prescribing for Elderly Patients   Edited by Stephen Jackson, Paul Jansen and Arduino Mangoni

Venous insufficiency accounts for at least 50 % of leg ulcers.

Combined Arterial and Venous Disease

Arterial insufficiency and venous hypertension commonly co-exist. A lack of exercise is a common causative factor in both conditions.

Skin Malignancy

Australia has the highest rate of skin cancer in the world. The incidence is three times that in the USA and six times that in the UK. Even in Europe however, the rate of skin cancer has increased dramatically and this is attributed to the popularity of holidays in the sun. Total deaths from skin cancer are higher in the UK than in Australia at about 2000 per year, largely due to malignant melanoma.

The most common types of skin cancer causing ulceration are squamous cell and basal cell carcinoma. Malignant melanoma is much less common and tends to form tumours rather than ulcers. There are 374 000 non-melanoma skin cancers diagnosed in Australia every year and incidence increases with age. Skin cancer accounts for at least 5 % of chronic leg ulcers (4).

Neuropathy

Peripheral neuropathy results in chronic ulcers due to repeated trauma which goes unheeded (Figure 41.1). Neuropathy is most commonly due to diabetes or alcohol but there are numerous other causes including pernicious anaemia, chronic renal failure and leprosy. There are frequently associated deformities of the foot, such as hammer toes or multiple fractures and bone destruction (Figure 41.2). These deformities alter the weight bearing area of the foot and pressure ulcers then occur due to excessive weight on abnormal points.

Pressure Ulceration

Pressure ulceration occurs as a result of an impairment of mobility which frequently occurs with age. Long periods of bed rest result in

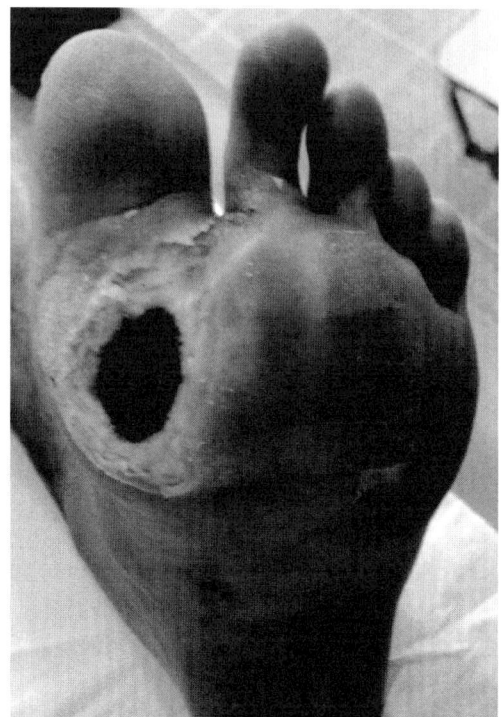

Figure 41.1. Pressure ulcer beneath the 1st metatarso-phalangeal joint of the left foot of a 42 year old diabetic with peripheral neuropathy. The ulcer is due to repeated trauma

damage to the skin over the heels and other bony prominences of the foot and ankle such as the lateral malleolus.

Once again deformity of the foot may also lead to pressure ulceration due to badly fitting shoes. Deformity of the toes, particularly hallux valgus (Figure 41.3), is extremely common due to decades of conforming to fashionable foot wear and this problem is therefore more common in women.

Mechanical Disruption

The foot and ankle are subject to continual movement and wounds subjected to continuous disruption may fail to heal. The problem is most commonly encountered in wounds at the back of the heel over the Achilles tendon (Figure 41.4) but this factor may also play a part in ulcers overlying medial and lateral malleoli.

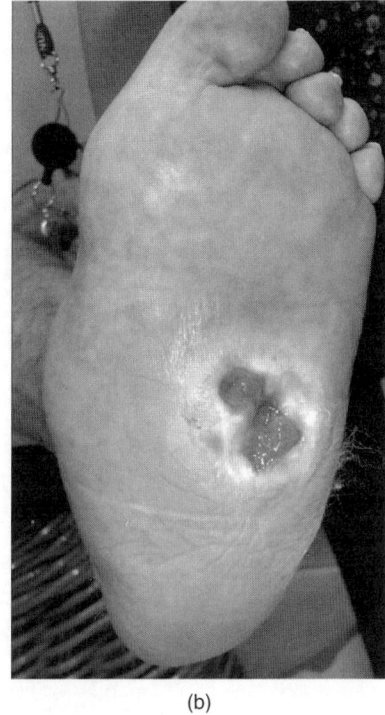

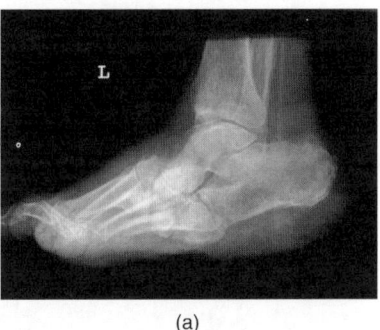

(a)   (b)

Figure 41.2. Ulcer on the plantar surface of the left foot in a 76 year old diabetic with peripheral neuropathy. Plain X ray of the foot revealed extensive fractures in the mid-foot resulting in complete loss of the arch with resulting "boat foot" deformity. Hammer toe deformity is also pronounced demonstrating how weight is taken on the heads of the metatarsals in diabetic patients

Haematological Disorders

Anaemias and myeloproliferative disease are relatively common in the elderly due to a variety of causes. These disorders adversely affect wound healing as do the drugs used in their treatment such as hydroxyurea (5).

SYMPTOMS AND SIGNS

Chronic leg ulcers most usually start with minor trauma. An inflammatory reaction occurs in response and if chronic inflammation becomes established wound healing will not occur until it is controlled.

Ulcers due to venous hypertension may start spontaneously. Large varicose veins may or may not be obvious. Venous eczema can be a precursor or else a lesion over a prominent varicosity at the ankle may develop and then break down into an ulcer.

Lipodermatosclerosis is frequently present and develops progressively over many years before ulceration occurs. It is an inflammatory condition though it is often misdiagnosed as infection and treated with antibiotics. The lower limb is invariably oedematous making palpation of distal pulses difficult but the foot and toes are warm and pink with good capillary return.

Venous ulcers may be quite painless but may also be associated with severe pain and this is most marked in the presence of atrophie blanche (due to infarction of small areas of the skin). The majority of patients however do not complain of pain at night waking them from sleep.

In contradistinction, those with arterial insufficiency complain bitterly of pain from their ulcers. The pain occurs particularly on going

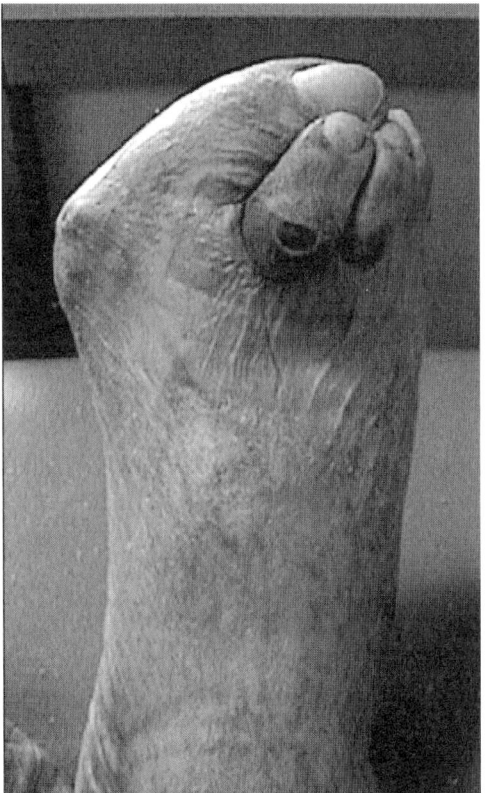

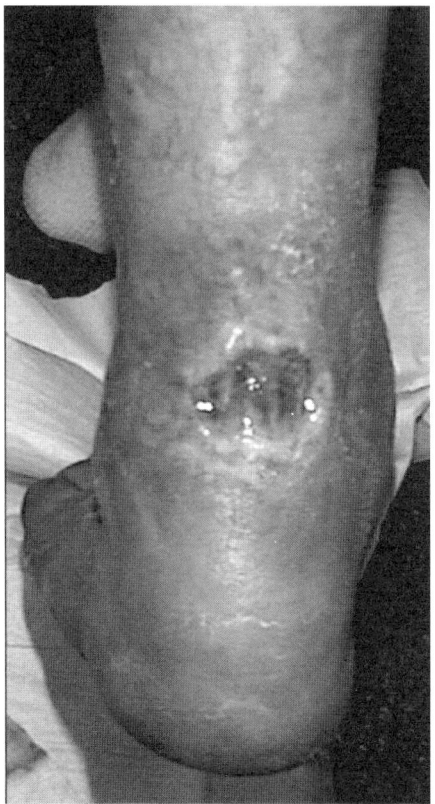

Figure 41.3. Pronounced hallux valgus deformity and crowding of the remaining toes due to foot wear in an 83 year old woman. Ulcer on the second toe is due to pressure from her shoe and the simplest solution in this case is amputation of the toe

Figure 41.4. Ulcer at the back of the heel overlying the Achilles tendon in a 65 year old retired footballer. The wound was originally caused by a new shoe and significant damage was allowed before he recognized the problem due to his alcoholic neuropathy. The wound failed to heal until the ankle was immobilized in plaster

to bed and wakes them from sleep in the early hours of the morning whereas during the day, when their legs are dependant, there is little pain. Patients with dementia or who are impaired by stroke may have trouble conveying their pain.

Arterial insufficiency is associated with trophic changes in the lower leg including loss of hair and thickening of the toenails. Pulses are often absent or reduced in volume not only at the ankle but in the popliteal fossa or even in the groin. The feet are often cool and the toes cyanosed. Pulses may occasionally be palpable at the ankle in diabetic patients despite arterial insufficiency in the foot or toes due to occlusion of distal arteries.

Ulcers due to arterial insufficiency are traditionally described on the most distal extremities such as the toes or heels but can also occur on the lower leg (Figure 41.5). Venous ulcers are almost invariably confined to the gaiter region of the leg (from ankle to knee) and are more common on the medial than the lateral side of the leg (Figure 41.6). Ulcers on the lateral or anterior aspects of the lower leg are more likely to have a component of arterial insufficiency involved (Figure 41.7).

Immobile patients often have toes and feet that are cyanosed when the legs are dependant despite a normal arterial supply. Venous hypertension due to a lack of activity results in pressure within the capillary bed causing the capillaries to become leaky (2). Fluid, fibrinogen and white blood cells pass into the

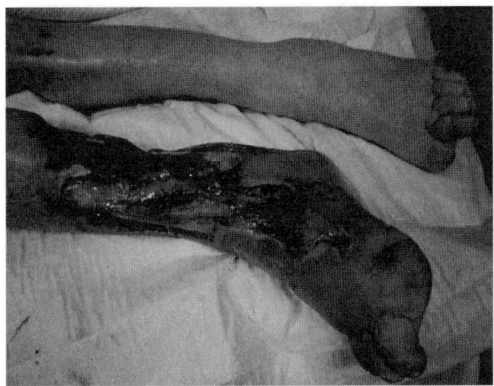

Figure 41.5. Ulceration of the lower leg of a 65 year old woman. The ulcer had started 18 months previously on the medial aspect of the leg and was unresponsive to dressings and antibiotics. She had previously undergone femoro-popliteal artery bypass grafting in the left leg and had required amputation of both great toes however despite this history arterial insufficiency was not recognised in time for limb salvage

interstitial tissue and the foot and lower leg thus become oedematous. In order to minimise this process the precapillary sphincters constrict causing arterio-venous shunts in the micro-circulation and hence there is cyanosis of the skin. This process is reversed by elevation of the legs and these patients will have warm, pink, well-perfused feet while in bed unlike patients with true arterial insufficiency.

Venous ulcers are highly exudative and the exudate causes maceration and inflammation of the surrounding skin. The edges of the ulcer are sloping and irregular. A heaped ulcer edge is suspicious of malignancy (Figure 41.8). Arterial ulcers usually have low levels of exudate and are characterised by punched out edges. The base consists either of necrotic tissue or else exposed underlying structures such as tendon (Figure 41.9). This appearance may also occur in neuropathic pressure ulcers. Pressure ulcers often have undermined edges with surface skin preserved but damage to deeper tissues hidden. The exudate is usually greater than that seen with arterial insufficiency and consequently the skin surrounding the ulcer is often macerated.

Ulcers due to pressure are located over obvious pressure areas such as the heel or else

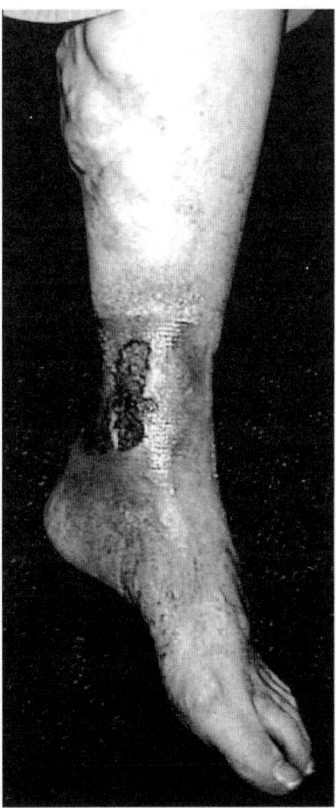

Figure 41.6. Classic venous ulcer situated in the medial gaiter region of the leg of a 72 year old woman. The ulcer has a serpiginous border and sloping edges and lies in the centre of an area of inflamed lipodermatosclerosis. Large varicose veins are obvious and excision of these veins is likely to result in cure of the ulceration as long as the deep veins are competent

over deformities of the foot. Sensation should be checked carefully to determine whether there is neuropathy.

Breathlessness at rest or on minor exertion should alert the clinician to the possibility of right heart failure or pulmonary hypertension. Other signs of these conditions include tachycardia, a raised JVP and enlargement of the liver.

DIAGNOSIS

A correct diagnosis can usually be established by a careful history and examination noting in

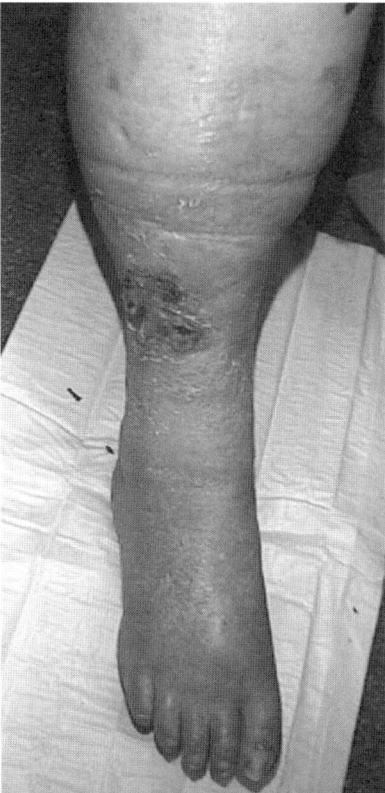

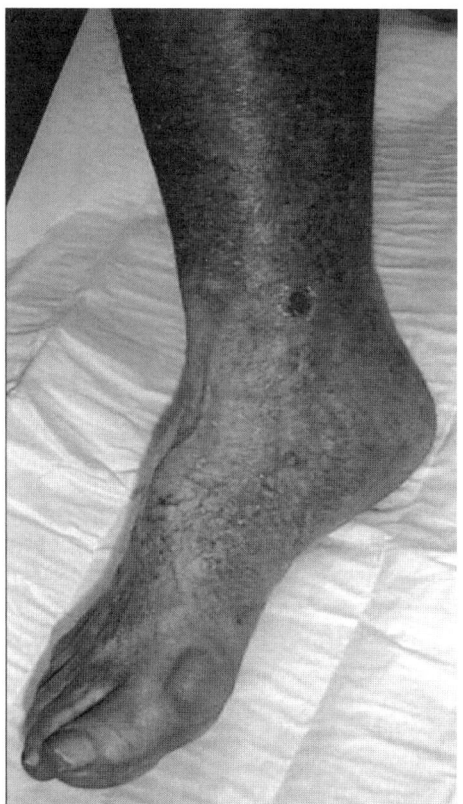

Figure 41.7. 77 year old woman with a 30 year history of intermittent leg ulceration. Although the ulcers were pure venous ulcers in earlier years she now has an occluded superficial femoral artery in addition to uncontrolled leg swelling. She had frequently been told to go home and sit with her legs up which exacerbated her inactivity and arterial disease

Figure 41.8. Small ulcer on the medial aspect of the ankle of a 75 year old man. Pronounced lipodermatosclerosis is evident however the ulcer has raised edges and excision biopsy proved it to be a basal cell carcinoma

particular the position of the ulcer, the arterial supply to the limb and deformities of the ankle or foot.

Assessment of the mobility of the patient is particularly important both in terms of establishing a diagnosis but also for the purpose of implementing effective treatment. Home circumstances and support services available to the patient is also vital information.

Blood tests including a full blood count, urea, creatinine and electrolytes should be taken.

Establishing whether the arterial supply is adequate is the most critical issue. If the limb has all pulses palpable and the toes are warm and well perfused then no further investigation of the arterial supply may be required.

Significant arterial insufficiency is evident when there are absent pulses and a positive Buerger's test. This clinical test is easily done while the patient lies supine. The leg is passively raised from the horizontal plane and the test is positive if the foot blanches due to a lack of arterial inflow. When the leg is then placed in a dependant position by sitting the patient up and hanging the legs over the edge of the bed, the leg becomes deeply suffused as it fills with blood. The angle from horizontal at which the foot blanches indicates the severity of arterial insufficiency, the smaller the angle the more pronounced the deficiency. When the test is positive an angiogram is the most effective means of investigation as this supplies the definitive answer as to definitive treatment possible in terms of angioplasty or arterial bypass

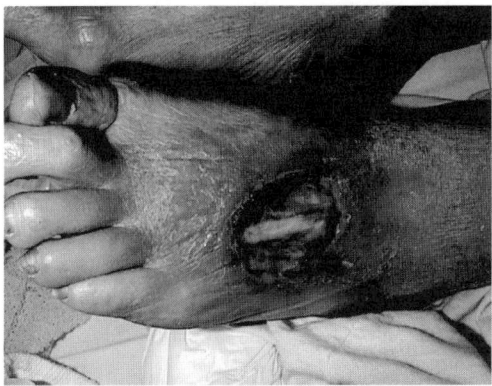

Figure 41.9. Classic arterial ulcer on the dorsum of the foot of a 92 year old woman. Edges of the ulcer are "punched out" and there is tendon exposed in the base. There was very little exudate. The angiogram is shown in Figure 41.11

surgery. Angiography involves risks of bleeding from the arterial puncture site and renal failure from the intravenous contrast required. If there is renal impairment, prehydration and treatment with acetyl cysteine are protective (6). Alternatively angiography can be performed with carbon dioxide at no risk to the kidneys though the images obtained are not as clear as those with contrast.

If there is doubt as to the diagnosis of arterial insufficiency then an ankle brachial pressure index can be measured using a hand held Doppler with a 5 to 8 MHz probe. Systolic brachial artery pressure is compared to the systolic pressure measured at the ankle (the best measurement from either the dorsalis pedis or posterior tibial arteries). The index should be >0.9 and any reduction indicates arterial insufficiency.

Unfortunately the measurement is frequently inaccurate in elderly patients as a result of heavily calcified arteries due to atherosclerosis. A raised index (>1.2) is highly suspicious of calcified arteries and the test result unreliable.

An arterial duplex scan supplies non-invasive information regarding the arterial supply. Lack of co-operation from a demented patient may make the examination impossible and obesity of the limb makes the results less reliable. Even when the examination is performed in ideal conditions there are areas in which arterial disease can be missed (Figure 41.10). This is most

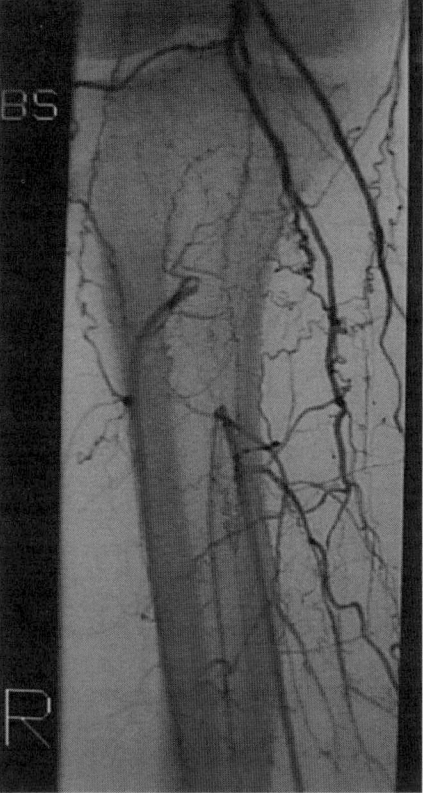

Figure 41.10. Duplex arterial scans frequently miss disease at the level of the knee where imaging is technically difficult. This angiogram reveals occlusion of the distal popliteal artery and tibio-peroneal trunk resulting in significant arterial insufficiency to the lower leg

common in the assessment of the tibio-peroneal trunk and the origin of the tibial arteries. Occlusion in these areas is critical and therefore despite an apparently clear arterial duplex scan if there are still significant clinical concerns regarding the adequacy of the arterial supply, an angiogram should be performed. CT angiography and MR angiography are increasingly accurate and have the advantage that they are non-invasive and utilize a minimal amount of contrast. Once adequacy of the arterial supply has been established then other causes for ulceration can be explored.

If there is any deformity of the foot then plain X-rays should be taken. Lateral and AP views of all bones of the foot and ankle should be requested.

Venous duplex scanning is not required for all patients with obvious venous ulcers. It should be performed if surgical intervention or sclerotherapy will be considered as treatment modalities. If there is significant deep vein occlusion then stripping of varicose veins is absolutely contra-indicated as it will exacerbate venous hypertension by removing outflow channels. If there are no obvious varicose veins but obvious skin changes of chronic venous insufficiency then a venous duplex scan will elucidate the venous pathology. Pulsatile flow in the deep veins is a strong indication of cardiac or pulmonary pathology causing high venous pressure in the right atrium. An echocardiogram is then required to confirm this and further cardiac and pulmonary investigations may subsequently be required. The absence of venous reflux or obstruction and an apparently normal venous system strongly suggests that the pathology is calf muscle pump dysfunction (a lack of exercise).

Biopsy of ulcers should be performed to exclude malignancy if there are suspicious features (such as heaped edges); if there is a history of previous skin cancer in the same position or if there is a history of many previous skin cancers. In addition, biopsies should be performed if there is failure of a supposed venous ulcer to decrease significantly in size within 12 weeks despite effective compression therapy.

THERAPY

Significant arterial insufficiency requires intervention to improve arterial inflow. This may mean arterial bypass grafting however angioplasty and stenting of the arteries of the lower limb are increasingly being performed instead of bypass surgery with good results (Figure 41.11). This approach is particularly appropriate in the elderly who often have concomitant medical problems making them high risk for anaesthesia. Angioplasty with or without stenting can be performed under local anaesthesia with sedation if required. Following the procedure it is now routine to prescribe low dose aspirin 100 mg in combination with

clopidogrel 75 mg daily. A high proportion of elderly patients take warfarin for atrial fibrillation or prosthetic cardiac valves but there is an increasing tendency to prescribe the anti-platelet agents in addition to warfarin even though this entails an increased risk of bleeding. The increase in blood flow following successful intervention is dramatic. Dry arterial ulcers become much more exudative and the limb becomes swollen. Compression therapy is therefore frequently needed to control oedema.

Venous ulcers require effective compression to allow healing to occur. This can be achieved with graduated compression stockings or with compression bandages. Graduated compression stockings must be properly fitted and usually require a pressure at the ankle of 30–40 mm Hg to be effective. They are often difficult to apply over dressings and therefore it is usually more appropriate to start with compression bandages. Layers of bandages have been shown to be far more effective than a single bandage and a four layer compression bandage can maintain adequate compression for up to one week without being changed. Graduated compression stockings must be removed at night and reapplied in the morning and therefore require more nursing input which adds to the attraction of compression bandages.

Dressings are largely immaterial to healing (7) but should aim to soak up the large amounts of exudate that are produced by venous ulcers. Bandages should be changed at a rate determined by the exudate and may have to be changed daily but can be left intact for up to a week if exudate is controlled.

There is a variety of bandages available ranging from high stretch to low stretch. High stretch bandages more efficiently reduce oedema however may be too painful and are not tolerated well particularly by elderly patients. Short stretch bandages are very much better tolerated at night. Some patients are unable to tolerate bandages or stockings and sequential compression pumps are an alternative for oedema control. These pumps must be used for six to10 hours a day to be effective and for mobile patients they are too cumbersome. For those confined to wheelchairs

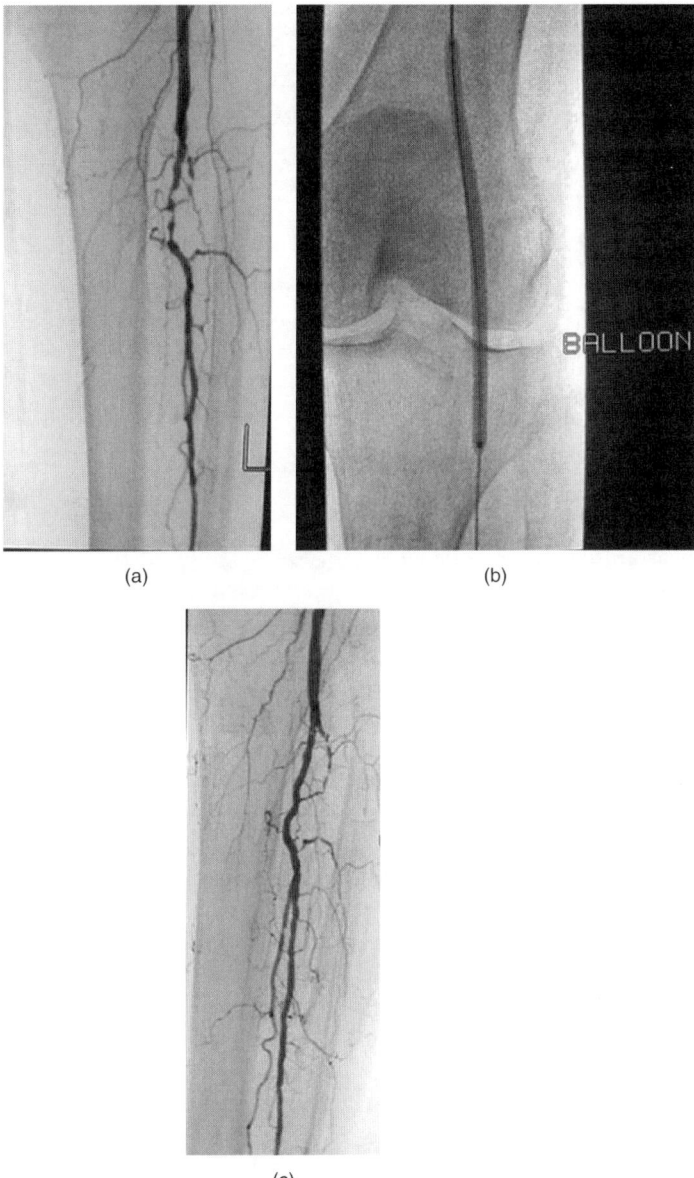

(a)

(b)

(c)

Figure 41.11. Angiogram of the leg of the 92 year old woman in Figure 41.9 revealed a critical stenosis of the tibio-peroneal trunk. Balloon angioplasty was performed under local anaesthetic and successfully improved the arterial supply to the foot allowing relief from rest pain and healing of the ulcer once tendon had been excised

they may be of very great benefit and they are particularly useful for patients with dependant cyanosis.

If there are obvious varicose veins as the cause for ulceration then intervention to treat these by surgical stripping or sclerotherapy will facilitate healing. If however there is also significant calf muscle pump dysfunction (lack of exercise) then venous surgery may not be successful at either healing the ulcer or preventing further ulceration. Where only compression techniques are used to heal venous ulcers then compression therapy must continue indefinitely or ulceration will recur. Graduated compression stockings are the preferred form of oedema control once ulcers have healed however elderly patients often have difficulty managing them. Arthritis of hips, knees or fingers; lower back pain; joint replacements; obesity and general frailty all result in the inability to get stockings on or off. Social circumstances then play an important role. A fit partner, carer or family member may be able to apply stockings daily. Those in hostels or nursing homes should have stockings applied on a daily basis by staff but this often proves problematic. A few community nursing services will attend to apply stockings in the morning and take them off at night.

Diuretics such as frusemide are often prescribed for the treatment of lower leg swelling but are mostly ineffective unless used in conjuction with compression therapy. If there are concomitant problems such as congestive heart failure or pulmonary hypertension then diuretics may play an important role. Electrolytes need to be monitored and potassium replacement may be required with long-term diuretic therapy.

Arterio-venous ulcers can sometimes be managed by a reduced level of compression therapy but the limiting factor is often pain. Ineffective control of oedema is the result and consequently there is lack of healing. Aggressive management to improve the arterial supply, as with arterial ulcers, is then the best option. A better arterial supply reduces pain and allows more effective compression to control oedema and obtain ulcer healing.

In those patients in whom joint movement is causing wound disruption and preventing healing, immobilisation of the ankle joint is required. A four layer compression bandage should be applied to the leg and then either a pneumatic walker or else a plaster cast applied. The plaster cast requires bi-valving so that dressings and bandages can be changed at intervals and the plaster cast reapplied and worn at all times between dressings (Figure 41.12). A pneumatic walker is probably as effective as a plaster cast but is more expensive and

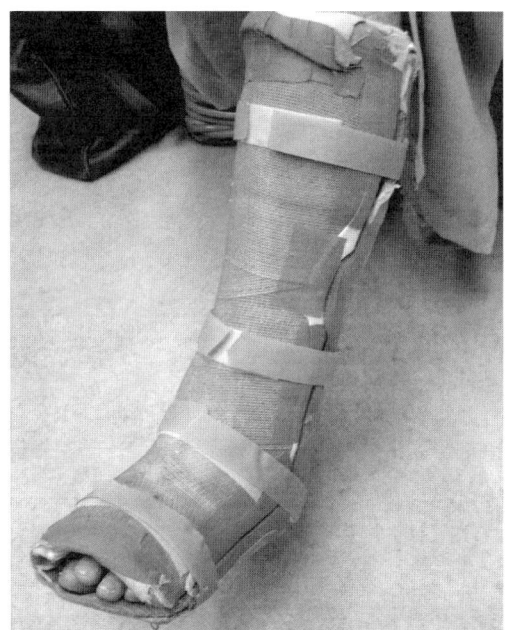

Figure 41.12. Total contact cast applied to the lower leg to immobilize the ankle joint and totally protect the foot. The cast allows ambulation instead of bed rest while ulcers heal. The cast has been bi-valved to allow the cast to be removed for dressings to be changed. Velcro straps then hold the cast in place

easier to tamper with. Demented or confused patients frequently interfere with dressings and bandages. Plaster casts in these patients are very effective as they ensure compliance.

Neuropathic ulceration can be treated successfully with complete bed rest but this is an expensive form of therapy and has associated risks including sacral pressure ulceration. It is far preferable to keep elderly patients mobile and the alternative is application of a total contact cast from the tips of the toes to the knee (8). The cast removes almost all pressure from the foot and prevents further damage. Where there are significant fractures of the bones of the foot (Charcot's neuropathic osteoarthropathy) then a total contact cast may be required for nine months or more to allow healing.

Less advanced disease may be treated by simple surgical procedures to correct deformities. These procedures include excision of a metatarsal head or the first

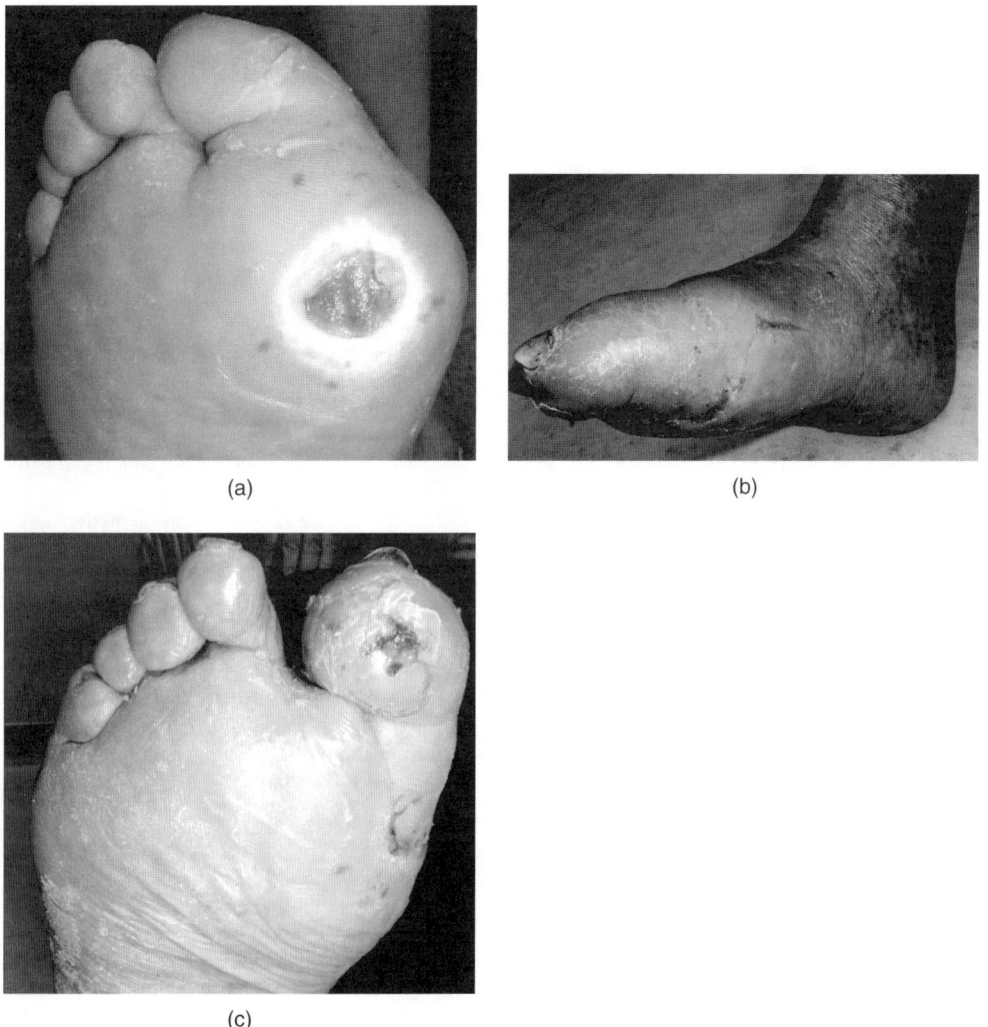

(a)

(b)

(c)

Figure 41.13. Neuropathic ulcer under the 1st metatarsophalangeal joint of an 83 year old man. An incision along the medial side of the foot was made and through this the joint was excised along with the ulcer and the wound closed primarily. A K wire was then placed down the length of the great toe to fix it to the 1st metatarsal. The incision healed within two weeks and the ulcer did not recur

metatarsophalangeal joint (Figure 41.13) and tendon transfers in the toes to correct hammer toe deformity. At times a simple amputation of a toe may be the simplest and easiest way to correct a deformity responsible for pressure ulceration. As long as the arterial supply is adequate then the surgical wounds heal well by primary intention. Finally, neuropathic feet and particularly those with deformities, require specially made footwear to prevent further damage and recurrent ulceration.

Pressure ulcers require relief from pressure and there are a variety of devices to protect heels and bony prominences for patients in bed. None of these are ideal and the most effective means of reducing pressure areas is with the use of pressure relieving mattresses. Pressure ulcers are particularly prevalent in the elderly and there are now several scoring systems (Waterlow, Braden, Norton) used to predict the likelihood of this complication. Appropriate preventative measures can then be taken.

Recognition of the early signs of pressure ulcers such as blistering or inflammation and prompt action to relieve the pressure will significantly reduce tissue loss and prevent the pain of established deep pressure ulcers.

Ulcers that are due to squamous cell or basal cell carcinoma require complete excision. If the resulting wound cannot be closed primarily then the wound will heal with compression bandaging. Alternatively skin grafting can be performed though this involves the creation of another (and often more painful) wound in terms of the donor site.

Antibiotics are frequently used in the treatment of chronic leg ulcers but have not been shown to increase rates of healing (9). Topical antibiotics are not recommended as they can cause sensitization (10). Antibiotics are only required if there is a florid cellulitis surrounding the ulcer or obviously progressing up the leg. The overuse of antibiotics in the treatment of ulcers has contributed to the dramatic increase in antibiotic resistance that is widely described.

KEY POINTS

- Leg ulcers require investigation as effective treatment depends on a correct diagnosis.
- Arterial supply is critical to healing and minimally invasive methods of arterial revascularisation are now available.
- Ulcers due to leg swelling (venous ulcers) require adequate compression therapy with either layered bandages or graduated compression stockings.
- Neuropathic and pressure ulcers require measures to relieve pressure.
- Skin malignancy should be excluded by biopsy.

GUIDELINES

Venous leg ulcers
http://www.rcn.org.uk/publications/pdf/
guidelines/leg_ulcer_implemen.pdf
Leg ulcers

http://www.sign.ac.uk/pdf/qrg26.pdf
Compression bandaging
http://www.worldwidewounds.com/1997/
september/Thomas-Bandaging/bandage-paper.
html
Pressure ulcers
http://www.epuap.org/glprevention.html

REFERENCES

1. London NJM. Donnelly R. ABC of arterial and venous disease. *BMJ* 2000; **320**: 1589–91.
2. Editors NL Browse, KG Burnand, M Lea-Thomas (Eds) *Diseases of the Veins*. London: Arnold, 1988. Chapter 3 Physiology and functional anatomy.
3. Raju S. Fredericks RK Late hemodynamic sequelae of deep venous thrombosis. *J Vasc Surg* 1986; **4**: 73–9.
4. Yang D. Morrison BD, Vandongen YK, Singh A, Stacey MC. Malignancy in chronic leg ulcers. *Med J Aust* 1996; **164**: 718–20.
5. Bader U, Banyai M, Boni R, Burg G, Hafner J. Leg ulcers in patients with myeloproliferative disorders: Disease or treatment-related? *Dermatology* 2000; **200**: 45–8.
6. Tepel m, Van der Giet M, Schwarzfeld C, Laufer U, Liermann D, Zidek W. Prevention of radiographic contrast agent induced reductions in renal function by acetylcysteine. *N Engl J Med* 2000; **343**: 180–4.
7. Stacey MC, Jopp-Mckay AG, Rashid P, Hoskin SE, Thompson PJ. The influence of dressings on venous ulcer healing—a randomised trial. *Eur J Vasc Endovasc Surg* 1997; **13**: 174–9.
8. Warren G Nade S. *The Care of Neuropathic Limbs*. Chapter 11 *Protecting neuropathic limbs*. New York, London: Parthenon Publishing Group, 1999..
9. Huovinen S, Kolitainen P, Jarvinen H, Malanin K, Sarna S, Helander I et al. Comparison of ciprofloxacin or trimethoprim therapy for venous leg ulcers: results of a pilot study. *J Am Acad Dermatol* 1994; **31**: 279–81.
10. Zaki I, Shell L, Dakiel KL. Bacitracin: a significant sensitiser in leg ulcer patients. *Contact Dermatitis* 1994; **31**: 92–4.

42 Xerosis and asteatotic eczema

Michael Yeung and Daniel Creamer

Department of Dermatology, King's College Hospital, London, UK

XEROSIS

Introduction

Xerosis is the term used to describe skin which has become dry and scaly. It is an inevitable consequence of skin ageing. Xerosis leads to asteatotic eczema which is extremely common in the elderly.

Aetiology

As well as ageing, excessive exposure to hot, dry environments (centrally-heated rooms) and water and soap can also cause xerosis. These factors decrease the intercellular lipid content of the stratum corneum. The water content of this layer is thus reduced, resulting in drying and cracking.

Symptoms and signs

The skin of the lower legs is usually affected first, appearing dull with a fine scale. The thighs and trunk may be involved, but the face, neck, soles and palms are usually spared. Mild pruritus may also be present. In asteatotic eczema there is fissuring of the dried-out stratum corneum which forms a 'crazy paving' pattern with redness apparent in the cracks.

Diagnosis

Diagnosis is usually made clinically.

Therapy

- Correct predisposing factors.
- Twice daily application of an emollient.
- The use aqueous cream as soap substitute.

Key Points

- Xerosis is very common in the elderly and if left untreated may progress to asteatotic eczema.
- Attending to triggering factors such as over-heated rooms and excessive exposure to soap and water is important.

Guidelines

Norman RA. Xerosis and pruritus in the elderly: recognition and management. *Dermatol Ther* 2003; **16**: 254–9.

References

Shenefelt PD, Fenske NA. Aging and the skin: recognising and managing common disorders. *Geriatrics* 1990; **45**: 57–66.

ACTINIC KERATOSES AND BOWEN'S DISEASE

Introduction

Both actinic keratoses and Bowen's disease are dysplastic lesions which usually occur on sun-damaged skin. Bowen's disease carries a risk of developing into invasive squamous cell carcinoma while actinic keratoses are probably best considered as markers of photodamage. The prevalence of both is greatly increased in the elderly population.

Aetiology

Actinic keratoses and Bowen's disease are a result of keratinocyte nuclear damage caused by ultra-violet radiation. Individuals with fair skin who have had an excessive lifetime's exposure to strong sunlight are at higher risk. Exposure to other forms of radiation or chemical carcinogens, such as arsenic, can also be causative.

Symptoms and signs

Actinic keratoses usually occur on chronically sun-exposed areas such as the face, scalp and hands. Other signs of photodamage are often present, such as freckling, xerosis and telangiectasiae. Actinic keratoses appear as mildly inflamed, well-demarcated, scaly macules usually 0.5–1.0 cm in diameter. Bowen's disease presents as a red, slightly scaly, patch usually on the face, bald scalp, hands and lower legs. Patches of Bowen's disease are usually larger than actinic keratoses.

Diagnosis

The diagnosis of actinic keratoses is usually made clinically, but a biopsy of Bowen's disease is necessary to exclude an inflammatory condition. Histopathology of actinic keratoses shows hyperkeratosis and parakeratosis with a variably thickened epidermis and epidermal dysplasia. Histopathology of Bowen's disease shows full-thickness epidermal dysplasia with large, abnormal keratinoctyes.

Therapy

Most actinic keratoses can be treated with applications of liquid nitrogen cryotherapy.

Zones of skin bearing multiple actinic keratoses (e.g. bald scalp) can be treated with topical applications of 5-fluorouracil or imiquimod. Alternatively such areas can be treated with photodynamic therapy.

Bowen's disease is best treated surgically, either excision or curettage. Small areas can also be treated with cryotherapy. Large areas of involvement can be treated with topical applications of 5-fluorouracil or imiquimod. Alternatively such areas can be treated with photodynamic therapy.

Key Points

- Both actinic keratoses and Bowen's disease represent areas of epidermal dysplasia.
- Bowen's disease possesses a potential to progress to invasive squamous cell carcinoma.
- Ablative therapy is commonly used: cryotherapy for actinic keratoses and surgery for Bowen's disease.

Guidelines

Cox NH, Eedy DJ, Morton CA. Guidelines for management of Bowen's disease. British Association of Dermatologists. *Br J Dermatol* 1999; **141**(4): 633–41.

Drake LA, Ceilley RI, Comelison RL et al. Guidelines of care for actinic keratoses: committee on guidelines of care. *J Am Acad Dermatol* 1995; **32**(1): 95–8.

References

Lee MM, Wick MM. Bowen's disease. *Clin Dermatol* 1993; **11**(1): 43–6.

Barnaby JW, Styles AR, Cockerell CJ. Actinic keratoses: differential diagnosis and treatment. *Drugs Aging* 1997; **11**(3): 186–205.

Links

http://www.bad.org.uk/patients/leaflets/actinic.asp

http://www.bad.org.uk/public/leaflets/bowens.asp

BULLOUS PEMPHIGOID

Introduction

Bullous pemphigoid is an autoimmune, sub-epidermal blistering dermatosis which mainly affects the elderly.

Aetiology

Autoantibodies are directed against two structural proteins found at the dermo-epidermal junction (BP antigens 180 and 230). Loss of these adhesion molecules results in detachment of the epidermis from underlying dermis with consequent blistering.

Symptoms and signs

Often there is an initial pre-bullous phase characterized by an eruption of itchy, red, urticated plaques. After this prodrome, which lasts from a few days to several weeks, the characteristic tense blisters develop. The blisters measure 1–5 cm in diameter and arise on red, inflamed skin usually on the limbs, lower abdomen and flexures. As well as being itchy, blistered skin can be painful. Extensive areas of epidermal detachment can lead to significant amounts of fluid and protein loss. Exposed dermis readily becomes colonized by bacteria, which can lead to local or systemic sepsis.

Diagnosis

Skin biopsy: Histopathology shows a subepidermal blister with an eosinophil-rich infiltrate. Direct immunofluorescence of perilesional skin shows a linear deposition of C3 and IgG along the dermo-epidermal junction.

Indirect immunofluorescence of patients' serum will demonstrate circulating antibodies directed against the basement membrane zone.

Therapy

- Super-potent steroid ointment twice daily to localized areas.
- Prednisolone 0.5–1 mg/kg/day, tapering dose with response.
- Steroid sparing agents such as azathioprine 100–150 mg daily or mycophenalate mofetil 0.5–1 g twice daily.

Key points

- The blistering phase of bullous pemphigoid is often preceded by a prodrome of itchy, urticated plaques.

- Patients almost always require moderate-to-high dose oral corticosteroids for a prolonged period of time.

Guidelines

Wojnarowska F, Kirtschig G, Highet A et al. Guidelines for the management of bullous pemphigoid *British Journal of Dermatology* 2002; **147**: 214–21.

References

Loo WJ, Burrows NP Management of autoimmune skin disorders in the elderly. *Drugs Aging* 2004; **21**(12): 767–77.

CANDIDIASIS

Introduction

Candidiasis can affect both cutaneous and mucosal surfaces. The elderly are prone to oral candidiasis (especially if they wear dentures), flexural candidiasis (intertrigo) and occlusion candidiasis if they are bed ridden. Vulvovaginal candidiasis is common in adult women, however the presence of cutaneous candidiasis at other body sites may be indicative of immunosuppression or diabetes.

Aetiology

In normal individuals, the yeast *Candida albicans* is relatively harmless, but once the immune system becomes weakened it can colonize skin and mucous membranes and cause superficial infections. It is most commonly found in areas which are warm and moist such as the mouth, submammary folds, axillae and anogenital skin.

Symptoms and signs

Initially there is erythema in the affected area, often a flexure, with soreness and itching. The redness then spreads to the surrounding skin with a leading, pustular margin. There may be central superficial desquamation. Tiny, pustular, satellite lesions are commonly seen beyond the eruption's margin.

Diagnosis

Often the diagnosis is made clinically, but skin swabs should be taken for microbiology.

Relevant investigations should be performed to investigate any possible underlying cause of immunosuppression, if suspected.

Therapy

- Oral candidiasis: Nystatin lozenges or suspension bd for one to two weeks. Dentures should be removed overnight and cleaned with saline before they are replaced.
- In immunocompromised patients use oral fluconazole 150 mg as a single dose or itraconazole 400 mg as a single dose.
- Vulvovaginal candidiasis: EITHER clotrimazole pessaries 200 mg for three nights, OR oral therapy with fluconazole 150 mg as a single dose or itraconazole 400 mg as a single dose.
- Candida intertrigo: Clotrimazole cream 1 % bd for one to two weeks. Keep macerated skin folds clean and dry.

Key Points

- Cutaneous candidiasis tends to occur in moist, warm environments such as the mouth and flexures. It occurs more commonly in the immunocompromised.
- Cutaneous candidiasis is characterized by areas of erythema with pustules.
- Muco-cutaneous candidiasis can usually be successfully treated with topical therapy.

Guidelines

Guidelines of care for superficial mycotic infections of the skin: mucocutaneous candidiasis. *J Am Acad Dermatol* 1996; **34**(1): 110–5.

References

Laube S. Skin infections and ageing *Ageing Res Rev* 2004; **3**(1): 69–89.

Hay DM. Yeast infections *Dermatol Clin* 1996; **14**(1): 113–23.

ERYSIPELAS AND CELLULITIS

Introduction

Erysipelas and cellulitis are common bacterial skin infections which frequently affect the elderly. The term erysipelas is used to describe superficial infections involving the dermis whereas in cellulitis infection also extends into the subcutis.

Aetiology

The causative bacteria are usually streptococci, mainly of the Group A subgroup. Less frequently, *Staphylococcus aureus* or other bacteria are causative. Portals of bacterial entry include ulcers, minor abrasions, or via tinea pedis. Lymphoedema, which occurs commonly in the elderly with chronically dependent, immobile legs, increases the susceptibility to erysipelas and cellulitis.

Symptoms and signs

Erysipelas usually affects the face with a unilateral, well-demarcated, red zone of hot, swollen skin. Cellulitis generally affects the lower legs, presenting in a similar manner, but often with more oedema. Cellulitis may blister and rarely may be associated with purpura when it is known as haemorrhagic cellulitis. There is regional lymphadenopathy. The patient is febrile and unwell.

Diagnosis

- Skin swabs and blood for bacterial culture.
- ASOT, FBC and CRP.

Therapy

- Mild involvement: oral penicillin V 500 mg qds + flucloxacillin 500 mg qds for seven days.
- Moderate-severe involvement: intravenous penicillin 500 mg qds + flucloxacillin 500 mg for five days. Use erythromycin or clarithromycin if allergic to penicillin.

- In patients with lymphoedema, who are at high-risk of developing cellulitis, low-dose antibiotics (e.g. penicillin V 500 mg od) may be helpful in preventing infection.

Key Points

- Mild cellulitis and erysipelas can be treated with oral antibiotics.
- Moderate-severe cases of cellulitis and erysipelas require intravenous antibiotics.

Guidelines

Weinberg J M, Scheinfeld NS. Cutaneous infections in the elderly: diagnosis and management. *Dermatol Ther* 2003; **16**(3): 195–205.

Laube S, Farrell AM. Bacterial skin infections in the elderly: diagnosis and treatment *Drugs Aging* 2002; **19**(5): 331–42.

References

O'Donnell J A, Hoffmann M T. Skin and soft tissues. Management of four common infections in the nursing home patient *Geriatrics* 2001; **56**(10): 33–8, 41

Laube S. Skin infections and ageing *Ageing Res Rev* 2004; **3**(1): 69–89.

Links

http://www.bad.org.uk/patients/leaflets/erysipelas.asp

CONTACT DERMATITIS

Introduction

Contact dermatitis occurs when the skin reacts to an exogenous substance. It is divided into allergic contact dermatitis, which is triggered following sensitization to specific chemicals, and irritant contact dermatitis which results from contact with substances which are pro-inflammatory in all individuals.

Aetiology

Allergic contact dermatitis (ACD) is a delayed hypersensitivity reaction to an exogenous allergen following initial sensitisation. Irritant contact dermatitis (ICD) occurs via direct inflammatory pathways without any prior sensitization. The tendency to all forms of eczema or dermatitis is increased in elderly skin due to cutaneous dryness (xerosis) which is a part of the normal ageing process.

Symptoms and signs

Contact dermatitis occurs at sites of contact with the offending substance, often hands, feet, face and lower legs. In the elderly, allergic contact dermatitis is perhaps most commonly encountered on the lower legs and, in this situation, may be caused by an allergy to a chemical present in bandages, dressings or topical medicaments. As with other forms of eczema contact dermatitis is red, itchy and slightly scaly. In acute contact dermatitis oedema, vesicles and exudation occurs, while chronic forms are characterized by lichenification. Irritant contact dermatitis is most commonly seen following excessive exposure to soap and water and is therefore usually encountered on the hands.

Diagnosis

The diagnosis is made clinically and is suspected by the recognition of eczema occurring in an unusual pattern. In allergic contact dermatitis the specific sensitizer(s) can be identified with patch testing.

Therapy

- Avoid the culprit chemical or offending substance.
- Frequent usage of emollient.
- Twice daily application of an appropriate corticosteroid ointment (mild for the face, moderately-potent for the trunk and limbs), weaning down to once daily with response and stop when dermatitis clear.

- If topical corticosteroid is contra-indicated, then a topical immune modulator (e.g. tacrolimus ointment 0.1%) can be used to clear active inflammation.
- Oral prednisolone 0.5 mg/kg daily for five to 10 days if the patient has severe allergic contact dermatitis.
- Secondary infection with *Staphylococcus aureus* is common; treat with flucloxacillin 500 mg four times a day for seven days.

Key Points

- Exclude contact with culprit substance.
- Irritant contact dermatitis is usually caused by excessive exposure to soap and water.
- Treat the eczema with topical corticosteroid of appropriate strength.

Guidelines

Bourke J, Coulson I, English J. Guidelines for care of contact dermatitis *Br J Dermatol* 2001; **145**(6): 877.

References

Nedorost ST, Stevens SR. Diagnosis and treatment of allergic skin disorders in the elderly. *Drugs Aging* 2001; **18**(11): 827–35.

Links

National eczema society http://www.eczema .org/.

HERPES ZOSTER (SHINGLES)

Introduction

Herpes zoster is an acute, vesicular eruption of the skin. It occurs most commonly in the elderly and immunocompromised. These individuals are also at risk of more extensive involvement.

Aetiology

Following an infection with chickenpox, the Varicella zoster virus lies dormant in the dorsal root ganglion. In shingles reactivated virus migrates down peripheral sensory nerves and causes a vesicular rash on the skin.

Symptoms and signs

Pain may be experienced in the area for one to three days prior to the eruption of shingles. The rash is characterized by vesicles which appear within a well-demarcated, unilateral dermatomal distribution. There is usually a sharp cut-off at the midline. The most common sites of involvement are facial (ophthalmic branch of trigeminal nerve) and mid-thoracic to upper lumbar dermatomes (T3–L2). As the eruption progresses, erosions and haemorrhagic blisters may develop. Pustular lesions indicate secondary bacterial infection. Once the skin eruption has settled, pain within the affected dermatome (post-herpetic neuralgia (PHN)) can be severe and long-lasting. There is a particularly high rate of PHN following ophthalmic zoster.

Diagnosis

Vesicular fluid and vesicle base swabs can be taken for viral culture and viral DNA PCR.

Electron microscopy of scrapings from a vesicle base or immunofluorescence of the same material may identify the virus more rapidly.

Therapy

- Aciclovir 800 mg five times per day for seven days. The severity of post-herpetic neuralgia may be reduced if active therapy is instituted within 72 hours of the first vesicle. Valaciclovir 1 g tds for seven days or famciclovir 500 mg tds for seven days may be superior to aciclovir.
- In immunocompromised patients give intravenous aciclovir 10 mg/kg tds for seven days.
- Patients with shingles require adequate analgesia.
- Usually post-herpetic neuralgia settles within six months, however patients may require pain relief with drugs such as amitriptyline or gabapentin.

Key Points

- Post-herpetic neuralgia affects 50% of patients who are older than 60 years.

- Anti-viral therapy should be instituted as soon as possible to limit complications, including neuralgia.

Guidelines

Gnann JW Jr, Whitley RJ. Clinical practice: Herpes zoster. *N Engl J Med* 2002; **347**(5): 340–6.

Johnson RW, Dworkin RH. Treatment of herpes zoster and postherpetic neuralgia. *BMJ* 2003; **326**(7392): 748–50.

References

Schmader K. Herpes zoster in older adults. *Clin Infect Dis* 2001; **32**(10): 1481–6.

Links

http://www.bad.org.uk/public/leaflets/shingles.asp

LICHEN PLANUS

Introduction

Lichen planus (LP) is a common, usually self-limiting, inflammatory disorder of the skin. The eruption can be localized or widespread. Some drug reactions (e.g. beta-blockers) can produce an eruption which resemble LP and are termed lichenoid.

Aetiology

The aetiology of LP remains unknown, but there are associations with autoimmune conditions such as myasthenia gravis and vitiligo. LP is also associated with hepatitis B and C.

Symptoms and signs

The eruption is usually pruritic and occurs commonly on the flexural aspects of the wrists, ankles and low back. The lesions are flat-topped, violaceous (blue-red) papules which have a shiny surface. A white lacy network is sometimes seen on the surface of these lesions (Wickham's striae). Commonly, the buccal mucosae are involved, usually with a white reticulate eruption on the inside of the cheeks. Scarring alopecia can occur if the scalp is involved. Nail dystrophy may also occur.

Diagnosis

Skin biopsy. Histopathology demonstrates a band-like lymphocytic infiltrate at the dermo-epidermal junction causing a 'saw-tooth' profile of the rete ridges. Apoptotic keratinocytes are seen in the basal layer of the epidermis.

Therapy

A potent or superpotent corticosteroid ointment applied twice daily to the affected areas usually results in clearance. In the elderly use potent and superpotent corticosteroid ointments with care. Areas prone to skin atrophy (face and flexures) should be treated with a mild or moderately-potent corticosteroid ointment. UVB phototherapy or psoralen-UVA photochemotherapy can be useful in widespread LP. In resistant LP, ciclopsorin 3–5 mg/kg/day will often induce a remission.

Key Points

- The eruption of lichen planus is usually pruritic and occurs commonly on the flexural aspects of the wrists, ankles and low back.
- Lichen planus is most commonly treated with potent or superpotent topical corticosteroid ointments.

Guidelines

Cribier B, Frances C, Chosidow O. Treatment of lichen planus. An evidence-based medicine analysis of efficacy. *Arch Dermatol* 1998; **134**(12): 1521–30.

References

Norman RA, Blanco PM. Papulosquamous diseases in the elderly. *Dermatol Ther* 2003; **16**(3): 231–42.

Links

http://www.bad.org.uk/patients/leaflets/lichen.asp

MALIGNANT MELANOMA

Introduction

Malignant melanoma (MM) is a tumour of melanocytes which predominantly develops in the skin. Although MM is increasingly being observed in younger adults it is not uncommon in the elderly, particularly in individuals who have had a high cumulative sun exposure over many years. In most cases MM passes through an initial radial growth phase prior to adopting an invasive, vertical growth phase when it possesses a greater potential to metastasise.

Aetiology

Risk factors for developing MM include a family history of MM, fair skin, a history of excessive strong sun exposure and the presence of many atypical moles.

Symptoms and signs

Any pigmented lesion which changes in size, shape or colour should be suspected of being a melanoma until proven otherwise. The most significant clinical features are an increase in diameter, the development of an irregular outline and a variation of the pigmentation within the lesion. The clinical sub-types of melanoma are superficial spreading, nodular, acral lentiginous, sub-ungual and lentigo maligna. The elderly are particularly prone to lentigo maligna which is an *in situ* melanoma usually occurring on the face. It is a dark, macular lesion with an irregular margin and variable pigmentation. A small proportion of MMs are not pigmented, so-called amelanotic melanoma.

Diagnosis

- If suspected, the lesion should be excised with a margin of normal skin.
- Skin biopsy. Histopathology shows cytologically malignant melanocytes invading the dermis. Ulceration, atypical mitoses, a lymphocytic infiltrate and a lack of maturation of melanocytes within the dermal component

are all features which indicate a tumour with a potentially aggressive behaviour. The thickness of the tumour (Breslow thickness) is the best prognostic guide to five year survival. In tumours which have ulcerated and/or have a Breslow thickness greater than 2 mm, perform the following investigations: chest X-ray, CT or PET scan of chest, abdomen and pelvis, blood count, basic chemistry, liver function tests, ESR, LDH.

Therapy

Primary excision and thereafter wide local excision of scar.

Sentinel node biopsy is currently being offered as a staging procedure of the melanoma if more than 1 mm in thickness.

High dose interferon or dacarbazine chemotherapy for disseminated disease.

Lentigo maligna may respond to topical imiquimod.

Key Points

- Malignant melanomas less than 1 mm thick when excised have a five year survival rate of 95–100 %.
- Five year survival for malignant melanomas more than 4 mm thick is 50 %.

Guidelines

Roberts DL, Anstey AV, Barlow RJ, Cox NH. UK Guidelines for the management of cutaneous melanoma. *Br J Dermatol* 2002; **146**(1): 7–17.

References

Keller KL, Fenske NA, Glass LF. Cancer of the skin in the older patient. *Clin Geriatr Med* 1997; **13**(2): 339–61.

Links

Cancer Research UK http://info.cancer researchuk.org

Skin Cancer Foundation http://www. skincancer.org/melanoma

MYCOSIS FUNGOIDES

Introduction

Mycosis fungoides is a cutaneous T-cell lymphoma. Incidence is highest in the 5th and 6th decades of life, but it may occur at any age. It usually remains localised to the skin, but some cases progress to systemic involvement.

Aetiology

MF is a malignant lymphoma characterized by the expansion of a clone of CD4+ memory T cells. The malignant clone frequently lacks normal T cell antigens but possesses adhesion molecules which result in preferential cell migration into the skin. Some cases are associated with HTLV-1 infection.

Symptoms and Signs

There are four stages to mycosis fungoides:

- Stage 1 (1A <10%, 1B >10% of body surface area)—patches of erythema, fine scale, atrophy and poikiloderma mainly around the buttock and breast areas.
- Stage 2—As for stage 1, but with non-malignant lymphadenopathy (2A) or cutaneous nodules (2B).
- Stage 3—Erythrodermic skin involvement.
- Stage 4—Malignant infiltration of lymph nodes (4A) and viscera (4B).

Sezary syndrome is a leukaemic variant of cutaneous T cell lymphoma characterized by erythroderma and a high proportion of circulating malignant Tcells (Sezary cells). It carries a poor prognosis.

Diagnosis

- Skin biopsy. Histopathology shows an infiltrate of cytologically atypical lymphocytes in the upper dermis displaying epidermotropism. Collections of atypical lymphocytes in the epidermis form Pautrier microabscesses.
- T-cell subsets and Sezary cells.
- HTLV-1 serology.

Therapy

- For stage 1 disease (which is the majority of patients) general emollient therapy and phototherapy (narrow-band UVB or PUVA).
- Relapse is common after MF has been cleared and therefore long-term control can be achieved using intermittent courses of phototherapy or topical chemotherapy (mechlorethamine, carmustine). Treatment options for disease advanced beyond stage 1 include: radiotherapy, immunotherapy (interferon), retinoids (bexarotene) and chemotherapy.
- Extra-corporeal photophoresis is indicated for Sezary syndrome and erythrodermic mycosis fungoides.

Key Points

- In most patients mycosis fungoides is a benign condition with modest skin morbidity.
- Phototherapy (either UVB or PUVA) is usually able to control mycosis fungoides.

Guidelines

Whittaker SJ, Marsden JR, Spittle M, Russell-Jones R. Joint British Association of Dermatologists and UK Cutaneous Lymphoma Group guidelines for the management of primary cutaneous T-cell lymphomas. *Br J Dermatol* 2003; **149**(6): 1095–1107.

References

Diamandidou E, Cohen P R, Kurzrock R. Mycosis fungoides and Sezary syndrome *Blood* 1996; **88**(7): 2385–2409.

Links

Cutaneous Lymphoma Foundation (Mycosis Fungoides Foundation) http://www.clfoundation.org/

BASAL CELL CARCINOMA AND SQUAMOUS CELL CARCINOMA

Introduction

Basal cell carcinomas (BCC), which are the commonest type of skin tumour, can be locally invasive and destructive. Squamous cell carcinomas (SCC) are tumours which have the potential to metastasise. Both forms of non-melanoma skin cancer occur predominantly in individuals with fair skin who have been exposed to excessive amounts of strong sunshine, particularly those who have worked outdoors or lived abroad. The burden of non-melanoma skin cancer occurs predominantly in the elderly population.

Aetiology

UV-induced DNA damage in cutaneous keratinocytes leads to oncogenic mutations which, in turn, induce SCCs and BCCs. Patients on immunosuppressive medication (e.g. solid organ transplant recipients) are at higher risk of developing non-melanoma skin cancers (SCC > BCC).

Symptoms and signs

Both SCCs and BCCs tend to develop on uncovered skin which has received a high amount of ultraviolet radiation exposure. The face and upper torso are sites of predilection for BCC, whereas SCCs occur most commonly on tips of the ear, nose, lips, bald scalp and the dorsal aspects of forearms and hands. BCCs occur as solitary, slow-growing, red or skin-coloured plaques or nodules. They often have a pearly, infiltrated margin. As they enlarge, they may ulcerate or become crusted. Pigment or telangiectasiae may also be present. SCCs arise as ulcers, nodules or plaques which are often firm, indurated and painful. Well-differentiated SCCs may possess a scaly, keratotic surface. Poorly-differentiated SCCs can be fleshy and friable.

Diagnosis

Clinical diagnosis should be supported by a biopsy. Histopathology of a BCC reveals aggregates of basophilic cells with peripheral pallisading which bud from the basal epidermal layer and invade the dermis. Histopathology of a SCC shows nests of pleiomorphic squamous cells with eosinophilic cytoplasm and vesicular nuclei arising from the epidermis and invading the dermis.

Therapy

- BCCs and SCCs should be excised with a 2–5 mm margin of clinically normal skin.
- Nodular BCCs at low-risk sites and superficial BCCs can be removed using curettage.
- Patients with BCC or SCC who cannot tolerate surgery can be treated with radiotherapy.
- Superficial BCCs can be treated with topical imiquimod 5 % cream applied five days per week for six consecutive weeks.

Key Points

- Non-melanoma skin cancer occurs on uncovered skin in fair skinned individuals who have received excessive, cumulative sun exposure.
- Surgery or radiotherapy is the treatment of choice for these tumours.
- Superficial BCCs can be treated with imiquimod cream.

Guidelines

Telfer NR, Colver GB, Bowers PW. Guidelines for the management of basal cell carcinoma *Br J Dermatol* 1999; **141**(3): 415–23.

Motley R, Kersey P, Lawrence C Multiprofessional guidelines for the management of the patient with primary cutaneous squamous cell carcinoma *Br J Dermatol* 2002; **146**(1): 18–25.

References

Keller KL, Fenske NA, Glass LF. Cancer of the skin in the older patient *Clin Geriatr Med* 1997; **13**(2): 339–61.

Campbell FA, Gupta G. The management of non-melanoma skin cancer *Hosp Med* 2005; **66**(5): 288–93.

Links

Cancer Research UK http://info.cancerresearch uk.org/cancerandresearch/cancers/ nonmelanoma/

Skin Cancer Foundation http://www .skincancer.org

PSORIASIS

Introduction

Psoriasis is a common inflammatory skin condition with a variety of clinical sub-types. Chronic plaque psoriasis can affect individuals of any age, whereas palmo–plantar pustular psoriasis mainly affects females in the 5th to 7th decades. Psoriasis at any site is symptomatic, disfiguring and can be functionally disabling.

Aetiology

There is a strong genetic basis for psoriasis. In palmo-plantar pustular psoriasis, female sex is a contributing factor, as is cigarette smoking.

Symptoms and signs

Active psoriatic plaques are red, well-demarcated and scaly. They can be both itchy and painful. The lesions are usually symmetrically distributed and typically involve the extensor surfaces of the limbs, the trunk and scalp. Dystrophy of fingernails and toenails is common and a symmetrical, sero-negative arthritis occurs in approximately one-third of patients. In palmo-plantar pustular psoriasis, red plaques appear on the palms and soles which are studded with sterile pustules which vary in colour from yellow to brown.

Diagnosis

Diagnosis is usually made clinically.

Therapy

- Emollients, topical corticosteroids and vitamin D analogues (e.g. calcipotriol) should be used as first-line topical treatment.
- UVB or PUVA is preferable if there is widespread skin involvement.
- If systemic therapy is needed, acitretin (10–25 mg once daily) has the least side effect profile. Methotrexate is very effective and has activity against psoriatic arthritis. The effective dose of methotrexate in the elderly (5–15 mg once weekly) is often less than that required in younger adults (10–20 mg once weekly). Ciclosporin (3–5 mg/kg/day) can be used with good efficacy if methotrexate is not tolerated.
- For severe intractable disease, consider biological agents (e.g. etanercept).

Key Points

- Chronic plaque psoriasis is a relapsing-remitting disease. Therapy needs to be initiated when the condition is active.
- Localized disease can be controlled with topical treatment.

Guidelines

Mason J, Mason AR, Cork MJ. Topical preparations for the treatment of psoriasis: a systematic review *Br J Dermatol* 2002; **146**(3): 351–64.

Marsland AM, Chalmers RJ, Hollis S, Leonardi-Bee J, Griffiths CE. Interventions for chronic palmoplantar pustulosis *Cochrane Database Syst Rev* 2006; **1**: CD001433.

References

Naldi L, Griffiths CE. Traditional therapies in the management of moderate-to-severe chronic plaque psoriasis: an assessment of the benefits and risks. *Br J Dermatol* 2005; **152**: 597–615.

Links

Psoriasis Association
http://www.psoriasis-association.org.uk
National Psoriasis Foundation
http://www.psoriasis.org

SCABIES

Introduction

Scabies is usually associated with an intensely distressing itchy rash caused by infestation with the *Sarcoptes scabiei* mite. Elderly patients are particularly prone to becoming heavily infested with mites yet may be asymptomatic except for a generalised, scaly eruption (crusted or Norwegian scabies). Crusted scabies is especially problematic in residential or nursing homes where transmission to other residents and members of staff can occur easily.

Aetiology

Direct physical contact with an infested individual allows transmission of the mite. Female mites burrow into the skin and lay eggs in the epidermis. Consequently, sensitisation to the mites and their faeces causes the itchy dermatosis of scabies.

Symptoms and signs

In ordinary scabies, affected individuals complain of intense, generalised pruritus, which is often worse at night. While excoriations can be found all over the skin the diagnostic burrows are usually observed in the finger webs, sides of fingers, wrists and the insteps of feet. Scabetic burrows are short, linear, scaly lesions; sometimes the mite can be observed as a black dot at one end. Large inflammatory nodules may be seen at various sites, especially the genital skin and waist. Crusted scabies is characterized by widespread scaling associated with often only minimal amounts of erythema.

Diagnosis

- Scrapings from a burrow may demonstrate mites or eggs if viewed microscopically with 10 % potassium hydroxide solution.

Therapy

- Application of a topical anti-scabetic lotion (permethrin or malathion) all over the body, including under the finger- and toe-nails. The application should be left for 24 hours before being washing off. Repeat the treatment one week later.
- Crusted scabies not responding to topical therapy can be treated with a single dose of oral ivermectin 200 mcg/kg (available on a named-patient basis).

Key Points

- Once the scabies has been treated the itching takes two or three weeks to settle.
- All close personal contacts need to be treated at the same time as the patient.
- In nursing homes, all staff and contacts need to be treated.

Guidelines

Choisdow O. Clinical practices: scabies. *N Engl J Med* 2006; **354**: 1718–27.

References

Johnston G, Sladden M. Scabies: diagnosis and treatment. *BMJ* 2005; **331**: 619–22.

TINEA

Introduction

Tinea is a term used to describe fungal (dermatophyte) infections of the skin, hair and nails.

Aetiology

Several dermatophyte species, such as *Trichophyton rubrum* and *Epidermophyton floccosum*, are causative in tinea infections of the skin. The pattern of the eruption and site of involvement vary according to the infecting species of dermatophyte. Dermatophyte infections are contagious through direct physical contact.

Symptoms and signs

- *Tinea corporis*. Involvement of the body: itchy, scaly, annular lesions with raised edges.
- *Tinea cruris*. Involvement of the flexures: itchy, well-demarcated, red plaques in the flexures.
- Tinea pedis. Involvement of the feet: in the toe-webs there is peeling and maceration (especially occurs in the lateral toe clefts), on the soles of the feet there is redness and scaling extending onto the foot margins ('mocassin'-type).
- *Tinea manum*. Involvement of the hands: there is diffuse scaling and erythema of, usually, one palm only.
- *Tinea capitis*. Involvement of the scalpand hair: there is itching, scalp redness, scaling and hair loss. Tinea capitis is rare in adults.
- *Onychomycosis*. Involvement of the nails. There is nail thickening, discolouration and dystrophy.

Diagnosis

- Skin scrapings, plucked hairs and nail clippings sent for microscopy and culture.

Therapy

- For limited tinea corporis, tinea cruris, tinea pedis and tinea manum treat topically with either an allylamine-derivative cream (e.g. terbinafine) or an azole cream (e.g. clotrimazole bd for two to three weeks).
- Oral therapy is needed in: tinea corporis with multiple sites of involvement, extensive tinea cruris, 'mocassin'-type tinea pedis and tinea capitis. Use terbinafine 250 mg od for 4 weeks. For onychomycosis treat with terbinafine 250 mg od for three months. If oral terbinafine is contra-indicated, use oral itraconazole: for tinea corporis and tinea cruris–100 mg od for 15 days or 200 mg od for seven days. For tinea pedis and tinea manum–100 mg od for 30 days or 200 mg bd

for seven days. For onychomycosis–200 mg daily for three months or a 'pulse' of 200 mg bd for seven days, subsequent pulses repeated after a 21-day interval; fingernails 2 pulses, toenails 3 pulses. If a prolonged course of oral antifungals for onychomycosis is contraindicated, try amorolfine nail lacquer applied to affected nails 1–2 times per week for 6 months for fingers and nine to 12 months for toes.

Key Points

- Limited skin involvement can be treated with a topical antifungal preparation (e.g. terbinafine).
- Extensive cutaneous involvement and any scalp or nail involvement requires oral therapy, either terbinafine or itraconazole.
- Onychomycosis generally requires a prolonged course of oral antifungal therapy.

Guidelines

Weinberg JM, Scheinfeld NS. Cutaneous infections in the elderly: diagnosis and management *Dermatol Ther* 2003; **16**: 195–205.

References

Loo DS. Cutaneous fungal infections in the elderly. *Dermatol Clin* 2004; **22**: 33–50.

URTICARIA AND ANGIO-OEDEMA

Introduction

Urticaria and angio-oedema are a common conditions characterized by dermal swellings. Clinically, these dermatoses may range from an eruption of transient weals to a life-threatening dermatosis characterized by deep-seated oedema.

Aetiology

Although in many cases the cause is unknown, urticaria can be triggered by drugs (eg. opiates, NSAIDs), foods (nuts, shellfish), infections (e.g. hepatitis B); angio-oedema can also be caused by drugs (e.g. ACE inhibitors, opiates,

NSAIDs); physical urticaria can be precipitated by a variety of stimuli such as heat, cold and pressure.

Symptoms and Signs

Urticaria consists of multiple, pink, pruritic weals (superficial dermal swellings), each with a surrounding red flare. Individual lesions can display a variety of shapes and may coalesce to produce large swellings with irregular outlines. Typically a weal persists for a few hours (they always disappear within 24 hours) before resolving to leave normal skin. Patients may display positive dermographism (the tendency to develop weals at the site of gentle scratching of the skin). In angio-oedema the swellings are deep and usually confined to one area (most commonly lips, eyelids, genitalia) and may be symmetrical or unilateral. Affected skin is often not red and itching is usually absent. Angio-oedema lasts for a few hours to two to three days. Urticaria and angio-oedema may occur in an anaphylaxis reaction.

Diagnosis

The diagnosis is made clinically from the physical signs or from the history.

Therapy

- H1 antihistamines (e.g. levocetirizine 5 mg od) are usually effective but sometimes need to be given in supranormal doses.
- A sedating antihistamine taken at night (e.g. hydroxyzine 25–50 mg) can also be helpful.
- In severe, widespread involvement a moderate dose of prednisolone (e.g. 0.5 mg/kg/day) can be used for a short period (less than two weeks).
- Treat anaphylaxis with: IM or SC epinephrine (adrenaline) 0.5–1.0 mg, slow IV injection of chlorpheniramine 10–20 mg, IV hydrocortisone sodium succinate 100–300 mg and oxygen.

Key Points

- Urticaria is characterized by transient weals which are often extremely itchy.

- Angio-oedema is characterized by deep-seated, non-itchy swellings often involving the skin of the eyelids or lips.
- Both urticaria and angio-oedema should be treated with antihistamines.

Guidelines

Grattan C, Powell S, Humphreys F Management and diagnostic guidelines for urticaria and angio-oedema. *Br J Dermatol* 2001; **144**: 708–14.

References

Kaplan A P Clinical practice. Chronic urticaria and angioedema. *N Engl J Med* 2002; **346**(3): 175–9.

VENOUS ECZEMA AND THE DEPENDENCY SYNDROME

Introduction

Venous eczema is one of the cutaneous sequelae to venous insufficiency in the lower legs. The dependency syndrome is also a vascular problem of the lower legs and affects individuals with poor mobility that are largely chair-bound. As a consequence these related conditions are more common in the elderly than in younger adults.

Aetiology

Venous eczema occurs secondary to venous hypertension, which is in turn caused by venous incompetence. A number of functional and structural problems in the venous circulation (e.g. previous deep venous thrombosis, varicose veins) lead to incompetence which can be exacerbated by the hydrostatic influence of prolonged leg dependency. In the dependency syndrome sustained hydrostatic down-force produces a combination of venous and lymphatic insufficiency and therefore the physical signs are a consequence of venous congestion and lymphoedema. The dependency syndrome is a particular problem in patients who are chronically immobile and who sleep in a chair overnight.

Symptoms and signs

In venous eczema the skin of the lower legs is itchy, red and scaly. Other signs of venous insufficiency are usually present, such as oedema, varicose veins, ulceration and haemosiderin deposition. Although often bilateral, venous eczema can be unilateral if venous insufficiency is limited to one leg. In the dependency syndrome the physical signs are usually symmetrical and are characterized by erythema, demonstrable 'pitting' oedema as well as fixed swelling (lymphoedema) of the lower legs and feet. Chronic swelling will result in a 'cobblestone' appearance of the shins and deep creases at the ankles and toes. The two conditions often co-exist.

Diagnosis

- Diagnosis is usually made clinically.
- Venous studies can be performed to identify venous insufficiency.

Therapy

- Treat eczema with twice daily application of emollients and a potent topical corticosteroid ointment.

- Once eczema controlled, wean off topical corticosteroid ointment, but continue with emollient.
- For the dependency syndrome encourage the patient to have his/her legs elevated as much as possible. Sleeping in a bed at night is essential.
- Compression bandaging will reduce the swelling (check the arterial circulation to ensure that compression will be tolerated).
- Once the legs have normalized encourage the patient to wear below-knee, class 2 compression hosiery.

Key Points

- Venous eczema and the dependency syndrome often co-exist in elderly patients who are chronically immobile.
- Improved mobility, leg elevation and compression are important therapeutic manouvres in both conditions.
- If venous eczema is poorly controlled with topical therapies, refer to vascular surgeons.

43 Age-related eye diseases

Genevieve Larkin

Department of Ophthalmology, Kings College Hospital, London, UK

The leading causes of vision impairment and blindness in the developed world are primarily age related eye diseases. These are cataract, glaucoma, age related macular degeneration and Diabetes. The number of people with age-related eye disease is expected to double within the next three decades.

Age-related eye diseases are costly to treat, threaten the ability of older adults to live independently, and increase the risk of accidents and falls. To prevent vision loss and support rehabilitative services for people with low vision, it is imperative for the public health community to address the issue through surveillance, public education, and coordination of screening, examination and treatment.

CATARACT

Introduction

Cataract is defined as loss of transparency of the crystalline lens and may present as a continuous spectrum from minimal to dense opacity of the lens causing different degrees of visual disability experienced by any individual patient.

Cataract remains the leading cause of visual impairment in all regions of the world, except in the most developed countries. A study performed in Britain looked at the causes of visual impairment in people aged 75 and older, cataract accounted for 35.9 % of cases of

loss of vision followed by age related macular degeneration (AMD) and refractive errors only (1).

Based on statistics from the Department of Health (2), cataract surgery is at present the most performed elective surgical procedure in the UK and with increasing life expectancy and expansion of the elderly population the demand for surgery will continue to rise.

The interference with visual function is the direct consequence of lens opacification, but additional factors contribute to the disabilities experienced by each individual patient. The loss of distance and reading vision may not only lead to loss of self confidence and independence, but also loss of driving capabilities and an increased risk of falling, all of which have important functional consequences in elderly patients.

Aetiology

Cataracts are a multifactorial disease process with numerous genetic and environmental factors associated with their development (3).

Diagnosis

The ophthalmological history and examination will assess the degree of visual impairment, the nature of the cataract and the presence of other ocular conditions affecting the prognosis for vision.

Prescribing for Elderly Patients Edited by Stephen Jackson, Paul Jansen and Arduino Mangoni
© 2009 John Wiley & Sons, Ltd

Therapy

The treatment of cataract is by surgery and is recommended when the lens opacity becomes visually significant.

Preoperative care

Pupil dilation—eye drops instilled into conjunctival sac.

Phenylephrine 2.5 % and 10 % is an $\alpha 1$-receptor agonist that stimulates the α-receptors and causes pupil dilatation without cycloplegia.

Dosage: One drop instilled every 15 minutes four times before surgery.

The side effects of phenylephrine 2.5 % and 10 % can include blurring of vision, clouding of the cornea with repeated administration and pigment release into the anterior chamber. In predisposed people, with a narrow anterior chamber angle, it may precipitate angle closure glaucoma. Contact allergy to phenylephrine has been reported (4).

Both 2.5 % and 10 % phenylephrine have been associated with cardiovascular effects and should be used with caution in patients on monoamine oxidase inhibitors, tricyclic antidepressant or atropine or in those with hypertension, advanced arteriosclerotic changes, aneurysms, orthostatic hypotension, long-standing insulin dependent diabetes and in children with low bodyweights (5).

Cyclopentolate 1 % is a parasympathetic antagonist, useful for short term dilatation of the pupil and cycloplegia with the maximum mydriasis reached within 60 min and completely resolves within 24 hours. The cycloplegic effect reaches a maximum in one hour and recovers fully in 24 hours.

Dosage: One drop instilled every 15 minutes four times before surgery.

The side effects of cyclopentolate can include allergy, acute angle closure glaucoma with elevation of the intraocular pressure in predisposed patients, and blurring of vision. Systemic side effects have been reported and include tachycardia, facial flush, tremor, dryness of mouth and skin. A reported but rare side effect in elderly patients as well as in very young children is the occurrence of a psychotic reaction and delirium (6).

Non-Steroidal Anti-inflammatory eye drops Flurbiprofen sodium ophthalmic solution is one of a series of phenylalkanoic acids with analgesic, antipyretic, and anti-inflammatory activity. Its mechanism of action is believed to be the inhibition of the cyclo-oxygenase enzyme, that is essential in the biosynthesis of prostaglandins. Prostaglandins appear to have a role in the miotic response during ocular surgery in addition to increased vasodilatation, vascular permeability and intraocular pressure. Based on this evidence flurbiprofen is indicated in the inhibition of intraoperative miosis.

Dosage: A total of four drops of sodium ophthalmic solution should be administered by instilling one drop approximately every half hour beginning one hour before surgery.

The most frequently reported side effects of flurbiprofen are transient burning and stinging upon instillation and minor symptoms of ocular irritation.

Increased bleeding tendency of ocular tissues during the surgical procedure has been reported. Interaction of flurbiprofen with other topical ophthalmic medications has not been fully investigated.

Wound healing may be delayed with the use of flurbiprofen solution. It is recommended that flurbiprofen be used with caution in patients with known bleeding tendency or receiving other medications that may prolong the bleeding time.

Anaesthesia for cataract surgery

Most cataract surgery is done under local anaesthesia as a day case outpatient procedure. This reduces risks and complications related to general anaesthesia and makes the operation suitable for a larger number of patients (7), (8), (9).

The most common methods of local anaesthesia are topical administration of drops in the conjunctival sac, intracameral administration of anaesthetic intraoperatively and sub Tenon's block. These methods are not associated with systemic complications and are suitable for the majority of patients.

Alternative methods of anaesthesia are peribulbar or retrobulbar block and general anaesthesia. A variety of local anaesthetic agents are used but are outside the scope of this chapter.

Post-operative care

At the end of the surgery topical antibiotic with or without steroid injection is administered into the subconjunctival space, antibiotic alone can be injected intracamerally (10). The most commonly used antibiotics is cefuroxime but gentamicin(never intracamerally) is used in patients allergic to penicillin. This is followed by a combination of topical antibiotic and steroid eye drops for a period of four weeks. Oral administration of a carbonic anhydrase inhibitor in the immediate post operative period can be given to avoid postoperative spikes of intraocular pressure.

Common combinations include neomycin and polymyxin B sulfates with dexamethasone ophthalmic suspension/tobramycin and dexamethasone. The antimicrobial component is active against: *Staphylococcus aureus, E coli, Haemophilus influenzae, Klebsiella, Enterobacteria, Neisseria* and *Pseudomonas aeruginosa.*

Dosage: instillation of one drop four to six times daily for one week, three times daily for one week, twice daily for one week, once daily for one week.

Side effects of the steroid component can include an increase in intraocular pressure and delayed wound healing. Side effects of the antimicrobial component are allergic rection to the antibiotic, corneal epithelial toxicity and the risk of secondary infections.

No information is available with regard to drug interactions and systemic absorption.

Key Points

- All medications for diabetes, cardiovascular and respiratory conditions should be continued as usual and aspirin and warfarin do not need to be stopped (11).
  The use of alpha receptor blockers for benign prostatic hypertrophy should be noted as they may cause a recently identified "floppy iris syndrome" with intraoperative complications (12).
- Adequate counselling must be given to patients with breathing difficulties as they might require oxygen and positioning of the operating table.
- Cataract is a common condition in elderly patients, surgical treatment is warranted when it represents a major cause of visual impairment.

Guidelines

The Royal College of Ophthalmologists, Cataract Surgery Guidelines 2004, updated in 2007 http://www.rcophth.ac.uk/docs/publications/published-guidelines/FinalVersionGuidelines April2007Updated.pdf

Links

National Eye Institute, "Cataract: What you should know" http://www.nei.nih.gov/health/cataract/cataract_facts.asp

Royal National Institute of the Blind: http://www.rnib.org.uk

Driver and Vehicle Licensing Agency: http://www.dvla.gov.uk/

The Royal College of Ophthalmologists, "Understanding cataract", http://www.rcophth.ac.uk/docs/publications/UnderstandingCataracts.pdf

REFERENCES

1. Evans JR, Fletcher AE, Wormald RP. Causes of visual impairment in people aged 75 years and older in Britain: an add-on study to the MRC Trial of Assessment and Management of Older People in the Community. *Br J Ophthalmol* 2004; **88**: 365–70.
2. Department of Health National Eye Care Plan. May 2004.
3. Hammond CJ, Sneider H, Spector TD, Gilbert CE. Genetic and environmental factors in age

related nuclear cataract in monzygotic and dizygotic twins. *N Engl J Med* 2000; **342**: 1786–90.

4. Resano A, Esteve C, Fernandez Benitez M. Allergic contact blepharoconjunctivitis due to phenylephrine eye drops. *J Investig Allergol Clin Immunol* 1999; **9**(1): 55–7.

5. Schlichtenbrede FC, Burkhardt KU, Bartram MC, Wiedemann R. [Biochemical stress monitoring during cataract surgery; phenylephrine 10 % shows no changes in serum-catecholamines in comparison with phenylephrine 5 %]. *Klin Monatsbl Augenheilkd*. 2001; **218**(7): 479–83.

6. Mirshahi A, Kohnen T. Acute psychotic reaction caused by topical cyclopentolate use for cycloplegic refraction before refractive surgery: case report and review of the literature. *J Cataract Refract Surg*. 2003; **29**(5): 1026–30.

7. Davis DB, Mandel MR. Efficacy and complication rate of 16,224 consecutive peribulbar blocks. A prospective multicenter study. *J Cataract Refract Surg* 1994; **20**(3): 327–37.

8. Frieman BJ, Friedberg MA. Globe perforation associated with subtenon's anesthesia. *Am J Ophthalmol* 2001; **131**(4): 520–1.

9. Norregard JC, Schein OD, Bellan L, Black C, Alonso J, Bernth-Petersen P, Dunn E, Anderson TF, Espellargues M, Anderson GF. International variation in anaesthesia care during cataract surgery: Results form the international cataract surgery outcomes study. *Arch Ophthalmol* 1997; **115**(10): 1304–8.

10. Ciulla TA, Starr MB, Masket S. Bacterial endophthalmitis prophylaxis for cataract surgery: an evidencebased update. *Ophthalmology* 2003; **109**: 13–24.

11. Konstantatos A. Anticoagulation and cataract surgery: a review of the current literature. *Anaesth Intensive Care* 2001; **29**(1): 11–8.

12. Chang DF, Campbell JR. Intraoperative floppy iris syndrome associated with tamulosin. *J Cataract Refract Surg* 2005; **31**(4): 664–73.

GLAUCOMA

Introduction

Glaucoma is a clinical syndrome consisting of a triad of signs:

1. High intraocular pressure, usually greater than or equal to 20 mmHg.
2. Characteristic visual field loss.
3. Atrophy of the optic nerve head.

The most common variety presents in adult life and is a chronic progressive condition that can cause severe loss of vision and loss of visual field if not treated. In this section we focus our discussion on treatment and management of chronic open angle glaucoma and acute angle closure glaucoma.

Glaucoma is an important cause of visual disability that accounts for 15 % of registered blindness in the United Kingdom. It may affect patients of all ages. The most common type is the adult chronic form, rarely presenting as an acute condition but more generally as a chronic progressive disease. It is estimated that a large number of glaucoma patients are still undiagnosed, due to the lack of symptoms until late in the disease, and this number is expected to rise with the increase of the elderly population (1).

Primary open angle glaucoma (POAG) affects 2 % of the white population over the age of 40. The majority of patients are elderly presenting with the chronic type of the disease, although glaucoma may also manifest in children and young adults. It is estimated that about 500 000 people suffer from glaucoma in England and Wales and an equivalent number remain undiagnosed.

The Afro-Caribbean race has a four-fold increased risk of glaucoma compared to whites, but the same risk as a white person with a first degree relative affected by the condition (2).

Aetiology and Terminology

The pressure of the eyeball is maintained by the presence of aqueous humour inside the anterior part of the eye. When the pressure rises because the outflow mechanism is impaired the globe becomes firmer and the nerve fibre layer and the optic nerve may be damaged irreversibly (3). There are also cases of glaucoma with normal or low intraocular pressure. Therefore there are three types of glaucoma relative to the value of the pressure: high, normal and low tension glaucoma.

There is also a group of patients in which the intraocular pressure measures more than two standard deviations above the mean without evidence of glaucomatous damage or field loss, in these cases the condition is known as ocular hypertension (OHT). Some of these subjects will later develop glaucoma so require long term follow-up.

Additional terminology refers to the clinical presentation of the condition (acute or chronic glaucoma, congenital or acquired), to the anatomical changes in the anterior segment of the eye (angle closure or open angle), and to the presence of causative factors (primary or secondary).

Symptoms and Signs

Primary open angle glaucoma (POAG)

POAG may not be detected until very advanced. This is due to the preservation of central fixation until late, the absence of pain and the compensatory effect of the contralateral eye masking presence of field loss. In advanced glaucoma the patient may be aware of tunnel vision and also the central visual field can be affected.

It is recommended that people over 40 years of age be checked by an optometrist once yearly.

Signs of POAG

1. Intraocular pressure greater than average in 60–70 % of patients.
2. Open anterior chamber angle.
3. Peripheral visual field loss.
4. Optic nerve appearance which can include all or some of—a) thinning of the neurosensory rim, b) notching of the rim, c) nerve fibre layer haemorrhage, d)cup-disc ratio asymmetry greater than 0.2.

Acute angle closure glaucoma (AACG)

AACG usually presents in one eye with acute vision loss, conjunctival injection, mydriasis, pain and may be associated with sickness and nausea. The patient usually presents to the attention of the ophthalmologist acutely unwell. Rarely acute angle closure glaucoma may involve both eyes at the same time or may have a recurrent-remittent course before presenting to the specialist.

Diagnosis

In the diagnosis of glaucoma a detailed patient history regarding family history, past medical history and past ocular history is very important in identifying risk factors as well as understanding the pathogenesis better.

The following are essential steps in examining a patient with suspect glaucoma:

- Snellen visual acuity measurement.
- Slit lamp examination of the anterior segment.
- Intraocular pressure measurement (Goldmann applanation tonometry).
- Formal visual field test (Humphrey automated perimeter).
- Dilated fundus exam and assessment of the optic nerve head.

The three fundamental steps in the diagnosis of glaucoma are the measurement of the intraocular pressure, the assessment of visual fields by Humphrey automated perimetry and the fundoscopy for the assessment of the optic disc.

Therapy

Treatment of Primary Open Angle Glaucoma (POAG)

The treatment of Primary Open Angle Glaucoma aims to lower the intraocular pressure (IOP) as close as possible to a "target IOP" which should represent the optimal IOP to prevent further damage to the optic nerve.

Medical treatment is usually the first line approach and can be administered as topical or systemic medication. Both of these medications may have important systemic side effects that may be life threatening, particularly in the elderly (4), (5). A detailed medical and drug history must be taken and adequate counselling should be given to the patient about possible side effects at the beginning of the treatment. It should also be made clear that the treatment will be life-long.

The main treatment options are:

1. Medical treatment.
2. Surgical treatment: argon laser trabeculoplasty (ALT), filtering surgery, ciliary body ablation procedures.

Medical treatment

First line topical medications: prostaglandin analogues latanoprost 0.005 %, bimatoprost, travoprost:

- Treatment is applied once each day, preferably in the evening.
- Mechanism of action: improves the uveoscleral outflow of aqueous humor.
- Side effects: possible change in eye colour (especially in those with mixed coloured irides) and lash growth. It is also essential to advise patients regarding other possible side effects which include: conjunctival hyperaemia; transient punctate epithelial erosions; and rarely macular oedema, iritis, and uveitis. Asthmatic patients should be advised not to use Latanoprost within five minutes of taking their asthma medication. Treatment with Latanoprost should not be commenced in pregnant or breast-feeding patients.

Beta blockers: timoptol, timolol, levobunolol, betaxolol, carteolol:(6)

- Treatment: twice daily (except the long acting timolol, once daily).
- Mechanism of action: reduced production of aqueous humor by the ciliary body.
- Side effects: worsening of COPD, asthma, depression, loss of libido, impotence. In diabetics the systemic absorption of beta blockers may decrease the sensitivity to the symptoms of hypoglycaemia, slow pulse rate. Other possible side effects are dizziness, tiredness or a reduction in exercise tolerance.

Second line topical medications

Carbonic anhydrase inhibitors: dorzolamide, brinzolamide: (7), (8)

- Treatment: two to three times daily.
- Mechanism of action: reduces the production of aqueous humor by the ciliary body.
- Side effects: tend to sting when first instilled into the eye. Possible side effects include a bitter taste.

Alpha-agonists: brimonidine, apraclonidine:

- Treatment: two or three times daily.
- Mechanism of action: reduces the production of aqueous humor from the ciliary body and increases the outflow from the eye.
- Side effects: dry mouth, allergic reaction and feeling of being generally unwell. It can also cause depression in susceptible people and it has been associated with nightmares in children.

Combination agents

Combination agents are used in patients needing more than one medication in order to control the intraocular pressure. The most commonly used combinations are:

- Carbonic Anhydrase inhibitors and beta blockers (trusopt and timolol).
- Prostaglandin analogues and beta blockers (latanoprost and timolol).

The possibility of systemic side effects from topical medication is rare, nonetheless it is good practice to apply a gentle pressure over the tear punctum after administration of the eye drops to minimize systemic absorption of the drug.Eye drops of first choice are prostaglandin analogues and beta-blockers, other preparations are used in association or second line treatment.

Where good pressure control cannot be achieved by medical treatment alone and with evidence of progressive visual field loss surgery is advocated.

Acute angle closure glaucoma (AACG)

The treatment of AACG depends on severity, duration of the attack, intraocular pressure at presentation and visual acuity. AACG is an ophthalmic emergency and delaying the referral to the specialist may cause severe permanent damage. Medications include topical pressure lowering agents and systemic pressure lowering agents. As soon as the attack is broken a YAG laser peripheral iridotomy is performed in both eyes as a prophylactic measure to prevent further attacks. Less commonly an angle closure attack may be the result of phacomorphic glaucoma, where the enlarging lens causes a forward displacement of the iris plane, in these cases cataract extraction should be planned when the pressure and inflammation are controlled.

- Topical medications:

    a. Topical beta blockers (e.g. levobunolol or timolol 0.5%) in one dose
    b. Topical carbonic anhydrase inhibitors (e.g. apraclonidine 1.0% or brimonidine 0.2% one dose.
    c. Topical steroids (e.g. prednisolone acetate 1%) every 15 min for four doses, then hourly
    d. Topical miotics (e.g. pilocarpine 1% to 2% every 15 min for two doses and pilocarpine 0.5% in the contralateral eye—which may also be at risk of angle closure- for one dose.

Miotics: cholinergic agonists, e.g. pilocarpine:

- Maintenance treatment: three or four times a day.
- Mechanism of action: improves the flow of fluid out of the eye through the conventional outflow pathway.
- Side effects: headache or eye ache, may cause accomodative spasm and blurred vision. It is usually not indicated in patients with high myopia as there is the risk of retinal detachment.
- Systemic medications -Intravenous acetazolamide 500 mg is administered when not contraindicated, the intraocular pressure and the visual acuity should be rechecked after one hour.

Pain and vomiting should be addressed with i.m. or i.v. medications. Systemic carbonic anhydrase inhibitors: acetazolamide:

- Intravenous Treatment: 250–500 mg i.v.
- Oral treatment: 125–250 mg p.o., two to four times daily, or 250 mg p.o. long acting twice daily.
- Mechanism of action: reduces the production of aqueous humor from the ciliary body.
- Side effects: is contraindicated in patients with allergy to sulfa drugs. Possible side effects are nausea, fatigue, metallic taste and paraesthesia. Very rarely aplastic anaemia, thrombocytopenia, agranulocytosis and Stevens Johnson syndrome have been reported. Patients on long term treatment with aspirin should be monitored closely for acid-base imbalance.

Key Points

- All patients should be instructed how to apply eye drops. It is recommended to practice punctal occlusion (blocking the tear duct) for three minutes after taking the drops in order to minimise systemic absorption and risk of systemic side effects.
- The medical treatment is life-long.
- The goal of the treatment is to prevent further damage to the optic nerve.

Guidelines

- The Royal College of Ophthalmologists "Guidelines for the management of open angle glaucoma and ocular hypertension 2004". http://www.rcophth.ac.uk/docs/publications/glaucoma2004.pdf.
- Gordon MO, Beiser JA, Brandt JD, et al. The Ocular Hypertension Treatment Study. Baseline factors that predict the onset of primary open-angle glaucoma. *Arch Ophthalmol* 2002; **120**: 714–20.
- The AGIS Investigators. The Advanced Glaucoma Intervention Study (AGIS), 7. the relationship between control of intraocular pressure and visual field deterioration. *Am J Ophthalmol* 2000; **130**: 429–40.

- Collaborative Normal-Tension Glaucoma Study Group. Comparison of glaucomatous progression between untreated patients with normal-tension glaucoma and patients with therapeutically reduced intraocular pressures. *Am J Ophthalmol* 1998; **126**: 487–97.

Links for Professionals

- International Glaucoma Association: http://www.iga.org.uk.
- Royal National Institute for the blind: http://www.rnib.org.uk.
- Driver and Vehicle Licensing Agency: http://www.dvla.gov.uk.

Links for Patients

- Patient information "understanding glaucoma": http://www.rcophth.ac.uk/docs/publications/UnderstandingGlaucoma.pdf.
- National Eye Institute: http://www.nei.nih.gov.
- Information for patients: http://www.patient.co.uk.
- "Glaucoma: what you should know" http://www.nei.nih.gov/health/glaucoma/glaucoma_facts.asp.

REFERENCES

1. Robinson R, Deutsch J, Jones HS, et al. Unrecognised and unregistered visual impairment. *Br J Ophthalmol* 1994; **78**: 736–40.
2. Sommer A, Tielsch JM, Katz J, Quigley HA, Gottsch JD. Relationship between intraocular pressure and primary open angle glaucoma among white and black Americans. *Arch Ophthalmol* 1991; **109**: 1090–5.
3. Araie M, Yamagami J, Suzuki Y. Visual field defects in normal-tension and high-tension glaucoma. *Ophthalmology* 1993; **100**: 1808–14.
4. Novack GD, O'Donnell MJ, Molloy DW. New glaucoma medications in the geriatric population: efficacy and safety. *I Am Geriatr Soc* 2002; **50**: 956–62.
5. Detry-Morel M. Side effects of glaucoma medications. *Bull Soc Belge Ophthalmol* 2006; **299**: 27–40.
6. Goldberg I, Goldberg H. Betaxolol eye drops. A clinical trial of safety and efficacy. *Aust N Z J Ophthalmol* 1995; **23**: 17–24.
7. Fraunfelder FT, Meyer SM, Bagby GC Jr, Dreis MW. Hematologic reactions to carbonic anhydrase inhibitors. *Am J Ophthalmol* 1985; **100**: 79–81.
8. Anderson CJ, Kaufman PL, Sturm RJ. Toxicity of combined therapy with carbonic anhydrase inhibitors and aspirin. *Am J Ophthalmol* 1978; **86**: 516–9.

AGE RELATED MACULAR DEGENERATION

Introduction

Age Related Macular Degeneration (AMD) is an age-related condition involving the macular area of the retina and causing loss of central vision. The condition accounts for almost 50 % of people registered as blind or partially sighted in England (1) and is the most common cause of irreversible visual loss in the western world in individuals over 50 years of age.

Aetiology

Age-related Macular Degeneration is a multifactorial disease, risk factors include environmental and genetic determinants. Epidemiological studies have shown that AMD is most prevalent in Caucasians although its prevalence is increasing in other communities. Cigarette smoking has emerged as a modifiable and consistent risk factor (2) and vascular disease and hypertension appear associated with the condition. Recent studies on genetic predisposition for AMD have successfully identified the complement factor H as the first major susceptibility gene for AMD identified in chromosome 1 (3). Other factors like light exposure, iris and skin colour as well as dietary antioxidant vitamin and mineral intake have not to date been shown to modify the risk (4, 5).

Symptoms and Signs

Definitions of the Epidemiological Study Group:

- Age Related Maculopathy (ARM): early changes in the macula in subjects after 50 years of age that may predispose to the progression towards late stage of Age Related Macular Degeneration (AMD) which is generally asymptomatic. Signs include, white yellow spots called drusen, clumps of hyperpigmentation and patches of hypopigmentation associated with drusen
- Age Related Macular Degeneration (ARMD) can be dry or atrophic in nature, it is the most common form making up about 90 % of cases. The condition generally is bilateral although it may be asymmetrical The more serious form is wet or neovascular in nature, the least common making up about 10 % of cases. The condition is treatable in a proportion of cases, depending on the stage of the lesion, its fluoroangiographic characteristics and the time from the onset of symptoms.
- Atrophic or dry AMD generally presents with gradual symptoms over months or years with difficulty in reading and recognising faces with patchy shadows around the central field of vision. A proportion of patients may remain asymptomatic and present to the ophthalmologist following an optician referral. On examination there is atrophy of the photoreceptors, RPE and choriocapillaris with the lesions frequently resembling a geographic map hence "geographic atrophy".
- Neovascular or wet AMD presents with rapid visual deterioration over days or weeks with distortions affecting distance and reading vision as well as obscurations of the visual target in activities involving fine detail. The symptoms are produced by the presence of sub-retinal fluid, exudate, haemorrhage or pigment epithelial elevation in the foveal and parafoveal region. The condition tends to be bilateral although the involvement of each eye can be separate in time. Examination reveals elevation of the retina in the macular region that may be associated with haemorrhage and retinal pigment epithelial (RPE) changes. A pigment epithelium detachment, if present, will give rise to fluid accumulation and pale colour of the neurosensory retina.

Two main types of neovascular AMD are classified on the basis of fluorescein angiography: These are Classic Neovascular membrane, a neovascular membrane that shows well defined margins on fluorescein angiography and Occult Neovascular membrane a "poorly defined" neovascular membrane whose margins cannot be easily drawn in all its components during a fluoroangiogram.

Diagnosis

- Distance and Near Visual acuity.
- Dilated slit lamp fundus examination.
- Fundus Fluorescein angiography (FFA), Ocular coherence tomography (OCT), Indocyanine green angiography (ICG).

Dilated fundus examination using Tropicamide 1 % and Phenyleprhine 2.5 % is diagnostic in most cases although fluorescein angiography is often necessary as confirmation of the findings, to provide evidence as to the location of the neovascular membrane and to detect the status of previously treated macular lesions.

Fluorescein angiography

This investigation is an excellent method for studying the retinal circulation.

Fluorescein is an orange water-soluble dye that binds to serum proteins in a proportion between 70 and 85 %. 5 ml of 2 % Fluorescein are injected intravenously and the transit through the retinal circulation is imaged by using a blue light (490 nm) and recording on film the green light (530 nm) emitted by fluorescein.

Side effects of Fluorescein angiography (FFA): The risks of undertaking fluorescein angiography must be assessed for every patient.

The clinical decision to proceed is made following careful history taking noting previous history of atopy or unusual reaction to the test in the past (8).

All patients should be informed about a yellow discolouration of skin and urine for the following 24 hours. About one in ten patients may experience nausea and retching. More serious complications such as anaphylaxis and collapse are much rarer accounting for less than one in 2000 cases. Death is an extremely rare complication, reported in one in 1:200 000. Staff attending the fluorescein angiography clinic should be trained in basic life support, emergency drugs and a defibrillator should be readily available.

Indocyanine Green angiography (ICG): This investigation is of particular value to study the choroidal circulation and is useful as an adjunct to fluorescein angiography in the investigation of age related macular degeneration.

The proportion of indocyanine molecules binding to serum proteins is about 98 %, producing excellent visualization of the choroidal vasculature with absence of leakage under normal conditions.

The molecules of the dye have an excitation peak and emission wavelength in the near-infrared spectrum (805 nm and 835 nm respectively).

Indocyanine (40 mg diluted in 2 ml of water for injections) is injected intravenously and serial photographs are taken using an infrared excitation light and barrier filters. ICG is a complementary test to FA used for studying abnormalities of the choroidal circulation.

Side effects of Indocyanine Green angiography: Adverse effects related to indocyanine are known to occur but the overall incidence is low. The indocyanine dye has been used for decades and the test is considered to have a high level of safety (9). Indocyanine angiography is contraindicated in patients allergic to iodine and shellfish as the preparation contains iodine 5 %.

Minor side effects have been reported in the literature and include mild nausea, pruritus and skin reactions. Rarer and more severe systemic reactions include syncope, pyrexia and skin necrosis. Patients should be informed about the staining of the stool in the 24–48 hours following the test.

Therapy

Photodynamic therapy

Photodynamic therapy with verteporfin can reduce the risk of vision loss in patients with subfoveal choroidal neovascularisation secondary to AMD. Photodynamic therapy (PDT) involves administration of verteporfin by intravenous injection and a non-thermal red light at a wavelength of 689 nm, the treatment can be repeated every three months.

Verteporfin, a benzoporphyrin derivative, is a photosensitising agent, approved for treating certain types of choroidal neovascularisation secondary to AMD.

Pharmacokinetics: Maximum concentration (Cmax) of the drug occurs at the end of the infusion and is proportional to the dose and rate of infusion. The drug is metabolized, to a small extent, to its diacid metabolite by liver and plasma esterases. Information concerning drug interactions is limited. The extent of formation of the metabolite benzoporphyrin derivative diacid (BPD-DA) is less than 10 %. Renal elimination is minimal (<0.01 % of the dose). The pharmacokinetics are bi-exponential with distribution in the first one to three hours and elimination t1/2 of five to six hours. Patients older than 65 years have a slightly higher average Cmax than patients younger than 65 years. There is no significant difference between Japanese and Caucasian individuals and between men and women. Verteporfin is rapidly eliminated in the bile, mainly as unchanged drug. Dose adjustments are not required for age, gender, race or mild hepatic or renal impairment. The drug is rapidly eliminated and reactions due to photosensitivity are unlikely after 24–48 hours (10).

Verteporfin side effects: The most frequently reported side effects (in more than 2 %) are visual disturbances, injection site reactions, photosensitivity reactions and infusion related back-pain. This may be mild to severe and may be associated with dyspnoea and precordial pain. It is probably due to high level of circulating thromboxanes induced by liposomal composition of verteporfin(12). Five per cent of patients reported deterioration of visual acuity within 7 days of treatment, with a recovery in later stages (11).

New pharmacological approaches to age-related macular degeneration: as a result of a better understanding of molecular mechanisms, a variety of new treatments have recently been developed for patients with AMD. The purpose of this section is to summarize the more recent pharmacological approaches. These may not be available in all units. In the UK they are still awaiting NICE guidance or being used off label.

Drugs targeting vascular endothelial growth factor (VEGF): Pegaptanib sodium (anti-VEGF aptamer) has been studied for nearly a decade to optimize and characterize its biological effects. It has been shown to be effective in treating choroidal neovascularisation associated with AMD. Recent studies have shown that VEGF (165) plays an important role in ocular neovascularization and vascular permeability secondary to AMD. Pegaptanib is an RNA aptamer that can selectively bind with VEGF (165) and inhibit the growth of blood vessels and vascular leakage. The drug was the first aptamer for therapeutic use in humans approved by the Food and Drug Administration in the United States for the treatment of all subtypes of neovascular AMD in December 2004. The two-year safety profile of pegaptanib sodium is favourable. The drug administered by ophthalmologists is by intravitreal injection, the doses are repeated every six weeks for 54 weeks. All doses were well tolerated in the study (13). The most common ocular adverse events were endophthalmitis, retinal detachment, and traumatic cataract. There were no reported serious systemic adverse effects associated with VEGF inhibition.

Bevacizumab (Avastin): Indications—this drug appears successful in the treatment of neovascular AMD, proliferative diabetic retinopathy and macular oedema secondary to diabetes and retinal vein occlusion. There is an emerging practice of utilizing bevacizumab for the treatment of neovascular AMD despite the lack of any phase III clinical trial data. Although the drug is still off label, it appears to be safe and produces similar outcomes to those seen with ranibizumab (see below), therefore generating considerable ethical controversy. The drug received FDA approval as an angiogenesis inhibitor in early 2005. In Europe it is currently used as first line treatment in combination with 5-FU for patients with metastatic colorectal cancer, breast cancer and lung cancer.

Dosage and administration: Bevacizumab is administered by injection of 1.25–2.5 mg into the vitreous cavity. No significant intraocular toxicity has been reported. The duration of action after intravitreal bevacizumab administration is currently unknown. Reinjections will be necessary to maintain a beneficial effect.

Contraindications: History of active of recent ocular inflammation, diagnosis of glaucoma.

The mechanism of action Bevacizumab is a humanized monoclonal antibody directed against a natural protein called vascular endothelial growth factor (VEGF) that stimulates new blood vessel formation, a process known as angiogenesis. The drug binds the VEGF receptor and blocks the growth of new vessels.

Adverse reactions: Systemic adverse reactions have been reported from its use in chemotherapy: severe allergic reactions, gastric bleeding, high blood pressure, fatigue, muscle cramps. Short-term safety and efficacy of bevacizumab has been assessed for a period of three months in a clinical trial for neovascular AMD. There are no data available with regard to long-term ocular and general safety and efficacy of the drug. There are no reported serious drug-related ocular or systemic adverse events with the doses used in ophthalmic treatment (14). Adverse events related to the intravitreal injection are possible: endophthalmitis, intraocular inflammation, increased intraocular pressure, retinal tears, retinal detachment. The observation of a possible therapeutic effect in the fellow eye raises concerns that systemic side effects are possible in patients receiving intravitreal injections (15). No clinical trials have been published to date.

Ranibizumab: Indications—this drug was approved by the FDA in June 2006 and the MHRA in January 2007 for the treatment of neovascular AMD (wet form). From clinical trials it appears that this drug maintains or improves vision in 95 % of patients treated for wet AMD at one year.

Dosage and administration: The drug is administered by intravitreal injection, two different doses have been used in trials: 0.3 mg and 0.5 mg. The actual number of injections needed will be physician directed, driven by patient's disease status and response to treatment. In one of the trials, administration was once monthly for three months, then every three months for two years, although the injections could be repeated at monthly intervals for 12 months.

Contraindications include history of active recent ocular inflammation and diagnosis of glaucoma. The drug is identified as FDA pregnancy category C, it is not known whether it passes into breast milk or if it could produce harm to a nursing baby.

Mechanism of action: Ranibizumab is an antibody fragment to Vascular Endothelial Growth Factor and derived from Bevacizumab. The molecule is designed to bind and inhibit VEGF-A, a protein playing a critical role in the formation of new blood vessels. The binding to VEGF-A prevents the interaction of VEGF-A with its receptors on the surface of endothelial cells, reducing endothelial cell proliferation, growth of new vessels and vascular leakage.

Adverse reactions: the following side effects have been reported by 6 % of patients: conjunctival haemorrhage, eye pain, vitreous floaters, increased intraocular pressure, intraocular inflammation. Serious adverse events related to the injection procedure occurred in less than 0.1 %, including endophthalmitis, retinal detachments and traumatic cataracts. Intraocular inflammation and increased intraocular pressure was observed in less than 2 % of treated patients.

Cost of ranibizumab: Each injection is expected to cost $1950. In the clinical trials that reported a gain in vision, it was used monthly for 12 months, costing $23 500 at the current selling price. In other trials the total number of injections ranged between five and seven per year.

Corticosteroids with anti-angiogenic properties

Anecortave acetate is an angiostatic agent and has been studied in randomized, placebo-controlled studies for treatment of subfoveal choroidal neovascularisation. The drug is administered as posterior juxtascleral depot under the Tenon's capsule. Each application uses a dose of 15 mg and can be repeated after a six months interval. The safety and efficacy outcomes of the study outweigh the risks associated with the drug and the injection (15). No serious adverse events related to the study drug have been reported.

Triamcinolone acetonide (4 mg intravitreally) is being used as monotherapy or combination therapy for age related macular degeneration. Reported ocular side effects are:

- Posterior subcapsular cataract formation becomes visually significant in almost half (45 %) of eyes by one year after injection and requires surgery (16).
- Increase of intraocular pressure occurs in 7–10 % of the eyes treated and the prevalence increases with repeated injections.
- Retinal detachment 1.8 %.
- Endophthalmitis 0.9 % (17).

Pharmacokinetics of Triamcinolone acetonide: The half-life of the injected amount in the vitreous appears to be 24 days for 4 mg preservative free TA and 23 days for 4 mg commercially available formulation TA (18). With regard to higher doses, 16 mg preservative free TA produced a longer vitreous half-life of 39 days. No signs of ocular toxicity were identfied. Due to limited experience there are no data available for long-term ocular or systemic adverse effects.

Key Points

- Fundoscopy is diagnostic in most cases of AMD but fluorescein angiography may be required to ascertain the best treatment of the lesion.
- If the patient is symptomatic an early referral to an Ophthalmology Department with treatment facilities should be organized.
- The condition tends to be bilateral, patients must look out for symptoms in the second eye.
- Certain types and stages of AMD are not suitable for any form of treatment and patients need adequate counselling, visual aids and social support.

- AMD does not lead to blindness, although the amount of central vision impairment can fulfil the criteria for registration as partially sighted or blind.

Guidelines

The Royal College of Ophthalmologists Guidelines "Age-related Macular Degeneration"

Verteporfin in photodynamic therapy (VIP) trial: VIP Report No. 4 *Arch Ophthalmol* 2006; **124**(17): 660–4.

Links

- Fighting Blindness, http://www.fightingblind ness.ie.
- The National Eye Institute, http://www.nei. nih.gov/health/maculardegen/armd-facts.asp.
- The Macular Disease Society, http://www. maculardisease.org.
- The Partially Sighted Society, info@part-sight.org.uk
- The Royal National Institute for the Blind, http://www.rnib.org.uk.
- Cassette library for the blind and anyone who cannot read ordinary print books, http://www.calibre.org.uk.

REFERENCES

1. Evans J. *Causes of blindness and partial sight in England and Wales 1990–1991. Studies on medical and population subjects No. 57*. London: Her Majesty's Stationery Office, 1995.
2. Khan JC, Thurlby DA, Shahid H et al. Smoking and age related macular degeneration: the number of pack years of cigarette smoking is a major determinant of risk for both geographic atrophy and choroidal neovascularisation. *Br J Ophthalmol* 2006; **90**: 75–80.
3. Hageman GS, Anderson DH, Johnson LV et al. A common haplotype in the complement regulatory gene factor H (HF1/CFH) predisposes individuals to age-related macular degeneration. *Proc Natl Acad Sci USA* 2005; **102**: 7227–32.
4. Khan JC, Shahid H, Thurlby DA et al. Age related macular degeneration and sun exposure, iris colour, and skin sensitivity to sunlight. *Br J Ophthalmol* 2006; **90**: 29–32.
5. Evans JR, Henshaw K. Antioxidant vitamin and mineral supplementation for preventing age related macular degeneration (Cochrane Review), In *The Cochrane Library*, Issue 4 1999. Oxford Update Software.
6. Fraunfelder FT, Meyer SM. Systemic reactions to ophthalmic drug preparations. *Med Toxicol Adverse Drug Exp* 1987; **2**: 287–9.
7. Resano A, Esteve C, Fernandez Benitez M. Allergic contact blepharoconjunctivitis due to phenylephrine eye drops. *J Investig Allergol Clin Immunol* 1999; **9**: 55–7.
8. Yannuzzi LA et al. Fluorescein angiography complication survey. *Ophthalmology* 1986; **93**: 611–17.
9. Hope-Ross M, Yannuzzi LA, Gragoudas ES et al. Adverse reactions due to indocyanine green. *Ophthalmology* 1994; **101**: 529–33.
10. Houle JM, Strong A. Clinical pharmacokinetics of verteporfin. *J Clin Pharmacol* 2002; **42**: 547–57.
11. Schnurrbusch UE, Jochmann C, Einbock W, Wolf S. Complications after photodynamic therapy. *Arch Ophthalmol* 2005; **123**: 1347–50.
12. Pece A, Vadala M, Manzi R, Calori G. Back pain after photodynamic therapy with verteporfin. *Am J Ophthalmol* 2006; **141**: 593–4.
13. D'Amico DJ. Pegaptanib sodium for neovascular age-related macular degeneration: two-year safety results of the two prospective, multicenter, controlled clinical trials. *Ophthalmol* 2006; **113**: 1001–6.
14. Rich RM, Rosenfeld PJ, Puliafito CA et al. Short-term safety and efficacy of intravitreal bevacizumab (avastin) for neovascular age-related macular degeneration. *Retina* 2006; **26**: 495–511.
15. D'Amico DJ. Anecortave Acetate Clinical Study Group. Anecortave acetate (15 milligrams) versus photodynamic therapy for treatment of subfoveal neovascularisation in age-relaed macular degeneration. *Ophthalmol* 2006; **113**: 3–13.
16. Thompson JT. Cataract formation and other complications of intravitreal triamcinolone for macular oedema. *Am J Ophthalmol* 2006; **141**: 629–37.
17. Konstantopoulos A, Williams CP, Newsom RS, Luff AJ. Ocular morbidity associated with intravitreal triamcinolone acetonide. *Eye* 2007; **21**(3): 317–20.

18. Kim H, Csaky KG, Gravlin L et al. Safety and pharmacokinetics of a preservative free triamcinolone acetonide formulation for intravitreal administration. *Retina* 2006; **26**: 523–30.

DIABETIC RETINOPATHY

Introduction

Diabetic retinopathy is the commonest cause of visual impairment in people of working age in the developed world and its prevalence is increasing in the developing nations (1).

The prevalence of retinopathy increases with the duration of diabetes and therefore its screening and management are particularly important in the elderly population. Epidemiological studies show that in patients with juvenile onset insulin dependent diabetes (Type I) the prevalence of retinopathy is minimal at 5 years from diagnosis but increases to 95 % 15 years from the diagnosis (2), (3), (4). In maturity onset, non-insulin dependent diabetes (NIDDM, Type II), up to 38 % of patients have signs of retinopathy at presentation, as from the UK Prospective Diabetes Survey (UKPDS) (5).

It is estimated that 8 % of blind registrations are secondary to the effects of diabetic retinopathy, this proportion of blind people represents a cost to society and could be prevented by early diagnosis and treatment, regular screening and control of collateral risk factors like smoking, high blood pressure, cholesterol, and weight loss (7).

The course of the disease is well known and population based screening programmes and early treatment have been effective in slowing down disease progression and preventing irreversible blindness (6–10).

The rate of sight threatening complications due to diabetic retinopathy is much higher in young patients although the overall proportion of visually impaired people is larger in elderly diabetics, due to the larger number of patients with NIDDM and as a result of a long period of undiagnosed and often asymptomatic hyperglycaemia in middle aged and elderly diabetic patients.

Aetiology

Diabetes mellitus is a disorder of glucose metabolism resulting from diminished availability or effectiveness of insulin, resulting in an increase in blood glucose concentration and damage to various tissues: large and small vessels, kidneys, neuromuscular junctions, eyes, skin and the immune system with an increased susceptibility to infections.

Symptoms and Signs

Diabetic retinopathy (DR) is classified as:

- Non proliferative diabetic retinopathy (NPDR) then graded depending on its severity into mild, moderate, severe or pre-proliferative and very severe or pre-proliferative.
- Proliferative diabetic retinopathy (PDR) is classified depending on the location of the new vessels into neovascularisation on the disc (NVD) and/or neovascularisation elsewhere (NVE).
- Diabetic maculopathy may coexist or be a separate entity and is classified as diffuse or focal maculopathy, ischaemic or non-ischaemic.

Diagnosis

Clinical examination includes measurement of visual acuity, intraocular pressure, slit-lamp biomicroscopy with iris and angle (gonioscopy) examination, dilated fundus exam of the posterior pole and peripheral retina and vitreous and fundus fluorescein angiography where necessary.

Therapy

Argon Laser Photocoagulation

Laser photocoagulation is a form of therapy based on the absorption of light energy by ocular pigments, its conversion to heat and the production of a retinal burn. In the treatment of diabetic retinopathy the aim of laser photocoagulation is to stop vascular leakage and to arrest neovascularisation (11).

Modalities of treatment:

- Focal treatment of microaneurysms and microvascular lesions in diabetic maculopathy.
- Grid treatment for diffuse macular oedema.
- Panretinal laser Photocoagulation (PRP) for proliferative diabetic retinopathy.

Delivery systems:

- Slit lamp delivery using a contact lens.
- Indirect ophthalmoscope: portable system used with the patient lying on a couch, can be used if the patient is unable to sit up, during general anaesthesia in theatre, when visualisation of the peripheral retina is necessary.
- Intraocular delivery is used during vitreoretinal procedures and delivered by fibre-optic probes.

Preparation of patients for Argon Laser Photocoagulation

All patients for retinal laser treatment need dilating drops and topical or local anaesthesia (12), (13). The procedure, the underlying benefits and risks of treatment should be carefully explained. Patients must be aware of risks of delaying treatments as well as the benefit of regular follow-up.

Multiple treatments may be needed and the effect of treatment is not immediately manifest to the patient. The aim of laser treatment in diabetic retinopathy is to prevent vision loss that may occur as a result of the changes at the level of the retinal vessels.

Pupillary dilatation

In elderly diabetic patients the administration of dilating drops (phenylephrine 2,5 % or 10 %, tropicamide 1 %) may need to be repeated every 10 minutes because of iris neuropathy causing slow dilatation.

Key Points

- Patients' education regarding the importance of:

  - maintaining near-normal glycaemic level
  - maintaining near-normal blood pressure level
  - lowering serum lipid level.
  - stopping smoking
  - reducing heavy alcohol consumption
  - avoiding rapid changes in blood glucose level
- Warning patients about possible temporary worsening of the retinopathy as a consequence of an improved control of the glycemia.
- Asymptomatic patients with diabetes mellitus and good visual acuity should be educated and motivated to maintain their annual dilated ocular examination to detect early signs of progression of diabetic retinopathy
- Prevention of visual loss depends on early diagnosis, early intervention and regular follow-up.
- Patients with visual impairment should be offered referral to low vision aid clinic, vision rehabilitation and social services.

Guidelines

- American Academy of Ophthalmology Retina Panel, Preferred Practice Patterns Committee. Diabetic Retinopathy. San Francisco (CA): American Academy of Ophthalmology (AAO); 2003.33p.
- The Royal College of Ophthalmologists, "Guidelines for Diabetic Retinopathy 2005", http://www.rcophth.ac.uk/docs/scientific/DiabeticRetinopathyGuidelines2005.pdf.
- UKPDS: United Kingdom Prospective Diabetes Study, *Annals of Internal Medicine* 1996; **124**: 136–45.
- DCCT: Diabetes Control and Complication Trial, http://diabetes.niddk.nih.gov/dm/pubs/control/.
- ETDRS: Early Treatment Diabetic Retinopathy Study, http://www.nei.nih.gov/neitrials/viewStudyWeb.aspx?id = 53.

Links

- Royal National Institute for the Blind: http://www.rnib.org.uk, "Understanding diabetes related eye conditions".

- American Diabetes Association: http://www. diabetes.org/type-1-diabetes/eye-complications.jsp.
- National Eye Institute: "Information for people with diabetes" http://www.nei.nih.gov/health/diabetic/ded_risk.asp.
- Driver and Vehicle Licensing Agency: http://www.dvla.gov.uk/.

REFERENCES

1. Evans J. *Causes of Blindness and Partial Sight in England and Wales 1990–1991*. HMSO, 1995.
2. Sparrow JM, McLeod BK, Smith TD, Birch MK, Rosenthal AR. The prevalence of diabetic retinopathy and maculopathy and their risk factors in the non-insulin-treated diabetic patients of an English town. *Eye* 1993; **7**: 158–63.
3. Klein R, Klein BEK, Moss SE: The Wisconsin epidemiologic study: II Prevalence and risk of diabetic retinopathy when age at diagnosis is less than thirty years. *Archives of Ophthalmology* 1984; **102**: 520–6.
4. Klein R, Klein BEK, Moss SE: The Wisconsin epidemiologic study: II Prevalence and risk of diabetic retinopathy when age at diagnosis is thirty or more years. *Archives of Ophthalmology* 1984: **102**: 527–33.
5. Early Treatment Diabetic Retinopathy Study Research Group. Photocoagulation for Diabetic Macular Edema. ETDRS Report No. 1. *Arch Ophthalmol* 1985; **103**: 1796–1806.
6. Burnett S, Hurwitz B, Davey C, Ray J, Chaturvedy N, Salzmann J et al. The implementation of prompted retinal screening for diabetic eye disease by accredited optometrists in an inner-city district of North London: a quality of care study. *Diabet Med* 1998; **15**: 538–43.
7. O'Hare JP, Hopper A Madhaven C, Chamy M, Purewal TS, Harney B et al. Adding retinal photography to screening for diabetic retinopathy: a prospective study in primary care. *Br Med J* 1996; **312**: 679–82.
8. Garvican L, Clowes J, Gillow T. Preservation of sight in diabetes: developing a national risk reduction programme. *Diabet Med* 2000; **17**: 627–34.
9. Ryder REJ, Close CF, Krentz AJ, Gray MD, Souten H, Taylor KG et al. A "fail-safe" screening programme for diabetic retonopathy. *J Royal Coll Physicians London* 1998; **32**: 134–137.
10. Diabetic retinopathy Study Research Group. Photocoagulation treatment of Proliferative Diabetic Retinopathy, Clinical application of Diabetic Retinopathy Study Findings, DRS Report No. 8, *Ophthalmology* 1981; **88**: 583–600.
11. Hay A, Flynn HW Jr, Hoffman JI, Rivera AH. Needle penetration of the globe during retrobulbar and peribulbar injections. *Ophthalmology* 1991; **98**: 1017–24.
12. Budd J, Hardwick M, Barber K, Prosser J. A single-centre study of 1000 consecutive peribulbar blocks. *Eye* 2001; **15**: 439–40.
13. Resano A, Esteve C, Fernandez Benitez M. Allergic contact blepharoconjunctivitis due to phenylephrine eye drops. *J Investig Allergol Clin Immunol* 1999; **9**: 55–7.

44 Ear disorders

Wynia Derks[1] and Gerrit Hordijk[2]

[1]Department of Ear, Nose, Throat, Onze Lieve Vrouwe Gasthuis, Amsterdam,
The Netherlands
[2]Department of Ear, Nose, Throat, University Medical Centre, Utrecht,
The Netherlands

INTRODUCTION

Ear disorders are very common in the elderly population and are of debilitating potential. Therefore, special care and attention is pivotal for this age-group. An ordinary but frequent problem relates to age-associated changes in cerumen, which becomes hard and dry and can block the ear canal more easily. External otitis is another infirmity of old age. Several cleaning methods and therapeutic options will be discussed in this chapter. Most importantly, more than half of the elderly suffers from presbyacusis and they are at great risk of becoming isolated, therefore, it is imperative to recognize hearing loss and prescribe hearing aids promptly. To prevent additional cochlear damage one must recognize the dangers of ototoxic medication, which is frequently prescribed in later life. Tinnitus is more widespread in the elderly population. Knowledge on this condition is necessary to reassure patients. In this chapter the symptoms, causes, and therapy of these ear disorders are portrayed.

HEARING LOSS

Hearing loss can be divided into three different types, based on the components of the auditory system affected. Conductive hearing loss is caused by inadequate functioning of the ear canal, tympanic membrane, or ossicular chain, so that sound is not transmitted into the inner ear. The most common cause of conductive deafness in older people is cerumen impaction; other causes include fluid in the middle ear, middle ear infection, choleasteatoma, and ossicular chain problems. Sensorineural hearing loss is caused by dysfunction of the cochlea or auditory nerve. The most common form of this type of hearing loss is presbyacusis. Mixed hearing loss is a combination of conductive and sensorineural hearing loss.

Cerumen impaction

Symptoms and diagnosis

Deafness occurs only when the external auditory canal is completely blocked. Other symptoms are itching, tinnitus and a sensation of fullness in the ear. Cerumen can easily be detected by inspection of the ear with an otoscope.

Causes

With aging the apocrine glands of the ear canal skin become atrophic, producing less of the watery component of cerumen, which becomes drier and harder. This less-fluid cerumen migrates more slowly within the ear canal. (10) In addition, especially in men, the tragic hairs in the ear canal become longer, thicker and coarser with age and trap dry cerumen more easily. The introduction and pressure of the earmold of a hearing aid may also contribute to cerumen accumulation.

Prescribing for Elderly Patients   Edited by Stephen Jackson, Paul Jansen and Arduino Mangoni
© 2009 John Wiley & Sons, Ltd

Therapy

Cerumenolytics

Wax-softening agents are often used to disperse the cerumen and reduce the need for syringing, or to facilitate it. Many substances can be used, such as water, saline, diluted table vinegar, baby or olive oil, and various special pharmaceutical ear drops; however, these products should be avoided if the status of the tympanic membrane is unknown. There is no consensus on the effectiveness of the various cerumenolytics in use, and the poor quality of clinical trials performed to date makes it difficult to offer definitive recommendations regarding effective cerumenolytics (1, 5).

Lavage

The efficacy of lavage for cerumen removal has not been investigated. Syringing is easily and direct visualization of the ear canal is not necessary. The ear should be irrigated with water at body temperature and the ear canal straightened by pulling up on the auricle. The tip of the syringe should not be placed past the lateral one-third of the ear canal. Direct otoscopy needs to be performed after lavage, in order to evaluate the success of the procedure. Before syringing, perforation of the tympanic membrane must be excluded by a careful history. If the tympanic membrane is perforated, an otolaryngologist should remove the wax manually. Hard wax can be softened first with a cerumenolytic. Local steroid or antibiotic eardrops can be prescribed if there is inflammation of the meatus.

Suction, cerumen spoons, etc

Suction tools, cerumen spoons, and curettes should be used only under direct visualization to prevent injury to the ear drum.

If any of the above-mentioned methods prove ineffective, the patient should be referred to an otolaryngologist.

Presbyacusis

Presbyacusis is a progressive, age-associated sensorineural hearing loss. Presbyacusis is very common in people older than 55 years, affecting a third of people between 65 and 75 years and up to a half of people older than 75 (4, 8). Because the loss of hearing is gradual, people with presbyacusis may not realize that their hearing is impaired.

Causes

The pathological basis for presbyacusis appears to be the gradual devascularization of the cochlea and the loss of functional hair cells. Secondary to hair cell loss, there may be progressive neuronal dropout along the cochlear nerve. Histopathological changes are most pronounced in the basal turn of the cochlea, where the high-frequencies are percepted (8, 12). Although the main cause of presbyacusis is aging, other factors should be considered. A genetic predisposition, ototoxic medication, a history of middle ear infections and exposure to noise in earlier life will hasten the onset of noticeable hearing loss.

Symptoms

Presbyacusis typically results in bilateral high-frequency hearing loss, which makes it difficult for affected individuals to understand speech. The loss is particularly disabling as most consonants are in the high frequency range, and people first experience difficulty in understanding women and children due to the high pitch of their voices. While affected individuals can usually cope with conversation on a one-to-one basis in quiet surroundings, in crowded rooms their limited high-frequency perception is overwhelmed by the barrage of low-frequency sound. As hearing further deteriorates the ability to understand speech becomes more severely affected. Discrimination loss occurs; even with sufficiently loud speech, 100 % comprehension can no longer be achieved, and even louder speech leads to poorer comprehension. A common phenomenon associated with presbyacusis is recruitment. The threshold of hearing increases as hearing declines, but the pain threshold remains the same, resulting in a much narrower dynamic range of hearing.

With this type of hearing loss it is easy to misinterpret what is being said, which may erode a person's self-confidence. Affected individuals may avoid socializing and risk becoming isolated and depressed.

Diagnosis

Otoscopy shows no abnormalities. The Weber and Rinne tuning fork tests help to distinguish between conductive and sensorineural hearing loss. The hearing impairment can be detected in the physician's office by means of a whispered voice test. The physician should stand an arm's length behind the patient and mask hearing in one ear by occluding the ear canal and rubbing the tragus with a circular motion. He of she should whisper a short sentence and ask the patient to repeat it. A systematic review of this technique showed a sensitivity for hearing impairment of 90–100 %, and a specificity of 70–87 % (13).

If hearing loss is suspected, audiologic assessment in a soundproof environment is obligatory. The severity of a patient's hearing loss is determined by audiometry. Audiograms provide a measurement of hearing thresholds for pure tones at frequencies of 250, 500, 1000, 2000, 4000 and 8000 hertz (Hz). The most important frequencies for understanding speech are 500–1000–2000 Hz. Pure tone average is the average of the hearing thresholds at these frequencies. The normal range for adult pure tone average is 0 to 25 dB. Normal conversational speech occurs at 40 to 60 dB. The ability to understand speech is more important than the ability to hear pure tones. Speech audiometry is carried out using uniform test material consisting of monosyllabic words.

Treatment

A hearing aid is indicated when the average hearing loss in the main speech frequencies exceeds 35 dB. Hearing aids can be adjusted so that the amplification varies depending on the frequency and intensity of the sound. To avoid disappointment, patients must realize that hearing aids cannot restore the user's hearing ability to normal. Results may be disappointing if there is a large loss in discrimination. It should be stressed that it does take time to get used to wearing a hearing aid; however, most people do get used to them and find them of great benefit. Therefore it is better not to wait too long with prescribing a hearing aid.

Hearing aids can be placed completely in the canal, in the ear, or behind the ear. Individuals with severe hearing loss who require a great deal of amplification and power should use 'behind the ear' hearing aids, which have the largest power sources. These hearing aids also have larger dials and controls, which make them easier to use by older people. Other hearing devices include loop systems, TV listening devices, amplified telephones, telephones that use text instead of sound, and flashing or vibrating alarm clocks and doorbells.

TINNITUS

Tinnitus is the awareness of sound that does not originate from an external source. Tinnitus is one of the most widespread disorders of the auditory system, affecting approximately 17 % of the general population with the frequency increasing to about 33 % in the elderly (15). Most people with tinnitus are not bothered by its presence and only about one fourth are annoyed to the extent that they actively seek help. Quality of life can be severely impaired by the psychological effects of tinnitus.

Causes

Tinnitus is commonly divided into two categories, sounds generated by para-auditory structures and sounds generated within the auditory pathway (otogenic). Tinnitus generated by sound sources external to the auditory system is theoretically audible to a listener. The sounds can be caused by vascular abnormalities or mechanical disorders. Vascular sounds are characterized by rhythmic pulsations that are coincident with the heartbeat (caused by hypertension, glomus jugulare, carotid stenosis, dehiscent jugular bulb, AV-malformations, or an aberrant vascular loop compressing the auditory nerve). Mechanical sounds can result from an abnormally patent Eustachian tube, palatal or stapecial muscle myoclonus (caused by multiple sclerosis, CVA, or intracranial neoplasms), or temporomandibular joint disorder. However, tinnitus generated by para-auditory structures, is rare, accounting for only 4% of all cases. The vast majority of tinnitus cases are subjective and only perceived by the patient (11).

Tinnitus of otogenic origin can be caused by ear wax or middle ear disorders such as middle ear effusion or otosclerosis. However, most elderly patients with tinnitus also have hearing loss at the cochlear level due to, for example, presbyacusis, noise-induced hearing loss, or Meniere's disease. Ototoxic drugs, (e.g. aminoglycoside antibiotics, loop diuretics, non-steroidal anti-inflammatory drugs, chemotherapeutic agents) may cause tinnitus. Sometimes tinnitus occurs after accidental or surgical trauma to the inner ear. Tinnitus can also be generated in the neural pathway. Little is known about the underlying physiological mechanisms that cause sensorineural tinnitus, but the latest pathogenetic theories target the central nervous system as the 'generator' of tinnitus, even in patients whose associated hearing loss is due to cochlear injury (7). The loss of input to neurons in the central auditory pathways can result in abnormal firing, thereby leading to the perception of tinnitus. The tone of the tinnitus often corresponds with the frequency of the hearing loss, and the perceived loudness is usually 0 to 20 dB above the hearing threshold.

Symptoms

Tinnitus can be constant or intermittent and is located unilaterally, bilaterally or generally in the head. A high-pitched continuous tone is the most commonly described type of tinnitus and is frequently a result of sensorineural hearing loss. Low-pitched tinnitus is often described in patients with Meniere's disease. An open Eustachian tube can cause sounds similar to ocean roar that may be synchronous with respiration. Tinnitus that is distinctly pulsing or described as rushing, flowing, or humming is usually vascular in origin and often increases in frequency and intensity with exercise. A rhythmic, clicking noise indicates myoclonus of the palatal muscles or middle ear structures.

Patients should be asked about previous ear disease, noise exposure, hearing status, and medication use. They should also be asked if they have experienced depression, anxiety and insomnia, conditions that can worsen the impact of tinnitus.

Otoscopic examination is necessary to exclude external and middle ear pathology and audiometric tests of both bone and air conduction should be performed. Tinnitus of non-otogenous origin may be heard by auscultation around the ear and neck, and a complete head and neck examination including the cervical spine and temporomandibular joint is required. If the tinnitus seems to be of vascular origin, angiography or MRA should be performed. In patients with an asymmetry in hearing function, imaging studies such as MRI are necessary to rule out neoplasms.

Treatment

Tinnitus associated with external canal disorders (e.g., external otitis, cerumen impaction) and middle ear space processes (e.g., otitis media and otosclerosis) often resolves after treatment of the underlying condition. If possible, all tinnitus-producing medications, such as aminoglycoside antibiotics, high-dose loop diuretics and non-steroidal anti-inflammatory drugs should be discontinued. If no modifiable factors are identified, patients should be reassured and told that they do not have a serious life-threatening condition. Special attention should be paid to stress, anxiety and depressive symptoms because these factors can exacerbate tinnitus.

A wide variety of pharmacological and complementary strategies have been tried, including antidepressants, neuromodulators (gabapentin), dietary supplements (B vitamins and zinc), herbal medications (ginkgo biloba), homeopathy, aromatherapy, craniosacral therapy, chiropractic manipulation, low-dose laser, ultraquiet ultrasonic therapy and low-dose electrical stimulation. No therapy is predictably associated with a cure or sustained tinnitus relief. Cognitive therapy, tinnitus-retraining therapy, and biofeedback have proven beneficial in some individuals, but definitive studies are lacking. Most studies performed so far have an inadequate design, have not been replicated, or yielded contradictory results and significant placebo effects. Additionally, these trials are hampered by the inability to measure tinnitus objectively. A review of 69 randomized clinical trials comparing drug and non-drug treatments showed that no treatment provided a long-term reduction of tinnitus in excess of the effect of placebo. Non-specific support and counselling may be helpful, and tricyclic antidepressants may be useful in severe cases (2, 11).

Surgery for subjective tinnitus is not recommended, though some cochlear implant recipients experience tinnitus relief. A preliminary study of direct neurostimulation of the cochlear nerve, by implanting an intracerebral electrode, has been performed, the results are promising (6).

If the patient suffers from hearing loss, a hearing aid can be used to introduce masking simply by amplifying environmental noise. A special tinnitus masking device can be used which delivers a constant or varied signal at a specified frequency. Overall, masking devices may improve tinnitus in only 10–15 % of patients (11).

EXTERNAL OTITIS

Causes

Anatomical and biochemical changes associated with ageing reduce the elasticity of the meatal skin and lead to atrophy of the ceruminous and sebaceous glands. This causes drying of the meatal skin, disturbance of its chemical balance, and increased susceptibility to bacterial or fungal infection. Shampoo and water exacerbate skin dryness and excessive cleaning or vigorous manipulations make it worse by removing the protective cerumen and by creating abrasions in the thin skin of the ear canal, which allow organisms to gain access to deeper

tissue. Hearing aids that occlude the ear canal also predispose their users to external otitis.

Symptoms and diagnosis

External otitis is inflammation, often with infection, of the external auditory canal. External otitis has acute (less than six weeks), chronic (longer than three months), and necrotizing (malignant) forms. Acute external otitis is very painful and may present as a single episode, or recur. The external auditory meatus is red and swollen and usually filled with fetid debris. Symptoms are otalgia, pruritus, discharge, and hearing loss. The most common organisms responsible for external otitis are *Staphylococcus aureus* and *Pseudomonas aeruginosa*.

In chronic external otitis the meatus becomes wider, the epithelial lining is atrophic, and dry scales of epidermis accumulate. There is intense itching, which causes the patient to scratch his external ear vigorously. In turn, this may cause damage and promotes the development of a superinfection.

Severe necrotizing inflammation can develop from external otitis, especially in older people with diabetes. The infection is generally caused by anaerobic gram-negative organisms, usually *Pseudomonas aeruginosa*. Necrotizing (malignant) external otitis is characterized by osteomyelitis and destruction of the temporal bone. It can be life-threatening.

Treatment

Avoidance

Patients should be told to avoid getting water in the ear and to resist scratching/itching their ear.

Cleaning

Cleaning the ear is the single most important aspect of treatment. The removal of desquamated skin and purulent material facilitates healing and improves the penetration of ear drops. Primary care practitioners can clean the ear canal with a cerumen wire loop or cotton swab to gently remove debris. There is a risk of pushing debris further, instead of removing it from the external meatus. The ear canal can also be irrigated with half strength hydrogen peroxide (1.5 %) if the tympanic membrane is intact. Otolaryngologists clean the ears under the binocular magnified vision of a microscope.

Topical agents

Numerous topical agents have been used to treat external otitis, including acidifying solutions, antiseptics, antibiotics, and anti-inflammatory drugs. Antiseptics (alcohol, gentian violet, m-resyl acetate, thymol) function as bacteriostatic agents. Although their precise mechanism is not fully understood, they render the ear canal less habitable for bacteria and provide mechanical debridement.

Acidifying solutions such as acetic acid, aluminium acetate, hydrochloric acid, etc. inhibit bacterial growth by lowering the pH. Mild acute otitis externa can be treated by cleaning of the ear canal and applying drops containing acetic acid for up to three days after symptoms have resolved (typically five to seven days total).

The addition of topical steroids to the acetic solution decreases inflammation, resulting in decreased pain and relief of pruritus. In a randomized trial of 213 adults, patients treated with acetic acid drops alone had a lower cure rate and longer duration of symptoms than patients treated with acetic acid plus steroid drops (17). Several prospective randomized studies have found similar cure rates among patients treated with steroid drops with or without antibiotics (3, 14, 16, 17). For this reason, non-antibiotic topical agents should be used in primary care settings.

Topical antibiotics with or without steroids are available in various formulations. Polymyxin and neomycin are often used in combination in ear drops. Neomycin is effective against *S. aureus* and polymyxin is effective against *P. aeruginosa*. Neomycin-induced contact dermatitis occurs in an estimated 5 % of recipients. Aminoglycoside antibiotics can be ototoxic. Ciprofloxacin and ofloxacin provide excellent bacterial coverage against *S. aureus* and *P. aeruginosa* and are less ototoxic.

However, the tendency for rapid development of resistance to quinolone antibiotics should temper enthusiasm for their use in the primary care setting.

In severe acute otitis externa, the ear canal may be so swollen that it is necessary to use a wick, which acts as a vehicle for the drops and can draw inflammatory fluid from the ear canal. The wick is removed 24 to 72 hours later and the ear is reinspected and cleaned.

In chronic otitis externa, the debris should be removed gently and steroid cream applied.

Systemic antibiotics

Systemic antibiotics are recommended for severe otitis externa. Necrotizing (malignant) external otitis requires long (weeks to months), and intensive antibiotic treatment and extensive surgery is often needed. The prognosis is poor.

Painkillers

The pain caused by otitis externa can be severe. Adequate pain medication is required.

DRUGS CAUSING HEARING PROBLEMS

Ototoxicity is defined as drug-induced damage to the inner ear, resulting in hearing loss, tinnitus and/or vertigo. Ototoxic medication is frequently prescribed in later life; moreover, the decline in renal function that occurs with advancing age leads to a decreased clearance of these drugs, increasing the risk of cochlear damage. Toxic substances can be delivered systemically or topically through perforations/ventilation tubes in the ear drum. The ototoxicity of a drug depends on the drug used, its dose, the patient's renal function, and other conditions. In some cases, there is full recovery after the drug has been discontinued. Ototoxicity begins in the ultra high frequencies (>8000 Hz) and sometimes goes undiagnosed initially when the hearing loss is slight and restricted to the higher frequencies.

Causes

At least 96 different agents have potential oto-toxic side effects (9). Among these, aminogly-coside antibiotics are perhaps the most common offending agents. This group of antibiotics includes streptomycin, neomycin, gentamicin and tobramycin. Hearing toxicity generally in-volves the high frequencies first. The hearing loss may by unilateral or asymmetric and can progress after cessation of therapy. Vestibulo-toxicity often occurs. Well-defined risk factors for aminoglycoside-induced hearing loss in-clude renal disease, longer duration of therapy, increased serum levels, advanced age, and con-comitant administration of other ototoxic drugs, particularly loop diuretics. Careful and regular monitoring of auditory function (especially in the ultra high frequencies) and serum antibiotic levels may help the physician identify ototoxi-city. Vancomycin has been associated with oto-toxicity when administered intravenously but not when given orally.

Neomycin-, gentamycin-, and tobramy-cin-containing topical preparations have long been used directly in the ear for the treatment of external otitis and chronic otitis media. The reduced permeability of the inflamed membranes of the round and oval windows, dilution of the toxic drugs by purulent fluids, and increased absorption into the vascular system by the hyperaemic mucosa probably account for the decreased toxicity of these drugs in the presence of otitis media. The use of these drops should be discontinued when the ear becomes dry.

Many elderly patients are on diuretics. Loop diuretics, such as, furosemide, acetazolamide, and bumetanide, are ototoxic, especially when prescribed in high doses. The diuretics may cause a hearing loss with a rapid onset; some-times vestibulotoxicity occurs. The hearing loss will usually, but not always, reverse itself when the drugs are stopped.

Aspirin and less often the non-steroidal anti-inflammatory drugs may cause tinnitus and sensorineural hearing loss. The hearing loss is dose dependent. On discontinuation of the drug, hearing usually, but not always, returns to normal and tinnitus disappears.

Platinum-based chemotherapeutic drugs in particular are well documented as causing dose-dependent sensorineural hearing loss. The hearing loss initially is worse at high frequen-cies, bilateral, and irreversible. It occasionally is accompanied by tinnitus and vertigo.

A number of other drugs, such as the an-timalarial drugs quinine and chloroquine may also cause ototoxicity.

Therapy

There are no current treatments to reverse the effects of ototoxicity. Since most ototoxicity occurs when the harmful drugs are used in high doses, careful dose calculations are the best method of prevention. Sometimes it is possible to replace the ototoxic drug with a drug with less-severe adverse effects. People who suffer permanent hearing loss may elect to use hearing aids; people with balance problems may require physical therapy.

REFERENCES

1. Burton, MJ, Doree, CJ Ear drops for the re-moval of ear wax. *Cochrane.Database.Syst.Rev* 2003; No. 3, p. CD004400.
2. Dobie, RA A review of randomized clinical trials in tinnitus *Laryngoscope* 1999; **109**(8): 1202–11.
3. Emgard, P, Hellstrom, S A group III steroid solution without antibiotic components: an ef-fective cure for external otitis *J Laryngol Otol* 2005; **119**(5): 342–7.
4. Gratton, MA, Vazquez, AE Age-related hearing loss: current research *Curr Opin Otolaryngol Head Neck Surg* 2003; **11**(5): 367–71.
5. Hand, C, Harvey, I The effectiveness of topical preparations for the treatment of earwax: a sys-tematic review *Br J Gen Pract* 2004; **54**(508): 862–7.
6. Holm, AF, Staal, MJ, Mooij, JJ, Albers, FW Neurostimulation as a new treatment for se-vere tinnitus: a pilot study *Otol Neurotol* 2005; **26**(3): 425–8.
7. Lockwood, AH, Salvi, RJ, Burkard, RF, Galan-towicz, PJ, Coad, ML, Wack, DS Neuroanatomy of tinnitus *Scand Audiol Suppl* 1999; **51**: 47–52.
8. Marcincuk, MC, Roland, PS Geriatric hearing loss. Understanding the causes and providing

appropriate treatment *Geriatrics* 2002; **57**(4): 44, 48–6.

9. Matz, G.J. Clinical perspectives on ototoxic drugs *Ann Otol Rhinol Laryngol Suppl* 1990; **148**: 39–41.

10. Meador, JA. Cerumen impaction in the elderly *J Geronto.Nurs* 1995; **21**(12): 43–5.

11. Noell, CA, Meyerhoff, W L Tinnitus. Diagnosis and treatment of this elusive symptom *Geriatrics* 2003; **58**(2): 28–34.

12. Ohlemiller, KK Age-related hearing loss: the status of Schuknecht's typology *Curr Opin Otolaryngol Head Neck Surg.* 2004; **12**(5): 439–43.

13. Pirozzo, Papinczak, Glasziou, P Whispered voice test for screening for hearing impairment in adults and children: systematic review *BMJ* 2003; **327**(7421): 967.

14. Ruth, M, Ekstrom, T, Aberg, B, Edstrom, S A clinical comparison of hydrocortisone butyrate with oxytetracycline/hydrocortisone acetate-polymyxin B in the local treatment of acute external otitis *Eur Arch Otorhinolaryngol* 1990; **247**(2): 77–80.

15. Sataloff, J, Sataloff, RT, Lueneburg, W Tinnitus and vertigo in healthy senior citizens without a history of noise exposure *Am.Otol* 1987; **8**(2): 87–9.

16. Tsikoudas, A, Jasser, P, England, RJ Are topical antibiotics necessary in the management of otitis externa? *Clin Otolaryngo.Allied Sci.* 2002; **27**(4): 260–2.

17. van Balen, FA, Smit, WM, Zuithoff, NP, Verheij, TJ Clinical efficacy of three common treatments in acute otitis externa in primary care: randomised controlled trial *BMJ* 2003; **327**(7425): 1201–5.

45 Pain

Albert J.M. van Wijck

University Medical Center, Utrecht, The Netherlands

INTRODUCTION

Pain is a common problem in the elderly. The prevalence is estimated to be at least 40 % in the general population, increasing to 80 % in nursing homes (1–3). Often, pain is unrecognized, misdiagnosed and untreated. Pain has a high impact on quality of life and affects physical, cognitive and social functioning. Pain induces distress, sadness, fear, depression and loss of control. Due to co-morbidity, drug interactions and increased sensitivity for side-effects of analgesic drugs pharmacologic treatment of pain can be difficult and disappointing. Therefore, attention should be given to the psycho-social aspect of pain. Concomitant psychiatric disorders such as depression must be treated at the same time.

AETIOLOGY

With ageing, the prevalence of pain increases due to age related painful conditions such as osteoarthritis. By general deterioration of health, pain often occurs due to e.g. pressure sores, contractures or constipation. Improvements in the management of cancer increase life expectancy, but are accompanied by a rise in the incidence of tumour-related pain syndromes such as radiation-induced neuropathy. Although the word "pain" is used to describe any feeling that is unpleasant and hurts, this does not mean that pain is a monolithic entity. Pain normally serves as an alarm system activated in response to actual or impending damage to the organism. Once the alarm has gone off, pain dominates the attention over other sensations and motivational drive. The threshold for eliciting pain has to be high enough that it does not interfere with normal activities but low enough that it can be evoked before frank tissue damage occurs. This threshold is not fixed and can be shifted either up or down, which may be adaptive ore maladaptive. The pain threshold may be decreased by emotions such as fear, depression, and decline.

Nociceptive pain is associated with actual or potential tissue damage. Once tissue has been damaged mechanically, physically, by infection, ischemia or tumour growth, multiple chemical mediators are released. The resulting 'inflammatory soup' is rich in cytokines, kinins, growth factors, purines and amines such as substance P. Some inflammatory mediators directly activate free nerve endings, the nociceptors. Others mediators produce sensitisation of the nervous system, which is characteristic for **inflammatory pain**, enabling easier activation of the pain pathway until the tissue heals. **Visceral pain** originates in the internal organs such as bowel, kidney and the heart. The autonomous nervous system plays a role in the pain pathway of visceral pain. **Somatic pain** originates from the bones, muscles or skin.

Neuropathic pain can be the consequence of damage to the central or peripheral nervous system. Examples are postherpetic neuralgia, trigeminal neuralgia, painful diabetic

Prescribing for Elderly Patients Edited by Stephen Jackson, Paul Jansen and Arduino Mangoni
© 2009 John Wiley & Sons, Ltd

neuropathy and phantom limb pain. Neuropathic painis much more difficult to treat than nociceptive pain and requires other drugs.

DIAGNOSIS

Before the start of treatment, a proper diagnosis should be made. Pain can be a symptom of an underlying disease. However, chronic pain can be a disease on its own. Is the pain nociceptive, neuropathic or both? History and physical examination are the most important tools for diagnosing pain. It is essential to obtain a detailed description of the location and distribution of the pain, quality of the pain, severity or intensity of the pain and periodicity and duration of the pain and the affective concomitants of pain. Superficial somatic pain is well localized, but pain arising from visceral structures can be referred remotely or localized with difficulty. Pain with a segmental distribution can arise from dysfunction of nerve roots. The quality of pain is a most important distinguishing characteristic because it indicates whether the causative factor is superficial or deep and nociceptive of neuropathic. Pain associated with superficial nociception is usual sharp whereas pain caused by deep somatic or visceral disease is dull, diffuse and poorly localizable. Burning or electric pain indicate neuropathy, as well as sensory abnormalities such as paresthesia, hypesthesia and allodynia. The severity of pain is perhaps the most difficult aspect of pain to evaluate because it cannot be measured precisely and objectively. In general, pain can be rated on a scale from 0 to 10, 0 being no pain and 10 being the most severe pain imaginable. The simplest approach is to use a verbal numeric scale (NRS), but a visual analogue scale, on which the patient marks a 100 mm line, is preferred by many. However, in the elderly the assessment of pain can be more time consuming than in younger adults. Avoid time pressure and adapt the instruments in patients with impairments in hearing, vision, dexterity, comprehension or articulation. Especially in patients with cognitive dysfunction, assessment of the intensity of pain by self report is not always possible. Measurement of pain intensity then depends more on observation of facial expression and other pain related behaviour. For this purpose, several rating scales have been developed. Elderly patients may be less inclined to acknowledge pain due to several reasons. (a) a belief that pain is normal and must be lived with as one ages (b) fear that pain may forebode serious illness or death (c) unfamiliarity with what others may consider common terms in pain language (d) concern that pain complaints will be dismissed as elderly hypochondriasis (e) concern that complaining may lead to people avoiding them (f) stoicism. However, pain perception does not decrease with age.

THERAPY

For the oral analgetic drugs see Table 45.1. Topical drugs are only applicable if a small area of the skin is involved. Capsaicin 0.025 % q6h induces depletion of substance P in sensitized free nerve endings. Pain may increase during first two weeks of application. Lignocaine 5 % cremor or patch in case of postherpetic neuralgia.

Treatment of pain depends on the cause of the pain and the individual needs of the patient. However, several basic principles can be kept in mind.

1. Show attention, respect and understanding to the patient and his or her family. Many patients with chronic pain suffer as much from the lack of understanding from others as from the pain itself.
2. The pain threshold may move upward by: undisturbed sleep; company; distraction; mobility; clear goals; independence. A multimodal or multi-disciplinary approach is superior to medication only.
3. Pain can be complex and difficult to treat. Therefore, careful explanation of diagnosis, goal of the treatment and planned steps in the treatment is important and can avoid non-compliance or disappointment. Use an algorithm (e.g. for neuropathic pain see Figure 45.1 or the algorithm in reference 4).
4. Start low and go slow with medication. However, each drug has to be taken in an

Table 45.1. Analgetic drugs in the elderly

Drug	Dose	Pharmaco-kinetics	Metabolism	Interactions	Important adverse events
paracetamol	500–1000 mg q6–8h	total clearance young adults: 4.1 ml/min/kg elderly : 3.4 ml/min/kg	hepatic	none	none
diclofenac	50 mg q8h	young adults: $t^1\!/_2$ 3.9 ± 4.4 hrs $t^1\!/_2$ 3.5 ± 3.3 hrs	hepatic	Diminish effect of diuretics and antihypertensives; Increases concentration of lithium, digoxin, methotrexate, aminoglycosides; increase bleeding risk with concomitant use of coumarines	Peptic ulcers, increased bleeding time, heart failure, renal failure, hypertension, Increased chance on early cardiovascular death.
ibuprofen	200–800 mg q8–12h	unbound clearance of S-enantiomer young: 15.9 ± 2.2 l/min elderly: 11.5 ± 4.1 l/min	Hepatic	See diclofenac	See diclofenac
naproxen	250–500 mg q12h	clearance of unbound drug young: 713 ± 164 l/h elderly: 281 ± 96 l/h	Hepatic	See diclofenac	See diclofenac, no increase of cardiovascular death.
celecoxib	100–200 mg q12–24h	young adults: $t^1\!/_2$ 11.8 ± 8.7 hrs elderly: $t^1\!/_2$ 11.2 ± 2.9 hrs	Hepatic	See diclofenac	See diclofenac, less peptic ulcers in comparison to non selective NSAIDs
tramadol	100 mg q6h drops may be useful, one drop = 2.5 mg slow release 200 mg q12h	Young adults: $t^1\!/_2$ 4.5–9.5 hrs	Renal and hepatic	carbamazepine decreases tramadol concentration	constipation, nausea, pruritus, sedation, delirium
codeine	10–20 mg q6h	Young adults: $t^1\!/_2$ 3–4 hrs	Renal and hepatic	Increase of sedation with use of alcohol and sedating drugs	constipation, nausea, pruritus, sedation
morphine oxycodone fentanyl	Start low, use slow release for daily dosing	Young adults: $t^1\!/_2$ 2–3 hrs renal impairment $t^1\!/_2$ 41–141 hrs (morphine)	Hepatic (active metabolite morphine-6-glucoronide) and renal	Increase of sedation with use of alcohol and sedating drugs	constipation, nausea, pruritus, sedation, respiratory depression only when administered intravenously.

(continued overleaf)

Table 45.1. (*continued*)

Drug	Dose	Pharmaco-kinetics	Metabolism	Interactions	Important adverse events
amitriptyline	10–75 mg qhs	Start low Young adults: $t^1/_2$ 12–25 hrs elderly: $t^1/_2$ hrs 31h	Hepatic (active metabolite nortriptyline) and renal	many. Combination with serotonine re-uptake inhibitors may increase plasma concentration	Anticholinergic: sedation, dry mouth, arythmias, bladder dysfunction, blurred vision. Not to be used after recent myocardial infarction.
nortriptyline	10–75 mg qhs	Start low Young adults: $t^1/_2$ hrs 26–36h elderly: $t^1/_2$ hrs 45–55h	Hepatic (CYP2D6) Genetic poly-morphism is possible with ultrarapid metabolism	many. Combination with serotonine re-uptake inhibitors may increase plasma concentration	less anticholergic side effects than amitriptyline.
Carbama-zepine	100–200 mg q8–12h	Clearance young adults: 74.6 ± 28.3 ml/h/kg elderly: 57.1 ± 20.6 ml/h/kg	hepatic and renal clearance	many (by induction of CYP2C9 and CYP 3A)	sedation, elevated liver enzymes, leukopenia
Gabapentin	100–1200 mg q8h	Clearance young adults: 130–230 ml/h/kg elderly: 65–115 ml/h/kg	renal clearance	none	sedation
Pregabalin	75–300 mg q12h	Clearance young adults: 45–75 ml/h/kg	renal clearance	none	sedation

adequate dose before it can be concluded that it is not working.

5. Medication should be taken in a daily schedule, not p.r.n. For incidental pain in cancer patients, e.g. before wound care, escape medication can be useful on top of the daily schedule.

6. Be aware of concomitant diseases and interactions with other drugs

7. Use drugs that are suited for the cause of the pain. For nociceptive pain, use the WHO Pain Relief Ladder (see Figure 45.2): paracetamol, NSAIDs and opioids. For neuropathic pain, use anti-epileptics or tricyclic antidepressants.

8. Opioids are not contra-indicated in the elderly, although side effects do occur. Addiction is not an issue.

KEY POINTS

- Pain in the elderly is often a complex problem that requires a multimodal strategy.
- Pharmacological treatment depends on the cause of the pain and the individual needs of the patient.
- Neuropathic pain needs other drugs than the analgesics suited for nociceptive pain.
- In general, start low and go slow.

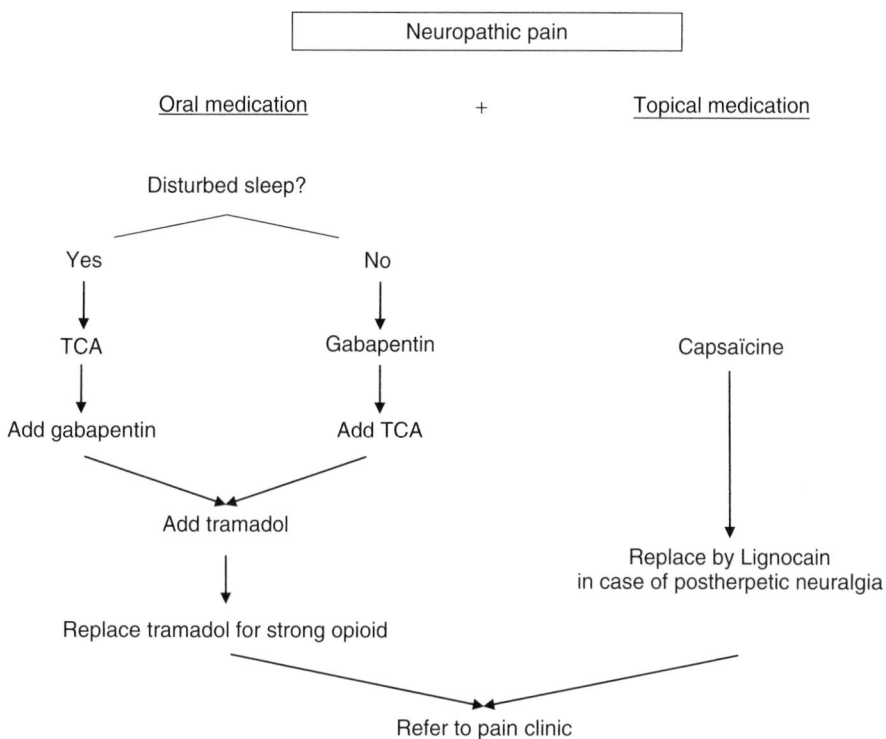

Figure 45.1. Algorithm for the treatment of neuropathic pain. TCA = tricylic antidepressant

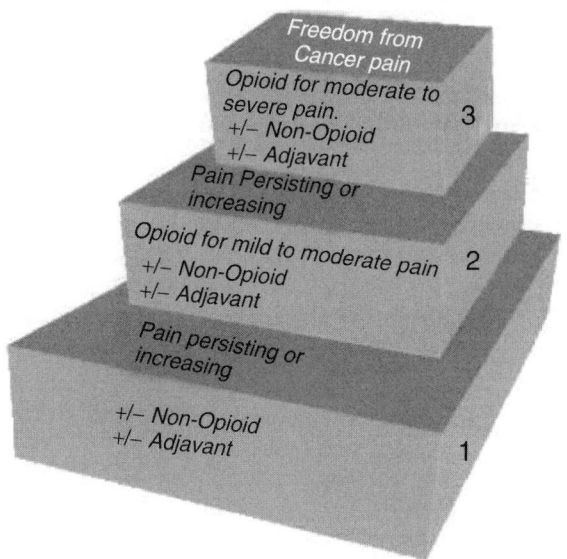

Figure 45.2. WHO's pain relief ladder (http://www.who.int/cancer/palliative/painladder/en/)

Standard scheme

Day 1	-	-	300 mg
Day 2	300	-	300
Day 3	300	300	300
Day 4	300	300	600
Day 5	600	300	600
Day 6	600	600	600

If sedation occurs, slow down by keeping the dose stable for 3 days.
Continue 600 mg tid for 4 weeks, then evaluate. The dose may be increased in steps to 3600 mg/day.
For this scheme, 275 capsules of 300 mg are needed.

Slow scheme

Day 1	-	-	100 mg
Day 2	100	100	100
Day 3	100	100	200
Day 4	200	200	200
Day 5	200	200	300
Day 6	300	300	300
Day 7	300	300	300
Day 8	300	300	400
Day 9	400	400	400

If sedation occurs, slow down by keeping the dose stable for 3 days.
Continue 400 mg tid for 4 weeks, then evaluate. If necessary increase to 600 mg tid.
For this scheme, 50 capsules of 100 mg and 100 capsule of 400 mg are needed.

Figure 45.3. Dose escalation schemes for gabapentin

REFERENCES

1. Leong IY, Nuo TH. Prevalence of pain in nursing home residents with different cognitive and communicative abilities. *Clin J Pain* 2007; **23**(2): 119–27.
2. Torrance N, Smith BH, Bennett MI, Lee AJ. The epidemiology of chronic pain of predominantly neuropathic origin. Results from a general population survey. *J Pain* 2006; **7**(4): 281–9.
3. Fox PL, Raina P, Jadad AR. Prevalence and treatment of pain in older adults in nursing homes and other long-term care institutions: a systematic review. *CMAJ* 1999; **160**(3): 329–33.
4. Finnerup NB, Otto M, McQuay HJ, Jenssen TS, Sindrup SH. Algorithm for neuropathic pain treatment: an evidence based proposal. *Pain* 2005; **118**(3): 289–305.

46 Palliative care in the elderly

Alexander de Graeff and Saskia Teunissen

Department of Medical Oncology, University Medical Centre, Utrecht, The Netherlands

INTRODUCTION

Palliative care is defined by the World Health Organization as 'an approach to care that improves the quality of life of patients and their families facing the problems associated with life-threatening illness, through the prevention and relief of suffering by means of early identification and impeccable assessment and treatment of pain and other problems, physical, psychosocial and spiritual' (1).

Palliative care:

- provides relief from pain and other distressing symptoms;
- affirms life and regards dying as a normal process;
- intends neither to hasten or postpone death;
- integrates the psychological and spiritual aspects of patient care;
- offers a support system to help patients live as actively as possible until death;
- offers a support system to help the family cope during the patients illness and in their own bereavement;
- uses a team approach to address the needs of patients and their families, including bereavement counselling, if indicated;
- will enhance quality of life, and may also positively influence the course of illness;
- is applicable early in the course of illness, in conjunction with other therapies that are intended to prolong life, such as chemotherapy

and radiotherapy, and includes those investigations needed to better understand and manage distressing clinical complications.

As indicated in the last bullet point, palliative care may be both disease-oriented and symptom-oriented. As the disease progresses, at some point it will not be possible any more to modify the course of the disease and treatment will be restricted to symptoms.

Palliative care may also be defined operationally as 'care for patients for whom cure is impossible and death due to their disease is unavoidable'. Survival after the moment when cure is not or no longer possible may vary enormously, from weeks to years. Thus, palliative care and terminal care (i.e., care for patients expected to die within one to two weeks or less) are not synonymous.

The majority of these patients have cancer, but many other diseases (e.g., heart failure, chronic obstructive pulmonary disease (COPD), AIDS, amyotrophic lateral sclerosis, muscle dystrophy) may be implicated. Patients with cancer often have a reasonably predictable decline in physical health over a period of weeks, months, or, in some cases, years (2). Patients with heart or lung failure have a much less predictable course of their disease, characterised by periods of exacerbations, which may or may not result in death; if a patient survives one or more of such episodes a gradual deterioration in health and functional status is typical. Estimation of life expectancy may be very

Prescribing for Elderly Patients Edited by Stephen Jackson, Paul Jansen and Arduino Mangoni

difficult in these patients. Elderly patients may die as a result of one of these diseases, but those who escape cancer and organ system failure are likely to die of either brain failure (such as Alzheimer's or other dementia) or generalized frailty of multiple body systems.

SYMPTOMS

Symptom control is a key issue in palliative care (3). Symptoms change over time and may manifest rapidly and unexpectedly. Symptoms are inherently subjective. The expression of the symptom, verbally or non-verbally, is the only dimension of the symptom that may be observed by others.

A wide variety of symptoms may occur in palliative care patients. (Table 46.1).

Symptom prevalence in elderly patients has not been studied systematically. There is some indication that confusion, drowsiness, dizziness, visual and auditory impairment and urinary incontinence occur more frequently, and pain, dysphagia, nausea, vomiting, dyspnoea, cough, headache, insomnia, anxiety and depression less frequently than in younger patients, but results of studies are sometimes conflicting (3, 5). In a retrospective study in family members, friends and officials of patients dying from

Table 46.1. Symptom prevalence in patients with incurable cancer (2)

Fatigue	74 % (63–83 %)(1)
Pain	71 % (67–74 %)
Lack of energy	69 % (57–79 %)
Weakness	60 % (51–68 %)
Appetite loss	53 % (48–59 %)
Nervousness	48 % (39–57 %)
Weight loss	46 % (34–59 %)
Dry mouth	40 % (29–52 %)
Depressed mood	39 % (33–45 %)
Constipation	37 % (33–40 %)
Worrying	36 % (21–55 %)
Insomnia	36 % (30–43 %)
Dyspnoea	35 % (30–39 %)
Nausea	31 % (27–35 %)
Anxiety	30 % (17–46 %)
Irritability	30 % (22–40 %)

[1]Figures are given as mean percentage (95 %-confidence interval)

cancer or other causes, the proportion of symptoms reported to have been 'very distressing' decreased with age (4).

Symptom burden is determined not only by the number and intensity of the symptoms, but also by their impact on mood, their meaning and by the interaction between the patient and others (family, friends, professional caregivers).

Despite a long tradition and experience in some countries (particularly in the United Kingdom) relatively little clinical research has been performed in the field of symptom control. Palliative care is to a large degree 'experienced based' and not 'evidence based'. However, over the past years expertise in the field of palliative care research has improved considerably and there are increasing numbers of publications in this field.

PALLIATIVE CARE IN THE ELDERLY

Elderly patients differ in a number of aspects from their younger counterparts. These differences may have implications for symptoms and their treatment in palliative care patients. As these changes with age are dealt with elsewhere in this book, they will only be mentioned briefly here:

1. Physical changes:
   - Degenerative changes in the central nervous system may lead to an increased proneness for drowsiness (e.g., as a side-effect of medication) and delirium and to decreased cognitive functioning.
   - Cardiovascular changes may lead to hypotension, particular as a side-effect of medication.
   - Decreased lung function may result in decreased exercise tolerance, dyspnoea, cough and pneumonia.
   - Decreased motility of the gastro-intestinal tract may lead to early satiety, nausea, vomiting and constipation.

   These and other changes lead to a greater degree of decrease in physical and cognitive functioning, a greater dependency on others for activities of daily living and increased use of health care resources, compared to the 'healthy' elderly.

2. Pharmacokinetic and pharmacodynamic changes leading to different handling of drugs and an increased prevalence of side-effects.

3. Higher prevalence of co-morbidity and polypharmacy, resulting in an increase in number and severity of symptoms, organ dysfunction and drug interactions.

4. Compliance with pharmacological or non-pharmacological treatment may be impaired by lack of mobility, visual impairment and decreased cognitive functioning.

5. Elderly patients are in a different phase of life. There may be a different attitude towards death and dying. This may be one of the explanations that elderly patients with advanced cancer have better quality of life compared to younger patients (6). Demands of seriously ill patients on family caregivers rise exponentially with age. However, these patients may have lost their partner and their children may be unable or unwilling to give support. Shortage of informal caregivers is a problem increasing with age (5). Depending on income, insurance, place of residence and country, the necessary health care resources may be unavailable.

All of these factors may lead to complex physical and/or psychosocial problems requiring intensive palliative care. Unfortunately, there is evidence showing underassessment and undertreatment of symptoms of older people and lack of access to palliative care resources, in particular home care and nursing homes (7, 8).

TREATMENT OF COMMON SYMPTOMS IN ELDERLY PATIENTS

Fatigue

Together with pain, fatigue (also described as lack of energy or weakness) is the most frequently occurring symptom in palliative care patients (9). It has a major effect on quality of life. Fatigue should be regarded as a multidimensional concept (encompassing physical, functional and psychological aspects), often caused by several factors:

- directly tumour-related;
- treatment-related;
- medication;
- uncontrolled symptoms;
- comorbidity.

In the assessment and treatment of fatigue, it is very important to recognise and treat reversible factors, such as anemia, dehydration, weight loss, infection, hypoxia, electrolyte disorders (hypercalcemia, hyponatremia), hypothyroidism, adrenal insufficiency or depression. Uncontrolled symptoms such as pain, dyspnoea or insomnia should be treated optimally.

Non-pharmacological treatment of fatigue itself includes advice about energy conserving and exercise. There is limited evidence that corticosteroids and methylfenidate are effective in reducing fatigue in advanced cancer patients.

Anorexia and weight loss

Anorexia (appetite loss) and cachexia (extreme weight loss and muscle atrophy) frequently occur in the final stages of disease (10). The anorexia-cachexia syndrome is often a hallmark of impending death and in many cases also a direct cause of it.

Anorexia and weight loss may be caused on the one hand by disease- and treatment-related symptoms and on the other hand by metabolic changes, caused by an increased production of cytokines, such as tumour necrosis factor (TNF), interleukin-1, interleukin-6 and gamma-interferon.

If weight loss is predominantly caused by a decreased intake of nutrients due to general or gastrointestinal symptoms, treatment should be aimed at those symptoms; nutritional interventions (sometimes including enteral nutrition) may be effective (11).

In some cases the occurrence of anorexia and weight loss is not (entirely) explained by the symptoms present. In those cases, the above mentioned metabolic changes may be the predominant factor. The classic model for this situation is the patient with pancreatic cancer, where anorexia and cachexia may occur relatively early in the course of the disease. Nutritional interventions have little or no influence on weight loss in this situation. In patients with a life expectancy of more than two to three months progestins (in particular megestrol acetate in relatively high dosages) are of proven value with regard to anorexia, weight loss and quality of life (12); however, they do not improve survival. For patients with a shorter life expectancy corticosteroids (e.g., dexamethasone) should be considered. They increase appetite and well-being, but do not have any influence on weight (13).

Nausea and vomiting

Nausea and vomiting may have a severe impact on quality of life. Severe vomiting may also lead to dehydration.

The physiology of nausea and vomiting involves the gastrointestinal tract and the central nervous system. Several neurotransmitters and receptors (among others, dopamine, serotonine, acetylcholine, histamine and neurokinin-1) may be involved; knowledge of these mediators directs drug therapy.

Nausea and vomiting may be caused by:

- impaired gastric emptying: due to drugs (e.g., opioids, drugs with anticholinergic (side-) effects), obstruction, paraneoplastic autonomic neuropathy or peptic disease;
- other abdominal/visceral causes: constipation, liver metastases, carcinomatous peritonitis, bowel obstruction;
- metabolic factors: drugs (e.g., opioids, chemotherapeutic drugs), hypercalcemia, acute renal insufficiency;
- disturbance of the vestibular system (rare in palliative care patients);
- brain metastases or carcinomatous meningitis.

Treatment is aimed primarily at the cause (if possible), e.g., change of medication or treatment of hypercalcemia. Non-pharmacological symptomatic treatment may include nasogastric suction (in case of gastric retention or bowel obstruction), administration of fluids and dietary advice.

Dopamine antagonists are usually the drugs of choice for pharmacological symptomatic treatment (14). Metoclopramide and domperidone (both dopamine antagonists) have the advantage of also being a prokinetic (and thus effective in cases of delayed gastric emptying) and are the drugs of first choice. Domperidone has not been studied systematically and never been compared to metoclopramide, but is preferred by some geriatricians because of its lack of central side effects (drowsiness, extrapyramidal side-effects, akathisia). Haloperidol (a pure dopamine antagonist) is also often used. Corticosteroids (e.g., dexamethasone) have proven value in the treatment for nausea and vomiting due to chemotherapy, but are also used for nausea and vomiting due to other causes. Serotonin antagonists (ondansetron, granisetron or tropisetron) are standard of care for chemotherapy-associated nausea and vomiting, but are also effective in refractory nausea due to other causes; an important disadvantage of their use in this situation is the frequent occurrence of constipation as a side-effect. Finally, levomepromazine and olanzapine are (very) effective in refractory nausea and vomiting and may be used as a treatment of last resort.

If vomiting is due to bowel obstruction, treatment with octreotide (a somatostatin analogue decreasing gastrointestinal secretions) or butylscopolamine (an anticholinergic agent) should be considered.

Constipation

Constipation is a major issue in elderly palliative care patients. General risk factors for constipation such as decreased intake of fibres and fluid, inactivity, suboptimal toilet facilities, dehydration, depression, drowsiness, confusion, the use of constipating medication (e.g. opioids, drugs with anticholinergic effects) and comorbidity are almost invariably present in these patients. Bowel obstruction, carcinomatous peritonitis, hypercalcemia or spinal cord compression may play a role.

Prevention of constipation is an important issue. If possible, care should be taken for optimal toilet facilities, exercise, intake of fluids and fibers and prophylactic use of laxatives in patients using opioids. However, some of these measures may not always be feasible.

Once constipation has occurred, the cause, if possible, should be treated, e.g. by changing medication, treating comorbidity, relieving bowel obstruction or spinal cord compression, chemotherapy for chemotherapy sensitive types of cancer (ovarian or colorectal cancer) or treatment of hypercalcemia.

Non-pharmacological treatment includes the same measures used for prevention (again, if feasible).

Little systematic research has been performed with regard to the use of laxatives (15). Bulk-forming laxatives are to be used only if adequate intake of fluids is guaranteed. Usually, an osmotic laxative (polyethylene glycol electrolyte solution, magnesium (hydr)oxide or lactulose) is given; if this is not effective in adequate doses, senna or bisacodyl should be added. In case of fecal impaction a sodium phosphate enema should be given first; high oral doses of polyethylene glycol electrolyte solutions may also be given orally in this situation.

Dyspnoea

Dyspnoea refers to the sensation of unpleasant breathing. It is often associated with hypoxia but may occur without it. It is a predominant symptom in patients with heart failure, COPD and lung cancer. Fear of suffocation is often present.

Dyspnoea may be caused by (16):

- major airways: obstruction by tumour, sputum, foreign object, bleeding;
- lung: pneumonia, COPD, extensive lung metastases, carcinomatous lymphangitis, pneumonitis due to chemotherapy or radiotherapy;
- pleural cavity: pleural effusion, pneumothorax;
- cardiovascular: pulmonary embolism, superior vena cava syndrome, heart failure, pericarditis, dysrhythmia;
- miscellaneous: anemia, ascites, amyotrophic lateral sclerosis, muscle dystrophy.

Whenever possible, the cause should be treated, e.g. by relief of airway obstruction, antibiotics, bronchodilator agents, radiotherapy or chemotherapy, pleural drainage, anticoagulants, placing of stent in superior vena cava, treatment of heart failure, correction of anemia and treatment of ascites.

Interventions combining breathing control, activity pacing, relaxation techniques and psychosocial support are of proven value in relieving dyspnoea. There is limited evidence for the use of oxygen, predominantly in patients with COPD; generally, oxygen therapy is recommended only in the presence of hypoxia. Facial cooling in itself may relieve dyspnoea.

Opioids are of proven value in the treatment of dyspnoea in COPD, lung cancer and heart failure. They should be administered orally or parenterally, often in low doses. If given proportionally, they do not induce respiratory depression.

Corticosteroids (dexamethasone or prednisone) are given for dyspnoea caused by COPD, superior vena cava syndrome, carcinomatous lymphangitis or pneumonitis due to radiotherapy or chemotherapy. Apart from COPD, their effectivity has not been proven by clinical research.

Dyspnoea may lead to severe agitation and anxiety. In these cases the adjunct use of benzodiazepines should be considered. In cases of severe and refractory dyspnoea in terminal patients, palliative sedation may be considered (17).

REFERENCES

1. World Health Organisation. Definition of palliative care. http://www.who.int/cancer/palliative/definition, 2006.
2. Murray SA, Kendall M, Boyd K, Sheikh A. Illness trajectories and palliative care. *Br Med J* 2005; **330**: 1007–11.
3. Teunissen SCCM, Wesker W, Kruitwagen C, de Haes H, Voest E, de Graeff A. Symptom prevalence in patients with incurable cancer. Accepted for *J Pain Symptom Manage*, 2007.
4. Addington-Hall J, Altmann D, McCarthy M. Variation by age in symptoms and dependency levels experienced by people in the last year of

life, as reported by surviving family, friends and officials. *Age Ageing* 1998; **27**: 129–36.

5. Teunissen SCCM, de Haes H, Voest E, de Graeff A. Does age matter in palliative care? *Crit Rev Oncol Hematol* 2006; **60**: 152–8.

6. Lundh Hagelin C, Seiger A, Fürst CJ. Quality of life in terminal care–with special reference to age, gender and marital status. *Supp Care Cancer* 2006; **14**: 320–8.

7. Cleary JF, Carbone PP. Palliative medicine in the elderly. *Cancer* 1997; **80**: 1335–47.

8. World Health Organization 2004. *Better Palliative Care for Older People*. Edited by E. Davies & I. Higginson ISBN 9289010924.

9. Mock V. Fatigue management: evidence and guidelines for practice. *Cancer* 2001; **15** (Suppl. 6): 1669–707.

10. Inui A. Cancer anorexia-cachexia syndrome: Current issues in research and management. *CA Cancer Journal for Clinicians* 2002; **52**: 72–91.

11. Bachmann P, Marti-Massoud C, Blanc-Vincent MP et al. Summary version of the standards, options and recommendations for palliative or terminal nutrition in adults with progressive cancer. *British Journal of Cancer* 2003; **89** (Supplement 1): S107–S110.

12. Maltoni M, Nanni O, Scarpi E et al. High-dose progestins for the treatment of cancer anorexia-cachexia syndrome: a systematic review of randomised clinical trials. *Annals of Oncology* 2001; **12**: 289–300.

13. Desport JC, Gory-Delabaere G, Blanc-Vincent MP et al. Standards, options and recommendations for the use of appetite stimulants in oncology. *British Journal of Cancer* 2003; **89** (Supplement 1), S98–S100.

14. Glare P, Pereira G, Kristjanson LJ, Stockler M, Tattersall M. Systematic review of the efficacy of antiemetics in the treatment of nausea and vomiting in patients with far-advanced disease. *Supportive Care in Cancer* 2004; **12**: 432–440.

15. Larkin PJ, Sykes NP, Centeno C et al. The management of constipation in palliative care: clinical practice recommendations. *Palliat Med* 2008; **22**: 796–807.

16. Dudgeon D, Lertzman M. Dyspnea in the advanced cancer patient. *J Pain Symptom Management* 1998; **16**: 212–219.

17. De Graeff A. Dean M. Palliative sedation therapy in the last weeks of life: a literature review and recommendations for standards. *J Palliat Med* 2007; **10**: 67–85.

INDEX

Note: Page numbers in *italics* refer to figures and tables.

5α-reductase inhibitors
  for bladder outflow tract obstruction 349
  for nocturnal frequencey in BPH 356–7
5-aminosalicylic acid (5-ASA) 305
5-fluorouracil (5-FU)
  for actinic keratoses 454
  chemotherapy for GI cancer *327*, *328*, *387*

abciximab 57, *115*, 119
abdominal malignancies 321
  aetiology 324
  epidemiology 321–3
  key points 329
  symptoms and signs 324–5
  therapy 325
    chemotherapy 327–9
    surgery 325–6
acarbose 68, *295*, 394, 395, *396*, 397
ACE inhibitors
  adverse effect on asthma *185*
  and ARBs 136
  drug interactions *5*, 55
  effects on continence *346*
  fewer adverse cardiovascular events 431
  heart failure therapy 129–30, *131*
  for hypertension *94*, 96, 97
  and PDE-5 inhibitors 364
  for post-ACS management 121
  preventing atrial fibrillation 146
acetazolamide, glaucoma treatment 475
achalasia 279, 286–7
acid suppression, GI disorders 283–6, 291, 293
acromegaly 392, 398
ACS *see* acute coronary syndrome
actinic keratoses 453–4
activated partial thromboplastin time (aPTT), heparin
    activity 59, 60, 161, 165
acute angle closure glaucoma (AACG) 473
  treatment of 474–5
acute asthma
  BTS/SIGN guidelines 191–2

  for treatment *193*
  features of *192*
acute coronary syndrome (ACS) 111
  aetiology 111–12
  diagnosis 112–13
  high risk criteria *122*
  key points and guidelines 121–2
  symptoms and signs 112
  therapy
    anti-thrombin therapy 119–20
    antiplatelet agents 113, 119
    drugs and dosages *114–18*
    post-ACS management 121
acute mesenteric ischaemia 309–11
acute urinary retention (AUR) 353, 355, 356
adherence 6
  important for heart failure patients 129
  methods of measuring 7
  reasons for impaired 501
  to anti-tuberculous regimens 219
  to antidepressant medication 31
adverse drug reactions (ADRs) 4–6, 7
age-related changes in pharmacokinetics 2–3
age related macular degeneration (AMD) 476
  aetiology 476
  diagnosis 477–8
  key points 480–1
  symptoms and signs 476–7
  therapy 478–80
agitation and behavioural problems 22
  diagnosis 23
  key points 25
  symptoms and signs 22–3
  therapy 23–5, 86
alcohol consumption
  and heart failure 128
  hyperlipidaemia-induced 101
  and hypertension 93
  and insomnia 45, 46, 47
  and liver diseases 335, 336–7, 338
  risk factor for abdominal cancers *324*

alcoholic liver disease 336–7
aldosterone antagonists 98, 129, *132*, 136
alendronate
    lowering risk of hip fractures 422
    for Paget's disease 424
alkaline phosphatase activity
    osteomalacia 426, 427
    Paget's disease 423, 424–5
allopurinol
    drug interactions 306, *327*, *387*, *406*, 407
    for gout *415*, 416
    for hyperuricemia 177
alpha adrenergic agonists
    effects on continence *346*
    glaucoma treatment 474
    phenylephrine 470
    vasoldiling drugs 97
alpha-blockers
    associated with risk of falls *431*
    benign prostatic hyperplasia 356, 357
    bladder outflow tract obstruction 349, 350
    effects on continence *346*
    for hypertension *94*, 98–9
alveolar osteitis 266
Alzheimer's disease (AD) 13
    aetiology 13–14
    diagnosis 14, *15*
    symptoms and signs 14
    therapy 14–18
        drug treatment *16–17*
        for secondary psychosis 39
AMD *see* age related macular degeneration
aminoglycosides (AG) 217, *328*, 488, 490, 491, *495*
aminosalicylates (5-ASA), ulcerative colitis 305
amiodarone
    for atrial fibrillation 143–5, *144*, *147*
    drug interactions 5, 48, 50, 103, *104*, *134*, *167*, 205
    hepatotoxicity 334, 335
amitriptyline *8*, *32*, *255*, 458, *496*
amoxicillin *153*, *204*, 291, 303
ampicillin 153, *155*, *204*
amputation, deformities causing pressure ulcers 444,
    445, 451
amyloid angiopathy 53
anaemia 171
    in breast cancer patients 384–5
    finding in abdominal cancers *324*, 325
    iron deficiency/administration 171–2
    refractory anaemia 175, 176
    transfusion 172
analgesic drugs *495–6*
anastrazole, for breast cancer *388*
androgen 356, 357, 398, 399–400
anecortave acetate, AMD treatment 480
angio-oedema 465–6
angiogenesis inhibitors 479

angiography 308, 310, 446–447, *449*, 477–8
angioplasty 448
angiotensin-2 receptor blockers (ARBs)
    for atrial fibrillation 146
    effect of diuretic usage 135
    heart failure 129, 136, 137
    for hypertension 94, 96, *97*
    for post-ACS management 121
angiotensin converting enzyme inhibitors *see* ACE
    inhibitors
angular cheilitis 268
anorexia of ageing 298–9
anorexia in palliative care patients 501–2
antiarrhythmics
    drug interaction with antiepileptics 87
    negative cardiovascular effects of 431
    treatment of AF 140, 143–5
antibiotics
    acute mesenteric ischaemia 311
    adverse effects *255*, *299*, 303, 304, 314, 471, 491
    cellulitis and erysipelas 457
    for community acquired pneumonia 202–5
    diverticulitis 308
    for eradication of H. pylori 291–2
    exacerbations of COPD 194
    for external otitis 490
    increase in resistance to 346, 439, 452
    for infective endocarditis 153–5
    leg ulcer treatment 452
    malabsorption 303
    mouth ulcers 270, 271
    odontogenic infections 266
    for post-operative cataract 471
    for pulmonary tuberculosis 215–18
anticholinergics
    adverse effects 4, *32*, 38–39, 77, *190*, 267, 431–2,
        496
    and bowel obstruction 502
    causing delirium 19
    causing insomnia *46*
    causing xerostomia 267, 278
    for chronic stable COPD *188*
    for detrusor overactivity 373–4
    and GI tract motility 301
    and increased fall risk *431*
    for myasthenia gravis 278–9
    and Parkinson's disease 80
anticoagulants 3
    following stroke 59–61
    for heart failure patients 136–7
    for infective endocarditis 155
    for patients with AF 148–9
    for patients with prosthetic cardiac valves 156–7
    in patients undergoing non-cardiac surgery 157–8
    for thrombosis and emobolism 161–8
    see also heparins; warfarin

anticonvulsants *see* antiepileptic drugs (AEDs)
antidepressants 30–1
  combination therapy 33
  and detrusor overactivity 374
  dosing guide *32*
  as hypnotics *46*, 48
  and increased risk of falls 421, 430, *431*
  mirtazapine, aiding weight gain 258
antidiarrhoeal therapy 316–17
antiemetics 246, 384, 422
antiepileptic drugs (AEDs) 85
  adverse effects/drug interactions 87
  causing osteomalacia 426, 427
  dosage *88–9*
  newer drugs 85–6
  safety of 86
  withdrawal 87, 90
antifungals 268, 269, 280, 465
antihistamines
  causing delirium *19*
  non-sedating, adverse effects of *185*
  sedative effects 46, 48
  for urticaria and angio-oedema 466
antihypertensives 93–4
  ACE inhibitors (ACEIs) 96, 97
  ARBs 96, 97
  CCBs 95–6
  centrally-acting vasodilators 97–8
  directly acting vasodilators 98–9
  exacerbating lower limb oedema 441
  and increased risk of falls 431
  indications/contraindications *94*
  perindopril reducing stroke recurrence 54
  thiazide/thiazide-like diuretics 94–5
  see also beta-blockers
antimicrobials *see* antibiotics
antimuscarinic agents
  and cognitive dysfunction 349
  detrusor overactivity 373–4
  urinary incontinence 347–8
antiplatelet therapy 54
  acute coronary syndrome 113, 119
  atrial fibrillation 149
  and bleeding risk 164
  for patients with prosthetic valves 156–7
  for stroke prevention 54–8
antipsychotics 33
  adverse effects in dementia *25*
  atypical
    for Alzheimer's related psychosis 39
    for anxiety and agitation 40
    for Parkinson's disease 80
    safety of 39
  increased fall risks 39, 430, *431*
  risks of conventional 39
  and swallowing disorders 279

antiseptics 439, 490
anxiety and agitation 36
  benzodiazepines for 39, 40
aortic valve disease 156
aphthous ulcerations 270–1
apomorphine
  erectile dysfunction 364
  Parkinson's disease *78*
appetite loss, palliative care patients 501–2
appetite regulation, effect of ageing on 298–9
apraclonidine, for glaucoma 474
argon laser photocoagulation 482–3
arterial duplex scanning 447
arterial insufficiency
  causing leg ulceration 441
  symptoms associated with 443–4
arthritis
  gouty arthritis and pseudogout 413–16
  osteoarthritis (OA) 408–11
  rheumatoid arthritis (RA) 403–8
asbestosis 233
aspirin
  for acute coronary syndrome 113, 119
  adverse effects of 55
  arterial insufficiency 448
  and bronchoconstriction 183
  causing tinnitus 491
  drug interactions 55, *415*
  and peptic ulcers 288, 289, 290
  for prevention of recurrent stroke 54–5, 163
    aspirin/dipyridamole combination 55
  reducing risk of thromboembolism 149, 156, 157,
    158
asteatotic eczema 453
asthma 183
  acute asthma
    BTS/SIGN guidelines for treatment *193*
    features of *192*
  definition of *185*
  distinguishing from COPD 186, *187*
  drugs for *192*
  management of 186–91
  presentation & diagnosis 184
  risk factors and triggers 183–4
  spirometry 184–6
atherosclerosis
  hyperlipidaemia as risk factor 101–9
  and poor arterial supply to lower leg 441
atorvastatin *118*
atrial fibrillation 139
  antithrombotic therapy 149
  causes of 142
  classification of 142
  cost of 140
  detection of with ECG 127
  diagnosis 140–2

atrial fibrillation (*continued*)
    drugs for acute cardioversion *144*
    electrophysiological mechanisms 140
    epidemiology 139
    key points 150
    management of 142–3
    rate control in permanent AF 146–8
    rate versus rhythm control 145–6
    and risk of stroke 54, 148–9
    suppression of paroxysms 143–5
    symptoms and signs 140
    treatment of acute onset 143
atrial flutter (AFL) 139, 140, 141, 143, 144
atrial tachycardia (AT) 139, 141
atypical antipsychotics
    augmenting agents for depression 33
    for Parkinson's disease 80
    for psychosis symptoms 39
    and swallowing disorders 279
augmentation cystoplasty 376
azathioprine
    immunosuppressant 229, 230, 231, 232
    inflammatory bowel disease 306
    interaction with allopurinol *415*, 416
    for rheumatoid arthritis *406*, 407
azytromycin, anti-tuberculous agent 217–18

B-type natriuretic peptide (BNP) 128
balance, assessment of 421
basal cell carcinoma 442, 452, 462–3
beclomethasone (BDP), inhaled steroid 187, *189*
behavioural and psychological symptoms of dementia
    (BPSD) 22–5
behavioural therapy
    for detrusor overactivity 372–3
    for weight loss 252
benign gynaecological disorders
    detrusor overactivity 370–3
    drug therapies 373–6
    lichen planus 377
    lichen sclerosis 377–8
    urinary incontinence 370
    urogenital atrophy 367
    urogenital prolapse 367–70
benign prostatic hyperplasia (BPH)
    assessment 353
    International Prostate Symptom Score (IPSS) *354*
    nocturnal frequency 355
    prostate specific antigen (PSA) testing 353
    treatment 355
        lifestyle changing 355
        medical 355–7
        surgical 357–8
    urinary retention 353, 355
benzodiazepines
    for anxiety and agitation 40
    delirium 20, *21*

hepatic clearance of 48, 333
    for insomnia 47
    side effects *255*
    withdrawal benefits 48
beta-blockers 96–7
    contraindications *94*
    eye drops 431
    glaucoma treatment 474
    properties of *97*
    rate control in AF 143, 146, *148*
    for unstable angina 120
    vasovagal collapse and carotid sinus
        hypersensitivity 431
beta cell insulin secretion 391, 392, 394
$beta_2$-agonists, asthma and COPD 187–190, 192–3,
    195
bevacizumab, for neovascular AMD 479
bile acid malabsorption 315, 317
bile acid sequestrants, LDL-C reduction 108
bisphosphonates
    breast cancer treatment 383–4, *388*
    Paget's disease 424–5
    prevention of hip fractures 422
'Black Triangle' drugs 8
bladder control 343–4
'bladder drill', for detrusor overactivity 372–3
bladder outflow tract obstruction 344–5
    treatment of 349–50
blood pressure, measurement of 92
body mass index (BMI) 249
    overweight and obese people 250–1
    risk factor for hip fractures 420
    under-nourished people 252–3, 256
bone marrow disease 173–4
bone mineral density (BMD)
    low BMD and risk of hip fractures 420
    measurement of 421
    and weight loss 251
botulinum toxin (Botox)
    for achalasia 279, 287
    for detrusor overactivity 350, 375–6
    swallowing disorder treatment 279
Bowen's disease 453–4
breast cancer 381
    drug dosages and interactions 385, *386–8*, 389
    key points 389
    management of early 382–3, *384*
    management of metastatic *385*
    presentation and diagnosis 381–2
    supportive care during treatment 384–5
    treatment of advanced 383–4
breath tests
    diagnosis of gastroparesis 297
    diagnosis of malabsorption 303
breathlessness, drug therapy for 188, 193, 194, 195
brimonidine and brinzolamide, for glaucoma 474

bronchiolitis obliterans organizing pneumonia (BOOP) 232–3

bronchodilators, chronic stable COPD 195

BTS (British Thoracic Society), guidelines
anti-TNF-α treatment 407
asthma 184, 186, 191, 193
pneumonia 201

bullous pemphigoid 454–5

burning mouth syndrome 269–70

cachexia 258, 501–2

calcitonin, for Paget's disease 424

calcium channel blockers (CCBs)
acute coronary syndrome 121
AF rate control 146
contraindicated for HF *130*
hypertension 94, 95–6
for incontinence *346*, 348
intrusor overactivity 374

calcium pyrophosphate disease (CPPD) 413–14
treatment 416

cancer
abdominal 321–9
breast 381–9
lung 237–47
skin 460–3
thyroid 399

candidiasis 267–268, 455–6

cannabinoids, for appetite stimulation 258

CAP (community acquired pneumonia) *see* pneumonia

capecitabine, cytotoxic drug *327*, 328, *386*, 389

capsaicin
improving swallowing 279
for neurogenic DO 374
for neuropathic pain 494, *497*
for osteoarthritis *410*

captopril 96, *97*, *117*, *133*, 278

carbamazepine
as an analgesic *496*
anti-epileptic agent 85, 86, 87, 89, *89*
drug interactions *167*, *216*, *495*

carbidopa-levodopa combination
adverse effects *255*
for parkinsonism 76–7, *78*
for restless leg syndrome 49–50

carbonic anhydrase inhibitors 471, 474, 475

carboplatin, lung cancer treatment 239–40, *241*, *243*, *245*, *246*

carcinoid tumour 323

cardiac resynchronization therapy (CRT) 136

cardiac troponin, elevation of 113, 119

cardiovascular drugs, and increased risk of falls 429–31

cardioversion
electrical 143, 149
pharmacological 143, 144, 146

carotid sinus hypersensitivity 429, 430, 431, 432

cataract 469–71

catheterization 358, 370, 376

celecoxib, analgesic 409, *495*

cellulitis 265–266, 456–7

cerebral infarction *see* stroke

cerumen impaction 485–6

chemo-radiotherapy, for NSCLC 241, *242*

chemotherapy
anti-tuberculous 214
for breast cancer 383–5
drugs used in 238–40
for mesothelioma 243, 245, *246*
protocols for NSCLC 240–2, *243*, *244*
for small cell carcinoma 243, *245*

chest pain
acute coronary syndrome 112–13
non-cardiac 287
postprandial hypotension 67

chest X-ray (CXR)
asthma-COPD differences *187*
heart failure diagnosis 127–8
pneumonia diagnosis 200–1

chlorhexidine, for dental problems 264, 265, 266, 271

cholesterol levels
drugs raising HDL-C 106
drugs reducing LDL-C 103, 106, 107, 108
measuring 102
and stroke prevention 54

cholestyramine, diarrhoea prevention 317

cholinesterase inhibitors (ChEIs)
adverse effects *255*
effects on continence *346*
treatment of dementia 14–15, *16–17*, 18

chondroitin sulphate, for osteoarthritis *410*, 411

chronic lymphocytic leukaemia (CLL) 178–9

chronic myelomonocytic leukaemia (CMML) 175

chronic obstructive pulmonary disease (COPD) 183
and asthma
differences in therapeutic approaches *192*
distinguishing from 186, *187*
definition of *185*
key points & guidelines 196–7
management of 186–91
exacerbations 192–4
stable 195–6
objective tests 184–6
presentation and diagnosis 184
risk factors and triggers 183, *184*

chronic pancreatitis *315*, *324*, *392*

cirrhosis 335–6

cisplatin
lung cancer treatment 239–40, *241*, *242*, *243*, *245*, *246*
toxicity and drug interactions 328

citalopram, antidepressant 31, *32*

'clam' cystoplasty 376

claritromycin, anti-tuberculous agent 217–18
clinical practice guidelines (CPGs) 9–10
clonazepam *47*, 50, 51, 85
clopidogrel
    acute coronary syndrome *114*, 119
    stroke prevention 56–7
codeine, analgesic *495*
coeliac disease 302, 303, *315*
cognitive behavioural therapy (CBT) 30, 46, 93
cognitive dysfunction
    and antimuscarincs 349
    comorbid with schizophrenia 37
    and depression 29
    and measurement of pain 494
    in Parkinson's disease 74
    screening tests 30
    see also dementia
colonography 313, 318, 325
colonoscopy 304, 308, 310–11, 313, 316, 317
colorectal cancer 321–2
    diagnosis 325
    risk factors and presentation 324–5
    treatment 325–9, *326*
compliance to medication *see* adherence
compression therapy, venous ulcers/ eczema 448–50,
    467
COMT-inhibitors, treatment of Parkinson's disease 75,
    79
Confusion Assessment Method (CAM) 20
constipation 311
    aetiology 311–12
    diagnosis 312–13
    key points, guidance and links 313
    major cause of urogential prolapse 369
    palliative care patients 502–3
    symptoms and signs 312
    therapy 313, *314*
contact dermatitis 457–8
COPD *see* chronic obstructive pulmonary disease
corticosteroids
    acute asthma 193
    adverse effects of long-term use 280, 412
    anti-angiogenic 480
    chronic stable COPD 195
    exacerbations of COPD *192*, 194
    for gout 414, *415*
    for lichen planus 459
    lung disease 229, 230, 232–4
    for nausea and vomiting 502
    for osteoarthritis *410*
    polymyalgia rheumatica 412
    rheumatoid arthritis 404, 407
    risk factor for hip fracture 420
    for silicosis 233
COX-2 selective NSAIDs
    adverse effects 409

preferred for GI disorders 288, 289, 290
cramps, nocturnal 50
creatine kinase (CK) measurement 102
Crohn's disease (CD) 303, 304–7
cryotherapy 454
crystal associated arthritis 413–16
CURB-65 criteria for CAP severity 201, *202*
cutaneous candidiasis 455–6
cutaneous T-cell lymphoma 461
cyanosis, in immobile patients 444–5
cyclopentolate, for pupil dilation 470
cyclophosphamide 229–30, 231, 232, *245*, *386*
cyclosporin 190, *406*, 407, 463
cystoplasty 376
cytotoxic drugs
    interstitial lung disease 229–30
    leading to swallowing problems 280
    toxicity and interactions *327–8*

dalteparin 60, 161, *166*
darifenacin, antimuscarinic agent 348, 374
deafness, causes of 485
deep vein thrombosis (DVT) 163, 165
degenerative valvular disease 158–9
deglutition
    changes with age 276–7
    medications affecting 278–80
    normal stages 275–6
delirium 18–19
    aetiology 19
    comorbidity with psychosis 35
    diagnosis 20
    key points and guidelines 22
    symptoms and signs 20, 37
    therapy 20–2
delusions
    in dementia 14, 22–3, 37
    in psychosis 35, 37, 38, 74, 80
dementia 13
    adverse effects of neuroleptics *25*
    aetiology 13–14
    diagnosis and assessment 14, *15*
    key points and guidelines 18
    major depression as a risk factor 29
    primary cause of psychosis 36
    symptoms and signs 14, 37
    therapy 14–18
dementia with Lewy bodies (DLB) 13, 14, 18, 22, 23,
    25
dental caries 264–5
denture stomatitis 268–9
dependency syndrome 466–7
depression 27
    aetiology 27–8
    and anorexia of ageing 298, 299
    diagnosis 29–30
    and Parkinson's disease 74

psychotic 37–8
signs and symptoms 28–9
    cognitive dysfunction 29, 37
therapy 30–3
    antidepressant dosing *32*
    treatment algorithm 31, 33
dermatitis 457–8
desmopressin, for nocturnal polyuria 350, 374
desquamative interstitial pneumonitis 233
detrusor muscle, normal working of 343–4
detrusor overactivity (DO) 344, 345, 370–1
    causes of 371
    drug therapy 373–4
    physiotherapy 372–3
    surgical solutions 375–6
dexamethasone 180, *244*, 245, *246*, 273, 384, 471,
        502, 503
diabetes mellitus
    diagnosis 392–3
    and gastroparesis 296, 297
    medication 393–5
        adverse effects 396–7
        drug-drug interactions 395–6
        interactions within diabetes drugs 396
    potential causes of 391–2
diabetic retinopathy 482–4
diarrhoea and faecal incontinence 314–17
    aetiology 314–15
    diagnosis 316
    symptoms and signs 315–16
    therapy 316–17
diastolic dysfunction/heart failure
    aetiology 127
    diagnosis of 128
    pharmacological treatment 137
    prevalence according to age *127*
diclofenac, analgesic *495*
diet
    and constipation 313
    guidelines for the elderly 257
    and hyperlipidaemia 101
    and hypertension 93
    and pressure ulcers 438
    and type 2 diabetes 391
    and weight loss 250–2
dietary supplements 85, 258, 337, 411, 422
diffuse oesophageal spasm 286, 287
digoxin
    adverse effects 19, 28, *255*, *299*, 301
    drug interactions *5*, *8*
    for heart failure 129, *131*, 136
    rate control in AF 143, 146, 147, *148*
dilated fundus examination 477
dipyridamole 56
    antithrombotic treatment *158*
    combined with aspirin 55, 149

prescribing guidelines 57
valvular heart disease *157*
Directly Observed Therapy (DOT) 219
disease modifying anti-rheumatic drugs (DMARDS)
        40–6, 404, 407
diuretics
    effects on continence *346*, 372
    for heart failure 135
    lower leg swelling 450
    thiazide 94–5
diverticulosis 307–9
    aetiology 307–8
    diagnosis 308
    symptoms and signs 308
    therapy 308–9
dizziness
    and anti-vertigo drugs 432
    symptom preceding falls 419, 421
    see also hypotension
DMARDS *see* disease modifying anti-rheumatic drugs
DO *see* detrusor overactivity
docetaxel 240, *243*, *244*, *246*, *386*
domperidone
    for gastroparesis 297
    for nausea and vomiting 502
    for Parkinson's disease 77, *79*
donepezil 16, 18
dopamine agonists
    improving swallowing 279
    Parkinson's disease 77, *80*
    for primary RLS/PLMS 49–50
    for prolactinomas 398
    for restless legs syndrome 49–50
dorzolamide, glaucoma treatment 474
doxazosin 98–9, 349, 356, 357
doxorubicin, cancer chemotherapy drug *386*
doxycycline, for pneumonia 203, *204*
dressings
    for leg ulcers 441, 448, 450
    for pressure ulcers 439
'drop attacks' 419–20
drug absorption, effect of ageing on 2
drug clearance by kidney and liver 3
drug distribution in the body 2
drug induced liver disease 334–5
drug interactions in the elderly *5*
duloxetine, for stress urinary incontinence in women
        350–1, 373
duodenal ulcer 288, 291
dutasteride, 5a-reductase inhibitor 349, 357
dyspepsia, non-ulcer 292–3
dysphagia *see* swallowing disorders
dyspnoea, causes and treatment 503

ear disorders 485
    drugs causing hearing problems 490–1
    external otitis 489–90

ear disorders (*continued*)
   hearing loss 485–7
   tinnitus 487–9
Eastern Cooperative Oncology Group (ECOG),
      performance status *240, 326*
echocardiography
   atrial fibrillation diagnosis 142
   endocarditis diagnosis 152
   heart failure diagnosis 128
eczema
   asteatotic eczema 453
   venous eczema 466–7
EGFR (epidermal growth factor receptor) inhibitors
      242
elderly onset rheumatoid arthritis (EORA) 403–4
electrocardiogram (ECG)
   acute coronary syndrome 112–13
   atrial arrhythmias 140–2, 145, 421
   heart failure 127
electroconvulsive therapy (ECT) 33
elimination half life, calculation of 2
EMB *see* ethambutol
embolic prophylaxis *157*
emesis *see* vomiting
enalapril *117*
endocarditis, infective 151–2
   diagnosis and prevention 152
   treatment 153–5
endocrine conditions 391
   hormone replacement 399–400
   hyperparathyroidism 399
   key points 400
   pituitary adenomas 397–8
   thyroid disease 398–9
   type 2 diabetes 391–7
endoprostatic stents 357
enoxaparin 16, *115, 166*
Enterococci, infective endocarditis 151–2, *155*
epidemiology 1–2
epilepsy 83
   aetiology 83, *84*
   diagnosis 84–5
   incidence 83, *84*
   key points 90
   symptoms and signs 83
   therapy 85–90
epirubicin, breast cancer drug *386*
eplerenone, for heart failure 129, *132*, 136
eptifibatide, for ACS *114*, 119, *120*
erectile dysfunction 361
   diagnosis and assessment 362–3
   key points 366
   prevalence and aetiology 361–2
   psychological impact 362
   treatment options 363–6
erysipelas 456–7

erythromycin syrup, for gastroparesis 297
ethambutol (EMB), tuberculostatic 214, 217
   adverse reactions *216*
   recommended dosage *215*
   within anti-tuberculous regimen 218–19
ethanol *see* alcohol
examestane, breast cancer drug *388*
exercise, lack of
   heart failure patients 137
   hypertensive patients 93
   for maintaining muscle mass 252
   patients with high risk of falls 422
   patients with type 2 diabetes 391–2
   and venous ulceration 441, 442, 448, 450
external otitis 489–90
eye diseases 469
   age related macular degeneration 476–81
   cataract 469–71
   diabetic retinopathy 482–4
   glaucoma 472–6
ezetimibe, drug lowering LDL-C *105*, 107

factor Xa inhibitors 119–20, 162
faecal incontinence 314–17
faecal osmotic gap, calculation of 315
fainting *see* syncope
falls 419
   causes 419–20, *420*
   diagnostic approach 420–1
   drug-related 429, 433
      assessment 432
      fall-risk-increasing drugs 430–2
      pathophysiology 429–30
      treatment by drug withdrawal 432–3
   key points 427
   and osteoporosis
      hip fracture 420, 422
   prevention and treatment 422
   risk factors 419–20
fatigue
   insomnia treatment 47, 48
   treatment of 501
fesoterodine, antimuscarinic drug 348
fibrates *104–5*, 106
finasteride, 5a-reductase inhibitor 349, 355, 356–7
flucloxacillin 153, *154*
fludrocortisone 65, 66, 422
fluorescein angiography, AMD 477–8
fluoride 264–5
fluoroquinolones (FQ) 203, 214, 217
fluoxetine, antidepressant 31, *32*
flurbiprofen sodium, eye drops 470
fluvoxamine, antidepressant 31, *32*
folic acid deficiencies 173
fondaparinux, factor Xa inhibitor 119–20, 162
food impaction 287
foot deformities 442–5

fosinopril *117*
fractures
    hip fractures 420, 422
    in Paget's disease 423
    pseudofractures in osteomalacia 426
frontotemporal dementia (FTD) 13, 14, 22, 23
functional incontinence 345, 371
fungal infections
    candidiasis 267–8
    denture stomatitis 268–9
    from prolonged steroid use 280
    skin, hair and nails 464–5

gabapentin
    anti-epileptic drug 85–6, 88
    dosage for pain relief *496*
    dose escalation schemes for *498*
    for neuropathic pain *497*
gait disorders, testing 421
galantamine 14–15, *17*, 18, *46*
gastric adenocarcinoma 322–3
    diagnosis 325
    risk factors and presentation 324–5
    treatment 325–9, *326*, *327*
gastric emptying 295–6
    and anorexia of ageing 298–9
    causes of delayed 296
    diagnosis of delayed 297
    drugs for prevention of 297, 502
    symptoms of delayed 296–7
gastritis 292
gastro-intestinal stromal tumour (GIST) 323
gastrointestinal (GI) disorders *see* lower GI disorders;
        upper GI disorders
gastrooesophageal reflux disease (GORD) 283
    acid suppression 283–5
    diagnosis via endoscopy 283
    and Helicobacter pylori infection 285
    key points 286
    risk of malignancy 285–6
    surgical treatment 285
    symptoms and signs 283
gastroparesis
    aetiology 296
    diagnosis and therapy 297
    symptoms and signs 296–7
gemicitabine 240, 242, *243*, *244*, 329, *329*, *387*
gentamicin 153, *153*, *154–5*
giant cell arteritis (GCA) 411
gingivitis 263–4, 272
glaucoma 472–6
glucosamine, role in management of osteoarthritis
        409
glyceryl trinitrate *116*
goitre 399
Gold, for rheumatoid arthritis *406*, 407
GORD (gastro-oesophageal reflux disease) 279–80

gout
    aetiology 413
    diagnosis 414
    signs and symptoms 413–14
    treatment 414, *415*, 416
growth hormone 158
    hypersecretion of 392, 398
    replacement therapy 258, 399–400
gynaecological disorders *see* benign gynaecological
        disorders

H_2-receptor antagonists (H2RAs) 284, 285
haematological disorders 171
    acute leukaemia 176–7
    adverse effect on wound healing 443
    anaemia 171–3
    lymphoproliferative conditions 177–80
    multiple myeloma 180
    myelodysplastic syndromes 175
    thrombocytopenia 173–4
    vitamin B12 & folic acid deficiencies 173
haemorrhoids 317–18
hallucinations 14, 22–3, 37, 38, 49, 50, 74, 80
Hamilton Depression Rating Scale (HDRS) 31
HDL-cholesterol 101, 102, 103, 107, 108
hearing aids 487
hearing loss 485–7
heart failure (HF) 125
    aetiology 125–7
    classification of symptoms *126*
    clinical presentation 127
    diagnosis 127–8
    epidemiology 125
    factors leading to worsening *129*
    incidence and prevalence *126*
    key points and guidelines 137
    therapy 128
        drug treatment 129–131, *132–4*, 135
            drugs to be avoided *130*
            guidelines for sequence of 129
        general measures 128–9
Helicobacter pylori
    acute gastritis 292
    gastrooesophageal reflux disease 285
    MALT lymphomas 323
    peptic ulcer disease 288–92
    risk factor for gastric carcinomas *324*
heparin induced thrombocytopenia (HITT) 173, 174
heparins 59
    low molecular weight heparins (LMWHs) 60, 119,
        161, *162*
    in older people 60
    pharmacokinetics 59–60
    unfractionated *115*, 119, 161, *162*
hepatitis
    alcoholic 336–7
    drug-induced *216*, 220

hepatitis (*continued*)
    hepatitis B 340
    hepatitis C 338–40
    in HIV-infected persons 222
    non-alcoholic 337–8
hepatotoxicity 220, 334–5
herpes simplex labialis 271–2
herpes zoster (shingles) 458–9
hip fractures
    prevention of 422
    risk factors 420
HIV infection and tuberculosis 211, 216, 220, 221,
    222
HMG-CoA reductase inhibitors *see* statins
Holmium laser enucleation of the prostate (HoLEP)
    358
hormonal treatments for breast cancer 383, *388*
hospital acquired pneumonia (HAP) 199, 200, 201
hydralazine
    for heart failure *134*
        with isosorbide dinitrate 136
    for hypertension 98
hypercapneic respiratory failure 192
hyperglycaemia 296, 392, 393, 394, 400
hyperlipidaemia 101
    aetiology 101
    diagnosis 102
    guidelines and key points 108–9
    risk factor for stroke 54
    symptoms and signs 102
    therapy 103
        bile acid sequestrants 108
        ezetimibe 107
        fibrates 106
        guidelines 108–9
        lipid-lowering drugs *104–5*
        nicotinic acid (niacin) 106–7
        omega-3 fatty acids 108
        statins 103
hyperosmolar coma, diabetes complication 392
hyperparathyroidism 399
hypersensitivity pneumonitis 233–4
hypertension 91
    aetiology 91–2
    diagnosis 92
    investigations 93
    pharmacology of antihypertensives 94–9
    risk factor for heart failure 126, 127
    risk factor for stroke 53–4
    symptoms and signs 92
    therapy 93
        drug treatment algorithm *95*
        non-pharmacological 93
        pharmacological 93–4
hyperthyroidism 142, 399
hyperuricemia 413, 414, 416

hypnotics 47–8
    drug interactions 48
    and increased fall risk 430
    pharmacokinetics of *47*
    withdrawal of 48, 432
hypocalcaemia 425
hypoglycaemia 393–7
hypopituitarism 398
hyposalivation 266–7
hypotension
    caused by alpha-blockers 356
    orthostatic hypotension 63–6
    postprandial hypotension 66–9
hypothyroidism
    cause of pure secondary hypercholesterolaemia 101
    testing for 102
    treatment of 398, 399

ibuprofen, analgesic *495*
idiopathic pulmonary fibrosis (IPF) 230–1
ILD *see* interstitial lung disease
imatinib, cancer drug 329
imipramine, role in detrusor overactivity 374
imiquimod cream, for skin diseases 454, 460, 462
immune thrombocytopenic purpura (ITP) 173, 174
immunosuppressants, COPD and asthma 190
incontinence
    faecal 314–17
    skin cleansing to prevent pressure sores 438–9
    urinary 343–351, 370–6
incretin drugs, type 2 diabetes 394
indocyanine green angiography (ICG) 478
infective endocarditis 151–2
    diagnosis and treatment 152–5
    prevention of 152
inflammatory bowel disease (IBD) 304
    aetiology 304
    diagnosis 304–5
    symptoms and signs 304
    therapy 305–7
INH *see* isoniazid
inhaled steroids, chronic asthma 187–90
insomnia 45–8
    drug treatment 47–8
    initial assessment 45
    non-drug treatment 46–7
insulin 394–5
    adverse effects of 397
    Glargine insulin 395
    inducing hypoglycaemia 394–5
    insulin sensitizers 394
    weight gain 394, 396
insulin resistance 391
    cause of mixed hyperlipidaemia 101
    causes of 391, 392
    risk factor for essential hypertension 92
    thiazide diuretics increasing risk of 95

International Prostate Symptom Score (IPSS) *354*
interstitial lung disease (ILD) 225
    aetiology of 226
    assessment of *227*
    clinical presentation 225–6
    forms of 226–7, *228*
    key points and links 234
    problems in the elderly 227
    therapy 229
    assessing response to 229
    drugs 229–30
    general measures 234
    for specific forms 230–4
intracerebral haemorrhage *see* stroke
intravenous thrombolysis, ischaemic stroke 58–9
ipratropium bromide, acute asthma *193*
irinotecan, cytotoxic drug *328, 329*
iron chelation therapy 176
iron deficiency
    and abdominal cancers *324, 325*
    cause of anaemia 171
    iron administration 172
    and restless leg syndrome 49
irritable bowel syndrome (IBS)
    cause of diarrhoea 316
    and diverticulosis 308
    Rome II criteria *312*
isoniazid (INH), tuberculostatic 214
    adverse reactions and drug interaction *216*
    and drug-induced hepatitis 220
    pharmacodynamics 215
    recommended dosage *215, 221*
    treatment of LTBI 221–2
    within anti-tuberculous regimen 218–19
isosorbide dinitrate, for heart failure *134*, 136
itraconazole, for tinea 465

kidney, rug clearance 3
kyphosis, in osteoporosis patients 421

L-Dopa *see* levodopa
lamivudine, for hepatitis B 340
lamotrigine, newer anti-epileptic drug 86, 87, 88
laparoscopic colposuspension, stress incontinence 374–5
laparoscopic fundoplication 285
laser photocoagulation therapy 482–3
laser prostatectomy 358
latent autoimmune diabetes of adults (LADA) 391
latent tuberculosis infection (LTBI) 221–2, 229
laxatives 313, *314*, 503
    abuse, testing for 316
LDL-Cholesteral
    drugs reducing levels of 103, 106, 107, 108
    measurement of 102
leflunomide, for rheumatoid arthritis *405*, 407

leg ulceration 441
    aetiology 441–3
    diagnosis 445–8
    key points 452
    symptoms and signs 443–5
    therapy 448–52
letrozole, breast cancer drug *388*
leukaemia 176–7
levetiracetam, newer anti-epileptic drug 86, *88*
levodopa (L-DOPA)
    causing psychotic symptoms 36
    and diagnosis of PD 75
    dyskinesias induced by 80
    improving swallowing 279
    for restless legs syndrome 49–50
    side effects *78*
    treatment of PD 76–7
levomepromazine, for nausea and vomiting 502
Lewy Body Disease
    dementia with 13, 14, 18, 22, 23, 25
    in Parkinson's disease 74, 75
    psychotic symptoms, treatment of 40
lichen planus 377, 459
lichen sclerosis 377–8
lipid lowering drugs 54, 101, *104–5*
    ezetimibe 107
    fibrates 106
    nicotinic acid 106–7
    statins 103
lipodermatosclerosis 443, *445, 446*
liposomal doxorubicin 383, *387*
lisinopril 96, *97, 118, 133*
lithium
    augmenting agent for depression 33
    drug interactions *21*, 95, *132–3*, 409, *410, 415, 495*
    effects on continence *346*
    side effects 278
liver
    age-linked physiological changes 333–4
    drug clearance by 3
    hepatotoxicity 220, 334–5
liver disease 333–4
    alcoholic 336–7
    cirrhosis 335–6
    drug induced 334–5
    hepatitis B 340
    hepatitis C 338–40
    non-alcoholic steatohepatitis 337–8
liver transplantation 340–1
long-acting beta2 agonist (LABA), asthma 188–90
long-term catheterization 358
long-term oxygen therapy (LTOT) 195–6
loop diuretics
    adverse effects *255*, 413, *488, 491*
    for heart failure 135

Looser's zones, diagnosis of osteomalacia 426
low molecular weight heparins (LMWHs) 60, 119,
        161, *162*, 165, *166*
lower gastrointestinal disorders
    constipation 311–14
    diarrhoea and faecal incontinence 314–17
    diverticulosis 307–9
    haemorrhoids 317–18
    inflammatory bowel disease (IBD) 304–37
    malabsorption 301–3

mesenteric ischaemia 309–11
lower urinary tract symptoms (LUTS)
    in benign prostatic hyperplasia 353–8
    gender differences in 345
    increased incidence of with age 343
    urinalysis 346
    urinary diary, keeping 371–2
    see also urinary incontinence
LTOT (long-term oxygen therapy) 195–6
lung cancer 237
    aetiology 237–8
    chemotherapeutic drugs 238–40
    diagnosis and staging 238
    ECOG performance status 238, *240*
    guidelines 247
    international staging system *239*
    key points 245, 247
    non cytotoxic agents 242
    symptoms and signs 238
    treatment 238
        anti-emetic therapy 245, *246*
        for mesothelioma 243, 245, *246*
        for non-small cell lung cancer (NSCLC) 240–2,
            243, *244*
        small cell carcinoma 243, *245*
lung disease *see* interstitial lung disease
lymphocytic interstitial pneumonitis (LIP) 233
lymphoma 323
macroadenomas 397–8
macrolides *5*, 48, 194, 203, 217–18
Macroplastique, for stress incontinence 375
magnesium, acute asthma *193*
malabsortion 301–3
    aetiology 301–2
    diagnosis 303
    of drugs 219
    symptoms and signs 302–3
    therapy 303
malignant melanoma 460
malnutrition
    role in development of pressure ulcers 437
    see also anorexia of ageing; obesity; under-nutrition
Malnutrition Universal Screening Tool (MUST) 256
MALT lymphomas 323
mammography 381–2
manic psychosis 37–8

MAO-B inhibitors, treatment of PD 77, 79
medication
    affecting swallowing 278–9
    alternative routes of administration 280–1
    causing hearing problems 490–1
    decreasing the lower oesophageal sphincter pressure
        279–80
    effect on continence *346*
    increasing risk of falls 429–32
    patients with swallowing disorders 280
    pill-induced oesophagitis 287–8
    reviews 9, 432, 433
meglitinides, drugs inducing increased beta cell
        insulin secretion 394, 397
melatonin, sleep-inducing 48
memantine *17*, 18, 23, *255*
mesenteric ischaemia 309
    aetiology 309
    diagnosis 310–11
    symptoms and signs 309–10
    therapy 311
mesothelioma, treatment of 243, 245, *246*
metabolic syndrome 101, 250, 337, 338
metastatic disease
    clinical presentation 382
    treatment of 383–4, *385*
metformin
    adverse effects *130*, 255
    and lactic acidosis, no evidence for 397
    type 2 diabetes treatment 393–5, *396*
methotrexate (MTX)
    for breast cancer treatment *387*
    for interstitial lung disease 230, 231, 232
    for psoriasis 463
    for rheumatoid arthritis 404, *405*, 406
metoclopramide
    for gastroparesis 297
    for nausea and vomiting 502
metoprolol 46, *97*, *116*, 130, *133*, *147*
micturation system 343–5
mid-urethral tape procedures, stress incontinence 375
midodrine, for orthostatic hypotension 65, *66*
Mini Mental State Examination (MMSE) 14, 30
minoxidil, directly acting vasodilator 98
miotics, glaucoma treatment 475
mirtazapine
    antidepressant *32*
    for weight gain 258
mitral valve disease 156
mobility
    causes of impaired 429
    drugs increasing risk of falls 430–2
    improved by withdrawal of fall-risk-increasing
        drugs 429–30
    testing 432
moclobemide *32*

monilial oesophagitis 287
monoamine oxidase inhibitors (MAOIs) 31
monoclonal antibodies 57, 179, 305, 383, 479
mood disorders 36
  symptoms and signs 37–8
morphine *495*
  for osteoarthritis 409, 410
mouth and dental disorders 263
  alveolar osteitis 266
  angular cheilitis 268
  burning mouth syndrome 269–70
  candidiasis 267–8
  dental caries 264–5
  denture stomatitis 268–9
  odontogenic infections 265–6
  oral liichen planus 272–3
  periodontal disease 263–4
  recurrent aphthous stomatitis 270–1
  recurrent herpes simplex 271–2
  xerostomia and hyposalivation 266–7
moxifloxacin, bactericidal agent 217
moxonidine, centrally-acting vasoldilator 97–8
multi-drug resistant TB (MDRTB) 213–14, 217, 219, 221
multinodular goitre 399
multiple myeloma 180
muscular pain, polymyalgia rheumatica 411–12
My Pyramid Plan, dietary advice 257
myasthenia gravis (MG) 278–9
Mycobacterium tuberculosis (MTB) 211–12, 213, 214, 215, 221
mycosis fungoides 461
mydriatic agents 470
myelodysplastic syndromes 175
myopathy
  in osteomalacia 425, 426
  in osteoporosis 421, 422
  statin-induced 102, 103
  tachycardia induced cardiomyopathy 146

naproxen, analgesic *495*
natriuretic peptides, diagnosis of HF 128
nausea, treatment of 502
necrotectomy, pressure ulcers 439
neuroleptics *see* antipsychotics
neuropathic pain 493–4
  algorithm for treatment of *497*
  diagnosis of 494
  gabapentin dose escalation schemes *498*
neuropathy, peripheral *442*, *443*, *444*
  causes and symptoms 442
  surgical procedures 451
  total contact cast 450
Neuropsychiatric Inventory (NPI) 23
neurotransmitters
  involved in nausia & vomiting 502
  in lower urinary tract 344

niacin *see* nicotinic acid
nicotinic acid, lipid-lowering drug *105*, 106–7
nociceptive pain 494
  diagnosis 494
  drugs for *495–6*
  WHO Pain Relief Ladder *497*
nocturia 46, *354*, 355
nocturnal leg cramps 50
non-adherence to medication *see* adherence
non-alcoholic steatohepatitis (NASH) 337–8
non-benzodiazepine hypnotics 48
non Hodgkin lymphoma (NHL) 179–80
non invasive ventilation (NIV) 192, 194, 196
non-REM sleep parasomnias 51
non-specific interstitial pneumonia (NSIP) 226, 233
non-steroidal anti-inflammatory drugs (NSAIDs)
  concerns about OTC use of 8
  drug interactions
    with aspirin 55
    with clopidogrel 57
    with thiazides 95
    with warfarin 5
  eye drops 470
  for gout *415*
  increasing risk of falls 431
  and malabsorption 301
  for osteoarthritis 409, *410*
  risk factor for peptic ulcers 288, 289–90, 291
  risk factor for tinnitus 488, 491
  side effects 409
non-ulcer dyspepsia 292–3
nortriptyline, analgesic *496*
NSCLC (non small cell lung cancer) 240–2, *244*
NSTE-ACS (non-ST elevation ACS) 113, 119–20
NSTEMI (Non-ST segment elevation myocardial infarction) 111, 120, 121
nucleic acid amplification, diagnosis of TB 211
nutritional disorders 249
  medication affecting nutritional health *255*
  nutritional frailty 252
  obesity 249–52
  under-nutrition 252–4
    management of 257–9
    screen and assessment of 254, 256

obesity 249–52
  drugs reducing 393, 395
  and risk of type 2 diabetes 391–2
occupational therapy
  for assistance in feeding 257
  for patients with risk of falls 422
octreotide, treatment for vomiting 502
ocular hypertension (OHT) 473
odontogenic infections 265–6
oedema control, compression therapy 448, 450
oesophageal cancer 322
  diagnosis 325

oesophageal cancer (*continued*)
  risk factors and presentation 324–5
  treatment 325–329, *326*, *327–8*
oesophageal dysphagia 275
oesophageal infections 287
oesophageal motility disorders 286–7
oesophagitis, medication-induced 287–8
oestrogen therapy
  for recurrent urinary tract infection 350
  for urogenital atrophy 367
olanzapine *24*, 39, 40, 65, 279, 502
olfactory dysfunction, early sign of PD 74
omega-3 fatty acids 108, 407–8
onychomycosis 465
opioid analgesics
effects on continence 346
and increased risk of falls 431
for osteoarthritis 409, *410*, 411
oral candidiasis 267–8
oral glucose tolerance test (OGTT) 393
oral liichen planus 272–3
orlistat, weight reduction drug 395
oropharyngeal dysphagia 275
orthostatic hypotension 63
  aetiology 63–4
  anticholinergics inducing 432
  diagnosis 64
  hypertension causing/increasing severity of 431
  improvement by withdrawal of fall-risk-increasing
        drugs 429–30
  key points 66
  methods of testing 432
  symptoms and signs 64
  therapy 64–6
orthostatic hypotension, advice to avoid falls 422
osteitis deformans *see* Paget's disease
osteoarthritis 408
  aetiology 408
  diagnosis 408
  key points 411
  non pharmacotherapies 409
  pharmacotherapies 409, *410*, 411
osteomalacia 425
  aetiology 425–6
  clinical signs 426
  diagnosis 426
  treatment 426–7
osteoporosis and risk of falls 420–2
otitis externa 489–90
ototoxicity 490–1
over-the-counter (OTC) drugs 2, 7–8
overactive bladder (OAB) 345
  antimuscarinic drugs 347–9
  topical oestrogens for women 350
oxaliplatin, cytotoxic drug *328*, 328–9
oxybutynin, antimuscarinic drug 347, 373, 374

oxygen therapy
  for acute asthma *193*
  for COPD 193, 194
  for hypersensitivity pneumonitis 234
  long-term *192*, 195–6

paclitaxel 240, *241*, *243*, *246*, *387*
Paget's disease 422–3
  clinical signs 423
  imaging 423–4
  laboratory investigation 424
  pathogenesis and localization 423
  treatment 424–5
pain 493
  aetiology 493–4
  diagnosis 494
  key points 496, 498
  therapy 494–6
palliative care 499
  elderly patients 500–1
  symptom prevalence 500
  treatment of symptoms
    anorexia and weight loss 501–2
    fatigue 501
    nausea and vomiting 502
pamidronate, biphosphanate *388*
pancreatic carcinoma 323
  diagnosis 325
  risk factors and presentation 324–5
  treatment 325–9, *326*
pancreatic endocrine tumours 323
pancreatitis, cause of diabetes mellitus 392
paracetamol *495*
  for osteoporosis 409, *410*
parathyroid hormone (PTH) 425, 426
Parkinson's disease (PD) 14, 73
  aetiology and pathology 75
  atypical antipsychotics for 39
  diagnostic criteria 75–6
  main causes of *76*
  psychotic symptoms 36
  and slow gastric emptying 296, 297
  symptoms and signs 74–5
    motor symptoms 74
    non-motor symptoms 74–5
  therapy 76–81
    neurosurgery 81
    non-drug 76
    pharmacological 76–81
paroxetine, antidepressant *32*
PDE-5 inhibitors, erectile dysfunction 363–4
peak expiratory flow (PEF), asthma diagnosis
        185–6
pegaptanib sodium, for neovascular AMD 479
pelvic floor exercises (PFE)
  for mild prolapse 369
  for stress incontinence 372

pelvic organ prolapse 367
    classification of 368
    management 368–9
    symptoms and diagnosis 368
    treatment
        intravaginal devices 369
        physiotherapy 369
        prevention 369
        surgery 369–70
pemetrexed, lung cancer treatment *244*, *246*
penicillin 153, *154*
peptic ulcer disease 288
    diagnosis 289
    symptoms and signs 288–9
    therapy
        for established ulceration 291
        Helicobacter pylori eradication 291–2
        prophylaxis 289–90
percutaneous coronary intervention (PCI), ACS 113,
        119–20
percutaneous enteral gastrostomy (PEG) feeding
        258–9
peri-urethral bulking agents, stress incontinence 375
perindopril *117*
periodic limb movements of sleep (PLMS) 48–50
periodontal disease 263–4
pharmacology of ageing 1–10
phenobarbitone, avoidance of 85, 87
phenylephrine, for pupillary dilation 470, 483
phenytoin, older anti-epileptic agent 85, 87, 89
photodynamic therapy (PDT), for AMD 478
phototherapy, skin conditions 459, 461
physiotherapy
    for patients with risk of falls 422
    for urodynamic stress incontinence 372–3
phytotherapy, benign prostatic hyperplasia 355–6
pill-induced oesophagitis 287–8
pilocarpine, glaucoma treatment 475
pituitary adenomas 397–8
platelet glycoprotein (GP) IIb/IIIa inhibitors, stoke
        management 57–8
platinum compounds, chemotherapeutic agents
        238–240, 328–9, 491
pneumonia 199
    aetiology and pathogenesis 199–200
    assessment of patient 201–2
    diagnosis 200–1
    epidemiology 199
    prevention 206
    symptoms and signs 200
    therapy 202–3
        important drug issues 202–6
Pneumonia Severity Index (PSI) 201, *202*
point of care (POC) devices 167
polymerase chain reaction (PCR), detection of TB 213
polymyalgia rheumatica (PMR) 411–12

polypharmacy vs. appropriate prescribing 7
population ageing, trends in 1
postprandial hypotension 66–7
    aetiology 67
    diagnosis and therapy 68
    key points 68–9
    symptoms and signs 67–8
prednisolone, alcoholic hepatitis 337
pregabalin, analgesic *196*
presbyacusis 486–7
prescribing audit, indicators for 8–9
pressure ulcers 435
    classification *436*
    costs associated with 435
    and deformity of the foot 442
    key points 439–40
    local treatment 439
    prevention 438–9
    risk assessment 437–8
    role of nutrition 437
    role of pressure in 435–7
primary open angle glaucoma (POAG) 473
    treatment of 473–4
procalcitonin, biomarker for antibiotic use 205
progestins, for appetite loss 502
prokinetics, constipation treatment 313
prolapse *see* urogenital prolapse
propiverine hydrochloride, for urinary incontinence
        348, 374
propranolol, beta-blocker 4, *97*, 336
proprioception, testing of 421
prostaglandin analogues, glaucoma treatment 474
prostaglandin E1, erectile dysfunction 365
prostate enlargement
    treatment using 5α-reductase inhibitors 349
prostate specific antigen (PSA) testing 353
prostate surgery 357–8
prosthetic valves 156–7
protein binding of drugs 3
protein and energy supplementation 258
proton pump inhibitors (PPIs) 279, *284*, 284–5, 289
'pseudodementia' 29, 37
pseudogout *see* calcium pyrophosphate disease
        (CPPD)
pseudohypertension 92
psoriasis 463–4
psychotic illness 35
    aetiology 35–6
    diagnosis 38
    key points 40
    in Parkinson's disease 74–5, 80
    symptoms and signs 37–8
    therapy 38–40
psychotropic drugs
    and increased fall risk 429, 430, *431*
    increased sensitivity to with age 4

pulmonary embolism 163–4
pulmonary fibrosis *see* idiopathic pulmonary fibrosis
pulmonary tuberculosis 211
    clinical presentation 212–13
    diagnosis 213
    key points 222
    pathogenesis 211–12
    treatment 213–14
        chemotherapy 214
        drugs 214–18
        regimen 218–19
        follow-up during 220
        initiation of therapy 219–20
        of latent tuberculosis infection 221–2
        WHO recommendations *218*
pyrazinamide (PZ), tuberculostatic 214, 216–17
    adverse reactions and drug interaction *216*
    and hepatotoxicity 220
    recommended dosage *215*
    within TB treatment regime 218–19

quality of life
    affected by tinnitus 487
    and erectile dysfunction 362
    and pain 493
    palliative care patients 499, 501
    and PEG feeding 258–9
    and urinary conditions *354*, 355, 370, 373, 374
quinapril *118*
quinine sulphate, nocturnal leg cramps 50

radiography, bone density imaging 423–4
radioiodine therapy, for hyperthyroidism 399
radiotherapy
    for abdominal cancers 321
    basal/squamous cell carcinomas 462
    for breast cancer 383, *384*
    for lung cancer 238
    for NSCLC 240
    small cell carcinoma 243
ramipril *117*
ranibizumab, treatment of neovascular AMD 479–80
reactivation TB 212, 221
reboxetine *32*
recurrent aphthous stomatitis 270–1
reflux disease 283–6
REM behaviour disorder 50–1
renal disease, contributor to osteomalacia 426
renal excretion of drugs 3, 385–9
renal failure, and gastroparesis 296
respiratory failure, features of 194
respiridone *24*, 25, 39, 40, 279
restless legs syndrome (RLS) 48–50
reteplase *116*
'reversible dementia' 29
review of patient's medication 9, 432, 433

rhabdomyolysis, risk factors for 101, 102, 103, 106, 107, 108
rheumatoid arthritis (RA) 403
    aetiology 403
    diagnosis 404
    key points 408
    prevalence 403
    symptoms and signs 403–4
    therapy 404, *405–406*, 407–8
rifampicin (RMP) , tuberculostatic 214
    adverse reactions and drug interactions *216*, 220
    pharmacodynamics of 215–16
    recommended dosage *215*, *221*
    treatment regimen for TB/LTBI 218–19, 221
risedronate *255*, 280, 422, 424
risk assessment, pressure ulcer scoring systems 437–438, 451–2
rivastigmine 14–15, *16*, 23, *79*, 80
RLS (restless legs syndrome) 48–50
RMP *see* rifampicin
Rome II criteria for IBS *312*

sacral neuromodulation 376
salicylic acid 55
sarcoidosis 231–2
sarcopenia 299
scabies 464
schizophrenia 36
    medication for 40
    symptoms and signs 37
sclerotherapy, varicose veins 351, 448, 449–50
screening
    breast cancer 381–2
    for cancer in patients with unprovoked VTE 161
    diabetes mellitus 392
    for HCC in cirrhotic patients 336
    latent tuberculosis infection 221
    for under-nutrition 249, 254, 256
sedatives
    avoidance of for delirium 20, 22
    effects on continence *346*
    negative effects 278, 430
    and risk of falls 422, 430, *431*
    withdrawal of 432
seizures *see* epilepsy
selective serotonin reuptake inhibitors (SSRIs) 31
    causing anxiety and agitation 31, 36
    effect on continence *346*
    and insomnia 46
    interaction with aspirin 55
    risk of falls and fractures 430
serotonin syndrome 33, 409, 411
sertraline, antidepressant 31, *32*, *255*
Sezary syndrome 461
shingles 458–9
sialorrhea (drooling), treatment of 279
sibutramine, weight reduction drug 395

SIGN (Scottish Intercollegiate Guidelines Network)
    guidelines for acute asthma treatment 186,
    191, 193
sildenafil, PDE-5 inhibitor 363, 364
silicosis 233
skin cancer
    and azathioprine treatment for IBD 306-7
    biopsy of ulcers to exclude 448
    causing ulceration 442
    malignant melanoma 460
    mycosis fungoides 461
    non-melanoma 442, 452, 462-3
sleep disorders
    insomnia 45-8
    nocturnal leg cramps 50
    in Parkinson's disease 74
    REM behaviour disorder 50-1
    restless legs syndrome 48-50
sleep hygiene 46-7
sleep restriction therapy 47
SM *see* streptomycin
small cell carcinoma 323
    treatment 243, *245*
small intestinal bacterial overgrowth (SIBO) 301-3
smoking
    cardiovascular risk factor 93
    risk factor for COPD 183
sodium fusidate *154*
sodium valproate 85, 87, 89
solifenacin, antimuscarinic agent 348, 374
spirometry
    diagnosis of asthma 184, *186*
    diagnosis of COPD 184-5, *186*
spironolactone 98, 136, 336
squamous cell carcinoma 442, 452, 462-3
St. John's wort, drug interactions 8
Standardised Nutritional Assessment (SNA) 256
Staphylococci 152, 200, 456, 458, 471, 489
    antibiotics for infective endocarditis *154*
statins
    adverse effects *255*
    following ACS 121
    lipid lowering 103, *104*
    treatment of AF 146
STEMI (ST segment elevation myocardial infarction)
    111, 119, 120, 121
steroids *see* corticosteroids
    antibiotics for infective endocarditis *154-5*
    causing erysipelas and cellulitis 456
    causing late prosthetic endocarditis 151, 152
    and community acquired pneumonia 200, 203
streptokinase 58, *115*, 120-1
streptomycin (SM), TB treatment 214, 215, 217, 218
stress urinary incontinence 350-1
    duloxetine 373
    surgical interventions 374-5

stroke 53
    aetiology 53
    key points 61
    modifiable risk factors 53-4
    therapy 54-61
        antiplatelet therapy 54-7
        heparins 59-60
        thrombolysis 58-9
        warfarin 60-1
strontium ranelate, lowering hip fracture incidence
    420
subjective global assessment (SGA), nutritional status
    256
suicide risk, depressed patients 30
sulfasalazine (SSZ) 305, 306
    for rheumatoid arthritis *406*, 407
sulphonyureas, for type 2 diabetes 393, 394, 395, 396,
    397
supplements, dietary 85, 258, 337, 411, 422
suprapubic arch sling procedure (SPARC) 375
swallowing disorders 275
    aetiology 277
    diagnosis 277
    key points and links 281
    and medication 278-81
    symptoms and signs 277
    therapy 277-8
syncope 69
    aetiology 69, 420
    diagnosis 70
    key points and guidelines 71
    symptoms and signs 69-70
    therapy 70-1
syringing (lavage) for ear wax removal 486
systolic dysfunction *127*, 128

tadalafil, PDE-5 inhibitor 363, 364
tamoxifen 57, 383, *388*
tardive dyskinesia 37, 39
taste impairment, drugs causing 278
taxanes, chemotherapeutic agents 240
TB *see* pulmonary tuberculosis
tegaserod, constipation treatment 313
tenecteplase *115*
tension free vaginal tape (TVT) 375
terbinafine, for tinea 465
testosterone therapy, risk of prostate cancer 400
theophylline
    for COPD 192, 195
    potential adverse effects of *190*
thiazide/thiazide-like diuretics 94-5
thiazolidenediones, for type 2 diabetes 394, 396,
    397
thioguanines, drug metabolism of 305-7
thiopurine S-methyltransferase (TPMT) 305-6
thrombocytopenia 173-4
thromboembolism, prevention of 155-8

thrombolysis
   acute coronary syndrome 120–1
   treatment for ischaemic stroke 58–9
thymidylate synthase inhibitors 328
thyroid disease 398–9
thyroid function test 102
thyroid hormone replacement 399
thyroid nodules and tumours 399
Timed Up and Go Test 432
tinea 464–5
tinnitus 487–9
tirofiban, for ACS *114*
tirofiban, glycoprotein (GP) IIb/IIIa inhibitor 57–8
TNF-α blockers, for rheumatoid arthritis 221, 407
tolterodine, antimuscarinic agent 348, 373, 374
tooth decay 264–5
tooth extraction, alveolar osteitis following 266
tophi, formation of in gout 413, 414, 416
topical analgesics, for osteoarthritis *410*
total contact cast 450
toxic multinodular goitre 399
tramadol, analgesic *495*
   for osteoarthritis 409–10
trandolapril *118*
transaminases, measuring 102
transcutaneous nerve stimulation (TENS), for
        osteoarthritis 409
transdermal therapy
   oxybutynin 373
transfusion
   acute leukaemia 177
   due to iron deficiency 172–3
   red blood cell (RBC) 176
   thrombocytopenia 174
transient ischaemic attack (TIA) *see* stroke
transobturator tapes (TOT) 375
transoesophageal echocardiography (TOE) 138–139,
        148–9
transphenoidal surgery 398
transurethral prostaglandin E1 365
transurethral resection of prostate (TURP) 357–8
trastuzumab, tumour antibody *387*
treatment-resistant depression 33
triamcinolone acetonide, for AMD 480
tricylic antidepressants (TCAs) 31
   and increased risk of falls *431*
   for neuropathic pain *497*
triglycerides, reduction of 103, 106, 107, 108
tropicamide, for pupillary dilation 477, 483
trospium chloride, for urinary incontinence 348, 374
tuberculosis *see* pulmonary tuberculosis
type 1 diabetes 391
type 2 diabetes
   aetiology 391–2
   dangers of unrecognized 392
   diagnosis 392–3

medication for 393–5
drug interactions within diabetes drugs 396
general adverse effects 396
risk of drug-drug interactions 395–6
specific adverse effects 397
secondary cause of hyperlipidaemia 101
symptoms and signs 392

ulcerative colitis (UC) 304–7
ulcers
   leg ulceration 441–52
   pressure ulcers 435–40
under-nutrition 252–4
    aetiology 298–9
    assessment of 254, 256
    non-drug management of 257
    pharmacological management of 258–9
undertreatment 9–10
unfractionated heparin (UFH) 119
unstable angina (UA) 111, 113, 120, 122
upper gastrointestinal disorders 283
   gastritis 292
   gastrooesophageal reflux disease 283–6
   non-cardiac chest pain 287
   non-ulcer dyspepsia 292–3
   oesophageal infections 287
   oesophageal motility disorders 286–7
   peptic ulcer disease 288–92
   pill-induced oesophagitis 287–8
upper oesophageal sphincter (UOS), role in
        swallowing 276
urease breath testing 292
urethra, control of 343–4
uricosuric agents, for gout *415*
urinalysis 346–7
urinary diary 371–2
urinary incontinence 343
   assessment/investigation 346–7, 371
   bladder outflow tract obstruction 349–50
   causes of 370, 371
   management 371–3
   pathophysiology 345
   pharmacological treatment 347–9, 350
   stress urinary incontinence 350–1, 370
   subtypes of 345
urinary retention, BPH 353, 355
urinary tract infection (UTI)
   testing for 246–7
   topical oestrogen therapy 350
urodynamic stress incontinence (USI) 370
   duloxetine for 373
   following prolapse surgery 368–9
   physiotherapy 372
   surgery 374–5
urodynamics 371
urogenital atrophy 367
urogenital prolapse 367–70

urologic disorders 343–51
usual interstitial pneumonitis (UIP) 226–7, 230
uticaria 465–6

vaccination, pneumococcal 206
vadenafil, PDE-5 inhibitor 363, 364
valproate sodium 85, 87, 89
valvular heart disease 151
    degenerative, prevention of 158–9
    infective endocarditis 151–2
        diagnosis and treatment 152–5
        prevention of 152
    link to cabergoline and pergolide 50, 80
    thromboembolism, prevention of 155–8
vancomycin 153, *154–5*
varicose veins and leg ulceration 441, 443, 445, 448,
        449–50
vascular dementia (VaD) 13, 14, 18, 22, 23
vascular endothelial growth factor (VEGF), drugs for
        479
vasodilators 97–9
    negative cardiovascular effects of 431
vasovagal collapse 429, 431, 432
venlafaxine, antidepressant 31, *32, 255*
venous eczema 466–7
venous hypertension 441–2
venous thromboembolism (VTE) 162–163, 163–6,
        168
venous ulcers 441, *445*
    compression therapy 448, 450
    lack of exercise causing 441
    position of 444
    symptoms and signs 443
ventilation 191–2, 194, 196
verapamil, increased sensitivity to 3–4
verteporfin, photodynamic therapy 478
vertigo 419
    anti-vertigo drugs 432
    and drug-induced hearing loss 491
vinblastine, vinca alkaloid 240, *246*
vinca alkaloids, chemotherapeutic agents 240
vincristine, vinca alkaloid 130, *245, 246*
vindesine, vinca alkaloid 240
vinorelbine, vinca alkaloid 240, *241, 242, 243, 244,
        387*
visco-supplementation, osteoarthritis *410*, 411
visual field defects
    sign of pituitary adenomas 398
    see also glaucoma
vitamin B12 deficiency 173
    and high risk of falls 421
vitamin D deficiency
    causing osteomalacia 425, 426
    and high risk of falls 421
    and hyperparathyroidism 399

vitamin D supplementation 258
    for osteomalacia 426–7
    for osteoporosis 422
vitamin K 60, 61
    for excessive INR 168
    intake of dietary, effect on INR 167
    vitamin K antagonists *162*, 165–7
    vitamin K1 for excessive INR 167–8
vitamin supplementation 167, 258
volume of distribution of drugs 2
vomiting
    anti-emetic agents for chemotherapy 245, *246*
    side effect of drugs *16–17, 241, 244, 255, 386*
    treatment in palliative care 502
VTE *see* venous thromboembolism (VTE)
vulvovaginal candidiasis 455, 456

warfarin 60
    adjusting dosage for age 166
    adverse effects 61
    and bleeding risk 164–5
    drug interactions 5, *167*
    following stroke 60–1
    heart failure 137
    patient education 167
    response to bleeding 167–8
    starting dosage 165–6
    underprescribed for AF 148
    vitamin K and alcohol 167
weight gain
    adverse effect of diabetes drugs 394, 396
    due to fluid retention 394
    symptom of hypothyroidism 399
weight loss
    advised for gout 414
    advised for reducing hypertension 93
    anorexia of ageing 298–9
    effect of dieting 251–2
    link to increased mortality 250
    and loss of bone mineral density 251
    palliative care patients 501–2
    symptom of abdominal cancer 325
'white coat hypertension' 92
WHO Pain Relief Ladder *497*
withdrawal of medication 432–3
wound dressings 439

xerosis 453
xerostomia 266–7
    medications causing 278

zoledronate, biphosphanate *388*, 389